LABORATORY MEDICINE
in Psychiatry and Behavioral Science

SECOND EDITION

LABORATORY MEDICINE
in Psychiatry and Behavioral Science

SECOND EDITION

Sandra A. Jacobson, M.D.

Research Associate Professor,
University of Arizona College of Medicine,
Phoenix, Arizona

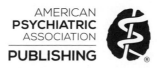

AMERICAN
PSYCHIATRIC
ASSOCIATION
PUBLISHING

If you wish to buy 50 or more copies of the same title, please go to www.appi.org/specialdiscounts for more information.

Second Edition

Manufactured in the United States of America on acid-free paper
27 26 25 24 23   5 4 3 2 1

American Psychiatric Association Publishing
800 Maine Avenue SW, Suite 900
Washington, DC 20024-2812
www.appi.org

Library of Congress Cataloging-in-Publication Data
Names: Jacobson, Sandra A., 1953- author. | American Psychiatric Association Publishing, issuing body.
Title: Laboratory medicine in psychiatry and behavioral science / by Sandra A. Jacobson.
Description: Second edition. | Washington, DC : American Psychiatric Association Publishing, [2023] | Includes bibliographical references and index.
Identifiers: LCCN 2022043652 (print) | LCCN 2022043653 (ebook) | ISBN 9781615374502 (paperback) | ISBN 9781615374519 (ebook)
Subjects: MESH: Mental Disorders--diagnosis | Clinical Laboratory Techniques | Psychotropic Drugs | Tables
Classification: LCC RC473.D54 (print) | LCC RC473.D54 (ebook) | NLM WM 16.1 | DDC 616.89/075--dc23/eng/20230118
LC record available at https://lccn.loc.gov/2022043652
LC ebook record available at https://lccn.loc.gov/2022043653

British Library Cataloguing in Publication Data
A CIP record is available from the British Library.

Contents

Chapter 2. Diseases and Conditions 327

Chapter 3. Psychotropic Medications: Laboratory Screening and Monitoring 575

About the Author

Sandra A. Jacobson, M.D., received her medical degree from the John A. Burns School of Medicine in her home state of Hawaii. After completing an internship in internal medicine at the University of Hawaii Integrated Medical Residency Program in Honolulu, she underwent psychiatry residency training and fellowship training in neurophysiology at UCLA Neuropsychiatric Institute. She has held faculty positions at UCLA, Tufts University School of Medicine, the Warren Alpert School of Medicine at Brown University, and the University of Arizona College of Medicine–Phoenix. Her work in consultation/liaison psychiatry, inpatient and outpatient psychiatry, geriatric psychiatry, nursing home consultation, and clinical neurophysiology (electroencephalography) informs the format, choice of tests and diseases, and comments on psychiatric relevance for the material included in *Laboratory Medicine in Psychiatry and Behavioral Science*, Second Edition.

Introduction

This second edition of *Laboratory Medicine in Psychiatry and Behavioral Science* is substantially revised from the first edition published in 2012. In the intervening decade, an explosion of research and publication related to laboratory science and psychiatry has left virtually no subject area untouched. As with the first edition, this manual is designed to assist psychiatrists and other behavioral health clinicians in the care of adult psychiatric patients across a wide range of settings. To facilitate its use as a reference manual, the book is divided into three main sections, each marked with a black tab at the edge of its title page:

- Laboratory Tests
- Diseases and Conditions
- Psychotropic Medications: Laboratory Screening and Monitoring

Among the thousands of laboratory tests available, tests that were selected for inclusion met one or more of the following criteria: a core or basic laboratory test for any patient; a test that is particularly pertinent to psychiatry or behavioral health; or a test that is new to medicine and potentially of interest in the field of behavioral health, including geriatrics. Diseases and conditions selected for inclusion were those for which laboratory tests are primary or important in diagnosis or differential diagnosis; those that are core or common conditions among psychiatric or geriatric patients; and those that have important psychiatric, cognitive, or behavioral consequences. The appendices contain several algorithms, tables, and figures that may be useful in understanding and interpreting various laboratory tests and their underlying biology.

Years of clinical practice and research in neuropsychiatry inform not only the choice of tests but also the rationale for their use. For this edition, the primary source of medical information was the published literature accessed through PubMed from the National Library of Medicine. A wide range of other resources were also consulted, including *Drug Information*, published annually by the American Society of Health-System Pharmacists, and the online laboratory references at ARUP Laboratories (www.aruplab.com) and the American Association for Clinical Chemistry (www.testing.com). A complete listing of references appears in the back matter of the book.

General Guidelines for Laboratory Testing

Judicious use of the laboratory improves patient care in psychiatry and behavioral science just as it does in internal medicine and other specialties. Laboratory testing is only one component of the complete psychiatric evaluation, which also includes a history, review of systems, functional assessment, and physical and mental status examinations. When lab results are reviewed in the context of the patient's family history, personal history, lifestyle, and particular exam findings, there is less likelihood of overreacting to a result that may turn out to be inconsequential or even spurious. For example, with an isolated elevation in one test such as alanine transaminase and in the absence of any clinical evidence of disease, the test should simply be repeated and further workup performed only if a twofold or greater elevation persists. When laboratory findings are unclear or present questions, clinical laboratory staff can be an excellent resource for clinicians in the interpretation of test data and in planning further diagnostics. The reference ranges cited in this manual are only general guides, as few reference ranges apply across laboratories and testing methods. Reference intervals supplied by the local laboratory always supersede the intervals suggested here.

Laboratory Testing in Psychiatry

What constitutes standard laboratory screening for psychiatric patients in general is not well established. There does appear to be general agreement that a screening laboratory evaluation is indicated for the following patients: those presenting for the first time with major psychiatric syndromes (e.g., psychosis or major mood disorders), elderly patients admitted to the hospital, patients who are undernourished or significantly dehydrated, those with alcohol or drug dependence, and those with delirium or initial presentation of dementia.

Patients admitted to inpatient psychiatry services may undergo the following laboratory evaluation upon admission:

- Complete blood count
- Comprehensive metabolic panel
- Urinalysis
- Urine drug screen with alcohol
- HIV testing (from which patients may "opt out")

For patients who are at risk of the metabolic syndrome, or those who are to be started on an atypical antipsychotic or other drug associated with this syndrome, the following may be added:

- Lipid panel
- Hemoglobin A1C

Thyroid-stimulating hormone may be checked for patients presenting with mood disorders or significant anxiety, and for all females age 50 years and older unless testing was done within the past year. Urine or serum pregnancy testing may be performed if there is any question of pregnancy. More extensive laboratory testing may be indicated for patients presenting with syndromes such as acute psychosis, as discussed in the *Diseases and Conditions* chapter.

Cardiac-Related Tests

Inpatient psychiatrists and those working in research settings may be required to obtain and provide preliminary interpretation of electrocardiogram (ECG) tracings. The ECG is therefore covered in some depth in the *Laboratory Tests* chapter (including indications, critical and abnormal findings, and typical ECG findings associated with psychotropic medications) and in Appendix C (which includes a table listing 10 rules for a normal ECG, a figure depicting ECG waves and intervals, a figure depicting different degrees of heart block, and a gateway to the evaluation of 10-year cardiac risk using a tool developed by the American College of Cardiology). Other cardiac-related entries appear in the *Diseases and Conditions* chapter.

Chemistries

The largest component of the *Laboratory Tests* chapter involves blood chemistries. These are the laboratory tests most often found to be abnormal in patients seen in psychiatric consultation in the general hospital. Abnormalities of blood chemistry often contribute to delirium, anxiety, depression, and other common psychiatric presentations. Chemistry tests that are not yet clinically available are not included.

Cerebrospinal Fluid Testing

Cerebrospinal fluid (CSF) tests include amyloid-β_{1-42}, CSF analysis, cell count and differential, cytology, glucose, lactate, protein, and tau protein. These tests may be useful in the diagnosis of Alzheimer's disease, encephalitis, meningitis, and other neuropsychiatric disorders. For those who may be interested, several excellent video presentations showing in detail how the lumbar puncture is performed are available online (e.g., on YouTube).

Genetic Testing

The number of genetic tests currently available is very large, but most test for relatively rare conditions and thus are not included here. Genetic tests that are covered include apolipoprotein E (ApoE) genotyping, cytochrome P450 (CYP450) genotyping, fragile X (*FMR1*) mutation analysis, *HTT* mutation analysis for Huntington's disease, and 5-HTTLPR polymorphism in the serotonin transporter gene *SLC6A4*. For most clinicians, genetic tests are laboratory send-outs. It is important to inquire directly with the receiving laboratory about costs before sending samples, because these tests may not be covered by insurance and can be prohibitively expensive.

Hematology

Basic hematology is relevant to psychiatric practice not only because hematological abnormalities may underlie symptoms such as fatigue, inattention, and restless legs but also because psychotropic medications may significantly affect hematological values. In addition to clozapine, many other psychotropic drugs can cause hematological abnormalities. DRESS (drug reaction with eosinophilia and systemic symptoms) is one example that is increasingly recognized with psychotropics such as valproate and lamotrigine.

Imaging

Structural imaging is a core component of the diagnostic workup for a variety of conditions, particularly those at the interface of psychiatry and neurology. Structural imaging is indicated when signs and symptoms of a major psychiatric disorder first become manifest, for atypical presentations, for atypical age at onset, or for psychiatric symptoms associated with a focal neurological examination.

Because behavioral health clinicians often work in tandem with neurologists, neurosurgeons, and internists, they may find themselves in a position to order or suggest a variety of imaging studies, to assist patients in understanding study results, and to facilitate tests and procedures. Thus, the information related to imaging in this manual covers an array of services—not only neuroimaging but also basic studies such as a chest X-ray and bone mineral density (DEXA) scan. Other imaging tests covered in this manual include angiography, carotid ultrasound, CT, CT angiography, functional MRI, mammography, magnetic resonance angiography, magnetic resonance spectroscopy, MRI, PET, and SPECT. Appendix B includes a table listing signal appearances for various tissues on CT and MRI T1 and T2 scans, along with a description of the steps involved in reading a head CT scan.

Infectious Disease Testing

Specific infectious diseases encountered in neuropsychiatric practice that are covered in the *Diseases and Conditions* chapter of this manual include brain abscess, Creutzfeldt-Jakob disease, encephalitis (including arbovirus encephalitis and herpes simplex encephalitis), hepatitis, HIV/AIDS, Lyme disease, meningitis, infectious mononucleosis, progressive multifocal leukoencephalopathy, syphilis and neurosyphilis, tuberculosis, and urinary tract infection. Related entries in the *Laboratory Tests* chapter include hepatitis panel, HIV testing, Lyme antibodies, syphilis testing, and tuberculosis testing.

Screening and Monitoring of Psychotropic Medications

The *Laboratory Tests* chapter of this manual includes information about drug level testing for a selected group of medications, including benzodiazepines, clozapine, and mood stabilizers. The *Psychotropic Medications: Laboratory Screening and Monitoring* chapter covers what have come to be called "safety labs" for monitoring adverse effects of psychotropic medications, as well as screening lab tests used to obtain baseline values and to ensure that medications can safely be started. Appendix A presents a table of therapeutic and toxic drug levels for commonly used psychotropic medications.

In general, drug levels can be obtained for any drug to confirm toxicity or document noncompliance (with very low levels). Therapeutic ranges are included in this manual for many drugs. Free drug levels may be used in place of total drug levels when the patient has hypoalbuminemia, which can affect the interpretation of total drug levels.

Stool Tests

Tests for blood in stool are included because certain psychotropic medications cause occult gastrointestinal bleeding, an underdiagnosed problem in psychiatry. In addi-

tion to the fecal occult blood test, a newer test for occult blood—the fecal immunochemical test—is described.

Urine Tests

Routine urinalysis provides a great deal of information about general health and gen-
itourinary function. Individual components of the urinalysis are discussed separately
to deal with the many implications of individual urine test abnormalities. These components include urine appearance, bilirubin, blood or hemoglobin, casts, color, crys-
tals, epithelial cells and casts, glucose, ketones, leukocyte esterase, microalbumin,
nitrite, pH, protein, red blood cell counts and casts, specific gravity, white blood cell
counts and casts, and urobilinogen.

CHAPTER 1
Laboratory Tests

Adrenocorticotropic hormone (ACTH)

Type of test	Blood
Background and explanation of test	ACTH produced in the pituitary acts on the adrenal glands to stimulate the production of cortisol. The ACTH level increases when systemic cortisol levels are low and decreases when cortisol levels are high. Cortisol regulation is a critical component of homeostasis, because this hormone functions to maintain blood pressure; control metabolism of glucose, protein, and lipids; and assist in regulating the immune response. A normal diurnal variation is seen with ACTH, with peak levels occurring before 8:00 A.M. and trough levels before 11:00 P.M. Diurnal variation of cortisol levels naturally follows this variation of ACTH levels, with a slight time lag.
	In patients with suspected adrenal insufficiency or suspected Cushing's syndrome, stimulation tests are given to confirm the diagnosis and to determine the cause.
	• ACTH stimulation test (also known as cosyntropin or Cortrosyn test): Cosyntropin is a compound that acts as an ACTH analogue, stimulating the adrenal glands to produce cortisol. If cortisol levels remain low with stimulation, the patient has primary adrenal failure (Addison's disease).
	• Dexamethasone suppression test: This steroid feeds back to the pituitary to stop ACTH production. If cortisol remains high, the adrenal glands themselves are producing too much cortisol.
Relevance to psychiatry and behavioral science	The ACTH level is increased when a person is under stress or using amphetamines, steroids, alcohol, or lithium. ACTH drives cortisol production and secretion, and excess or deficient cortisol causes symptoms that could be mistaken for a primary psychiatric condition.
Preparation of patient	The patient should follow a low carbohydrate diet for 48 hours before testing and should avoid stress for 12 hours before testing.
Indications	ACTH level is checked to diagnose and monitor disorders involving abnormal cortisol levels. This test is indicated for the following patients:
	• Those with signs and symptoms of *hypercortisolism*, including hypertension, hypokalemia, hyperglycemia, truncal obesity, moon facies, abdominal striae, hirsutism, skin thinning, acne, and weakness
	• Those with signs and symptoms of *hypocortisolism*, including hypotension, hyperkalemia, hypoglycemia, hyponatremia, hypercalcemia, fatigue, loss of appetite, weight loss, and skin hyperpigmentation in nonexposed areas

Adrenocorticotropic hormone (ACTH) *(continued)*

Indications (*continued*)	• Those with signs and symptoms of *hypopituitarism*, including fatigue, weight loss, frequent nocturia, menstrual irregularities, hypogonadism, and decreased libido
Reference range	8:00 A.M. (peak): 25–100 pg/mL 6:00 P.M. (trough): 0–50 pg/mL For ACTH stimulation test, cortisol >20 μg/dL See **Dexamethasone Suppression Test** entry for that reference range.
Critical value(s)	None
Increased levels	• Addison's disease (with low cortisol) • Pituitary Cushing's syndrome (with high cortisol) • Ectopic ACTH production (with high cortisol) • Pituitary adenoma • Stress
Decreased levels	• Adrenal tumor (with high cortisol) • Hypopituitarism (with low cortisol)
Interfering factors	Drugs that increase the ACTH level include amphetamines, steroids, alcohol, lithium, insulin, levodopa, metoclopramide, and RU 486. Drugs that decrease the ACTH level include dexamethasone, other cortisol-like drugs (including prednisone, hydrocortisone, prednisolone, and methylprednisolone), and megestrol acetate.
Cross-references	**Adrenal Insufficiency** **Cortisol** **Cushing's Syndrome** **Dexamethasone Suppression Test**

American Association for Clinical Chemistry: Testing.com. Available at: https://www.testing.com. Accessed May 2021.

Dorin RI, Qualls CR, Crapo LM: Diagnosis of adrenal insufficiency. Ann Intern Med 139:194–204, 2003

Garcia C, Biller BM, Klibanski A: The role of the clinical laboratory in the diagnosis of Cushing syndrome. Am J Clin Pathol 120(suppl):S38–S45, 2003

Karaca Z, Grossman A, Kelestimur F: Investigation of the hypothalamo-pituitary-adrenal (HPA) axis: a contemporary synthesis. Rev Endocr Metab Disord 22(2):179–204, 2021

Khare S, Anjum F: Adrenocorticotropic hormone test, in StatPearls. Treasure Island, FL, StatPearls Publishing, 2021. Available at: https://www.statpearls.com/ArticleLibrary/viewarticle/20072. Accessed May 2021.

Malabanan AO, Meikle AW, Swenson L: Endocrine Disorders: Choose the Right Tests. The Primary Care Guide to Diagnostic Testing. Columbus, OH, Anadem, 2004

Thomas Z, Fraser GL: An update on the diagnosis of adrenal insufficiency and the use of corticotherapy in critical illness. Ann Pharmacother 41:1456–1465, 2007

Alanine transaminase (ALT)

Type of test	Blood
Background and explanation of test	ALT is one of two transaminases—liver enzymes involved in amino acid metabolism and cellular energy production. Unlike AST, ALT is primarily localized to the liver. Under normal conditions, ALT levels in blood are low. When the liver is injured, ALT is released into the circulation and provides an early sign of this injury before clinical symptoms develop. Extreme elevations of ALT (>10 times normal) usually suggest acute hepatitis, often viral in origin. In this condition, ALT levels can remain high for as long as 6 months. In chronic hepatitis, on the other hand, ALT levels may be only minimally elevated (<4 times normal) or even high-normal. The most common cause of mild ALT elevation in the Western hemisphere is non-alcoholic fatty liver disease. In liver disease such as cirrhosis or biliary obstruction, ALT levels may be normal.
	ALT values are usually considered in relation to other LFTs such as AST and ALP. In alcoholic liver disease, the ratio of AST to ALT is high (2:1 or more), even when neither value is elevated. AST is more sensitive to alcoholic liver disease, but ALT is more specific. In extrahepatic biliary obstruction, ALT is usually more elevated than AST. In acute MI, AST is always elevated, but ALT is not unless there is also liver injury.
Relevance to psychiatry and behavioral science	ALT is one of the tests of liver health (liver "function") that is closely monitored in psychiatric practice, mainly because of the potential hepatotoxicity of psychotropic drugs. ALT is also monitored in patients with alcohol use disorder (AUD), substance-induced liver disease, and hepatitis.
	Elevation of ALT may be found on routine screening. If the patient has no clinical symptoms and no risk factors for liver disease, and ALT is <3 times the upper limit of normal (ULN), a recheck is indicated after 1–3 months. If the elevation persists, further investigation is needed.
	If ALT is >3 times the ULN on a single measurement, further investigation is needed.
	Elevation of ALT may occur with initiation of a new psychotropic medication. In most cases, that ALT increase is benign, and the laboratory value will revert to baseline within weeks of dosage stabilization. Further investigation is needed if the value does not normalize or when ALP or bilirubin is also elevated.
	Pathological elevation of ALT may occur with AUD, substance-induced liver disease, or hepatitis. It is important not to be misled by a normal ALT value in a patient with established cirrhosis.
	In patients with cirrhosis due to hepatitis C who have a normal ALT result, active hepatitis may be present, such that they would benefit from antiviral therapy, β-blockers to prevent variceal bleeding, and other treatments.

Alanine transaminase (ALT) *(continued)*

Relevance to psychiatry and behavioral science *(continued)*	AST and ALT levels may also be normal in patients with hemochromatosis, in those receiving methotrexate, or after jejunoileal bypass surgery despite advanced liver disease. In all cases, the patients' history should be considered and an effort made to identify other evidence of liver disease.
Preparation of patient	None needed
Indications	• Component of LFT panel • Component of CMP • Monitoring medication effects on the liver • Clinical symptoms of liver disease such as jaundice, abdominal pain, ascites, nausea, vomiting, or darkening of urine • Distinguishing hemolytic jaundice from jaundice due to liver dysfunction • Evaluating patients with hepatitis exposure or symptoms of hepatitis • Evaluating patients with AUD or other substance abuse • Monitoring effects of treatment for liver disease
Reference range	Males: 10–40 U/L Females: 7–35 U/L Normal values may vary with testing method.
Critical value(s)	>300 IU/L indicates acute hepatic injury.
Increased levels	• Acute viral, infectious, ischemic, or toxic hepatitis (30–50 times normal) • Hepatic necrosis due to drugs (e.g., acetaminophen) • Hepatocellular disease (moderate to marked increase) • Alcoholic cirrhosis (mild increase) • Metastatic liver disease (mild increase) • Biliary obstruction (mild increase) • Fatty liver (mild increase) • Mild increase (<1.5× ULN) can be normal for sex, ethnicity, or BMI
Decreased levels	Certain drugs can falsely decrease levels, as noted below.
Interfering factors	Levels are normally slightly higher in males and Blacks. Many psychotropic drugs can falsely elevate ALT values. Aspirin, interferon, phenothiazines, and simvastatin can falsely reduce ALT values.
Cross-references	**Alcohol Use Disorder** **Aspartate Transaminase** **Cirrhosis** **Fatty Liver Disease** **Hepatitis, Viral** **Liver Function Tests**

Alanine transaminase (ALT) *(continued)*

American Association for Clinical Chemistry: Testing.com. Available at: https://www.testing.com. Accessed May 2021.

Fischbach FT, Fischbach MA: A Manual of Laboratory and Diagnostic Tests, 10th Edition. Philadelphia, PA, Wolters Kluwer Health/Lippincott Williams and Wilkins, 2018

Gopal DV, Rosen HR: Abnormal findings on liver function tests: interpreting results to narrow the diagnosis and establish a prognosis. Postgrad Med 107:100–102, 105–109, 113–114, 2000

Schreiner AD, Rockey DC: Evaluation of abnormal liver tests in the adult asymptomatic patient. Curr Opin Gastroenterol 34(4):272–279, 2018

Theal RM, Scott K: Evaluating asymptomatic patients with abnormal liver function test results. Am Fam Physician 53:2111–2119, 1996

Albumin

Type of test	Blood
Background and explanation of test	The most abundant protein in plasma, albumin serves primarily to maintain oncotic pressure inside blood vessels to keep them from becoming "leaky." It has a similar function in the urinary tract and for CSF. In addition, albumin transports various drugs and nutrients, provides a source of nourishment for tissues, and contributes to an acid-base buffer system in the blood. Albumin is normally reabsorbed in the kidneys, so undetectable levels are found in urine. The presence of albumin in the urine (as microalbumin or protein) presages or indicates kidney dysfunction. Albumin may also be lost from the blood through the GI tract or the skin or because of hemorrhage.
	The serum albumin level is highly correlated with future morbidity and mortality, not only in ill patients but also in seemingly healthy patients. It is such a strong predictor of poor surgical outcome that surgery may be postponed or canceled in the face of low values. Even so, attempts to improve nutritional status and thus raise serum albumin levels have not been successful. In fact, it is now known that serum albumin concentration correlates poorly with general nutritional status, such that serum albumin is no longer considered a reliable marker of undernutrition.
Relevance to psychiatry and behavioral science	Although serum albumin is routinely checked as part of the CMP, its clinical value has been questioned. The albumin level may be low in numerous disease states, most prominently liver disease, but the finding of low albumin helps little with differential diagnosis. Contrary to previous teachings, the albumin level does not decline significantly in chronic anorexia nervosa, possibly because of replacement by protein released from muscle breakdown.
	The albumin level can assist in the interpretation of borderline-normal calcium levels, as discussed in other tables. In addition, low albumin is of importance in psychopharmacology, in the interpretation of drug levels for highly protein-bound drugs. When the albumin level is low, the unbound percentage of these drugs is higher, and the measured concentration of total drug may underestimate the amount of drug acting on the target organ. In this case, the patient could develop symptoms of toxicity at apparently therapeutic levels. Free drug levels, which are available for many psychotropics, can be helpful in this situation.
Preparation of patient	None needed
Indications	Routine component of CMP
Reference range	Adults: 3.5–5.2 g/dL
	Recent research suggests that the lower limit of normal for serum albumin may more appropriately be set at 4.3 g/dL than the accepted value of 3.5 g/dL because values between 3.5 g/dL and 4.3 g/dL are still associated with relatively high mortality rates.

Albumin *(continued)*

Critical value(s)	<1.5 g/dL (<15 g/L) Levels of 2.0–2.5 g/dL may be associated with edema.
Increased levels	Dehydration
Decreased levels	• Schizophrenia, major depression • Liver damage, cirrhosis, alcohol use disorder • Nephrotic syndrome, renal disease • Inflammatory bowel disease • Heart failure • Burns • Severe skin disease • Low-protein, normal calorie diet (Kwashiorkor) • Acute inflammation • Chronic inflammation • Thyroid disease: Cushing's disease, thyrotoxicosis • Prolonged hospitalization or bed rest
Interfering factors	Level declines slowly after age 40 years. Decreased albumin levels occur in the last trimester of pregnancy. Drugs that increase albumin levels include anabolic steroids, androgens, growth hormones, and insulin. Drugs that decrease albumin levels include estrogens. IV fluids may invalidate results because of dilutional effects.
Cross-references	**Alcohol Use Disorder** **Comprehensive Metabolic Panel** **Protein, Serum**

American Association for Clinical Chemistry: Testing.com. Available at: https://www.testing.com. Accessed May 2021.

Boldt J: Use of albumin: an update. Br J Anaesth 104:276–284, 2010

Fischbach FT, Fischbach MA: A Manual of Laboratory and Diagnostic Tests, 10th Edition. Philadelphia, PA, Wolters Kluwer Health/Lippincott Williams and Wilkins, 2018

Levitt DG, Levitt MD: Human serum albumin homeostasis: a new look at the roles of synthesis, catabolism, renal and gastrointestinal excretion, and the clinical value of serum albumin measurements. Int J Gen Med 9:229–255, 2016

Aldosterone

Type of test	Blood
Background and explanation of test	Aldosterone is a steroid hormone produced in the adrenal cortex that regulates sodium retention and potassium excretion by the kidneys along with blood volume and blood pressure. Renin is an enzyme released by the kidneys when blood pressure drops that initiates a chain of events resulting in aldosterone production. In healthy individuals, when the renin level increases, the aldosterone level also increases. In primary aldosteronism, aldosterone secretion is independent of renin secretion and is not suppressible. To differentiate conditions associated with aldosterone abnormalities, renin and cortisol levels are checked along with aldosterone.
Relevance to psychiatry and behavioral science	When patients presenting with vague complaints of chronic fatigue and muscle weakness in the context of refractory hypertension and hypokalemia are treated only symptomatically, the underlying diagnosis of hyperaldosteronism may be missed.
Preparation of patient	Patients should avoid stress and strenuous exercise before testing. They can be supine or sitting upright but should remain in this position for 15–30 minutes before blood is drawn. Salt intake for 2 weeks before testing should be normal. If patient is hypokalemic, potassium should be replaced before testing.
Indications	• Signs and symptoms of hyperaldosteronism, including hypertension, fatigue, weakness, and low potassium • Suspected adrenal insufficiency
Reference range	Upright position, adults: 7–30 ng/dL Supine position, adults: 3–16 ng/dL Values are 3–5 times higher with a low-sodium diet.
Critical value(s)	None
Increased levels	• Primary aldosteronism or Conn's syndrome: high aldosterone, low renin, and normal cortisol • Secondary aldosteronism: high aldosterone, high renin, and normal cortisol
Decreased levels	• Cushing's syndrome: aldosterone low to normal, renin low, and cortisol high • Adrenal insufficiency or Addison's disease: aldosterone low, renin high, and cortisol low
Interfering factors	Factors affecting test results include salt intake, licorice ingestion, time of specimen collection, stress, posture, strenuous exercise, severe illness, and certain drugs (NSAIDs, diuretics, β-blockers, steroids, ACE inhibitors, and oral contraceptives).
Cross-references	**Adrenal Insufficiency** **Cortisol** **Cushing's Syndrome**

Aldosterone *(continued)*

American Association for Clinical Chemistry: Testing.com. Available at: https://www.testing.com. Accessed May 2021.

Fischbach FT, Fischbach MA: A Manual of Laboratory and Diagnostic Tests, 10th Edition. Philadelphia, PA, Wolters Kluwer Health/Lippincott Williams and Wilkins, 2018

Torpy DJ, Stratakis CA, Chrousos GP: Hyper- and hypoaldosteronism. Vitam Horm 57:177–216, 1999

Vaidya A, Carey RM: Evolution of the primary aldosteronism syndrome: updating the approach. J Clin Endocrinol Metab 105(12):3771–3783, 2020 [published correction appears in J Clin Endocrinol Metab 106(1):e414, 2021]

White PC: Disorders of aldosterone biosynthesis and action. N Engl J Med 331:250–258, 1994

Alkaline phosphatase (ALP)

Type of test	Blood
Background and explanation of test	ALP is an enzyme concentrated in osteoblasts (bone-forming cells) and cells that form the bile canaliculi in the liver. Smaller amounts of ALP are found in the placenta and bowel. Each of these organs elaborates a different isoenzyme of ALP, which can be distinguished by fractionation. Total ALP levels are used to evaluate liver and bone disease, with high levels indicating injury to one of these tissues.
	When ALP is elevated in tandem with other LFTs such as AST, ALT, or bilirubin, the cause of the ALP elevation is usually hepatic. In liver disease such as biliary obstruction, ALP and bilirubin are increased out of proportion to increases in AST or ALT. In hepatocellular liver injury such as occurs in hepatitis, ALT and AST are increased out of proportion to ALP.
	If the ALP level is high and the source of the elevation is unknown, ALP can be fractionated or GGT can be assayed. GGT is another enzyme produced in the liver that is not made by bone. GGT elevation then indicates a hepatic source.
	If ALP is elevated and calcium and phosphate levels are abnormal, the source is usually bone. Cancer metastatic to bone or liver can cause elevation in ALP. With treatment, ALP levels may decline. In some bone diseases such as Paget's disease, ALP may be the only laboratory abnormality, and the elevation seen can be up to 25 times the normal value. ALP is elevated in osteomalacia (bone softening) but not in osteoporosis, so the value can help distinguish these conditions.
Relevance to psychiatry and behavioral science	Numerous psychotropic drugs are associated with increased ALP levels. (See *Interfering Factors* section below.) A cholestatic drug reaction can be suggested by elevated ALP and GGT along with either elevated transaminases or bilirubin with a normal liver ultrasound. Alcohol overuse and cirrhosis are both associated with ALP elevation. In alcohol-related hepatitis, the ALP elevation is <2 times the upper limit of normal (ULN), and this does not correlate well with the bilirubin level.
Preparation of patient	Overnight fasting before the test is preferred because enzyme activity is affected by eating, especially fatty food.
Indications	• Component of the LFT panel • Signs/symptoms of liver disease • Signs/symptoms of bone disease
Reference range	Adults: 25–100 U/L ALP elevation may be found on routine screening. • If ALP is <1.5 times the ULN, recheck in 1–3 months. • If ALP is ≥1.5 times the ULN on two measurements 6 months apart, further investigation is needed. • If ALP is >3 times the ULN on a single measurement, further investigation is needed.
Critical value(s)	None

Alkaline phosphatase (ALP) *(continued)*

Increased levels *(continued)*	• Liver disease: cirrhosis, alcohol use disorder, hepatitis, cholestasis, cancer (primary or metastatic), infectious mononucleosis, diabetes, Gilbert's syndrome
	• Bile duct obstruction
	• Gallbladder disease
	• Bone disease: cancer (primary or metastatic), Paget's disease, osteomalacia, rickets, osteogenesis imperfecta
	• Hyperparathyroidism (with elevated calcium)
	• Hyperthyroidism
	• Infarction (myocardial or pulmonary)
	• Hodgkin's disease
	• Lung or pancreatic cancer
	• Ulcerative colitis
	• Peptic ulcer disease
	• Amyloidosis
	• Sarcoidosis
	• Bowel infarction or perforation
	• Chronic renal failure
	• Congestive heart failure
	• Hepatotoxic drugs
Decreased levels	• Hypothyroidism
	• Pernicious anemia and other anemias
	• Malnutrition
	• Magnesium or zinc deficiency
	• Milk-alkali syndrome
	• Celiac sprue
	• Congenital hypophosphatasia
Interfering factors	ALP levels increase at room temperature and in refrigeration; tests should be run the same day as collection.
	ALP levels decrease if blood is anticoagulated.
	People older than 50 years may have 1.5 times the normal level of ALP without pathology.
	Elevated ALP levels are seen in pregnancy and after menopause.
	ALP levels increase after fatty meals.
	Elevation in ALP is seen for several days after albumin infusion.
	A very large number of drugs are associated with ALP elevation, including all psychotropic drug classes and nearly all members of each class.
Cross-references	**Alcohol Use Disorder**
	Cirrhosis
	Liver Function Tests

Alkaline phosphatase (ALP) *(continued)*

American Association for Clinical Chemistry: Testing.com. Available at: https://www.testing.com/tests. Accessed May 2021.

Fischbach FT, Fischbach MA: A Manual of Laboratory and Diagnostic Tests, 10th Edition. Philadelphia, PA, Wolters Kluwer Health/Lippincott Williams and Wilkins, 2018

Giannini EG, Testa R, Savarino V: Liver enzyme alteration: a guide for clinicians. CMAJ 172:367–379, 2005

Reust CE, Hall L: Clinical inquiries: what is the differential diagnosis of an elevated alkaline phosphatase (AP) level in an otherwise asymptomatic patient? J Fam Pract 50:496–497, 2001

Alprazolam level

Type of test	Blood
Background and explanation of test	Benzodiazepines are Schedule IV sedative-hypnotic drugs used to treat anxiety and insomnia. Alprazolam is a fast- to intermediate-acting drug with a half-life that varies considerably among individual patients. In general, levels are checked when either overdose or noncompliance is suspected or to detect use without a prescription.
Relevance to psychiatry and behavioral science	On postmortem study, brain alprazolam levels were more than twice those in blood in cases in which alprazolam was judged not to have been a contributing cause of death. Toxicity with chronic benzodiazepine ingestion may be manifested as confusion, disorientation, memory impairment, ataxia, decreased reflexes, and dysarthria. With acute overdose, the patient may exhibit somnolence, confusion, ataxia, decreased reflexes, vertigo, dysarthria, respiratory depression, and coma. More serious consequences usually involve co-ingestion of alcohol or other sedatives.
Preparation of patient	None needed
Indications	• Screening for drug use • Suspicion of overdose • Signs of toxicity in a treated patient • Suspected noncompliance with prescribed therapy
Reference range	10–40 ng/mL with low-dose therapy (1–4 mg/day) 50–100 ng/mL with high-dose therapy (6–9 mg/day)
Critical value(s)	Above upper limits noted
Increased levels	• Overdose • Overuse • Poor metabolism • Hepatic encephalopathy
Decreased levels	Noncompliance
Interfering factors	None
Cross-references	Benzodiazepines

ARUP Laboratories: Alprazolam, in Lab Test Directory. Salt Lake City, UT, ARUP Laboratories, 2021. Available at: https://ltd.aruplab.com/Tests/Pub/0090010. Accessed May 2021.

Skov L, Holm KM, Johansen SS, Linnet K: Postmortem brain and blood reference concentrations of alprazolam, bromazepam, chlordiazepoxide, diazepam, and their metabolites and a review of the literature. J Anal Toxicol 40(7):529–536, 2016

Ammonia

Type of test	Blood
Background and explanation of test	Ammonia is a waste product made by intestinal bacteria and other cells during protein digestion. Under normal conditions, ammonia is transformed in the liver to urea, which can be excreted by the kidneys. If this cycle malfunctions, ammonia can build up in the blood, affecting acid-base balance and brain function. In acute hepatic failure, with a rapid rise in ammonia levels, there is a reasonable correlation of venous ammonia levels with arterial ammonia levels and of arterial ammonia with brain glutamine levels. In chronic hepatic insufficiency, correlations are much less robust.
Relevance to psychiatry and behavioral science	Routine blood tests do not include ammonia assays, in part because of the unreliability of ammonia sampling. Unless there is clinical suspicion of ammonia elevation based on the patient's history or exam findings, the ammonia level is not checked. For this reason, hyperammonemia may be underdiagnosed in some settings. Elevated ammonia levels can be found in hepatic failure due to alcoholic cirrhosis, hepatitis, and Wilson's disease, among other conditions. Acute hyperammonemia is associated with delirium and other mental status changes as well as seizures. In severe cases, coma and death from brain herniation can supervene. When acute hyperammonemia is suspected, the ammonia level should be ordered and checked *stat* because this represents a medically urgent situation. This order is also critical to the accuracy of the test, because ammonia levels increase with the breakdown of proteins during blood storage. Chronic hyperammonemia has less severe symptoms because of compensatory changes in ammonia metabolism and dampening of excitatory effects on the brain.
Preparation of patient	If possible, patients should fast for 8 hours except for water and should not smoke for 2 hours before testing.
Indications	<ul><li>Workup for mental status changes</li><li>Workup for lethargy and vomiting in a child after viral illness</li><li>Diagnosing hepatic encephalopathy</li><li>Diagnosing Reye's syndrome</li><li>Monitoring severity of hepatic disease and response to treatment</li><li>Evaluating genetic urea cycle disorders</li><li>Monitoring patients on hyperalimentation</li></ul>
Reference range	Dependent on what is measured: <ul><li>*Measured as NH_3, adults:* 15–60 µg/dL</li><li>*Measured as N, adults:* 15–45 µg/dL</li></ul>
Critical value(s)	$NH_3 > 200$ µmol/L

Ammonia *(continued)*

Increased levels	• Liver disease, especially after a precipitant such as GI bleeding or electrolyte imbalance
	• Decreased blood flow to the liver
	• GI hemorrhage
	• GI tract infection with distention and stasis
	• Reye's syndrome (with decreased glucose levels)
	• Renal failure
	• Total parenteral nutrition
	• Heritable defects in urea cycle enzymes (can appear at any age)
	• Use of valproic acid (especially in patients with carnitine deficiency)
	• Other drugs, including barbiturates, diuretics, and opioids
Decreased levels	• Hypertension
	• Antibiotics such as neomycin
Interfering factors	Sampling techniques greatly affect ammonia values.
	Hemolysis, use of a tight tourniquet, clenching fist, or allowing sample to sit increases ammonia levels, as does exercise or other muscular exertion and smoking.
Cross-references	**Alcohol Use Disorder**
	Cirrhosis
	Hepatic Encephalopathy
	Hepatitis, Viral

Blanco Vela CI, Bosques Padilla FJ: Determination of ammonia concentrations in cirrhosis patients: still confusing after all these years? Ann Hepatol 10(Suppl 2):S60–S65, 2011

Cohn RM, Roth KS: Hyperammonemia, bane of the brain. Clin Pediatr (Phila) 43:683–689, 2004

Fischbach FT, Fischbach MA: A Manual of Laboratory and Diagnostic Tests, 10th Edition. Philadelphia, PA, Wolters Kluwer Health/Lippincott Williams and Wilkins, 2018

Kundra A, Jain A, Banga A, et al: Evaluation of plasma ammonia levels in patients with acute liver failure and chronic liver disease and its correlation with the severity of hepatic encephalopathy and clinical features of raised intracranial tension. Clin Biochem 38:696–699, 2005

Amylase

Type of test	Blood
Background and explanation of test	Amylase is an enzyme produced by the parotid glands and the pancreas that facilitates digestion of complex carbohydrates. It enters the circulation in large amounts when the salivary glands or pancreas is inflamed and is excreted by the kidneys. The most important use of amylase testing is to diagnose acute pancreatitis, although lipase is more specific for this condition. In acute pancreatitis, the serum amylase level begins to rise 2 hours after onset, peaks at 24 hours, and persists for 2–4 days. Amylase appears in the urine with a lag time of 6–10 hours and persists for 7–10 days.
	Amylase can also be high in *macroamylasemia*. In this condition, amylase is bound to immunoglobulin, forming a molecule that is poorly filtered by the kidney because of its large size. Macroamylasemia does not cause symptoms but is associated with other diseases such as ulcerative colitis, celiac disease, HIV infection, and rheumatoid arthritis. It is also seen in apparently healthy patients. Macroamylasemia can be distinguished from acute pancreatitis by measuring urine amylase, which is low in macroamylasemia and high in acute pancreatitis.
Relevance to psychiatry and behavioral science	Amylase is elevated along with lipase in pancreatitis, and certain populations are at particular risk, including patients with alcoholism (especially males), gallstones (especially females), and hyperlipidemia and those treated with medications such as valproate, corticosteroids, or isoniazid. Amylase of salivary origin may be elevated in patients with eating disorders that include purging behaviors.
Preparation of patient	Patients should fast for ≥2 hours before testing.
Indications	Diagnosis and monitoring of patients with acute pancreatitis, although lipase alone may be sufficient for this purpose
Reference range	Adults ≤60 years: 25–125 U/L
	Adults >60 years: 24–151 U/L
Critical value(s)	Amylase ≥3 times the upper limit of normal is one criterion for acute pancreatitis.
Increased levels	• Pancreatitis • Other pancreatic disease or trauma • Eating disorder with purging • Partial gastrectomy • Appendicitis, peritonitis • Perforated peptic ulcer • TBI • Shock • Mumps or other salivary gland/duct inflammation or obstruction

Amylase *(continued)*

Increased levels *(continued)*	• Acute cholecystitis (stone in the common bile duct) • Intestinal obstruction • Ruptured ectopic pregnancy • Macroamylasemia
Decreased levels	• Pancreatic insufficiency, pancreatectomy • Liver disease, hepatitis • Cystic fibrosis
Interfering factors	Anticoagulated blood and lipemic serum interfere with results. Pregnancy and diabetes increase levels. Drugs that increase amylase levels include clozapine, desipramine, donepezil, mirtazapine, risperidone, valproate, and numerous non-psychotropic medications, including NSAIDs, acetaminophen, many opioids, and steroids. Drugs that decrease amylase levels include anabolic steroids, cefotaxime, propylthiouracil, zidovudine, and others.
Cross-references	**Lipase** **Pancreatitis, Acute**

American Association for Clinical Chemistry: Testing.com. Available at: https://www.testing.com. Accessed May 2021.

Boxhoorn L, Voermans RP, Bouwense SA, et al: Acute pancreatitis. Lancet 396 (10252):726–734, 2020

Fischbach FT, Fischbach MA: A Manual of Laboratory and Diagnostic Tests, 10th Edition. Philadelphia, PA, Wolters Kluwer Health/Lippincott Williams and Wilkins, 2018

Ghio L, Fornaro G, Rossi P: Risperidone-induced hyperamylasemia, hyperlipasemia, and neuroleptic malignant syndrome: a case report. J Clin Psychopharmacol 29:391–392, 2009

Ismail OZ, Bhayana V: Lipase or amylase for the diagnosis of acute pancreatitis? Clin Biochem 50(18):1275–1280, 2017

Angiography, computed tomography (cerebrovascular)

Type of test	Imaging
Background and explanation of test	In CT angiography, cerebral vasculature and tissues are examined using CT technology along with administration of contrast dye. This modality is used in the acute setting to evaluate new-onset headache, TIA, suspected stroke, bleeding from a cerebral aneurysm or arteriovenous malformation, and other events (as noted in the *Indications* section below). Compared to magnetic resonance angiography (MRA), CT angiography is superior in the detection of acute blood.
Relevance to psychiatry and behavioral science	Patients with stenotic lesions, aneurysms, vascular malformations, and other cerebrovascular conditions may exhibit associated psychiatric signs and symptoms, and CT angiography may be helpful in the diagnostic workup. Psychiatrists should be familiar with this modality and be able to explain what is involved to patients under their care, even though the test may be ordered by other specialists. Extremely detailed and lifelike images can now be obtained via an image processing technique—three-dimensional cinematic rendering—that facilitates exploration of and teaching about cerebral vasculature.
Preparation of patient	See **Computed Tomography Scan, Head**
Indications	• Sudden-onset severe or unilateral headache • Suspected carotid or vertebral dissection • Ipsilateral Horner syndrome • Suspected carotid vascular disease: asymptomatic cervical bruit and/or risk factors • TIA involving carotid or vertebrobasilar territories (combined with head CT) • New focal neurological deficit (combined with head CT) • Risk of unruptured aneurysm with positive family history (combined with noncontrast head CT) • Known subarachnoid hemorrhage • Known parenchymal hemorrhage • Acute ataxia (head and neck; combined with CT)
Reference range	No vascular stenosis, occlusion, dissection, dilatation, abnormal communication, or extravasated blood
Abnormal test	• Atherosclerotic stenosis or occlusion • Disease or aneurysm of the aorta • Aneurysm or arteriovenous malformation in the brain • Intracerebral or intracranial hemorrhage • Vascular injury from trauma • Hypervascular tumor or tumor invasion of vasculature

Angiography, computed tomography (cerebrovascular) *(continued)*

Interfering factors	Any motion artifact results in poor imaging. Patients who are agitated or unable to comprehend instructions to minimize motion from swallowing and breathing cannot be studied.
	Carotid artery overlap (internal with external on each side) makes it difficult to view an individual vessel.
Cross-references	**Computed Tomography Scan, Head**
	Stroke

Caton MT Jr, Wiggins WF, Nunez D: Three-dimensional cinematic rendering to optimize visualization of cerebrovascular anatomy and disease in CT angiography. J Neuroimaging 30(3):286–296, 2020

Fauci AS, Braunwald E, Kasper DL, et al (eds): Harrison's Principles of Internal Medicine, 17th Edition. New York, McGraw-Hill, 2008

Hopyan J, Ciarallo A, Dowlatshahi D, et al: Certainty of stroke diagnosis: incremental benefit with CT perfusion over noncontrast CT and CT angiography. Radiology 255:142–153, 2010

Angiography, magnetic resonance (cerebrovascular)

Type of test	Imaging
Background and explanation of test	Magnetic resonance angiography (MRA) is an application of MRI that images blood flow and highlights pathology of blood vessels. It can be performed with or without contrast medium, although contrast can aid visualization. The scan takes 15–30 minutes. Compared with CT angiography, MRA is superior in the resolution of adjacent tissues.
Relevance to psychiatry and behavioral science	Patients with stenotic lesions, aneurysms, vascular malformations, and other cerebrovascular conditions may exhibit associated psychiatric signs and symptoms. MRA may be helpful in the diagnostic workup.
Preparation of patient	No pretest preparation is needed. MRA is not performed on patients with implanted metal devices, including pacemakers, defibrillators, cochlear implants, metal heart valves, pumps, neurostimulators, certain prostheses, and certain intrauterine devices. For surgical implants reported to be MRI compatible, the brand, style, and serial number should be requested to confirm compatibility. MRA is not advised for pregnant patients or patients with epilepsy.
Indications	• Sudden-onset severe or unilateral headache • Suspected carotid or vertebral dissection • Ipsilateral Horner syndrome • Suspected vascular disease in carotid or vertebrobasilar arteries • Surgical planning for carotid artery disease (with carotid duplex study) • TIA involving carotid or vertebrobasilar territories (combined with head MRI) • New focal neurological deficit (combined with head MRI) • Risk of unruptured aneurysm with positive family history • Follow-up study for a known arteriovenous malformation or aneurysm • Known parenchymal hemorrhage • Ataxia, acute (head and neck; with MRI) • Evaluation of pulsatile tinnitus
Reference range	No vascular stenosis, occlusion, dissection, dilatation, abnormal communication, or extravasated blood seen
Abnormal test	• Atherosclerotic stenosis or occlusion • Aneurysm or arteriovenous malformation in the brain • Intracerebral or intracranial hemorrhage • Vascular injury from trauma • Hypervascular tumor or tumor invasion of vasculature

Angiography, magnetic resonance (cerebrovascular) *(continued)*

Interfering factors	Motion artifact results in unsatisfactory images. Patients who are agitated or unable to comprehend instructions to minimize motion from swallowing and breathing cannot be studied.
	Carotid artery overlap (internal with external on each side) makes it difficult to visualize individual vessels.
Cross-references	**Angiography, Computed Tomography (Cerebrovascular)**
	Magnetic Resonance Imaging

American College of Radiology: ACR Appropriateness Criteria: Cerebrovascular Disease. Reston, VA, American College of Radiology, 1996. Available at: https://acsearch.acr.org/docs/69478/Narrative. Accessed August 2021.

Bowen BC, Quencer RM, Margosian P, et al: MR angiography of occlusive disease of the arteries in the head and neck: current concepts. AJR Am J Roentgenol 162:9–18, 1994

Brant-Zawadzki M, Heiserman JE: The roles of MR angiography, CT angiography, and sonography in vascular imaging of the head and neck. AJNR Am J Neuroradiol 18:1820–1825, 1997

Cure JK: Imaging of vascular lesions of the head and neck. Facial Plast Surg Clin North Am 9:525–549, 2001

Patel MR, Edelman RR: MR angiography of the head and neck. Top Magn Reson Imaging 8:345–365, 1996

Zhang XH, Liang H: Systematic review with network meta-analysis: diagnostic values of ultrasonography, computed tomography, and magnetic resonance imaging in patients with ischemic stroke. Medicine (Baltimore) 98(30):e16360, 2019

Antidiuretic hormone (ADH)

Type of test	Blood
Background and explanation of test	ADH—also known as arginine vasopressin—is a hormone secreted by the posterior pituitary gland that controls the amount and concentration of urine that is produced by the kidneys.
	The concentration of dissolved particles in circulating blood is termed *serum osmolality*. When serum osmolality is low (serum is relatively dilute), ADH secretion is inhibited. In the absence of ADH, large volumes of dilute urine are excreted. When serum osmolality is high, more ADH is secreted, and small volumes of concentrated urine are excreted. These processes help maintain homeostasis. However, recent evidence suggests that not all actions of ADH are beneficial; high ADH secretion has been associated with progression of chronic kidney disease and adverse cardiovascular outcomes.
	ADH measurement is used in the diagnosis of conditions involving large amounts of urine (polyuria) or low serum sodium (hyponatremia), including diabetes insipidus, psychogenic polydipsia, SIAD, and syndromes of ectopic ADH production.
Relevance to psychiatry and behavioral science	Schizophrenia and other psychotic disorders are associated with psychogenic polydipsia. Lithium treatment can result in nephrogenic diabetes insipidus. SSRIs and many other psychotropic medications can cause SIAD.
Preparation of patient	Fasting for 12 hours before the test is preferred. Patients should refrain from strenuous activity before testing and should sit calmly for the blood draw.
Indications	• Polyuria • Hyponatremia
Reference range	<2.5 pg/mL
Critical value(s)	None
Increased levels	• Nephrogenic diabetes insipidus • SIAD • Acute intermittent porphyria • Brain lesions: tumor, trauma, neurosurgery • Guillain-Barré syndrome • Pulmonary disease (e.g., tuberculosis) • Ectopic ADH production (cancer)
Decreased levels	• Central diabetes insipidus (neurogenic or hypothalamic) • Psychogenic polydipsia • Nephrotic syndrome

Antidiuretic hormone (ADH) *(continued)*

Interfering factors	High platelet values invalidate results.
	Drugs associated with increased ADH include lithium, furosemide, and thiazide diuretics.
	Drugs associated with decreased ADH include chlorpromazine, clonidine, and guanfacine.
Cross-references	**Diabetes Insipidus**
	Hyponatremia
	Psychogenic Polydipsia
	Syndrome of Inappropriate Antidiuresis

American Association for Clinical Chemistry: Testing.com. Available at: https://www.testing.com. Accessed November 2021.

Fischbach FT, Fischbach MA: A Manual of Laboratory and Diagnostic Tests, 10th Edition. Philadelphia, PA, Wolters Kluwer Health/Lippincott Williams and Wilkins, 2018

Kanbay M, Yilmaz S, Dincer N, et al: Antidiuretic hormone and serum osmolarity physiology and related outcomes: what is old, what is new, and what is unknown? J Clin Endocrinol Metab 104(11):5406–5420, 2019

Kounin G, Bashir Q: Mechanism and role of antidiuretic hormone. Surg Neurol 53:508–510, 2000

Robertson GL: Antidiuretic hormone: normal and disordered function. Endocrinol Metab Clin North Am 30:671–694, 2001

Robinson AG: Disorders of antidiuretic hormone secretion. Clin Endocrinol Metab 14:55–88, 1985

Antinuclear antibody (ANA) testing

Type of test	Blood
Background and explanation of test	ANA testing screens for systemic rheumatic diseases including SLE, rheumatoid arthritis, polymyositis/dermatomyositis, mixed connective tissue disease, Sjögren's syndrome, scleroderma, and CREST syndrome.
	In the ANA test performed by indirect fluorescent antibody, the result is reported as a titer, along with the immunofluorescence pattern when the titer is high enough to be considered positive. Different threshold titers are used for diagnosis; for SLE, an ANA titer of 1:80 or more is accepted as positive. For other conditions, a titer of 1:160 or more is considered positive.
	When a high titer is obtained with screening, an extractable nuclear antigen (ENA) antibody panel can help to identify the specific disease:
	• Presence of anti–double-stranded DNA and anti-Smith antibodies in SLE
	• Anti-histone antibodies in drug-induced lupus
	• Anti–single-stranded-A antibodies (Ro) and anti–single-stranded-B antibodies (La) in Sjögren's syndrome
	• Positive anticentromere test, presence of anti–Scl-70 antibodies in scleroderma
	The immunofluorescence pattern may also be helpful in identifying the specific disease:
	• Homogeneous (diffuse) pattern: SLE and mixed connective tissue disease
	• Speckled pattern: SLE, Sjögren's syndrome, scleroderma, polymyositis, rheumatoid arthritis, and mixed connective tissue disease
	• Nucleolar pattern: scleroderma and polymyositis
	• Outline (peripheral) pattern: SLE
	The diagnosis of a systemic rheumatic disease is based on clinical signs and symptoms, and these tests are used only to confirm the diagnosis and identify the specific disease.
Relevance to psychiatry and behavioral science	ANA testing is most often used to diagnose SLE (lupus). Common neuropsychiatric symptoms of lupus include headaches, anxiety disorders, mood disorders, psychosis, cognitive dysfunction, and delirium. Seizures, abnormal movements (chorea, dystonia, hemiballismus), and stroke can occur. Drug-induced lupus can also cause a positive test and is important to rule out because this condition will subside when the offending drug is discontinued. Psychotropic medications associated with drug-induced lupus include carbamazepine, oxcarbazepine, phenytoin, and sertraline.
Preparation of patient	None needed

Antinuclear antibody (ANA) testing *(continued)*

Indications	• Symptoms suggestive of autoimmune disease: low-grade fever, joint pain, fatigue, rash • Suspicion of a second autoimmune disease in an affected patient • Unexplained neuropsychiatric symptoms
Reference range	≥1:160 on immunofluorescence antibody testing >3 on enzyme-linked immunosorbent assay (ELISA) testing
Critical value(s)	None
Positive test	• SLE • Drug-induced lupus • Sjögren's syndrome • Scleroderma • Rheumatoid arthritis • Raynaud's disease • Dermatomyositis • Mixed connective tissue disease
Negative test	Patient is unlikely to have one of the autoimmune disorders, although the test may need to be repeated later because of the intermittent nature of disease activity.
Interfering factors	False positives (more likely when titer is ≤1:160) are seen in 3%–5% of Whites, in 10%–37% of patients older than 65 years, and with certain drugs and infections. False-positive result can be seen in primary antiphospholipid syndrome. Drug-induced lupus can be caused by hydralazine, isoniazid, procainamide, and the psychotropic medications noted above.
Cross-references	**Systemic Lupus Erythematosus**

American Association for Clinical Chemistry: Testing.com Available at: https://www.testing.com. Accessed June 2021.

Benseler SM, Silverman ED: Neuropsychiatric involvement in pediatric systemic lupus erythematosus. Lupus 16:564–571, 2007

Hanly JG, Urowitz MB, Siannis F, et al: Autoantibodies and neuropsychiatric events at the time of systemic lupus erythematosus diagnosis: results from an international inception cohort study. Arthritis Rheum 58:843–853, 2008

Hussain HM, Zakaria M: Drug-induced lupus secondary to sertraline. Aust N Z J Psychiatry 42:1074–1075, 2008

Katz U, Zandman-Goddard G: Drug-induced lupus: an update. Autoimmun Rev 10:46–50, 2010

Ling M, Murali M: Antinuclear antibody tests. Clin Lab Med 39(4):513–524, 2019

Pisetsky DS: Antinuclear antibody testing: misunderstood or misbegotten? Nat Rev Rheumatol 13(8):495–502, 2017

Antiphospholipid (aPL) antibodies

Type of test	Blood
Background and explanation of test	The aPL syndrome (APS) is a systemic autoimmune disease characterized by thrombotic or obstetrical events that occur in patients with persistent aPL antibodies. The syndrome is often found in association with other autoimmune diseases such as SLE but can also be seen in the absence of other autoimmune symptoms. aPL antibodies include lupus anticoagulant, anticardiolipin, and anti-β-2 glycoprotein 1. Of the three tests, lupus anticoagulant correlates best with clinical events, but all three tests are performed to facilitate risk stratification. Persistence of antibodies is determined by testing on two or more occasions ≥12 weeks apart. If a patient with autoimmune symptoms does not test positive, the test is repeated because antibodies can develop at any time. Moreover, aPL antibodies are not just diagnostic markers for APS but also a risk factor for thrombosis and obstetrical events that are multifactorial. For this reason, non–aPL antibody risk factors for thrombosis (e.g., smoking, use of birth control pills or hormone replacement therapy) also must be considered. aPL antibodies have been identified in patients with COVID-19 infection, but it is not known whether they are involved in thrombotic events. At present, aPL antibodies have no role in COVID-19 diagnosis or management. Moreover, side effects of the mRNA vaccines for COVID appear to be well tolerated in patients with aPL antibodies or aPL syndrome.
Relevance to psychiatry and behavioral science	Neurological presentations of APS are well recognized. These include stroke/TIA, cognitive dysfunction, subcortical white matter changes, dementia, delirium, seizures, headaches, chorea, transverse myelitis, and motor neuropathy. Stroke occurring in a child or young adult should raise suspicion for APS. Headaches are often recurrent and refractory to usual treatments but may respond well to anticoagulation. In general, psychiatric presentations are not as well recognized, but psychosis and depression have been reported. Phenothiazine drugs can cause a transiently positive aPL test.
Preparation of patient	None needed
Indications	• Evaluation of recurrent thrombotic events • Thrombotic event in the absence of risk factors • Evaluation of repeated miscarriage in pregnancy • Investigation of thrombocytopenia, prolonged PTT, or inappropriate clotting • Confirmation of suspected Sneddon's syndrome (livedo reticularis accompanied by stroke/temporary ischemic event)
Critical value(s)	None

Antiphospholipid (aPL) antibodies (continued)

Positive test	The best use of aPL antibodies is for risk stratification, but a positive test is defined by the following:
	• Lupus anticoagulant present in plasma on two or more occasions ≥12 weeks apart, or
	• Anticardiolipin antibody of IgG and/or IgM isotype in serum or plasma, present in medium to high titer (>40 GPL or MPL or >99th percentile) on two or more occasions ≥12 weeks apart, or
	• Anti-β-2 glycoprotein 1 antibody of IgG and/or IgM isotype in serum or plasma (in titer >99th percentile) on two or more occasions ≥12 weeks apart
	The differential diagnosis for a positive test includes the following:
	• APS
	• SLE, other autoimmune disorders
	• HIV
	• Certain cancers
	• Advanced age
	• Infections (transient)
	• Certain drugs (transient): phenothiazines, procainamide
	• COVID-19 infection
Interfering factors	Anticoagulants, current infection, and prior syphilis infection may yield false-positive results.
Cross-references	**Antiphospholipid Syndrome**

Devreese KMJ: COVID-19-related laboratory coagulation findings. Int J Lab Hematol 43(Suppl 1):36–42, 2021

Favaloro EJ, Henry BM, Lippi G: COVID-19 and antiphospholipid antibodies: time for a reality check? Semin Thromb Hemost 48(1):72–92, 2022

Garcia D, Erkan D: Diagnosis and management of the antiphospholipid syndrome. N Engl J Med 378(21):2010–2021, 2018

Gezer S: Antiphospholipid syndrome. Dis Mon 49:696–741, 2003

Giannakopoulos B, Passam F, Ioannou Y, et al: How we diagnose the antiphospholipid syndrome. Blood 113:985–994, 2009

Sammaritano LR: Antiphospholipid syndrome. Best Pract Res Clin Rheumatol 34(1):101463, 2020

Sciascia S, Costanzo P, Radin M, et al: Safety and tolerability of mRNA COVID-19 vaccines in people with antiphospholipid antibodies. Lancet Rheumatol 3(12):e832, 2021

Apolipoprotein E (ApoE) genotyping

Type of test	Blood
Background and explanation of test	ApoE genotype is a major risk determinant of late-onset Alzheimer's disease (AD), with the ApoE ε4 allele promoting amyloid deposition and clinical symptoms of AD about 15 years earlier per ε4 allele. The ApoE ε2 allele confers reduced risk of AD compared to the more common ApoE ε3 allele. In addition to its effect on amyloid-β clearance from the brain, ApoE genotype is known to significantly influence tau pathology and neurodegeneration as well as microglial activity.
	ApoE also is suspected of being pathogenic itself, affecting critical brain homeostatic processes such as synaptic integrity and plasticity, lipid efflux and endocytosis, and cerebrovascular function. For these reasons, ApoE itself is now considered an important target of AD therapies, particularly in young, presymptomatic individuals.
	ApoE genotype also is known to influence the odds of attaining extreme longevity, with the ε4 allele significantly decreasing the odds and the ε2/ε2 and ε2/ε3 genotypes significantly increasing the odds.
	The rare ApoE Christchurch mutation (ApoEch) was found to greatly delay the onset of AD in a patient with autosomal dominant AD (presenilin-1 mutation).
Relevance to psychiatry and behavioral science	ApoE testing can help increase the specificity of diagnosis in patients who meet clinical criteria for AD, but it does not predict whether the disease will develop in asymptomatic individuals. In patients with the clinical diagnosis of AD, the presence of the ε4/ε4 genotype increases the probability that AD is the correct diagnosis to about 97%. On the other hand, ~42% of patients with AD do not have an ε4 allele. The test, therefore, is used in a specific context and not for screening or in the early stages of the diagnostic evaluation for dementia. Although it is possible to obtain ApoE testing through an online portal such as 23andMe, it is recommended that this testing be done through and in collaboration with a qualified health care provider.
Preparation of patient	Patient counseling is mandatory. The patient's expectations, the value of a positive or a negative test, out-of-pocket cost, implications for blood relatives, and the potential for discrimination in employment, insurability, and educational opportunities should be discussed. A plan for a follow-up discussion of test results should be made.
Indications	• Increasing specificity of diagnosis in a patient who meets clinical criteria for AD • Determining eligibility for clinical trials • Not useful for presymptomatic testing
Reference range	No ε4 allele present Possible genotypes: ε3/ε3; ε3/ε2; ε2/ε2

Apolipoprotein E (ApoE) genotyping *(continued)*

Critical value(s)	None
Abnormal test	Genotypes: ε4/ε4; ε4/ε3; ε4/ε2
Interfering factors	None
Cross-references	**Alzheimer's Disease**
	Cerebrospinal Fluid Amyloid β_{1-42}
	Cerebrospinal Fluid Tau Protein
	Dementia

Arboleda-Velasquez JF, Lopera F, O'Hare M, et al: Resistance to autosomal dominant Alzheimer's disease in an APOE3 Christchurch homozygote: a case report. Nat Med 25(11):1680–1683, 2019

McConnell LM, Sanders GD, Owens DK: Evaluation of genetic tests: APOE genotyping for the diagnosis of Alzheimer disease. Genet Test 3:47–53, 1999

Petersen RC, Waring SC, Smith GE, et al: Predictive value of APOE genotyping in incipient Alzheimer's disease. Ann N Y Acad Sci 802:58–69, 1996

Rebeck GW: The role of APOE on lipid homeostasis and inflammation in normal brains. J Lipid Res 2017 58(8):1493–1499, 2017

Sebastiani P, Gurinovich A, Nygaard M, et al: APOE alleles and extreme human longevity. J Gerontol A Biol Sci Med Sci 74(1):44–51, 2019

Selkoe DJ, Hardy J: The amyloid hypothesis of Alzheimer's disease at 25 years. EMBO Mol Med 8(6):595–608, 2016

Yamazaki Y, Zhao N, Caulfield TR, et al: Apolipoprotein E and Alzheimer disease: pathobiology and targeting strategies. Nat Rev Neurol 15(9):501–518, 2019

Aspartate transaminase (AST)

Type of test	Blood
Background and explanation of test	AST is an enzyme found in liver cells and other metabolically active tissues including the heart, skeletal muscle, kidney, brain, pancreas, lungs, RBCs, and WBCs. AST levels rise with cellular injury. AST is used with other liver enzyme tests such as ALT and ALP to evaluate liver function and detect liver damage. The pattern and degree of abnormality in each of these tests can be helpful in determining etiology.
	Extreme elevations in AST (>10 times the upper limit of normal [ULN]) are consistent with acute hepatitis, often of viral origin. As with ALT, the AST level in this condition can remain high for as long as 6 months. In chronic hepatitis, on the other hand, AST levels may be only minimally elevated (<4 times the ULN) or even high-normal. In liver disease such as cirrhosis, cancer, or biliary obstruction, AST levels may be nearly normal, but they are elevated more often than ALT. In liver damage due to alcohol, AST is usually significantly more elevated than ALT, a pattern unlike that seen in other causes of liver injury. In severe cirrhosis, the paradoxical finding of low AST may be seen, which is attributed to the loss of hepatocyte mass with a corresponding reduction of enzyme levels. In extrahepatic biliary obstruction, AST elevation is not as great as ALT elevation. Although AST does increase in response to muscle or heart injury, troponins are used instead in the workup of these conditions. The most common cause of mild AST elevation in the Western hemisphere is non-alcoholic fatty liver disease.
Relevance to psychiatry and behavioral science	AST is one of the tests of liver health (liver "function") that is closely monitored in psychiatric practice, mainly because of the potential hepatotoxicity of psychotropic drugs. AST is also monitored in patients with alcoholism, substance-induced liver disease, and hepatitis.
	Elevation of AST may be found on routine screening. If the patient has no clinical symptoms and no risk factors for liver disease, and AST is <3 times the ULN, a recheck is indicated after 1–3 months. If the elevation persists, further investigation is needed. If AST is >3 times the ULN on a single measurement, further investigation is needed. Elevation of AST may occur with initiation of a new psychotropic medication. In most cases, this AST increase is benign, and the lab value will revert to baseline within weeks of dosage stabilization. Further investigation is needed if the value does not normalize or when ALP or bilirubin is also elevated.
	Pathological elevation of AST may occur with alcohol use disorder, substance-induced liver disease, or hepatitis. It is important not to be misled by a normal AST value in patients with established cirrhosis. In patients with cirrhosis due to hepatitis C who have a normal AST result, active hepatitis may be present, such that they would benefit from antiviral therapy, β-blockers to prevent variceal bleeding, and other treatments.

Aspartate transaminase (AST) *(continued)*

Relevance to psychiatry and behavioral science *(continued)*	AST and ALT levels may also be normal in patients with hemochromatosis, in patients receiving methotrexate, or after jejunoileal bypass surgery, despite advanced liver disease. In all cases, the patient's history should be central to the diagnosis, and an effort should be made to identify other evidence of liver disease.
Preparation of patient	None needed
Indications	• Component of LFT panel • Component of CMP • Monitoring medication effects on the liver • Evaluating patients with clinical symptoms of liver disease, including jaundice, abdominal pain, ascites, nausea, vomiting, or darkening of the urine (bilirubinuria) • Distinguishing hemolytic jaundice from jaundice due to liver dysfunction • Evaluating patients with hepatitis exposure or symptoms of hepatitis • Evaluating patients with alcoholism or other substance abuse • Monitoring effects of treatment for liver disease
Reference range	Males: 14–20 U/L Females: 10–36 U/L The ratio of AST to ALT is also useful in the differential diagnosis of the cause of liver dysfunction.
Critical value(s)	>200 U/L indicates acute hepatic injury.
Increased levels	• Active cirrhosis (alcohol or drug-induced) • Hepatitis, acute or chronic • Infectious mononucleosis • Hepatic necrosis • Primary or metastatic carcinoma • Reye's syndrome • MI (with AST increase paralleling that of creatine kinase) • Numerous other conditions including hypothyroidism, muscle trauma, muscle inflammation, toxic shock syndrome, cardiac catheterization, recent brain trauma, stroke, surgery, muscular dystrophy, pulmonary embolism, malignant hyperthermia, shock, exhaustion, and heat stroke • Drugs metabolized in the liver, including most psychotropics
Decreased levels	• Uremia in kidney failure • Chronic dialysis

Aspartate transaminase (AST) *(continued)*

Decreased levels *(continued)*	• Vitamin B_6 (pyridoxine) deficiency • Pregnancy • *Drugs:* vitamin C, ibuprofen, naltrexone, pindolol, and trifluoperazine
Interfering factors	Diabetic ketoacidosis, severe liver disease, uremia, and sample hemolysis may give spurious results.
Cross-references	**Alanine Transaminase** **Alcohol Use Disorder** **Cirrhosis** **Hepatitis, Viral** **Liver Function Tests**

Agrawal S, Dhiman RK, Limdi JK: Evaluation of abnormal liver function tests. Postgrad Med J 92(1086):223–234, 2016

Fischbach FT, Fischbach MA: A Manual of Laboratory and Diagnostic Tests, 10th Edition. Philadelphia, PA, Wolters Kluwer Health/Lippincott Williams and Wilkins, 2018

Giboney PT: Mildly elevated liver transaminase levels in the asymptomatic patient. Am Fam Physician 71:1105–1110, 2005

Gopal DV, Rosen HR: Abnormal findings on liver function tests: interpreting results to narrow the diagnosis and establish a prognosis. Postgrad Med 107:100–114, 2000

Theal RM, Scott K: Evaluating asymptomatic patients with abnormal liver function test results. Am Fam Physician 53:2111–2119, 1996

Basic metabolic panel (BMP)

Type of test	Blood
Background and explanation of test	The BMP includes the following eight tests: • Creatinine • Glucose • Calcium • Sodium • Potassium • Carbon dioxide • Chloride • BUN
Relevance to psychiatry and behavioral science	Although the BMP is often used in the emergency setting as a means of rapidly assessing metabolic status, it is not the panel of choice for most patients with psychiatric presentations. In these cases, when general laboratory testing is considered necessary, the panel of choice would be the CMP, which includes LFTs.
Preparation of patient	Ideally, the patient should be fasting overnight before testing, although this is rarely done. Mineral-containing supplements should be held for 12 hours before testing, and vigorous exercise should be avoided.
Indications	• Rapid workup in the emergency setting • Monitoring specific lab values in a hospitalized patient
Reference range	See entries for individual tests.
Critical value(s)	See entries for individual tests.
Increased levels	See entries for individual tests.
Decreased levels	See entries for individual tests.
Interfering factors	See entries for individual tests.
Cross-references	**Comprehensive Metabolic Panel** See entries for individual tests.

Bile acids

Type of test	Blood
Background and explanation of test	Bile acids are produced in the liver, stored in the gallbladder, and secreted into the intestines after a meal. They facilitate digestion by emulsifying fats and are reabsorbed with the products of digestion. Under normal conditions, the liver is very efficient at clearing bile acids from the blood, and serum concentrations are low in the fasting state and increase only slightly after meals. With liver dysfunction, however, levels are elevated in the fasting state and may be markedly elevated after meals. Liver diseases that cause bile acid elevations include hepatitis (acute and chronic), cirrhosis, liver cancer, cholestasis, cholangitis, portal vein thrombosis, Budd-Chiari syndrome, Wilson's disease, and hemochromatosis. It is not possible to distinguish among these diseases using bile acid testing.
Relevance to psychiatry and behavioral science	Bile acids are a sensitive measure of liver dysfunction in certain disease states of relevance to psychiatry, as listed above. In addition, recent evidence suggests that bile acids have a role in mediating the effects of therapies used to treat metabolic disorders, including metformin, bile acid sequestrants, and bariatric surgery.
Preparation of patient	Patients should fast for ≥8 hours before the test.
Indications	• Early evaluation of liver dysfunction • Evaluating hepatic impairment from chemical and environmental toxins • Monitoring effects of interferon treatment for hepatitis C • Evaluating suspected intrahepatic cholestasis of pregnancy
Reference range	Patients 7 years of age and older: • Total bile acids: 0–7.0 µmol/L • Cholic acid (CA): 0–1.9 µmol/L • Chenodeoxycholic acid (CDC): 0–3.4 µmol/L • Deoxycholic acid (DCA): 0–2.5 µmol/L • Ursodeoxycholic acid (UDC): 0–1.0 µmol/L
Critical value(s)	None
Increased levels	• Hepatitis (acute and chronic) • Cirrhosis • Liver cancer • Cholestasis • Cholangitis • Budd-Chiari syndrome • Wilson's disease

Bile acids *(continued)*

Increased levels *(continued)*	• Hemochromatosis
	• Intrahepatic cholestasis of pregnancy
Decreased levels	Not applicable
Interfering factors	Gross hemolysis or lipemia of specimen invalidates results.
Cross-references	**Cirrhosis**
	Hemochromatosis
	Hepatitis, Viral
	Liver Function Tests
	Wilson's Disease

ARUP Laboratories: Bile acids, total, in Lab Test Directory. Salt Lake City, UT, ARUP Laboratories, 2021. Available at https://ltd.aruplab.com/Tests/Pub/0070189. Accessed June 2021.

Xie C, Huang W, Young RL, et al: Role of bile acids in the regulation of food intake, and their dysregulation in metabolic disease. Nutrients 13(4):1104, 2021

Bilirubin

Type of test	Blood
Background and explanation of test	When RBCs degrade, the hemoglobin component is broken down to unconjugated ("indirect") bilirubin. This form of bilirubin is transformed in the liver to conjugated ("direct") bilirubin, which is excreted into the GI tract, where it is reduced by bacteria to urobilinogen. This compound may be excreted in feces or reabsorbed, in the latter case reappearing in urine or bile. The bilirubin cycle is shown in Appendix D.
	When bilirubin levels are high, patients may appear jaundiced. High levels may be a consequence of overproduction (usually due to hemolysis) or underexcretion (due to liver or biliary tract disease). Routine bilirubin measurement is of total bilirubin; if this is not elevated, no further testing is needed. If level is elevated, the next step is fractionation, to determine whether bilirubin is primarily conjugated or unconjugated.
	When ≥30% of the bilirubin in a sample is in the conjugated (direct) form, conjugated hyperbilirubinemia exists; the differential diagnosis for this condition is shown in the *Increased Levels* section below. A positive urine dipstick test for bilirubin is also consistent with conjugated hyperbilirubinemia. In addition, other LFT abnormalities are usually seen with conjugated hyperbilirubinemia.
	In general, patients with conjugated hyperbilirubinemia should be evaluated for hepatobiliary disease, while those with unconjugated hyperbilirubinemia should be evaluated for causes of RBC destruction such as hemolytic anemia. Isolated elevation of unconjugated bilirubin levels is most often caused by Gilbert's syndrome, a common and usually benign genetic polymorphism associated with reduced glucuronidation of bilirubin. Establishing this diagnosis avoids costly and unnecessary testing for patients with intermittent jaundice. Any degree of bilirubinuria confirms the presence of conjugated hyperbilirubinemia, excludes hemolysis, and indicates the presence of hepatobiliary disease.
	Elevation of bilirubin may be found on routine screening. If total bilirubin is <1.5 times the upper limit of normal (ULN), recheck in 1–3 months unless there is clinical suspicion of disease. If total bilirubin is ≥1.5 times the ULN, determine the percentage that is indirect. If >70%, the diagnosis is probably Gilbert's syndrome. If not, further investigation is needed. If total bilirubin is >3 times the ULN, consultation is indicated because clinical disease is probable.
Relevance to psychiatry and behavioral science	Bilirubin may be elevated in alcohol use disorder, cirrhosis, pernicious anemia, and cancer of the head of the pancreas and as a drug reaction (e.g., to chlorpromazine or other phenothiazines).

Bilirubin (continued)

Preparation of patient	Patients should fast for 4 hours before test and should refrain from eating yellow foods (e.g., carrots, yellow beans, yams, pumpkin) for 3–4 days before test.
Indications	• Component of CMP • Presence of jaundice • History of alcohol overconsumption • Exposure to hepatitis • Signs of liver injury (e.g., from drugs) • Signs of liver disease such as cirrhosis or hepatitis • Evidence of bile duct obstruction • Hemolytic anemia (e.g., sickle cell disease)
Reference range	Total bilirubin 0.3–1.0 mg/dL Conjugated (direct) bilirubin 0.0–0.2 mg/dL
Critical value(s)	Adults: >12 mg/dL
Increased levels	*Elevation of total bilirubin* • Hepatocellular jaundice (viral hepatitis, cirrhosis, infectious mononucleosis, drug reactions) • Obstructive jaundice (gallstones, cancer) • Hemolytic jaundice (posttransfusion, pernicious anemia, sickle cell anemia, transfusion reactions, Crigler-Najjar syndrome) • Gilbert's syndrome • Dubin-Johnson syndrome • Pulmonary embolism • Congestive heart failure *Elevation of unconjugated (indirect) bilirubin* • Hemolytic anemia due to large hematoma • Trauma with large hematoma • Hemorrhagic pulmonary infarcts • Crigler-Najjar syndrome • Gilbert's syndrome *Elevation of conjugated (direct) bilirubin* • Blockage of liver or bile ducts • Cancer of the head of the pancreas • Gallstones • Hepatitis • Liver trauma • Cirrhosis

Bilirubin *(continued)*

Increased levels *(continued)*	• Long-term alcohol overconsumption • Drug reaction • Dubin-Johnson syndrome
Decreased levels	Not applicable
Interfering factors	Bilirubin levels are slightly higher in males than females. Blacks tend to have lower bilirubin values. Strenuous exercise may increase bilirubin levels. Fractionation tends to be unreliable in mild hyperbilirubin-emia using standard "diazo" methods; newer, more precise methods may be required in these cases. Elevated bilirubin levels may be caused by alcohol, morphine, theophylline, ascorbic acid, aspirin, chlordiazepoxide, chlorpromazine, and other phenothiazines.
Cross-references	**Alcohol Use Disorder** **Cirrhosis** **Hepatitis, Viral** **Liver Function Tests** **Urobilinogen**

American Association for Clinical Chemistry: Testing.com. Available at: https://www.testing.com. Accessed June 2021.

Fischbach FT, Fischbach MA: A Manual of Laboratory and Diagnostic Tests, 10th Edition. Philadelphia, PA, Wolters Kluwer Health/Lippincott Williams and Wilkins, 2018

Gopal DV, Rosen HR: Abnormal findings on liver function tests: interpreting results to narrow the diagnosis and establish a prognosis. Postgrad Med 107:100–114, 2000

Johnston DE: Special considerations in interpreting liver function tests. Am Fam Physician 59:2223–2230, 1999

Blood alcohol level (BAL)

Type of test	Blood
Background and explanation of test	Alcohol is rapidly absorbed from the GI tract when it is consumed on an empty stomach, with peak levels reached within 1 hour of ingestion. A small amount of alcohol is exhaled from the lungs and excreted in urine, but most is metabolized by the liver to acetaldehyde and subsequently to carbon dioxide and water.
	A healthy liver has the capacity to metabolize about one drink per hour (i.e., 12 oz of beer, 4–5 oz of wine, or 1–1.5 oz of hard liquor). When more than one drink per hour is consumed, the alcohol level in the circulation rises. In the measurement of the BAL, different systems of measurement yielding different units cause some confusion as to the meanings of particular values; see the *Reference Range* section below. In general, a level equivalent to ≥0.08% is consistent with legal intoxication in most U.S. jurisdictions.
Relevance to psychiatry and behavioral science	Psychiatrists may be consulted for the evaluation of patients in the emergency room who are intoxicated or withdrawing from alcohol, and familiarity with the BAL is critical in this context. Alcohol is also often involved in suicide attempts. BAL may be used to monitor patients who are in treatment for alcohol dependence.
Preparation of patient	None needed
Indications	• Diagnosing alcohol intoxication • Diagnosing alcohol withdrawal • Determining cause of coma • Providing legal evidence in motor vehicle accident cases or other events that may be related to intoxication • Monitoring employees suspected of drinking on the job • Monitoring patients who are in treatment for alcohol dependence or abuse • Monitoring ethanol level in patients treated for methanol poisoning
Reference range	Negative: <10 mg/dL, <2.00 mmol/L, <0.010% Negative by U.S. Department of Transportation (DOT): <20 mg/dL, <4.35 mmol/L, <0.020% Positive by U.S. DOT: >40 mg/dL, >8.68 mmol/L, >0.040% Positive under state laws: >80 mg/dL, >17.4 mmol/L, ≥0.08%
Critical value(s)	• BAL >300 mg/dL is consistent with severe alcohol toxicity and requires immediate treatment for overdose. • BAL >400 mg/dL can be fatal.

Blood alcohol level (BAL) *(continued)*

Critical values *(continued)*	• Symptoms of alcohol intoxication in the presence of a low BAL may signal a risk of serious impending withdrawal.
Increased levels	• BAL 50–100 mg/dL: slowing of reflexes and impaired visual acuity • BAL >100 mg/dL: CNS depression
Decreased levels	Not applicable
Interfering factors	Ingestion of other alcohols (e.g., isopropanol or methanol) can confound ethanol measurement.
Cross-references	**Alcohol Use Disorder**

Fischbach FT, Fischbach MA: A Manual of Laboratory and Diagnostic Tests, 10th Edition. Philadelphia, PA, Wolters Kluwer Health/Lippincott Williams and Wilkins, 2018

National Institute on Alcohol Abuse and Alcoholism: Biomarkers of heavy drinking, in Assessing Alcohol Problems: A Guide for Clinicians and Researchers. Edited by Allen JP, Wilson VB. Available at: https://pubs.niaaa.nih.gov/publications/assessingalcohol/allen.pdf. Accessed June 2021.

Blood gases

Type of test	Blood (arterial)
Background and explanation of test	A sampling of blood gases reveals the amount of dissolved oxygen and carbon dioxide (CO_2) in arterial blood along with information on acid-base status and a measure of how well oxygen is carried to the body. The partial pressure of carbon dioxide ($PaCO_2$) reflects the degree of alveolar ventilation. The partial pressure of oxygen (PaO_2) reflects the status of alveolar gas exchange with inspired air. Oxygen saturation (SaO_2) is the percentage of oxygen bound to hemoglobin and thus available for transport.
Relevance to psychiatry and behavioral science	Several psychiatric and psychotropic-related conditions result in blood gas abnormalities. Patients with CO_2 retention because of chronic obstructive pulmonary disease (COPD) can develop severe somnolence or confusional states, particularly after a sedative such as a benzodiazepine is given. In anxiety states, hyperventilation is both a cause of respiratory alkalosis and a symptom of the condition and can be accompanied by paresthesias, muscle twitching and spasm, dizziness, palpitations, and seizures. Understandably, patients may become panicked, with further escalation of symptoms. Salicylate overdose causes overbreathing and respiratory alkalosis. Opioid or barbiturate overdose causes underbreathing and respiratory acidosis.
Preparation of patient	Potential complications of arterial puncture (bleeding, hematoma, infection, nerve damage, occlusion) should be explained to the patient. A test for collateral circulation such as a modified Allen test is recommended prior to the procedure.
Indications	• Evaluating oxygenation or acid-base status • Evaluating patients with dyspnea or respiratory distress • Evaluating patients with head or neck trauma that could compromise breathing • Monitoring the effectiveness of oxygen therapy or artificial ventilation • Monitoring the effects of prolonged anesthesia • Workup of delirium or other mental status changes • Workup of hyperventilation in patients with severe anxiety • Workup of hypoventilation in overly sedated patients
Reference ranges	pH 7.35–7.45 $PaCO_2$ 35–40 mmHg PaO_2 80–100 mmHg HCO^{3-} 22–31 mEq/L SaO_2 96%–100%
Critical value(s)	pH ≤7.2 or >7.6 $PaCO_2$ <20 mmHg

Blood gases *(continued)*

Critical value(s) *(continued)*	$PaO_2 < 40$ mmHg $HCO^{3-} < 10$ mEq/L $SaO_2 < 60\%$
Abnormal test	*Respiratory acidosis:* pH low, $PaCO_2$ high; due to underbreathing or poor gas exchange. Causes include COPD, pneumonia, COVID-19 infection, asthma, airway obstruction, myasthenia gravis, and oversedation by medications such as benzodiazepines or opioids. *Respiratory alkalosis:* pH high, $PaCO_2$ low; due to hyperventilation. Causes include anxiety or emotional distress, TBI, pain, aspirin overdose, and certain lung diseases. *Metabolic acidosis:* pH low, HCO^{3-} low; due to metabolic or renal disease causing acidity of the blood. Causes include shock, renal failure, ethanol intoxication, aspirin overdose, and diabetic ketoacidosis. *Metabolic alkalosis:* pH high, HCO^{3-} high. Causes include heart failure, cirrhosis, chronic vomiting, hypokalemia, and overdose of sodium bicarbonate.
Interfering factors	Improper specimen handling invalidates results. Fever causes decreased SaO_2. Leukocytosis causes a rapid decline in pH.
Cross-references	None

American Association for Clinical Chemistry: Testing.com. Available at: https://www.testing.com. Accessed June 2021.

Fauci AS, Braunwald E, Kasper DL, et al (eds): Harrison's Principles of Internal Medicine, 17th Edition. New York, McGraw-Hill, 2008

Fischbach FT, Fischbach MA: A Manual of Laboratory and Diagnostic Tests, 10th Edition. Philadelphia, PA, Wolters Kluwer Health/Lippincott Williams and Wilkins, 2018

Blood urea nitrogen (BUN)

Type of test	Blood
Background and explanation of test	Urea produced in the liver as a product of protein metabolism circulates in the bloodstream and is eliminated by the kidneys. When the kidneys are not functioning normally, urea levels in the blood increase, and this increase can be measured by the BUN test. This increase in BUN is called azotemia and, when severe enough to produce clinical symptoms, uremia. The ratio of BUN to creatinine level may be increased when renal blood flow is compromised, as with dehydration or congestive heart failure. Excessive protein intake and GI bleeding are other causes of an increased ratio.
Relevance to psychiatry and behavioral science	Elevation of the BUN level in renal failure is associated with psychiatric signs and symptoms ranging from fatigue, lassitude, and somnolence to acute confusional states and delirium. Seizures can occur. In chronic renal disease, the BUN level correlates more closely with these uremic symptoms than does the creatinine level.
Preparation of patient	No fasting necessary. Dietary history may be needed to evaluate recent protein intake.
Indications	• Component of metabolic panels (BMP and CMP) • Evaluating renal function (with creatinine) • Monitoring adequacy of dialysis and other interventions for kidney disease
Reference range	Adults ≤60 years: 6–20 mg/dL Adults >60 years: 8–23 mg/dL BUN-to-creatinine ratio normally between 10:1 and 20:1
Critical value(s)	>100 mg/dL indicates severe impairment of renal function
Increased levels	• Renal disease (acute or chronic) • Renal injury • Decreased renal blood flow in the context of congestive heart failure, dehydration, shock, stress, burns, or acute MI • Rapid protein breakdown in the context of fever, burns, or cancer • Urinary tract obstruction • Hemorrhage into the GI tract • Diabetic ketoacidosis • Excessive protein intake • Anabolic steroid use • Pregnancy

Blood urea nitrogen (BUN) *(continued)*

Decreased levels	• Hepatic failure • Malnutrition, with low protein intake • Celiac disease with impaired absorption • SIAD • Overhydration • Pregnancy Ratio of BUN to creatinine may also be decreased (<10:1) in liver disease or malnutrition.
Interfering factors	Low-protein, high-carbohydrate diets result in lower BUN level. High-protein diets result in elevated levels. BUN is decreased in late pregnancy. Higher BUN levels are found in elderly adults and in males. Many drugs cause increased or decreased BUN levels.
Cross-references	**Basic Metabolic Panel** **Comprehensive Metabolic Panel** **Creatinine** **Syndrome of Inappropriate Antidiuresis** **Uremic Syndrome**

American Association for Clinical Chemistry: Testing.com. Available at: https://www.testing.com. Accessed June 2021.

Fauci AS, Braunwald E, Kasper DL, et al (eds): Harrison's Principles of Internal Medicine, 17th Edition. New York, McGraw-Hill, 2008

Fischbach FT, Fischbach MA: A Manual of Laboratory and Diagnostic Tests, 10th Edition. Philadelphia, PA, Wolters Kluwer Health/Lippincott Williams and Wilkins, 2018

Bone mineral density scan

Type of test	Imaging
Background and explanation of test	This scan—also known as bone densitometry or a DEXA scan—is an X ray of several body areas (e.g., spine, hip, forearm) to determine bone mineral density and thereby assist in diagnosing osteoporosis and osteopenia. The latter is a milder condition that may presage the development of osteoporosis. Several types of scans are available, but the DEXA scan is preferred because of its low radiation exposure and precision of results. Test results are reported using a T-score (density compared with that of healthy young adults) or a Z-score (density compared with that of healthy age-peers).
Relevance to psychiatry and behavioral science	Psychiatric disorders associated with reduced bone mineral density include substance abuse, schizophrenia, dementia, and depression. Psychotropic medications may also be implicated; for example, there is some evidence that SSRIs confer an increased risk of osteoporosis and fracture. Smoking is a well-known risk factor for reduced bone density. The DEXA scan is a commonly used test in the preventive care for adult and geriatric patients, particularly females. It is probably underutilized by psychiatrists who provide primary care to patients, particularly in geriatrics.
Preparation of patient	None needed
Indications	• Evaluation of bone density in females ≥65 years, postmenopausal females with risk factors such as smoking, males ≥70 years, and younger males with risk factors • Prediction of fracture risk
Reference range	T-score <1.0 SD below normal
Critical value(s)	None
Abnormal test	T-score 1.0–2.5 SD below normal: osteopenia T-score >2.5 SD below normal: osteoporosis
Interfering factors	Nuclear medicine imaging within past 72 hours (longer for gallium or indium) interferes with bone mineral density scanning. Any barium study within past 10 days interferes with spine imaging. Prosthetic devices or metal implants in areas being imaged interfere with scanning.
Cross-references	**Osteoporosis**

Anam AK, Insogna K: Update on osteoporosis screening and management. Med Clin North Am 105(6):1117–1134, 2021

ARUP Consult: Osteoporosis, in ARUP Consult: The Physician's Guide to Laboratory Test Selection and Interpretation. Salt Lake City, UT, ARUP Laboratories, 2018. Available at: https://arupconsult.com/content/osteoporosis. Accessed June 2021.

Lane NE: Epidemiology, etiology, and diagnosis of osteoporosis. Am J Obstet Gynecol 194:S3–S11, 2006

Brain natriuretic peptide (BNP)

Type of test	Blood
Background and explanation of test	BNP and N-terminal pro B-type natriuretic peptide (NT-proBNP) are hormones produced in the ventricles of the heart (primarily the left ventricle) that increase in abundance when the ventricle stretches or suffers pressure overload. BNP measured in plasma is used to diagnose congestive heart failure (CHF) and gauge its severity. When BNP is ordered, the lab will perform either BNP or NT-proBNP testing, depending on instrument availability, although the two tests are not interchangeable. These tests are very accurate in distinguishing heart failure from other causes of shortness of breath.
Relevance to psychiatry and behavioral science	This test may be indicated in older patients reporting excessive fatigue and inability to perform usual activities, symptoms that could be related to CHF but are sometimes mistaken for depression. The presence of shortness of breath is a critical feature.
Preparation of patient	Patients should fast overnight before testing. If the sample is nonfasting, this should be noted on the lab request form.
Indications	• Evaluating symptoms of ventricular dysfunction: fatigue, shortness of breath, cough, palpitations, and hypertension • Diagnosing CHF • Determining the severity of CHF • Monitoring the effects of therapy for heart failure
Reference range	Normal result* • BNP <125 pg/mL for patients <75 years • BNP <450 pg/mL for patients ≥75 years Levels will greatly exceed these reference values in most patients with CHF. Levels of 100–500 pg/mL are said to be inconclusive and require clinical correlation and further testing. BNP >500 pg/mL represents a positive test for CHF in patients <75 years. Threshold values for NT-proBNP depend on age and sex. See reference range for your laboratory.
Critical value(s)	>500 pg/mL
Increased levels	• CHF • Decrease in left ventricular ejection fraction • Diastolic dysfunction
Decreased levels	Patients taking medications used to treat heart failure, including ACE inhibitors, β-blockers, and diuretics

Brain natriuretic peptide (BNP) *(continued)*

Interfering factors	Improper sampling invalidates BNP results; samples must be collected in EDTA tubes. No special handling is needed for NT-proBNP (serum or plasma). Levels may be increased with age and kidney disease, and levels are generally higher in females.
Cross-references	**Chest X-Ray** **Echocardiogram**

*BNP levels are significantly lower in obese individuals, so 50% lower cutoff values should be used to determine abnormality.

American Association for Clinical Chemistry: Testing.com. Available at: https://www.testing.com. Accessed June 2021.

Fauci AS, Braunwald E, Kasper DL, et al (eds): Harrison's Principles of Internal Medicine, 17th Edition. New York, McGraw-Hill, 2008

Fischbach FT, Fischbach MA: A Manual of Laboratory and Diagnostic Tests, 10th Edition. Philadelphia, PA, Wolters Kluwer Health/Lippincott Williams and Wilkins, 2018

Mueller C, McDonald K, de Boer RA, et al: Heart Failure Association of the European Society of Cardiology practical guidance on the use of natriuretic peptide concentrations. Eur J Heart Fail 21(6):715–731, 2019

Calcium

Type of test	Blood
Background and explanation of test	Calcium has essential roles in neurotransmission, cardiac function, muscle contraction, blood clotting, and bone formation. The calcium level is maintained within a physiological range through the actions of PTH and vitamin D. Most calcium is stored in the bones and teeth; only 1% circulates in blood, half bound to albumin and half free (ionized form).
	When the albumin level drops, the total calcium level drops as well, but the concentration of free calcium is unaffected. For this reason, the total calcium value is corrected when the albumin level is low, using the following formula:
	$[4 \text{ g/dL} - \text{plasma albumin}] \times 0.8 + \text{total serum calcium}$
	Alternatively, free calcium can be measured directly, but in this case, the specimen requires special handling and expedited processing.
Relevance to psychiatry and behavioral science	An abnormal calcium level may be found during routine health screening and in the workup of various psychiatric signs and symptoms. Abnormal calcium levels may be associated with irritability, anxiety, depression, fatigue, lethargy, weakness, apathy, loss of appetite, delirium, nausea, vomiting, constipation, polyuria, polydipsia, bone pain, cardiac toxicity (including QTc prolongation and dysrhythmias), seizures, and coma. In patients with eating disorders, low calcium levels may result from chronic laxative abuse. Lithium increases the calcium level.
Preparation of patient	Patients should avoid taking lithium, antacids, thiazide diuretics, and vitamin D before testing. In drawing blood, application of the tourniquet should be as brief as possible.
Indications	• Routine screening (BMP and CMP)
	• Evaluation of parathyroid function
	• Evaluation of renal function
	• Symptoms of hypocalcemia: skeletal muscle cramps, abdominal cramps, paresthesias
	• Symptoms of hypercalcemia: upset stomach, constipation, nausea, vomiting
	• Workup for kidney stones
	• Workup for Paget's disease and other bone diseases
	• Calcium monitoring after kidney transplant
	• Calcium monitoring in certain cancers (breast, lung, multiple myeloma, kidney, or head/neck)
	• Monitoring treatment for abnormal calcium levels

Calcium *(continued)*

Reference range	*Total serum calcium*
	• Adults <60 years: 8.6–10.0 mg/dL
	• Adults 60–90 years: 8.8–10.2 mg/dL
	• Adults >90 years: 8.2–9.6 mg/dL
	Ionized serum calcium
	• Adults: 4.64–5.28 mg/dL
Critical value(s)	*Total serum calcium*
	• <6 mg/dL: tetany, seizures
	• >13 mg/dL: cardiac toxicity, dysrhythmias, coma
	Ionized serum calcium
	• <2 mg/dL: tetany, seizures
	• >7 mg/dL: coma
Increased levels	*Total serum calcium >12 mg/dL*
	• Hyperparathyroidism
	• Malignancy
	• Granulomatous disease (tuberculosis, sarcoidosis)
	• Prolonged immobilization with fracture (in children)
	• Excessive vitamin D intake
	• Paget's disease (with elevated ALP)
	Other diseases that can cause hypercalcemia but rarely severe enough to be symptomatic include thyrotoxicosis, milk-alkali syndrome, and adrenocortical insufficiency.
	Increased ionized calcium
	• Hyperparathyroidism
	• Cancer
	• PTH-producing tumors
	• Excessive vitamin D intake
Decreased levels	*Total serum calcium <4.0 mg/dL*
	• Hypoalbuminemia (causing pseudohypocalcemia)
	• Hypoparathyroidism
	• Increased phosphorus level due to laxative abuse, renal failure, or cytotoxic drugs
	• Acute pancreatitis
	• Renal failure
	• Malabsorption due to GI disease
	• Malnutrition, extreme dietary deficiency
	• Severe osteomalacia

Calcium *(continued)*

Decreased levels *(continued)*	• Vitamin D deficiency, rickets
	• Magnesium deficiency
	• Alkalosis
	• Alcoholism, cirrhosis
	• Heritable resistance to PTH
	Decreased ionized calcium levels
	• Hyperventilation to treat increased intracranial pressure (total calcium may be normal)
	• Bicarbonate administration to treat metabolic acidosis
	• Hypoparathyroidism
	• Acute pancreatitis
	• Vitamin D or magnesium deficiency
	• Toxic shock syndrome
	• Syndrome of multiple organ failure
Interfering factors	Lithium and thiazide diuretics increase the calcium level.
	Calcium-containing antacids or vitamin D taken just before testing could transiently increase the calcium level.
	Fluctuations in serum protein levels affect the interpretation of total calcium levels but not ionized calcium levels.
Cross-references	**Anxiety Disorder Due to Another Medical Condition**
	Delirium
	Depressive Disorder Due to Another Medical Condition
	Hypercalcemia
	Hypocalcemia
	Psychotic Disorder Due to Another Medical Condition
	Seizures

American Association for Clinical Chemistry: Testing.com. Available at: https://www.testing.com. Accessed June 2021.

Barstow C, Braun M: Electrolytes: calcium disorders. FP Essent 459:29–34, 2017

Carrick AI, Costner HB: Rapid fire: hypercalcemia. Emerg Med Clin North Am 36(3):549–555, 2018

Fischbach FT, Fischbach MA: A Manual of Laboratory and Diagnostic Tests, 10th Edition. Philadelphia, PA, Wolters Kluwer Health/Lippincott Williams and Wilkins, 2018

Pepe J, Colangelo L, Biamonte F, et al: Diagnosis and management of hypocalcemia. Endocrine 69(3):485–495, 2020

Zagzag J, Hu MI, Fisher SB, Perrier ND: Hypercalcemia and cancer: differential diagnosis and treatment. CA Cancer J Clin 68(5):377–386, 2018

Carbamazepine level

Type of test	Blood
Background and explanation of test	Carbamazepine is an antiepileptic drug used for a range of psychiatric indications, including bipolar disorder, aggression, agitation in the context of dementia and TBI, mood stabilization in patients with personality disorders, neuropathic pain, and adjunctive treatment for patients with depression, schizophrenia, and schizoaffective disorder.
	Therapeutic drug monitoring with carbamazepine is required because of the drug's narrow therapeutic index. It has numerous significant drug interactions and adverse effects, the latter including Stevens-Johnson syndrome/toxic epidermal necrolysis, which can be fatal. This syndrome particularly affects patients of Asian descent carrying the HLA-B*1502 allele, and this has prompted the FDA to recommend genotyping of all Asian patients before carbamazepine is used. The HLA-A*3101 allele, which is more widely distributed in the world population, has also been associated with hypersensitivity reactions.
	Carbamazepine's major active metabolite carbamazepine-10,11-epoxide has the same potency as the parent drug and contributes to both therapeutic and adverse effects. If carbamazepine toxicity is suspected, levels of both the parent drug and the epoxide should be checked. Further information about this drug can be found in the *Psychotropic Medications* chapter.
Relevance to psychiatry and behavioral science	See above.
Preparation of patient	Patients should be instructed to hold the dose of medication until blood is drawn for testing. Trough level is checked just before morning dose.
Indications	• Therapeutic drug monitoring • Signs and symptoms of toxicity • Question of noncompliance
Reference range	Total carbamazepine: 4–12 µg/mL Free carbamazepine: 1–3 µg/mL % free carbamazepine: 8%–35% (calculated) Carbamazepine-10,11-epoxide: 0.5–2 µg/mL
Critical value(s)	Total carbamazepine >15 µg/mL Free carbamazepine >3.8 µg/mL
Increased levels	• Renal failure increases the level of carbamazepine-10,11-epoxide. • *Drugs:* many, particularly coadministered drugs that are CYP3A4 inhibitors

Carbamazepine level *(continued)*

Decreased levels	• Noncompliance • *Drugs:* many, particularly coadministered drugs that are CYP3A4 inducers
Interfering factors	None
Cross-references	**Bipolar and Related Disorder Due to Another Medical Condition**

ARUP Laboratories: Carbamazepine, total, I Lab Test Directory. Salt Lake City, UT, ARUP Laboratories, 2021. Available at: https://ltd.aruplab.com/Tests/Pub/0090260. Accessed November 2021.

Brahmi N, Kouraichi N, Abderrazek H, et al: Clinical experience with carbamazepine overdose: relationship between serum concentration and neurological severity. J Clin Psychopharmacol 28(2):241–243, 2008

Ferrell PB Jr, McLeod HL: Carbamazepine, HLA-B*1502 and risk of Stevens-Johnson syndrome and toxic epidermal necrolysis: US FDA recommendations. Pharmacogenomics 9(10):1543–1546, 2008

Hiemke C, Bergemann N, Clement HW, et al: Consensus guidelines for therapeutic drug monitoring in neuropsychopharmacology: update 2017. Pharmacopsychiatry 51(1–2):9–62, 2018 [published correction appears in Pharmacopsychiatry 51(1–2):e1, 2018]

Karazniewicz-Łada M, Główka AK, Mikulska AA, Główka FK: Pharmacokinetic drug-drug interactions among antiepileptic drugs, including CBD, drugs used to treat COVID-19 and nutrients. Int J Mol Sci 22(17):9582, 2021

Petit P, Lonjon R, Cociglio M, et al: Carbamazepine and its 10,11-epoxide metabolite in acute mania: clinical and pharmacokinetic correlates. Eur J Clin Pharmacol 41(6):541–546, 1991

Carbohydrate-deficient transferrin (CDT)

Type of test	Blood
Background and explanation of test	Transferrin is a protein that carries iron through the circulation to the bone marrow, where RBCs are produced. Several forms of transferrin exist, with differing numbers of residues of the carbohydrate *sialic acid* attached. Normally, each transferrin molecule has four sialic acid chains attached. In people who drink significant amounts of alcohol (more than four or five drinks daily for several weeks or more), the number of transferrin molecules with only one, two, or three sialic residues is increased. These CDTs can be measured in the blood, providing a useful indicator of problem drinking.
	Studies have shown the CDT test to be positive in people drinking 50–80 g of ethanol daily for a minimum of several weeks. In general, the specificity of the test is high (97%), but the sensitivity is variable (65%–95%). Sensitivity can be improved without loss of specificity when GGT is measured in conjunction with CDT, because the combined test is positive in people drinking ≥40 g of ethanol daily.
	CDT value normalizes with 2–4 weeks of abstinence because the abnormal transferrin has a half-life of 14–17 days.
Relevance to psychiatry and behavioral science	This is a useful test to supplement other measures in the evaluation of drinking behavior when the patient has not admitted a problem. It can also be used to detect relapse in patients who are in treatment for alcohol dependence. In the latter case, the patient's own serial CDT values can provide a sensitive indicator of change in drinking status.
Preparation of patient	None needed
Indications	Detection of recent heavy alcohol consumption
Reference range	≤2.5%
Critical value(s)	≥2.6% suggests active drinking
Increased levels	• Recent heavy drinking • Transferrin D protein variant • Glycoprotein disorders • Primary biliary cirrhosis • Chronic active hepatitis
Decreased levels	Not applicable
Interfering factors	Differences in testing methods may render CDT results difficult to compare between laboratories.
Cross-references	**Alcohol Use Disorder**

Bortolotti F, Sorio D, Bertaso A, Tagliaro F: Analytical and diagnostic aspects of carbohydrate deficient transferrin (CDT): a critical review over years 2007–2017. J Pharm Biomed Anal 147:2–12, 2018

Chrostek L, Cylwik B, Szmitkowski M, et al: The diagnostic accuracy of carbohydrate-deficient transferrin, sialic acid and commonly used markers of alcohol abuse during abstinence. Clin Chim Acta 364:167–171, 2006

Carbohydrate-deficient transferrin (CDT) *(continued)*

National Institute on Alcohol Abuse and Alcoholism: Biomarkers of heavy drinking, in Assessing Alcohol Problems: A Guide for Clinicians and Researchers. Edited by Allen JP, Wilson VB. Available at: https://pubs.niaaa.nih.gov/publications/assessingalcohol/allen.pdf. Accessed June 2021.

Niemelä O: Biomarker-based approaches for assessing alcohol use disorders. Int J Environ Res Public Health 13(2):166, 2016

Rinck D, Frieling H, Freitag A, et al: Combinations of carbohydrate-deficient transferrin, mean corpuscular erythrocyte volume, gamma-glutamyltransferase, homocysteine and folate increase the significance of biological markers in alcohol dependent patients. Drug Alcohol Depend 89:60–65, 2007

Carbon dioxide (CO$_2$)

Type of test	Blood
Background and explanation of test	This test is also known as bicarbonate, CO$_2$ content, and total CO$_2$. Although CO$_2$ exists in the body as a dissolved gas and as an ion, >95% of the total CO$_2$ content in normal plasma comes from bicarbonate, which is regulated by the kidneys. Only a small fraction of total CO$_2$ content is contributed by dissolved CO$_2$ gas, which is regulated by the lungs. Total CO$_2$ provides a measure of the buffering capacity of the blood.
Relevance to psychiatry and behavioral science	This lab result may provide a clue to the presence of purging behaviors in patients with eating disorders. In addition, it may be increased in alcoholism and decreased in alcoholic ketosis, dehydration, head injury, or liver disease.
Preparation of patient	None needed
Indications	• Component of blood panel used for routine screening purposes • Used with blood gas values to determine whether an acid-base imbalance is primarily respiratory or metabolic in origin • Signs/symptoms of fluid/electrolyte imbalance • Monitoring chronic kidney disease
Reference range	Adults ≤60 years: 23–29 mEq/L Adults >60 years: 23–31 mEq/L Adults >90 years: 20–29 mEq/L
Critical value(s)	<6.0 mEq/L
Increased levels	• Recurrent vomiting • Chronic obstructive pulmonary disease (emphysema) • Aldosteronism • Cushing's syndrome
Decreased levels	• Recurrent diarrhea • Acute renal failure • Ethylene glycol or methanol poisoning • Starvation • Metabolic acidosis • Diabetic ketoacidosis • Addison's disease • Salicylate overdose • Use of chlorothiazide diuretics

Carbon dioxide (CO_2) *(continued)*

Interfering factors	Drugs that increase bicarbonate levels include fludrocortisone, barbiturates, bicarbonates, hydrocortisone, loop diuretics, and steroids.
	Drugs that decrease bicarbonate levels include methicillin, nitrofurantoin, tetracycline, thiazide diuretics, and triamterene.
Cross-references	**Blood Gases**

American Association for Clinical Chemistry: Testing.com. Available at: https://www.testing.com. Accessed June 2021.

Chernecky CC, Berger BJ: Laboratory Tests and Diagnostic Procedures, 5th Edition. St. Louis, MO, WB Saunders, 2008

Fischbach F, Dunning MB: A Manual of Laboratory and Diagnostic Tests, 8th Edition. Philadelphia, PA, Wolters Kluwer Health/Lippincott Williams and Wilkins, 2009

U.S. National Library of Medicine: CO2 blood test. MedlinePlus, 2021. Available at: https://medlineplus.gov/ency/article/003469.htm. Accessed June 2021.

Carotid ultrasound

Type of test	Imaging/Ultrasound
Background and explanation of test	Ultrasound technology utilizes the reflections from high-frequency sound waves to create images of the internal anatomy and structural pathology. Doppler analysis provides information about blood flow velocity and disturbance. These technologies are combined in the carotid duplex study, which evaluates the carotid vessels and, to a lesser extent, the vertebral vessels.
	In color duplex ultrasound, vascular lesions (e.g., plaque, stenosis, occlusion) are visualized in grayscale simultaneous with color-encoded images of flow patterns. When pathological findings are demonstrated, quantification can be achieved by analysis of Doppler spectral waveforms. The carotid arteries are examined in transverse and longitudinal section, with particular attention paid to the carotid bifurcation where pathology is most likely to occur. The vertebral arteries, because of their smaller size and partial inaccessibility, are examined only in longitudinal section.
Relevance to psychiatry and behavioral science	Patients with carotid or vertebral artery stenosis may present with intermittent or nonspecific symptoms that appear to be psychiatric in nature. For example, patients with TIAs are sometimes diagnosed as having panic attacks, and those with vertebrobasilar insufficiency may present with "dizziness" and be referred for evaluation of suspected somatic symptom disorder or illness-related anxiety.
Preparation of patient	A certain degree of patient cooperation required. Patients will be supine for test, asked to breathe quietly and evenly, and requested to remain silent and minimize swallowing so artifact can be minimized. Exam takes ~30 minutes.
Indications	• Suspected vascular disease in carotid or vertebral distribution • Cervical bruit • Risk factors for cerebrovascular disease (e.g., diabetes) • History of stroke or TIA • Light-headedness, dizziness, or blackouts • Headaches • Memory impairment • Follow-up after carotid vascular surgery or stenting • Follow-up for known asymptomatic carotid disease
Normal test	• Normal vascular anatomy and course of arteries • No evidence of stenosis or occlusion • No kinking or coiling of the carotid artery • Normal flow patterns • Normal thickness of arterial walls

Carotid ultrasound *(continued)*

Critical value(s)	≥60% occlusion of a carotid artery may be an indication for surgery or stenting, even in patients who are asymptomatic.
Abnormal test	• Stenosis • Occlusion • Dissection • Aneurysm • Carotid body tumor • Arteritis • Subclavian steal syndrome
Interfering factors	Extreme obesity, patient movement, and cardiac dysrhythmias may all affect test results.
Cross-references	**Stroke**

Fauci AS, Braunwald E, Kasper DL, et al (eds): Harrison's Principles of Internal Medicine, 17th Edition. New York, McGraw-Hill, 2008

Fischbach FT, Fischbach MA: A Manual of Laboratory and Diagnostic Tests, 10th Edition. Philadelphia, PA, Wolters Kluwer Health/Lippincott Williams and Wilkins, 2018

Saxena A, Ng EYK, Lim ST: Imaging modalities to diagnose carotid artery stenosis: progress and prospect. Biomed Eng Online 18(1):66, 2019

Cerebrospinal fluid amyloid-β_{1-42} (CSF Aβ_{1-42})

Type of test	CSF
Background and explanation of test	The processes of accumulation, aggregation, and deposition of the amyloid-β peptide Aβ_{1-42} are believed to be central to the pathogenesis of Alzheimer's disease (AD). CSF Aβ_{1-42} levels are lower in AD patients compared with age-matched cognitively healthy patients, although a considerable overlap in values is noted between AD, mild cognitive impairment, and control groups. In addition, the correlation of Aβ_{1-42} level and severity of dementia is not strong. For these reasons, CSF Aβ_{1-42} is of limited value in the individual clinical patient. The ratio of Aβ_{1-42} to Aβ_{1-40} in CSF is a better measure, with significant differences found between AD and control groups. Even better is the combination of this ratio with other measures, such as CSF phosphorylated tau and neuroimaging (amyloid PET, tau PET).
Relevance to psychiatry and behavioral science	This test is used for selected cases in the workup of cognitive impairment to provide evidence for or against a diagnosis of AD.
Preparation of patient	See **Cerebrospinal Fluid Analysis**
Indications	Aiding in the differential diagnosis of AD
Reference range	See laboratory reference range.
Critical value(s)	See laboratory reference.
Increased levels	Not applicable
Decreased levels	A decreased Aβ_{1-42}-to-Aβ_{1-40} ratio is a biomarker of a pathological state in AD and other diseases involving cognitive impairment, such as Parkinson's disease.
Interfering factors	CSF specimen requires special handling.
Cross-references	**Alzheimer's Disease** **Cerebrospinal Fluid Analysis** **Cerebrospinal Fluid Tau Protein**

Blennow K, Zetterberg H: Biomarkers for Alzheimer's disease: current status and prospects for the future. J Intern Med 284(6):643–663, 2018

Hansson O, Lehmann S, Otto M, et al: Advantages and disadvantages of the use of the CSF amyloid β (Aβ) 42/40 ratio in the diagnosis of Alzheimer's disease. Alzheimers Res Ther 11(1):34, 2019

Jack CR Jr, Bennett DA, Blennow K, et al: NIA-AA research framework: toward a biological definition of Alzheimer's disease. Alzheimers Dement 14(4):535–562, 2018

Lim EW, Aarsland D, Ffytche D, et al: Amyloid-β and Parkinson's disease. J Neurol 266(11):2605–2619, 2019

Selkoe DJ, Hardy J: The amyloid hypothesis of Alzheimer's disease at 25 years. EMBO Mol Med 8(6):595–608, 2016

Cerebrospinal fluid analysis

Type of test	CSF sampling by lumbar puncture (LP)
Background and explanation of test	In psychiatric settings, an LP is usually performed for diagnostic indications. Information is obtained regarding CSF protein, glucose, cellular elements (RBCs and WBCs), antigens, immunoglobulin, and other disease biomarkers. Opening pressure may or may not be measured. The report returned from the lab includes cell counts (with differential for WBCs if count is >5), total protein, albumin, glucose, IgG, IgA, IgM, oligoclonal bands if present, specific antibodies if present (e.g., measles or rubella), lactate if requested, and the appearance of a yellow color of CSF by visual inspection.
Relevance to psychiatry and behavioral science	As noted in the *Indications* section below, certain psychiatric and neuropsychiatric presentations may necessitate LP with CSF analysis.
Preparation of patient	Anticoagulant therapy should be held, or the effects reversed, before the procedure is started so INR is <1.2. Patients should be questioned regarding any history of lumbar spinal surgery, stenosis, or deformity such as scoliosis that might limit direct access to the subarachnoid space. Brain CT or MRI must be performed before LP in patients presenting with focal neurological deficits, new-onset seizures, altered level of consciousness, or papilledema. MRI may also be indicated for immunocompromised patients, to look for occult masses. Patients should be informed about possible adverse effects of LP, which include headache, back pain, infection, bleeding, and radicular symptoms. Rare adverse effects include cranial neuropathies (diplopia, facial numbness, hearing loss) and, potentially, brain herniation.
Indications	• Delirium or mental status change of unknown etiology • Seizures of unknown etiology • Acute, severe, or persistent headache or stiff neck • Suspected CNS infection • Unexplained fever in an immunocompromised patient • Suspected subarachnoid hemorrhage with negative CT scan • Multiple sclerosis • Transverse myelitis • Neurosarcoidosis • Guillain-Barré syndrome • Pseudotumor cerebri • Carcinomatous meningitis • CNS lymphoma
Contraindications to LP	• Mass lesion in the posterior fossa • Intracranial lesion with mass effect (seen on CT or MRI)

Cerebrospinal fluid analysis *(continued)*

Contraindications to LP *(continued)*	• Midline shift on CT or MRI • Poor visualization of the fourth ventricle or quadrigeminal cistern on CT or MRI • INR >1.5 • Platelet count <50,000/mm^3 • Lumbar skin or tissue infection
Reference range	See entries for individual CSF tests.
Critical findings	See entries for individual CSF tests.
Abnormal findings	See entries for individual CSF tests.
Interfering factors	*Specimen handling*: Samples should be examined as soon as possible or frozen until examination. Freeze/thaw cycles may interfere with special tests such as amyloid-β.
Cross-references	**Encephalitis, Viral** **Meningitis** **Multiple Sclerosis** See entries for individual CSF tests.

Irani DN: Cerebrospinal Fluid in Clinical Practice. Philadelphia, PA, Saunders Elsevier, 2009

Seehusen DA, Reeves MM, Fomin DA: Cerebrospinal fluid analysis. Am Fam Physician 68:1103–1108, 2003

Cerebrospinal fluid cell count and differential

Type of test	CSF sampling by lumbar puncture
Background and explanation of test	CSF cell counts include the number of RBCs, number of WBCs, and cell types. Normally, the CSF is acellular, containing only a small number of lymphocytes and monocytes in a ratio of 7:3 in adults. The total cell count is a sensitive indicator of acute inflammation in the CNS. An increase in the number of WBCs in the CSF is called *pleocytosis*.
Relevance to psychiatry and behavioral science	The CSF cell count and differential is an essential component of the workup for mental status changes, delirium, and seizures in cases in which an infectious or inflammatory cause is suspected. Specific causative agents can be identified in tuberculosis, neurosyphilis, and Lyme disease, among many other conditions.
Preparation of patient	See **Cerebrospinal Fluid Analysis**.
Indications	See **Cerebrospinal Fluid Analysis**.
Reference range	Adults: 0–5 WBCs/µL • 40%–80% lymphocytes • 15%–45% monocytes • 0%–6% neutrophils RBCs: normally not present, although they may be found in a traumatic tap
Critical value(s)	>20 neutrophils (polymorphonuclear leukocytes)
Abnormal findings	*Increased neutrophils*: meningitis (bacterial, early viral, early tubercular, fungal), amoebic encephalomyelitis, early cerebral abscess, reaction to CNS hemorrhage, injection of foreign substances into the subarachnoid space (chemotherapeutic agents, contrast dye), CSF infarct, metastatic tumor in contact with CSF, reaction to repeated lumbar puncture *Increased lymphocytes*: meningitis (viral, tubercular, unusual bacteria such as *Listeria*), meningoencephalitis (syphilis), CNS parasites, multiple sclerosis (with reactive lymphocytes), encephalopathy of drug abuse, Guillain-Barré syndrome, acute disseminated encephalomyelitis, meningitic sarcoidosis, human T-lymphotropic virus type III (HTLV-III), aseptic meningitis, fungal meningitis, polyneuritis *Increased monocytes*: chronic bacterial meningitis, toxoplasmosis, amoebic meningitis, multiple sclerosis, brain abscess rupture *Increased plasma cells*: acute viral infection, multiple sclerosis, sarcoidosis, meningoencephalitis (syphilis), subacute sclerosing panencephalitis, tubercular meningitis, parasitic infestation, Guillain-Barré syndrome, lymphocytic reactions *Presence of eosinophils*: certain infections (parasitic, fungal, rickettsial), idiopathic hypereosinophilic syndrome, reaction to foreign materials in CSF such as shunts or drugs, sarcoidosis

Cerebrospinal fluid cell count and differential *(continued)*

Abnormal findings *(continued)*	*Presence of malignant cells*: primary or metastatic cancers
	Presence of blast cells: acute leukemia
	Presence of macrophages: meningitis (tubercular or viral), reactions to blood, foreign materials, or lipids in CSF
Interfering factors	Traumatic tap, improper specimen handling
Cross-references	**Encephalitis, Viral**
	Lyme Disease
	Meningitis
	Syphilis
	Tuberculosis

Irani DN: Cerebrospinal Fluid in Clinical Practice. Philadelphia, PA, Saunders Elsevier, 2009

Reiber H, Peter JB: Cerebrospinal fluid analysis: disease-related data patterns and evaluation programs. J Neurol Sci 184:101–122, 2001

Seehusen DA, Reeves MM, Fomin DA: Cerebrospinal fluid analysis. Am Fam Physician 68:1103–1108, 2003

Cerebrospinal fluid cytology

Type of test	CSF sampling by lumbar puncture
Background and explanation of test	This test detects and characterizes malignant cells present in the CSF.
Relevance to psychiatry and behavioral science	CSF cytology is requested when CNS malignancy is suspected to underlie mental status changes, delirium, or seizures.
Preparation of patient	See **Cerebrospinal Fluid Analysis**.
Indications	• Clinical signs of carcinomatous meningitis • Radiographic evidence of brain metastases
Reference range	No malignant cells
Critical value(s)	None
Increased levels	Primary or metastatic malignancy
Decreased levels	Not applicable
Interfering factors	Improper specimen handling
Cross-references	**Brain Tumor** **Cerebrospinal Fluid Analysis** **Meningitis**

Irani DN: Cerebrospinal Fluid in Clinical Practice. Philadelphia, PA, Saunders Elsevier, 2009

Reiber H, Peter JB: Cerebrospinal fluid analysis: disease-related data patterns and evaluation programs. J Neurol Sci 184:101–122, 2001

Seehusen DA, Reeves MM, Fomin DA: Cerebrospinal fluid analysis. Am Fam Physician 68:1103–1108, 2003

Cerebrospinal fluid glucose

Type of test	CSF sampling by lumbar puncture
Background and explanation of test	Many diseases are associated with decreased CSF glucose because it is consumed during the pathological process. The normal range of CSF glucose is related to the serum glucose level in the 1–4 hours before the procedure.
Relevance to psychiatry and behavioral science	CSF glucose is an essential component of basic CSF analysis in the workup of mental status changes, delirium, or seizures.
Preparation of patient	See **Cerebrospinal Fluid Analysis**.
Indications	See **Cerebrospinal Fluid Analysis**.
Reference range	Adults: 45–80 mg/dL (about two-thirds of serum glucose level)
Critical value(s)	Levels <40 mg/dL are always pathological in adults.
Increased levels	• Cerebral hemorrhage • TBI • Hyperglycemia or diabetic coma • Hypothalamic lesion • Increased intracranial pressure • Uremia
Decreased levels	*CNS infection:* abscess, coccidioidomycosis, encephalitis, meningitis, neurosyphilis, toxoplasmosis, tuberculoma *CNS cancer:* tumor, leukemia, lymphoma, melanomatosis, meningeal carcinomatosis *CNS inflammatory/autoimmune disease:* sarcoidosis, lupus myelopathy, rheumatoid arthritis *Other CNS diseases:* GLUT1 deficiency syndrome, hypoglycemia, increased intracranial pressure, subarachnoid hemorrhage
Interfering factors	Hyperglycemia raises CSF glucose. Specimen must be examined by the lab immediately to avoid spurious results from glycolysis.
Cross-references	**Cerebrospinal Fluid Analysis** **Encephalitis, Viral** **Meningitis**

Irani DN: Cerebrospinal Fluid in Clinical Practice. Philadelphia, PA, Saunders Elsevier, 2009

Reiber H, Peter JB: Cerebrospinal fluid analysis: disease-related data patterns and evaluation programs. J Neurol Sci 184:101–122, 2001

Seehusen DA, Reeves MM, Fomin DA: Cerebrospinal fluid analysis. Am Fam Physician 68:1103–1108, 2003

Cerebrospinal fluid lactate

Type of test	CSF
Background and explanation of test	CSF lactate, which is independent of blood lactate, is a product of anaerobic metabolism. It reflects the degree of oxygen deprivation in brain tissue.
Relevance to psychiatry and behavioral science	This test is usually ordered when a lumbar puncture is performed on an inpatient, often in the critical care setting. The result can be used in the differential diagnosis of meningitis etiology and in gauging the severity of TBI.
Preparation of patient	See **Cerebrospinal Fluid Analysis**.
Indications	• Distinguishing bacterial meningitis from other causes of meningitis • Monitoring severe head injury
Reference range	Adults: 10–22 mg/dL
Critical value(s)	Increased CSF lactate after TBI suggests poor prognosis.
Increased levels	• Bacterial meningitis (>38 mg/dL) • Viral meningitis: lactate level generally lower • Brain abscess or tumor • Cerebral ischemia • TBI • Seizure • Stroke • Increased intracranial pressure
Decreased levels	Not applicable
Interfering factors	Because RBCs contain significant amounts of lactate, a traumatic tap may yield false-positive results. Specimens cannot be hemolyzed or xanthochromic.
Cross-references	**Cerebrospinal Fluid Analysis** **Meningitis** **Stroke**

Irani DN: Cerebrospinal Fluid in Clinical Practice. Philadelphia, PA, Saunders Elsevier, 2009

Reiber H, Peter JB: Cerebrospinal fluid analysis: disease-related data patterns and evaluation programs. J Neurol Sci 184:101–122, 2001

Seehusen DA, Reeves MM, Fomin DA: Cerebrospinal fluid analysis. Am Fam Physician 68:1103–1108, 2003

Cerebrospinal fluid protein

Type of test	CSF by lumbar puncture
Background and explanation of test	Under normal circumstances, CSF contains only a small amount of protein, and the finding of elevated protein reliably indicates a pathological process. This process can involve changed permeability of the blood-brain barrier, increased protein production within the CNS, problems with resorption of CSF at the level of the arachnoid villi, or blockage of CSF flow. Special protein studies may be used to determine the composition of protein (protein electrophoresis or oligoclonal bands by high-resolution serum protein electrophoresis, isoelectric focusing/ immunofixation) or to identify pathological processes such as myelin breakdown (myelin basic protein).
Relevance to psychiatry and behavioral science	Mean CSF protein levels are elevated in several conditions of interest to neuropsychiatrists, including bacterial meningitis (mean protein level 418 mg/dL), cerebral hemorrhage (270 mg/dL), brain tumor (115 mg/dL), aseptic meningitis (77 mg/dL), brain abscess (69 mg/dL), neurosyphilis (68 mg/dL), multiple sclerosis (43 mg/dL), acute alcoholism (32 mg/dL), and epilepsy (31 mg/dL).
Preparation of patient	See **Cerebrospinal Fluid Analysis**.
Indications	See **Cerebrospinal Fluid Analysis**.
Reference range	Adults ≤40 years: 15–45 mg/dL
	Adults 40–50 years: 20–50 mg/dL
	Adults 50–60 years: 20–55 mg/dL
	Adults >60 years: 30–60 mg/dL
Critical value(s)	Values >60 mg/dL in the absence of diabetes or recent stroke should be thoroughly investigated.
	Values >1,000 mg/dL suggest subarachnoid obstruction of CSF flow; the lower the block, the higher the value.
Increased levels	• Alzheimer's disease
	• Increased permeability of the blood-CSF barrier
	• Meningitis (bacterial, mycobacterial, fungal, or viral)
	• Hemorrhage (subarachnoid or intracerebral)
	• Stroke
	• Endocrine disorders (e.g., diabetes)
	• Metabolic disorders
	• Drug or alcohol toxicity
	• Obstruction to CSF circulation (from tumor, abscess, herniated disc, loculated effusion)
	• Increased protein synthesis (IgG): multiple sclerosis, subacute sclerosing panencephalitis, neurosyphilis

Cerebrospinal fluid protein *(continued)*

Increased levels *(continued)*	• Increased IgG synthesis with changed permeability of blood-CSF barrier: Guillain-Barré syndrome, SLE, periarteritis, chronic inflammatory demyelinating polyneuropathy (CIDP)
Decreased levels	Low values usually have little clinical significance but may be seen in CNS trauma with CSF leakage, CSF volume removal, intracranial hypertension, or hyperthyroidism.
Interfering factors	False elevation of protein may be seen with a traumatic tap, wherein protein level is highest in first tube and progressively lower in second through fourth tubes. Can be corrected if same tube is used for protein and cell counts by subtracting 1 mg/dL of protein for every 1,000 RBCs/mm^3.
Cross-references	**Alcohol Use Disorder** **Brain Abscess** **Brain Tumor** **Cerebrospinal Fluid Analysis** **Cerebrospinal Fluid Glucose** **Meningitis** **Multiple Sclerosis** **Stroke** **Syphilis**

Irani DN: Cerebrospinal Fluid in Clinical Practice. Philadelphia, PA, Saunders Elsevier, 2009

Reiber H, Peter JB: Cerebrospinal fluid analysis: disease-related data patterns and evaluation programs. J Neurol Sci 184:101–122, 2001

Seehusen DA, Reeves MM, Fomin DA: Cerebrospinal fluid analysis. Am Fam Physician 68:1103–1108, 2003

Cerebrospinal fluid tau protein

Type of test	CSF
Background and explanation of test	Tau is a microtubule-associated protein that, when elevated in CSF, is thought to reflect axonal injury. Tau can be assayed in CSF as total tau (T-tau) or phosphorylated tau (P-tau), with levels of the two closely correlated. In the CSF of patients with TBI or stroke, there is a marked increase in T-tau in proportion to the brain injury, with no change in P-tau. Similarly, with CJD, there is an increase in T-tau up to 20 times that seen in Alzheimer's disease (AD), with minimal or no change in P-tau. The only disease characterized by an increase in P-tau is AD, in which excessive phosphorylation at serine and threonine sites facilitates tau aggregation, leading to the formation of neurofibrillary tangles. CSF P-tau is a special study available only through designated labs. It is usually performed in tandem with CSF amyloid-β. Tau protein is reported as T-tau and P-tau.
Relevance to psychiatry and behavioral science	This test is used for selected cases in the workup of cognitive impairment to provide evidence for or against a diagnosis of AD. It can distinguish cognitive decline of AD from normal aging and from alcohol-related cognitive impairment. The ratio of tau to amyloid-β_{1-42} level appears to be superior to either test alone in differentiating these conditions.
Preparation of patient	See **Cerebrospinal Fluid Analysis**.
Indications	Ancillary test used to support diagnosis of AD
Reference range	Mean T-tau in control subjects: 212 pg/mL P-tau <61 pg/mL consistent with non-AD
Critical value(s)	Mean T-tau in AD: 534 pg/mL P-tau >61 pg/mL consistent with AD
Increased levels	AD
Decreased levels	Not applicable
Interfering factors	Not known
Cross-references	**Alzheimer's disease** **Cerebrospinal Fluid Amyloid β_{1-42}** **Cerebrospinal Fluid Analysis**

Dean RA, Shaw LM: Use of cerebrospinal fluid biomarkers for diagnosis of incipient Alzheimer disease in patients with mild cognitive impairment. Clin Chem 56:7–9, 2009

de Leon MJ, DeSanti S, Zinkowski R, et al: MRI and CSF studies in the early diagnosis of Alzheimer's disease. J Intern Med 256:205–223, 2004

Mitchell AJ: CSF phosphorylated tau in the diagnosis and prognosis of mild cognitive impairment and Alzheimer's disease: a meta-analysis of 51 studies. J Neurol Neurosurg Psychiatry 80:966–975, 2009

Mounsey AL, Zeitler MR: Cerebrospinal fluid biomarkers for detection of Alzheimer disease in patients with mild cognitive impairment. Am Fam Physician 97(11):714–715, 2018

Chest X-ray (CXR)

Type of test	Imaging
Background and explanation of test	Routine CXR consists of two views: posteroanterior and left lateral. Upright films are preferred because supine films do not show fluid levels. Each film is taken at full inspiration. The entire procedure takes only a few minutes. Exposure to radiation is minimal unless the procedure is often repeated. Although chest CT is superior to CXR in detecting lung disease related to COVID-19, CXR has been used when CT is unavailable or where infection control or decontamination issues have limited its use. CXR findings may be described as irregular, patchy, hazy, reticular, or ground glass opacities. The volume of involved lung can also be determined from CXR.
Relevance to psychiatry and behavioral science	Many of the conditions that can be diagnosed by CXR have an association with delirium. In the case of chronic conditions such as tuberculosis, depression may be prominent. In acute exacerbations of chronic obstructive pulmonary disease (COPD), anxiety may be the most pressing symptom. Chronic changes consistent with emphysema are common among psychiatric patients, in large part because of the prevalence of smoking. Aspiration pneumonia is common among patients with dementia, particularly in later stages.
Preparation of patient	Clothing and jewelry covering the chest are removed. The patient wears a hospital gown. Female patients should be asked about pregnancy. The thyroid gland may be covered with a lead shield.
Indications	• Delirium of unexplained etiology in an elderly patient • Dyspnea • Acute respiratory illness in any of the following patients: HIV-positive, age >40 years, age <40 years with positive physical exam, dementia, suspected severe acute respiratory syndromes (COVID-19, SARS) or anthrax exposure, febrile neutropenic patient, acute asthma with suspected pneumonia or pneumothorax, acute COPD exacerbation with one or more of the following: leukocytosis, pain, history of coronary artery disease, or history of congestive heart failure (CHF)
Abnormal findings	Foreign body, pneumonia, CHF, emphysema, abscess, cysts, pneumothorax, pleural effusion, TB, sarcoidosis, asbestosis, coccidioidomycosis, pulmonary embolus. May also detect bony abnormalities such as scoliosis, osteomyelitis, or osteoporosis. COVID-19 findings on CXR include lung tissue consolidation and ground-glass opacities. Latter may be difficult to detect on CXR.
Interfering factors	Conditions that interfere with patients' ability to achieve full inspiration interfere with a complete exam. These include obesity, pain, CHF, and restrictive lung disease.

Chest X-ray (CXR) *(continued)*

Interfering factors *(continued)*	If patients are unable to travel to the radiology department, an anterior-to-posterior film is obtained in bed, in the upright position. This view is much less likely to reveal pathology, particularly in area blocked by heart.
Cross-references	**Delirium**
	Tuberculosis

Fauci AS, Braunwald E, Kasper DL, et al (eds): Harrison's Principles of Internal Medicine, 17th Edition. New York, McGraw-Hill, 2008

Jacobi A, Chung M, Bernheim A, Eber C: Portable chest X-ray in coronavirus disease-19 (COVID-19): a pictorial review. Clin Imaging 64:35–42, 2020

Chlordiazepoxide level

Type of test	Blood
Background and explanation of test	Benzodiazepines are Schedule IV sedative-hypnotic drugs used to treat anxiety and insomnia. Chlordiazepoxide (Librium and others) is a benzodiazepine that is also commonly used to treat alcohol withdrawal. It is an intermediate-acting drug with a long half-life and with active metabolites. In general, levels of the parent drug and its metabolite nordiazepam are checked either when overdose or noncompliance is suspected or to detect use without a prescription. In the latter case, a urine drug screen would more likely be used to detect the metabolite oxazepam.
Relevance to psychiatry and behavioral science	Toxicity with chronic benzodiazepine ingestion may manifest as confusion, disorientation, memory impairment, ataxia, decreased reflexes, and dysarthria. With acute overdose, the patient may exhibit somnolence, confusion, ataxia, decreased reflexes, vertigo, dysarthria, respiratory depression, and coma. More serious consequences usually involve co-ingestion of alcohol or other sedatives. The administration of flumazenil does not affect the drug level.
Preparation of patient	None needed
Indications	• Screening for drug use • Suspicion of overdose • Signs of toxicity in a treated patient • Suspected noncompliance with prescribed therapy
Reference range	Chlordiazepoxide 500–3,000 ng/mL Nordiazepam 100–1,500 ng/mL
Critical value(s)	Chlordiazepoxide >5,000 ng/mL Nordiazepam >2,500 ng/mL
Increased levels	• Overdose • Overuse • Poor metabolism • Hepatic encephalopathy
Decreased levels	Noncompliance
Interfering factors	None
Cross-references	**Benzodiazepines** **Urine Drug Screen**

ARUP Laboratories: Benzodiazepines, urine, quantitative, in Lab Test Directory. Salt Lake City, UT, ARUP Laboratories, 2021. Available at: https://ltd.aruplab.com/Tests/Pub/2008291. Accessed June 2021.

Galanter M, Kleber HD (eds): The American Psychiatric Publishing Textbook of Substance Abuse Treatment, 4th Edition. Washington, DC, American Psychiatric Publishing, 2008

Wu AHB: Tietz Clinical Guide to Laboratory Tests, 4th Edition. St. Louis, MO, WB Saunders, 2006

Chloride

Type of test	Blood
Background and explanation of test	Chloride is an anion found in high concentration in the extracellular fluid, where it works to maintain osmotic pressure and water balance and acts as a buffer to maintain acid-base balance. Usually, chloride concentration rises and falls with sodium, but the chloride level can change independently when an acid-base imbalance occurs as the ion moves into and out of cells to maintain electrical neutrality.
	Chloride is ingested in food and table salt, with most absorbed in the GI tract and the excess excreted in urine. Normal blood levels are stable, with a slight decrease after meals, when the stomach produces acid to aid digestion using chloride from blood. When a massive diuresis occurs (e.g., with diabetes insipidus), chloride is lost through the urinary system. With significant vomiting or diarrhea, chloride is lost directly from the GI tract.
	Chloride is measured as a routine component of electrolyte panels because it is useful in the diagnosis of acid-base and water balance problems. The results of the blood test may be followed up with a blood gas, urine chloride testing, or blood or urine sodium measurement.
Relevance to psychiatry and behavioral science	Chloride levels are affected by any process that involves loss of fluid from the GI tract, changes in acid-base balance, or changes in sodium concentration. Neuropsychiatric conditions that may be associated with chloride derangements include diabetes insipidus, lithium intoxication, SIAD, psychogenic polydipsia, porphyria, TBI, eating disorders with purging behaviors, and hyperventilation.
Preparation of patient	Patient should fast for ≥8 hours before testing.
Indications	• Routine component of blood panels (electrolyte panel, BMP, CMP)
	• Suspicion of acidosis or alkalosis
	• Respiratory distress
	• Prolonged vomiting or diarrhea
	• Massive diuresis
Reference range	96–106 mEq/L
	Values may be higher in patients >90 years.
Critical value(s)	<70 mEq/L or >120 mEq/L
Increased levels	• Dehydration
	• Cushing's syndrome (with high sodium level)
	• Metabolic acidosis (with prolonged diarrhea)
	• Respiratory alkalosis (with hyperventilation)
	• Primary hyperparathyroidism

Chloride *(continued)*

Increased levels *(continued)*	• Certain kidney diseases (e.g., renal tubular acidosis) • Diabetes insipidus • Salicylate intoxication • TBI with hypothalamic injury • Eclampsia
Decreased levels	• Prolonged vomiting • Gastric suction • Salt-wasting diseases (e.g., SIAD, nephritis) • Chronic respiratory acidosis • Burns • Metabolic alkalosis • Overhydration or water intoxication • Addison's disease • Congestive heart failure • Acute intermittent porphyria
Interfering factors	Medications containing bromide can produce a positive reaction with some ion-selective electrode assays for chloride. Drugs that affect sodium level also affect chloride level. Ingestion of large amounts of baking soda or antacids can lower chloride level. Excessive IV saline infusion causes elevated chloride level.
Cross-references	**Bulimia Nervosa** **Diabetes Insipidus** **Lithium** **Porphyria** **Psychogenic Polydipsia** **Syndrome of Inappropriate Antidiuresis**

Ahmadi L, Goldman MB: Primary polydipsia: update. Best Pract Res Clin Endocrinol Metab 34(5):101469, 2020

American Association for Clinical Chemistry: Testing.com. Available at: https://www.testing.com. Accessed June 2021.

Fischbach FT, Fischbach MA: A Manual of Laboratory and Diagnostic Tests, 10th Edition. Philadelphia, PA, Wolters Kluwer Health/Lippincott Williams and Wilkins, 2018

Germon K: Fluid and electrolyte problems associated with diabetes insipidus and syndrome of inappropriate antidiuretic hormone. Nurs Clin North Am 22:785–796, 1987

Sailer C, Winzeler B, Christ-Crain M: Primary polydipsia in the medical and psychiatric patient: characteristics, complications and therapy. Swiss Med Wkly 147:w14514, 2017

Siragy HM: Hyponatremia, fluid-electrolyte disorders, and the syndrome of inappropriate antidiuretic hormone secretion: diagnosis and treatment options. Endocr Pract 12:446–457, 2006

Cholinesterase

Type of test	Blood
Background and explanation of test	Cholinesterase levels are used to confirm organophosphate poisoning. Organophosphate compounds are found in insecticides (e.g., malathion and parathion) and nerve gases (e.g., soman and sarin). These compounds inhibit the enzyme acetylcholinesterase, which breaks down acetylcholine. Symptoms of toxicity are attributable to cholinergic excess. Exposure can occur by inhalation, ingestion, or skin contact. Those at risk of exposure include farmworkers, gardeners, manufacturers, fumigators, military personnel, and children.
	Both RBC cholinesterase and plasma cholinesterase assays are available. RBC cholinesterase is more accurate, but plasma cholinesterase is easier to perform and more readily available. Blood should be drawn before treatment commences, but treatment should not wait until results are returned. Cholinesterase levels do not always correlate with severity of clinical symptoms.
Relevance to psychiatry and behavioral science	Initial psychiatric symptoms of acute organophosphate exposure include anxiety and emotional lability, poor concentration, insomnia, and nightmares. With more serious exposure, apathy, depression, anorexia, decreased libido, restlessness, hyperactivity, suicidal ideation, confusion, memory problems, hallucinations, paranoid ideation, and dissociation may be seen. Motor symptoms include tremor, ataxia, and seizures. Many of the same symptoms can be seen with chronic exposure. Genetic susceptibility has been described and can account for toxicity with relatively low-level exposure in some cases.
Preparation of patient	None needed
Indications	Clinical suspicion of organophosphate poisoning
Reference range	Plasma cholinesterase: 2.9–7.1 U/mL
	RBC cholinesterase: 7.9–17.1 U/mL
	RBC cholinesterase-to-hemoglobin ratio: 25–52 U/g hemoglobin
Critical value(s)	None
Increased levels	Acute or chronic organophosphate exposure
Decreased levels	Not applicable
Interfering factors	Spuriously reduced RBC cholinesterase levels may be found in patients with pernicious anemia or hemoglobinopathies and in those taking antimalarial drugs.
	Spuriously reduced plasma cholinesterase may be found in patients with liver disease, pregnancy, hypoproteinemia, neoplasia, hypersensitivities, or certain genetic deficiency syndromes and in those taking specific drugs (e.g., morphine, codeine, succinylcholine).

Cholinesterase *(continued)*

Interfering factors *(continued)*	*Specimen handling*: Frozen, clotted, or hemolyzed specimens invalidate results; use of oxalate blood tubes invalidates results.
Cross-references	**Organophosphate Poisoning**

ARUP Laboratories: Cholinesterase, RBC: ratio to hemoglobin, in Lab Test Directory. Salt Lake City, UT, ARUP Laboratories, 2021. Available at: https://ltd.aruplab.com/Tests/Pub/0020174. Accessed June 2021.

Brown JS: Environmental and Chemical Toxins and Psychiatric Illness. Washington, DC, American Psychiatric Publishing, 2002

Katz KD, Brooks DE: Organophosphate toxicity clinical presentation. Medscape, December 31, 2020. Available at: https://emedicine.medscape.com/article/167726-clinical. Accessed June 2021.

Clonazepam level

Type of test	Blood
Background and explanation of test	Clonazepam (Klonopin, Rivotril) is a member of the class of drugs known as benzodiazepines, which are Schedule IV sedative-hypnotics used to treat anxiety and insomnia. In general, benzodiazepine levels are checked when either overdose or noncompliance is suspected or to detect use without a prescription. For the latter indication, a urine drug screen would more likely be used than a blood level.
Relevance to psychiatry and behavioral science	Toxicity with chronic benzodiazepine ingestion may manifest as confusion, disorientation, memory impairment, ataxia, decreased reflexes, and dysarthria. There is some evidence that use of long-acting benzodiazepines such as clonazepam is associated with an increased risk of motor vehicle accidents and falls in elderly patients, even when levels are within the therapeutic range. With acute benzodiazepine overdose, patients may exhibit somnolence, confusion, ataxia, decreased reflexes, vertigo, dysarthria, respiratory depression, and coma. More serious consequences usually involve co-ingestion of alcohol or other sedatives. Administration of flumazenil does not affect the drug level.
Preparation of patient	None needed
Indications	• Suspected noncompliance with prescribed therapy • Screening for drug use • Suspicion of overdose • Signs of toxicity in a treated patient
Reference range	20–70 ng/mL (for dosages of 1–8 mg/day)
Critical value(s)	>80 ng/mL
Increased levels	• Overdose • Overuse • Poor metabolism • Hepatic encephalopathy
Decreased levels	Noncompliance
Interfering factors	None
Cross-references	**Benzodiazepines** **Urine Drug Screen**

ARUP Laboratories: Clonazepam, in Lab Test Directory. Salt Lake City, UT, ARUP Laboratories, 2021. Available at: https://ltd.aruplab.com/Tests/Pub/0090055. Accessed June 2021.

Chernecky CC, Berger BJ: Laboratory Tests and Diagnostic Procedures, 5th Edition. St. Louis, MO, WB Saunders, 2008

Wu AHB: Tietz Clinical Guide to Laboratory Tests, 4th Edition. St. Louis, MO, WB Saunders, 2006

Clozapine level

Type of test	Blood
Background and explanation of test	Clozapine (Clozaril and others) is an atypical antipsychotic drug used to treat patients with schizophrenia and related illnesses who have had a poor response to other drugs, particularly patients with recurrent suicidal ideation. The threshold level for clinical response is generally taken as 350 ng/mL. The dose-concentration relationship is affected by several variables, including ethnicity; Asian individuals require only 50% of the usual dosage to achieve the target level.
Relevance to psychiatry and behavioral science	Clozapine is the prototype atypical antipsychotic drug—the first to be marketed and still widely considered the most efficacious. Use of clozapine is limited by its potential to cause severe neutropenia and other serious adverse effects. In addition to schizophrenia, clozapine is used in the treatment of schizoaffective disorder, bipolar disorder, Parkinson's disease with psychosis, dementia with Lewy bodies, and psychosis in patients with tardive dyskinesia. Clozapine blood levels are routinely monitored during treatment and should also be checked when interacting drugs are started or discontinued and in the event of infection, which can be associated with increased clozapine levels.
Preparation of patient	Blood should be drawn at steady state (5–7 days after the last change in dosage), 12±2 hours after the last dose.
Indications	• Clozapine dosage >600 mg/day* (higher risk of seizures) • Signs/symptoms of toxicity • Expected drug interactions when other medications are used • Suspected noncompliance • Poor response to treatment
Reference range	350–600 ng/mL for major psychiatric disorders such as schizophrenia For psychosis arising in the context of medical conditions and for elderly patients, lower drug levels may be appropriate. Some patients with treatment-refractory schizophrenia benefit from higher drug levels.
Critical value(s)	≥1,000 ng/mL
Increased levels	Toxicity
Decreased levels	Influenced by many variables, including noncompliance with treatment. See **Clozapine** in the *Psychotropic Medications* chapter for more information.
Interfering factors	None
Cross-references	**Clozapine** **Therapeutic and Toxic Drug Levels at a Glance** (Appendix A)

*A lower threshold would apply to Asian patients.

Clozapine level *(continued)*

American Society of Health-System Pharmacists: AHFS Drug Information. Bethesda, MD, American Society of Health-System Pharmacists, 2016

Clark SR, Warren NS, Kim G, et al: Elevated clozapine levels associated with infection: a systematic review. Schizophr Res 192:50–56, 2018

de Leon J, Ruan CJ, Schoretsanitis G, De Las Cuevas C: A rational use of clozapine based on adverse drug reactions, pharmacokinetics, and clinical pharmacopsychology. Psychother Psychosom 89(4):200–214, 2020

de Leon J, Schoretsanitis G, Kane JM, Ruan CJ: Using therapeutic drug monitoring to personalize clozapine dosing in Asians. Asia Pac Psychiatry 12(2):e12384, 2020

Complete blood count (CBC)

Type of test	Blood
Background and explanation of test	The CBC is an automated count of blood cells that reports the following information: WBC, RBC, and platelet counts per volume, platelet volume, hemoglobin content, hematocrit, and red cell indices (MCV, mean corpuscular hemoglobin [MCH], mean corpuscular hemoglobin concentration [MCHC], and red cell distribution of width [RDW]).

MCH is a calculation of the amount of oxygen-carrying hemoglobin in a single RBC. Macrocytic RBCs have higher MCH values, and microcytic RBCs have lower MCH values.

MCHC is a calculation of the average concentration of hemoglobin in RBCs. Low MCHC, or hypochromia, is seen with diseases such as iron deficiency anemia or thalassemia, in which hemoglobin is diluted. High MCHC, or hyperchromia, is seen with conditions such as burns, in which hemoglobin is concentrated.

RDW is a calculation of the variance in size (anisocytosis) and shape (poikilocytosis) of RBCs.

If a *differential* is ordered with the CBC, types of WBCs are identified either manually or by automated means.

For any of the blood cells, unusual cell types or morphologies are explored through examination of a blood smear and are reported with the routine CBC. Other components of the CBC are discussed in separate entries in this chapter. |
| Relevance to psychiatry and behavioral science | This is a basic screening test that aids in the diagnosis of numerous medical conditions that can cause symptoms resembling primary psychiatric diseases. The CBC is a high-yield, low-cost test. |
| Preparation of patient | Fasting is not required. Physiological stress should be avoided just prior to testing. |
| Indications | • Basic screening panel for hospital admission and general health status

• Presurgical evaluation

• Monitoring after surgery

• Clinical signs/symptoms such as fever, fatigue, weakness, or abnormal bleeding or bruising

• Clinical suspicion of infection or inflammation |
| Reference range | MCH: 28–34 pg/cell

MCHC: 32–36 g/dL

RDW: 11.5%–14.5%

For all other values, see individual test components. |
Critical value(s)	See entries for test components.
Increased levels	See entries for test components.
Decreased levels	See entries for test components.

Complete blood count (CBC) *(continued)*

Interfering factors	See entries for test components.
Cross-references	See entries for CBC components.

American Association for Clinical Chemistry: Testing.com. Available at: https://www.testing.com. Accessed November 2021.

Chernecky CC, Berger BJ: Laboratory Tests and Diagnostic Procedures, 5th Edition. St. Louis, MO, WB Saunders, 2008

Fauci AS, Braunwald E, Kasper DL, et al (eds): Harrison's Principles of Internal Medicine, 17th Edition. New York, McGraw-Hill, 2008

Fischbach FT, Fischbach MA: A Manual of Laboratory and Diagnostic Tests, 10th Edition. Philadelphia, PA, Wolters Kluwer Health/Lippincott Williams and Wilkins, 2018

Comprehensive metabolic panel (CMP)

Type of test	Blood
Background and explanation of test	The CMP includes 14 tests: • Glucose • Calcium • Albumin • Protein (total protein) • Sodium • Potassium • Carbon dioxide • Chloride • BUN • Creatinine • ALT • AST • Bilirubin • ALP
Relevance to psychiatry and behavioral science	In patients presenting with psychiatric signs/symptoms, the CMP may be useful for rapid assessment of metabolic status. In psychiatry and behavioral medicine, this panel is used in preference to the BMP because it includes LFTs. The CMP is a high-yield, low-cost test.
Preparation of patient	Usually none, although overnight fasting yields a more meaningful glucose measurement in many cases. For optimal testing, see preparations recommended for individual tests.
Indications	• Metabolic screen for patients presenting with psychiatric signs/symptoms • Routine health screen • Monitoring specific lab values in a hospitalized patient
Reference range	See entries for individual tests.
Critical value(s)	See entries for individual tests.
Increased levels	See entries for individual tests.
Decreased levels	See entries for individual tests.
Interfering factors	See entries for individual tests.
Cross-references	**Basic Metabolic Panel** See entries for individual tests.

Computed tomography scan, head

Type of test	Imaging
Background and explanation of test	In a head CT scan, the attenuation of X-ray beams by tissues of differing density distinguishes gray and white matter, bone, CSF, and blood. Different "windows" can be requested in addition to the standard brain window (e.g., bone window, or subdural window to improve detection of a suspected subdural hematoma). A CT study can be performed nonenhanced ("without" contrast), or it can be enhanced with iodinated dye administered intravenously ("with" contrast). Contrast improves visualization of lesions such as stroke, tumor, and abscess.
	CT is preferred to MRI in the detection of calcified lesions, meningeal tumors, and acute blood. CT is less degraded by motion artifact than is MRI. It is inferior to MRI in the detection of ischemia or demyelination and is not as well able to visualize the brainstem, cerebellum, or temporal lobes due to artifact created at the bone-tissue interface.
	CT slice thickness ranges from 1 mm to 10 mm. Thicker cuts reduce the time of the study but also reduce sensitivity because smaller lesions may be missed. Even with thin slices, CT is a shorter study than MRI, and the cost is about half that of MRI. Spatial resolution of structures in CT is inferior to that of MRI.
	The axial CT scan image is presented as if one were viewing the brain from the foot of the bed while the patient lies supine, so the right side of the brain appears on the viewer's left. Brightness on the CT scan is proportional to the density of the tissue, so bone and calcium are very bright (white), CSF and fat are black, and gray matter is lighter gray than white matter. Appendix B contains further information.
Relevance to psychiatry and behavioral science	CT is a relatively low-cost, high-yield testing modality in certain patient populations, including those with new-onset headaches or new neurological deficits. In addition, CT (or MRI) is indicated for patients with a first episode of psychosis, prolonged catatonia, or first onset of psychosis, mood disorder, or personality changes after age 50 years.
Preparation of patient	The scan takes about 10 minutes. Radiation exposure is little more than that of plain films of the skull, but cumulative effects can be significant. CT contrast agent more likely than MRI gadolinium to cause an allergic reaction, which can be serious; anaphylaxis can occur. Allergic reactions are more common in patients with asthma or seafood allergies.
Indications	• Headache (sudden-onset severe or unilateral headache, new headache in a pregnant patient [without contrast]), new headache in suspected meningitis or encephalitis [without contrast, to evaluate intracranial pressure])
	• Ipsilateral Horner syndrome
	• New focal neurological deficit
	• Ataxia of acute onset

Computed tomography scan, head *(continued)*

Indications *(continued)*	• TIA (combined with CT angiography) • Suspected subarachnoid hemorrhage, brain parenchymal hemorrhage • Suspected carotid or vertebral dissection • First episode of psychosis with atypical presentation • First onset of psychosis, mood disorder, or personality changes after age 50 years • Prolonged catatonia
Normal test	• Normal anatomical landmarks identified • No midline shift • No extracerebral fluid accumulation (subdural or epidural) • No abnormal hypodense or hyperdense areas • If atrophy is present, it is generalized and mild, or moderate in a patient of advanced age
Abnormal test	The following appear dark (less dense) on CT due to accumulation of extravascular fluid: • Infarction • Demyelination • Inflammation • Gliosis • Most cancers • Cysts The following appear light (more dense) on CT: • Acute blood • Meningiomas • Thrombosis • Calcified masses • Calcified tubers • Colloid cysts • Certain primary lymphomas
Interfering factors	Motion artifact interferes with image acquisition.
Cross-references	**Additional Information on Neuroimaging** (Appendix B) **Angiography, Computed Tomography (Cerebrovascular)** **Magnetic Resonance Imaging** **Stroke**

Computed tomography scan, head *(continued)*

American College of Radiology: Appropriateness Criteria: Acute Mental Status Change, Delirium, and New Onset Psychosis. Reston, VA, American College of Radiology, 2018. Available at: https://acsearch.acr.org/docs/3102409/Narrative. Accessed June 2021.

Holt RE: The role of computed tomography of the brain in psychiatry. Psychiatr Med 1:275–285, 1983

Pearlson GD, Veroff AE, McHugh PR: The use of computed tomography in psychiatry: recent applications to schizophrenia, manic-depressive illness and dementia syndromes. Johns Hopkins Med J 149:194–202, 1981

Cortisol

Type of test	Blood, saliva, urine
Background and explanation of test	Cortisol is a steroid hormone released by the adrenal glands in response to stimulation by ACTH from the anterior pituitary gland. Cortisol has significant physiological effects, particularly on carbohydrate metabolism. Its level in the circulation normally peaks in the morning hours, drops in the evening, and reaches a nadir around midnight. In conditions involving excessive release of cortisol, the peak serum level may be normal, but the diurnal drop may not be seen. In testing for these conditions, levels might be drawn at 8:00 A.M. and 4:00 P.M., and sometimes also at 8:00 P.M. In testing for conditions involving decreased cortisol release, a single morning sample is used. In distinguishing Cushing's syndrome from simple obesity, a 24-hour urine free cortisol level might be used. Urine free cortisol is proportional to serum free cortisol and is the most sensitive and specific test for initial screening for Cushing's syndrome. Salivary cortisol reflects unbound cortisol and its diurnal variation in serum. Morning salivary cortisol levels are decreased in adrenal insufficiency, and evening salivary cortisol levels—drawn between 11:00 P.M. and midnight—are increased in Cushing's syndrome.
Relevance to psychiatry and behavioral science	HPA axis abnormalities are associated with a range of psychiatric disorders, including mood disorders, PTSD, schizophrenia, substance use disorders, and dementia. Glucocorticoids such as cortisol have regulatory effects on serotonergic function and stimulant-like effects on dopamine neurotransmission. Excessive glucocorticoid activity likely contributes to symptoms of psychotic mood disorders. In general, cortisol levels are elevated along with corticotropin-releasing factor (CRF) from the hypothalamus in major depression and stress, whether short-lived or sustained. In contrast, in PTSD, studies have found that cortisol levels are low, although CRF levels in CSF are increased. This pattern is consistent with increased sensitivity of the negative feedback loop of the HPA axis. Further supporting this idea is the exaggerated suppression of cortisol in response to dexamethasone in PTSD. In major depression, cortisol suppression is reduced in response to dexamethasone. In schizophrenia, cortisol levels are elevated, and nonsuppression of cortisol in response to dexamethasone is associated with negative symptoms and cognitive impairment. Stress and cortisol elevation have been implicated in numerous studies of relapse in substance-dependent patients. Drugs such as cocaine, amphetamines, alcohol, nicotine, and naloxone are associated with increased cortisol levels.

Cortisol (continued)

Preparation of patient	Patients should fast from food and fluids for 4–8 hours before testing and should refrain from physical activity for 10–12 hours before testing. They should relax in the recumbent position for 30 minutes before blood is drawn.
Indications	• Diagnosing Cushing's syndrome (hypercortisolism) • Diagnosing Addison's disease (hypocortisolism) • Monitoring treatment for hypercortisolism or hypocortisolism • Evaluating stress-related conditions
Reference range	*Total cortisol* • 8:00 A.M. 5–23 µg/dL • 4:00 P.M. 3–16 µg/dL • 8:00 P.M. <50% of 8:00 A.M. values *Free cortisol* • 8:00 A.M. 0.6–1.6 µg/dL • 4:00 P.M. 0.2–0.9 µg/dL *Saliva free cortisol* • 7:00 A.M. 1.4–10.1 ng/mL • 10:00 P.M. 0.7–2.2 ng/mL *Urine free cortisol, 24-hour* • By radioimmunoassay: ≥21 years: 20–90 µg/day • By high-performance liquid chromatography: ≤50 µg/day
Critical value(s)	Extreme cortisol elevation in the morning coupled with lack of diurnal variation suggests presence of carcinoma.
Increased levels	• Cushing's syndrome/disease • Ectopic ACTH production • High stress (thermal, traumatic, or psychological) • Metabolic syndrome (with hypertension, obesity) • Burns, trauma, shock • Postoperative state (e.g., post–coronary artery bypass grafting) • Severe disease (liver or kidney) • Acute infectious or inflammatory disease • Hyperpituitarism • Hyperthyroidism • Pregnancy • Strenuous exercise • Hypoglycemia

Cortisol *(continued)*

Increased levels *(continued)*	• Depression • *Drugs*: corticotropin, estrogens, oral contraceptives, yohimbine, and vasopressin
Decreased levels	• Adrenal insufficiency (Addison's disease) • Chromophobe adenoma • Craniopharyngioma • Hypophysectomy/Hypopituitarism • Hypothyroidism • Liver disease • Postpartum pituitary necrosis (Sheehan's syndrome) • PTSD • Rheumatoid arthritis • *Drugs:* dexamethasone
Interfering factors	Cortisol level increases with bright light exposure. Delay in spinning sample may give spuriously decreased result. Certain drugs can cause false elevations: interferon-γ, metoclopramide, quinacrine, and spironolactone. Other drugs can cause decreased cortisol levels: lithium, levodopa, phenytoin (in females), morphine, etomidate, and ketoconazole.
Cross-references	**Adrenal Insufficiency** **Cushing's Syndrome**

American Association for Clinical Chemistry: Testing.com. Available at: https://www.testing.com. Accessed May 2010.

Fauci AS, Braunwald E, Kasper DL, et al (eds): Harrison's Principles of Internal Medicine, 17th Edition. New York, McGraw-Hill, 2008

Fischbach F, Dunning MB: A Manual of Laboratory and Diagnostic Tests, 8th Edition. Philadelphia, PA, Wolters Kluwer Health/Lippincott Williams and Wilkins, 2009

Sadock BJ, Sadock VA, Ruiz P (eds): Kaplan and Sadock's Comprehensive Textbook of Psychiatry. Philadelphia, PA, Lippincott Williams and Wilkins, 2009

Wu AHB: Tietz Clinical Guide to Laboratory Tests, 4th Edition. St. Louis, MO, WB Saunders, 2006

C-reactive protein (CRP)

Type of test	Blood
Background and explanation of test	CRP is an acute-phase reactant secreted by the liver in response to inflammation or tissue injury when cytokines such as interleukin-6 are present in the circulation. CRP levels are very low or undetectable in the serum of healthy individuals. CRP levels rise within hours when the inflammatory response is stimulated and fall rapidly when inflammation subsides. Two separate CRP assays are available, both measuring the same molecule in blood, although using different assays: • CRP measures the molecule in the range 10–1,000 mg/L. • High-sensitivity C-reactive protein (hsCRP) measures the molecule in the range 0.5–10 mg/L. The hsCRP test is used in the assessment of risk for vascular events (e.g., heart attack, stroke), whereas CRP is used in the evaluation of patients at risk of bacterial infections or major inflammatory processes. CRP is analogous to the ESR, with the latter reflecting conditions involving increased plasma protein/fibrinogen levels such as autoimmune disease, and CRP reflecting inflammation from infection or trauma. High CRP levels have been identified in severe COVID-19 infection, even though CRP elevation is not usually found with viral infections. CRP is strongly associated with the severity and prognosis of COVID-19 infection.
Relevance to psychiatry and behavioral science	CRP can be helpful in the evaluation of conditions such as bacterial meningitis, SLE, or pancreatitis. Elevation of CRP is associated with delirium and the metabolic syndrome. There is some evidence that CRP might be useful as a marker of the phases of illness in schizophrenia.
Preparation of patient	None
Indications	*CRP* • Assessing activity of autoimmune disease • Assessing activity of inflammatory disease • Assessing severity and monitoring treatment of bacterial infection • Evaluating pancreatitis • Detecting infection after surgery • Detecting transplant rejection *hsCRP* • Stratification of risk for cardiovascular disease
Reference range	CRP <10 mg/L generally accepted as normal In most healthy adults, CRP <3 mg/L

C-reactive protein (CRP) *(continued)*

Reference range *(continued)*	hsCRP cardiovascular risk stratification: • Low risk: <1.0 mg/L • Average risk: 1.0–3.0 mg/L • High risk: 3.1–9.9 mg/L • Very high risk: >9.9 mg/L
Critical value(s)	CRP >50 mg/L is strongly associated with bacterial infection See risk stratification above for hsCRP.
Increased levels	*Large increase:* active inflammation, cancer, serious bacterial infection, burns *Minor increase:* mucosal infection (e.g., sinusitis, periodontitis), obesity, insulin resistance, pancreatitis, smoking, uremia, cardiac ischemia, oral hormone replacement therapy, sleep disturbance, chronic fatigue, alcohol use, depression, aging
Decreased levels	Not applicable
Interfering factors	Obesity and late-stage pregnancy affect results. Chronic inflammatory conditions such as arthritis may interfere with the evaluation of new inflammatory process. Recent illness may invalidate hsCRP risk stratification.
Cross-references	**Delirium** **Erythrocyte Sedimentation Rate** **High-Sensitivity C-Reactive Protein** **Meningitis** **Metabolic Syndrome** **Systemic Lupus Erythematosus** **Cardiovascular Risk Assessment** (Appendix C)

Abi-Saleh B, Iskandar SB, Elgharib N, et al: C-reactive protein: the harbinger of cardiovascular diseases. South Med J 101:525–533, 2008

American Association for Clinical Chemistry: Testing.com. Available at: https://www.testing.com. Accessed November 2021.

ARUP Laboratories: C-reactive protein, in Lab Test Directory. Salt Lake City, UT, ARUP Laboratories, 2021. Available at: https://ltd.aruplab.com/Tests/Pub/0050180. Accessed November 2021.

Ben-Yehuda O: High-sensitivity C-reactive protein in every chart? The use of biomarkers in individual patients. J Am Coll Cardiol 49:2139–2141, 2007

Bray C, Bell LN, Liang H, et al: Erythrocyte sedimentation rate and C-reactive protein measurements and their relevance in clinical medicine. WMJ 115(6):317–321, 2016

NACB LMPG Committee Members, Myers GL, Christenson RH, et al: National Academy of Clinical Biochemistry Laboratory Medicine Practice Guidelines: emerging biomarkers for primary prevention of cardiovascular disease. Clin Chem 55(2):378–384, 2009

Creatine kinase (CK)

Type of test	Blood
Background and explanation of test	CK, the enzyme that catalyzes the metabolism of creatine to creatinine, is found in the heart and skeletal muscles and in smaller concentrations in brain tissue. Three isoforms exist: CK-MM, localized mainly to skeletal muscle, CK-MB, localized mainly to heart muscle, and CK-BB, localized mainly to brain tissue. CK-BB from the CNS rarely enters the circulation; CNS injury may be reflected in only a slight elevation of total CK. CK-MB has been replaced by troponin testing for the diagnosis of heart attack.
	Small amounts of CK-MM in the circulation are normal. Most cases of elevated CK are either normal variants or the effects of exercise, particularly when coupled with dehydration.
	Persistent elevation of CK warrants investigation as a marker of muscle injury, which could be caused by endocrine, autoimmune, genetic, or drug-related factors. *Myalgia* is muscle pain in the absence of CK elevation, *myopathy* is muscle pain with CK elevation, and *rhabdomyolysis* is muscle pain, weakness, or swelling with CK elevation and myoglobinuria.
	Statin drugs, macrolide antibiotics (e.g., azithromycin), and antifungals (e.g., ketoconazole) are common causes of CK elevation. Among statins, simvastatin and pravastatin are associated with more muscle-related effects than are atorvastatin and rosuvastatin.
	COVID-19 infection is associated with a viral myositis (muscle inflammation) that ranges from mild to severe and may or may not be accompanied by CK elevation.
Relevance to psychiatry and behavioral science	CK elevation can be seen in patients with NMS, abrupt withdrawal of clozapine, Parkinsonism-hyperpyrexia syndrome, seizure, stroke, TBI, delirium tremens, carbon monoxide poisoning, or dystonic reactions. CK (and CK-MM) elevation can be induced by ECT, use of physical restraints, or recent intramuscular injections.
	Both typical and atypical antipsychotic drugs can be associated with an elevation of CK and CK-MM with or without muscle pathology. In most cases, CK normalizes when the drug is withdrawn, and renal function is unaffected.
Preparation of patient	Patients should avoid strenuous physical activity for 24 hours before testing.
Indications	• A patient reporting muscle pain or weakness
	• Suspicion of NMS
	• Evaluating muscle injury in chronic muscular diseases, such as muscular dystrophy
	• Evaluating muscle injury in acute or subacute conditions, such as myositis
	• Detecting muscle injury from statins and other drugs, including antipsychotic medications

Creatine kinase (CK) *(continued)*

Reference range	Males: 20–200 U/L
	Females: 20–180 U/L
Critical value(s)	None
Increased levels	• NMS
	• Parkinson-hyperpyrexia syndrome
	• Dystonic reaction
	• Seizure
	• ECT
	• TBI
	• Eosinophilia-myalgia syndrome
	• Cocaine intoxication with rhabdomyolysis
	• Myositis (e.g., with COVID-19)
	• Myocarditis
	• Stroke
	• Delirium tremens
	• Acute psychosis or mania
	• Recent surgery
	• Malignant hyperthermia
	• Cardioversion
	• Carbon monoxide poisoning
	• Recent EMG or electric shock
	• Subarachnoid hemorrhage
	• Muscular dystrophy
	• Hypothyroidism
	• Late pregnancy
	• Cancer (e.g., prostate, bladder, GI tract)
Decreased levels	Small muscle mass
Interfering factors	Benign elevations may be seen in Blacks and those with large muscle mass.
	Heavy or prolonged exercise increases CK levels.
	Intramuscular injections and use of physical restraints elevate CK levels.
Cross-references	**Myocardial Infarction**
	Neuroleptic Malignant Syndrome

ARUP Laboratories: Creatine kinase, total, serum or plasma, in Lab Test Directory. Salt Lake City, UT, ARUP Laboratories, 2021. Available at: https://ltd.aruplab.com/Tests/Pub/0020010. Accessed November 2021.

Belteczki Z, Ujvari J, Dome P: Clozapine withdrawal-induced malignant catatonia or neuroleptic malignant syndrome: a case report and a brief review of the literature. Clin Neuropharmacol 44(4):148–153, 2021

Creatine kinase (CK) *(continued)*

Dos Santos DT, Imthon AK, Strelow MZ, et al: Parkinsonism-hyperpyrexia syndrome after amantadine withdrawal: case report and review of the literature. Neurologist 26(4):149–152, 2021

Fischbach FT, Fischbach MA: A Manual of Laboratory and Diagnostic Tests, 10th Edition. Philadelphia, PA, Wolters Kluwer Health/Lippincott Williams and Wilkins, 2018

Kim EJ, Wierzbicki AS: Investigating raised creatine kinase. BMJ 373:n1486, 2021

Meltzer HY, Cola PA, Parsa M: Marked elevations of serum creatine kinase activity associated with antipsychotic drug treatment. Neuropsychopharmacology 15:395–405, 1996

Saud A, Naveen R, Aggarwal R, Gupta L: COVID-19 and myositis: what we know so far. Curr Rheumatol Rep 23(8):63, 2021

Creatinine

Type of test	Blood, 24-hour urine
Background and explanation of test	Creatinine is a waste product continually produced in skeletal muscle by the breakdown of creatine phosphate, with the amount produced dependent on the muscle mass of the individual. All creatinine that is filtered by the kidneys is eliminated, so the level of creatinine in the blood is inversely related to the GFR. Serum creatinine is used with BUN to evaluate kidney function, as both are elevated in kidney disease.
	Traditionally, creatinine clearance (and corresponding GFR) was estimated by the Cockcroft-Gault formula, but this was replaced by the more accurate Modification of Diet in Renal Disease (MDRD) Study formula, which has in turn been replaced by the Chronic Kidney Disease Epidemiology Collaboration (CKD-EPI) equation. This latest formula takes age, sex, and serum creatinine into account in a formula that many find unwieldy to use directly, but these values can be plugged into an open-access calculator at www.mdcalc.com/calc/3939/ckd-epi-equations-glomerular-filtration-rate-gfr.
	Importantly, the CKD-EPI formula does not use race or ethnicity as a factor. This is in recognition of the fact that the multiplier used to correct eGFR for Blacks resulted in inequitable and delayed care for chronic kidney disease in this population.
	The CKD-EPI formula is now used by many laboratories, and an eGFR is reported along with serum creatinine. If this estimate is not provided or if the laboratory used the MDRD equation, an estimate can be obtained at the website noted above.
	The ratio of BUN to creatinine is sometimes helpful in the differential diagnosis of the cause of kidney dysfunction. A normal ratio is between 10:1 and 20:1. An increased ratio suggests reduced blood flow to the kidney from conditions such as congestive heart failure or dehydration, or increased protein (urea nitrogen) from GI bleeding or dietary sources. A decreased ratio suggests malnourishment or liver disease, with decreased urea formation.
Relevance to psychiatry and behavioral science	Delirium is associated with various conditions in which creatinine is elevated. Creatinine is a component of the laboratory evaluation for newly hospitalized patients with suspected eating disorders. The level may be increased, or it may be normal despite significant renal dysfunction because of decreased muscle mass. Lithium may cause true creatinine elevation, with compromise of renal function and reduced clearance of other drugs and waste products.
Preparation of patient	None needed
Indications	• Component of BMP and CMP • Evaluating general health status

Creatinine *(continued)*

Indications *(continued)*	• Suspicion of kidney disease or dysfunction • Monitoring known kidney disease • Monitoring renal function on nephrotoxic drugs (e.g., lithium, aminoglycosides) • Preoperative assessment • Preparing for administration of contrast agents for imaging

Reference range	*Adults 18–60 years*
	  Males: 0.9–1.3 mg/dL
	  Females: 0.6–1.1 mg/dL
	Adults 61–90 years
	  Males: 0.8–1.3 mg/dL
	  Females: 0.6–1.2 mg/dL
	Adults >90 years
	  Males: 1.0–1.7 mg/dL
	  Females: 0.6–1.3 mg/dL

Critical value(s)	Planning for dialysis often begins when eGFR by CKD-EPI (or MDRD) declines to <30 mL/min/1.73m^2. Dialysis is usually started when eGFR declines to <15 mL/min/1.73m^2
Increased levels	*Kidney diseases* • Glomerulonephritis • Pyelonephritis • Acute tubular dysfunction • Nephrotic syndrome • Interstitial nephritis • Amyloidosis *Other conditions* • Reduced blood flow to kidneys (e.g., atherosclerosis) • Urinary tract obstruction (e.g., kidney stones or prostate enlargement) • Dehydration • Congestive heart failure • Shock • Hemorrhage • Muscle injury, rhabdomyolysis • Myasthenia gravis • Gigantism or acromegaly

Creatinine *(continued)*

Decreased levels	• Liver disease • Pregnancy • Small or decreased muscle mass • Burns • Carbon monoxide poisoning
Interfering factors	Serum creatinine varies with muscle mass. In body builders, measurement of cystatin C to reflect kidney function may be more appropriate. In older persons with declining muscle mass, creatinine level may remain stable in the face of significantly reduced renal function. For this population, serial creatinine measurements should be used. High-protein foods such as red meat may significantly increase serum creatinine levels. Creatine supplementation used by athletes slightly increases creatinine levels without apparent harm to kidney function. Many drugs falsely elevate creatinine levels, including ascorbic acid, barbiturates, some cephalosporins, clonidine, and levodopa.
Cross-references	**Blood Urea Nitrogen** **Lithium**

CKD-EPI Equations for Glomerular Filtration Rate (GFR). Available at: https://www.mdcalc.com/calc/3939/ckd-epi-equations-glomerular-filtration-rate-gfr.

Delanaye P, Cavalier E, Pottel H: Serum creatinine: not so simple! Nephron 136(4):302–308, 2017

Fischbach FT, Fischbach MA: A Manual of Laboratory and Diagnostic Tests, 10th Edition. Philadelphia, PA, Wolters Kluwer Health/Lippincott Williams and Wilkins, 2018

Raman M, Middleton RJ, Kalra PA, Green D: Estimating renal function in old people: an in-depth review. Int Urol Nephrol 49(11):1979–1988, 2017

Cystatin-C

Type of test	Blood
Background and explanation of test	Cystatin-C is a protein produced by nucleated cells that is filtered by the kidney and whose concentration rises with declining GFR, in a manner analogous to that of creatinine. Cystatin-C is a larger molecule than is creatinine, and its filtration rate is affected earlier than that of creatinine, so this protein may provide an earlier warning of renal impairment. In fact, the relationship of both cystatin-C and creatinine with GFR is not linear, such that small initial increases in either laboratory value may represent a significant decline in GFR.
	Both cystatin-C and creatinine blood values are affected by factors other than GFR. Unlike creatinine, cystatin-C is not affected by muscle mass or diet but is affected by age, obesity, diabetes, and inflammation. Because cystatin-C is also a prognostic indicator of cardiovascular risk, it may be of particular use in patients with chronic kidney disease (CKD). Cystatin-C is thought to be superior to creatinine in estimating GFR in patients with COVID-19. Specialists who estimate GFR using both creatinine and cystatin-C report that those estimates can differ, and when the cystatin-C-predicted GFR is lower than the creatinine-predicted GFR, prognosis tends to be worse.
	Cystatin-C testing is not yet universally available. It is also more costly and has a slower turnaround than creatinine.
Relevance to psychiatry and behavioral science	This test is superior to creatinine in monitoring early renal injury in patients undergoing chemotherapy, in renal transplant recipients, in those treated with lithium, and in those with cirrhosis, rheumatoid arthritis, or IgA nephropathy. A developing indication is the prescreening of patients scheduled to undergo imaging with contrast dye, which can be harmful to marginally functioning kidneys.
Preparation of patient	None needed
Indications	• Early detection of CKD • Monitoring known kidney disease • Prescreening for contrast-enhanced imaging
Reference range	0.5–1.2 mg/L
Critical value(s)	None noted
Increased levels	• CKD • Renal injury from toxins such as chemotherapy, lithium, or aminoglycosides
Decreased levels	Not applicable
Interfering factors	Hemolyzed or lipemic specimens invalidate results.
Cross-references	**Creatinine**

Cystatin-C *(continued)*

ARUP Laboratories: Cystatin C, serum with reflex to estimated glomerular filtration rate (eGFR), in Lab Test Directory. Salt Lake City, UT, ARUP Laboratories, 2021. Available at: https://ltd.aruplab.com/Tests/Pub/0095229. Accessed November 2021.

Benoit SW, Ciccia EA, Devarajan P: Cystatin C as a biomarker of chronic kidney disease: latest developments. Expert Rev Mol Diagn 20(10):1019–1026, 2020

Chen S, Li J, Liu Z, et al: Comparing the value of cystatin C and serum creatinine for evaluating the renal function and predicting the prognosis of COVID-19 patients. Front Pharmacol 12:587816, 2021

Ferguson TW, Komenda P, Tangri N: Cystatin C as a biomarker for estimating glomerular filtration rate. Curr Opin Nephrol Hypertens 24(3):295–300, 2015

Luo J, Wang LP, Hu HF, et al: Cystatin C and cardiovascular or all-cause mortality risk in the general population: a meta-analysis. Clin Chim Acta 450:39–45, 2015

Pasala S, Carmody JB: How to use…serum creatinine, cystatin C and GFR. Arch Dis Child Educ Pract Ed 102(1):37–43, 2017

Cytochrome P450 (CYP450) genotyping

Type of test	Genetic
Background and explanation of test	Many laboratories now offer CYP450 genotyping that includes the two isoenzymes most involved in psychotropic drug metabolism: CYP2D6 and CYP2C19. Although the literature on the clinical utility of CYP450 genotyping remains mixed, the FDA has published a Table of Pharmacogenetic Associations that can be useful to consult regarding testing for specific drugs. That list is included in the references below. Whole blood is optimal for testing.
Relevance to psychiatry and behavioral science	Psychotropic drugs metabolized by CYP2D6 include risperidone, venlafaxine, aripiprazole, brexpiprazole, deutetrabenazine, duloxetine, and atomoxetine, among numerous others. Poor metabolism resulting in higher drug concentrations is thought to underlie many of the adverse effects of these drugs. The poor metabolizer phenotype occurs in 7% of Whites and 1%–3% of those in other ethnic groups. Drugs metabolized by CYP2C19 include citalopram, escitalopram, diazepam, and doxepin. Poor metabolism resulting in higher drug concentrations is thought to underlie many of the adverse effects of these drugs. The poor metabolizer phenotype at 2C19 is found in 3%–4% of Whites and 14%–21% of Asians.
Preparation of patient	None needed
Indications	Clinical suspicion of poor metabolizer or ultrarapid metabolizer status, based on adverse effects or lack of efficacy
Abnormal test	Report returned indicating that the patient's genotype represents poor metabolizer or ultrarapid metabolizer status.
Normal test	Report returned indicating that the patient's genotype represents extensive metabolizer status (two copies of the active allele)
Interfering factors	None
Cross-references	None

ARUP Laboratories: Cytochrome P450 genotyping panel, in Lab Test Directory. Salt Lake City, UT, ARUP Laboratories, 2021. Available at: https://ltd.aruplab.com/Tests/Pub/3001524. Accessed June 2021.

de Leon J, Armstrong S, Cozza K: Clinical guidelines for psychiatrists for the use of pharmacogenetic testing for CYP450 2D6 and CYP450 2C19. Psychosomatics 47:75–85, 2006

Flockhart DA: Drug interactions and the cytochrome P450 system: the role of cytochrome P450 2C19. Clin Pharmacokinet 29(Suppl):45–52, 1995

Jessel CD, Mostafa S, Potiriadis M, et al: Use of antidepressants with pharmacogenetic prescribing guidelines in a 10-year depression cohort of adult primary care patients. Pharmacogenet Genomics 30(7):145–152, 2020

U.S. Food and Drug Administration: Table of Pharmacogenetic Associations. FDA.gov, 2021. Available at: https://www.fda.gov/medical-devices/precision-medicine/table-pharmacogenetic-associations. Accessed June 2021.

Dexamethasone suppression test (DST)

Background and explanation of test	The DST is used medically to screen for excess cortisol production from Cushing's syndrome and related conditions affecting the HPA axis. Normally, when exogenous cortisol is administered, the production of cortisol is reduced through a process of negative feedback to the pituitary gland and hypothalamus known as HPA axis suppression. In patients with Cushing's syndrome, this suppression is reduced or absent, and this is known as HPA axis nonsuppression. There are several protocols for performing the DST, using different doses of steroid and times of blood draw. A commonly used "low-dose" protocol involves administration of oral dexamethasone 1 mg between 11:00 P.M. and midnight, followed by a blood draw for cortisol measurement between 7:00 A.M. and 9:00 A.M. the following day. Normally, the morning cortisol level will be low or undetectable. In cases in which the cortisol level exceeds a certain threshold, the test is said to be positive. A dexamethasone level is drawn simultaneously to ensure that the dexamethasone was taken and that its level represents an adequate challenge.
Relevance to psychiatry and behavioral science	Dysregulation of the HPA axis has been found in patients with depression, especially melancholic and psychotic depression, and in PTSD. The DST may be useful in predicting response to treatment for these conditions and in distinguishing psychotic depression (nonsuppression) from schizophrenia (suppression). The DST remains an area of active research interest.
Preparation of patient	Patients should abstain from caffeine and physical activity and should not fast before the test.
Indications	• Screening for Cushing's syndrome • Aiding in diagnosis of depression, PTSD, and current anxiety disorders • Predicting response to treatment for depression and PTSD
Reference range	Depends on testing protocol; discuss with local laboratory
Critical value(s)	Depends on testing protocol
Increased levels	Nonsuppression in the following: • Cushing's syndrome/disease • Other adrenal disorders • Major depression (melancholic, psychotic) Variable findings in other psychiatric disorders
Decreased levels	PTSD
Interfering factors	False-positive results can be seen with acute illness, fasting, caffeine ingestion, dehydration, uncontrolled diabetes, fever, malnutrition, nausea, obesity, pregnancy, severe stress, and temporal lobe disease.

Dexamethasone suppression test (DST) *(continued)*

Interfering factors *(continued)*	Drugs that can cause false-positive results include aspirin overdose, barbiturates, carbamazepine, estrogen, meprobamate, methyprylon, phenytoin, rifampin, and tetracycline.
	False-negative results can be seen with adrenal failure, hypopituitarism, and poor metabolism of dexamethasone.
	Drugs that can cause false-negative results include high-dose benzodiazepines, corticosteroids, and cyproheptadine.
Cross-references	**Adrenocorticotropic Hormone**
	Cortisol
	Cushing's Syndrome

Nijdam MJ, van Amsterdam JG, Gersons BP, Olff M: Dexamethasone-suppressed cortisol awakening response predicts treatment outcome in posttraumatic stress disorder. J Affect Disord 184:205–208, 2015

Scherf-Clavel M, Wurst C, Nitschke F, et al: Extent of cortisol suppression at baseline predicts improvement in HPA axis function during antidepressant treatment. Psychoneuroendocrinology 114:104590, 2020

Vinkers CH, Kuzminskaite E, Lamers F, et al: An integrated approach to understand biological stress system dysregulation across depressive and anxiety disorders. J Affect Disord 283:139–146, 2021

Diazepam level

Type of test	Blood
Background and explanation of test	Benzodiazepines are Schedule IV sedative-hypnotic drugs used to treat anxiety and insomnia. Diazepam is a highly lipophilic benzodiazepine with a short transit through the circulation before being deposited in fatty tissue, where it can accumulate. It is then released erratically back into the circulation. Both diazepam and its active metabolite nordiazepam have long elimination half-lives. Diazepam levels generally have little clinical significance unless they are extremely high or low. Levels are rarely checked except to confirm overdose, noncompliance, or use without a prescription. In the latter case, a urine drug screen is more often used than a blood level.
Relevance to psychiatry and behavioral science	Toxicity with chronic benzodiazepine ingestion may manifest as confusion, disorientation, memory impairment, ataxia, decreased reflexes, and dysarthria. With acute overdose, the patient may exhibit somnolence, confusion, ataxia, decreased reflexes, vertigo, dysarthria, respiratory depression, and coma. More serious consequences usually involve co-ingestion of alcohol or other sedatives. Administration of flumazenil does not affect the drug level. Activated charcoal is no longer recommended as a treatment because of the high risk of aspiration. Supportive care, including intubation as indicated, is the mainstay of treatment.
Preparation of patient	None needed
Indications	• Screening for drug use • Suspicion of overdose • Signs of toxicity in treated patient • Suspected noncompliance with prescribed therapy
Reference range	Diazepam 200–1,000 ng/mL Nordiazepam 100–1,500 ng/mL
Critical value(s)	Nordiazepam >2,500 ng/mL *Note:* Administration of flumazenil does not affect drug level.
Increased levels	• Overdose • Overuse • Poor metabolism • Hepatic encephalopathy
Decreased levels	Noncompliance with prescribed drug
Interfering factors	None noted
Cross-references	**Benzodiazepines** **Urine Drug Screen**

ARUP Laboratories: Benzodiazepines, urine, quantitative, in Lab Test Directory. Salt Lake City, UT, ARUP Laboratories, 2021. Available at: https://ltd.aruplab.com/Tests/Pub/2008291. Accessed November 2021.
Wu AHB: Tietz Clinical Guide to Laboratory Tests, 4th Edition. St. Louis, MO, WB Saunders, 2006

Echocardiogram

Type of test	Imaging
Background and explanation of test	The echocardiogram is a noninvasive means to evaluate the position and size of the heart, movement of valves and chamber walls, and blood flow velocity. It can be performed at the bedside or in the laboratory. In transthoracic echocardiography (TTE), the transducer is placed on the chest, and pulsed high-frequency sound waves are transmitted through the chest wall and heart structures. For patients who are obese or who have chronic obstructive pulmonary disease, visualization may be poor by this method, so transesophageal echocardiography (TEE) is used, in which the transducer is inserted into the esophagus after the posterior pharynx is anesthetized. Different modes of echocardiographic study are now available, including stress echocardiography. The usual examination takes 30–45 minutes.
Relevance to psychiatry and behavioral science	Severe left ventricular dysfunction (left ventricular ejection fraction [LVEF] <35%) may be associated with fatigue, apparent loss of motivation, and depression. When the LVEF is ≤25%, the patient is prone to develop delirium with minor precipitants. Certain psychotropic medications (e.g., clozapine) are associated with pericardial effusion that can be seen on echocardiogram.
Preparation of patient	For routine echocardiography, no preparation is needed. For specialized procedures such as TEE or stress echocardiography, lab will provide patient instructions.
Indications	• Evaluating heart valve function • Evaluating velocity and direction of cardiac blood flow • Pericardial effusion • Monitoring patients with known cardiac disease • Monitoring patients with left ventricular assist devices
Normal result	Normal position, size, and movement of heart valves and chamber walls Normal heart structures
Abnormal result	• Valvular disease: stenosis, insufficiency, prolapse, regurgitation • Cardiomyopathy • Pericardial disease: effusion, tamponade, pericarditis • Endocarditis • Cardiac neoplasm • Intracardiac thrombus • Coronary artery disease • Prosthetic valve dysfunction • Congenital heart disease

Echocardiogram *(continued)*

Interfering factors	Cardiac rhythm disturbance, lung hyperinflation from mechanical ventilation, and transducer positioning for Doppler study all affect results.
Cross-references	**Medical Evaluation for Electroconvulsive Therapy** (Appendix C)

Fauci AS, Braunwald E, Kasper DL, et al (eds): Harrison's Principles of Internal Medicine, 17th Edition. New York, McGraw-Hill, 2008

Rose VL: American College of Cardiology and American Heart Association address the use of echocardiography. Am Fam Physician 56:1489–1490, 1997

Electrocardiogram

Type of test	Electrophysiology
Background and explanation of test	The ECG (or EKG) records the electrical activity of the heart, including voltages generated and the time it takes for these voltages to flow from one area of the heart to another. The ECG tracing can be used to identify the anatomical source of abnormal rhythms, presence of inadequate blood flow (ischemia), destruction of heart muscle (infarction), enlargement of heart chambers (atrial and ventricular hypertrophy), delays in conduction of electrical current, and inflammation of the tissue surrounding the heart (pericarditis). The ECG can also be helpful in evaluating the effects of electrolyte disturbances, systemic diseases, and medications or drugs that act on the heart and can assist in the evaluation of implanted pacemaker and defibrillator functions. As shown in Appendix C, a normal heart cycle consists of a P wave, QRS complex, and T wave; a U wave may also be seen. This cycle is repeated at regular intervals. The P wave occurs with atrial depolarization, the QRS complex with ventricular depolarization, and the T wave with ventricular repolarization. The U wave represents nonspecific recovery afterpotentials. The ECG is analyzed to determine rate, rhythm, intervals, voltages, axis, and presence of abnormal waveforms.
Relevance to psychiatry and behavioral science	ECG tracings for many patients in psychiatric care show changes suggestive of ischemia, even in the absence of any clinical correlates of disease. For example, anxiety and hyperventilation can be associated with sinus tachycardia and ST-segment depression with or without T-wave inversion, possibly mediated by autonomic function. More significant ECG abnormalities are seen in patients with eating disorders with associated electrolyte derangements. In addition, many psychotropic medications cause ECG abnormalities. Lithium, for example, is associated with T-wave flattening or inversion in most treated patients, and clozapine can be associated with ST-segment changes as well as T-wave inversion. These psychotropic-related findings are of uncertain significance. On the other hand, many psychotropics are known to cause prolongation of the QT interval, which can result in sudden cardiac death due to polymorphic ventricular tachycardia (*torsades de pointes*). Overdose of medications such as TCAs and dual-acting antidepressants may also cause significant ECG changes.
Preparation of patient	Patients should abstain from smoking and avoid heavy meals for ≥30 minutes and should rest for ≥15 minutes before testing.
Indications	• Routine admission testing for older patients • Preoperative screening before general anesthesia • ECT screening in patients older than 50 years or with previous abnormal ECG or known heart disease

Electrocardiogram *(continued)*

Indications *(continued)*	• Chest pain or other signs of possible MI • Syncope • Irregular pulse • Initiation of a psychotropic drug that affects cardiac conduction (e.g., TCA or antipsychotic)
Reference ranges	*Rate*: 60–100 beats per minute *Rhythm*: Normal sinus rhythm or sinus arrhythmia Intervals: • PR interval: 120–200 ms • QRS interval: 80–120 ms • QT interval: 350–430 ms (varies with heart rate [HR], sex, time of day) *Voltages*: • Top of R wave to bottom of S wave: 1 mV • P wave: 0.1–0.3 mV • T wave: 0.2–0.3 mV *Axis*: +90° to −30° in adults
Critical findings	*Ventricular tachycardia:* HR >100 with at least three irregular heartbeats in a row *Ventricular fibrillation:* very rapid HR, uncoordinated, fatal unless treated immediately *Torsades de pointes:* bradycardia, prolonged QT, and QRS that rotates around the isoelectric baseline *Idioventricular rhythm:* sustained rhythm with pacemaker localized to the ventricles, with HR 20–50 Severe bradycardia with HR <40 is often symptomatic. *Acute MI*: See **Myocardial Infarction** in the *Diseases and Conditions* chapter.
Abnormal findings	• *Bradycardia:* HR <60 • *Tachycardia:* HR >100 • *Atrial fibrillation:* HR rapid, rhythm irregular; ECG shows absence of P waves that normally precede QRS complexes • *Atrial flutter:* HR rapid (ventricular rate ~150), QRS narrow, ECG baseline has "sawtooth" appearance • *Junctional rhythm:* Atrioventricular node takes over as pacemaker; P waves absent or inverted on ECG or may appear after QRS complex • *First-degree heart block:* PR interval >200 ms; each P wave followed by QRS

Electrocardiogram *(continued)*

Abnormal findings *(continued)*	• *Second-degree heart block:* Some P waves blocked at atrioventricular node and have no following QRS
	• *Third-degree heart block* (complete heart block): complete dissociation between P waves and QRS
	• *Bundle branch block (BBB):* QRS >120 ms; right BBB prolongs last part of QRS and shifts axis right; left BBB prolongs the whole QRS and shifts the axis to the left.
	• *Left anterior fascicular block* (left anterior hemiblock): QRS <120 ms, left axis deviation ($-45°$ to $-90°$), qR in I and augmented Vector Left (aVL) and rS in II, III, and augmented Vector Foot (aVF)
	• *QTc prolongation:* >450 ms for men and >470 ms for women; results from delayed repolarization, which enables early afterdepolarizations and sets the stage for extrasystoles and possibly *torsades de pointes*
	• *Premature ventricular contractions (PVCs) or ventricular premature depolarizations (VPDs):* wide QRS that follows closely a normal QRS; when PVC occurs after every normal QRS, pattern is called *bigeminy*. When it occurs after every other normal QRS, pattern is called *trigeminy*. When three or more occur in a row, pattern is *ventricular tachycardia*.
	• *ST-segment changes:* normal ST segment serves as isoelectric line on ECG tracing. ST-segment depression (below baseline) may indicate ischemia. ST-segment elevation may indicate infarction.
Interfering factors	*Age:* T-wave inversion in leads V1–V3 may be normal finding into second decade (third decade in Blacks).
	Sex: Females often exhibit slight ST-segment depression.
	Race: ST-segment elevation and T-wave inversion that disappears with maximal exercise may be seen in Blacks.
	QRS axis shifts leftward with obesity, ascites, and pregnancy.
	Variations of normal anatomical heart position may affect axis.
	Inaccurate lead placement affects test results.
	Reversal of limb leads may suggest infarction or dextrocardia (heart in right chest).
	Deep breathing shifts position of heart.
Cross-references	**Additional Cardiac-Related Information** (Appendix C)
	Myocardial Infarction

Dubin D: Rapid Interpretation of EKGs, 3rd Edition. Tampa, FL, Cover, 1984
Fauci AS, Braunwald E, Kasper DL, et al (eds): Harrison's Principles of Internal Medicine, 17th Edition. New York, McGraw-Hill, 2008

Electroencephalogram (EEG)

Type of test	Neurophysiology
Background and explanation of test	The EEG records electrical potential differences between electrode pairs on the scalp or between a scalp electrode and a reference electrode. These potentials reflect underlying electrical activity in the cerebral cortex and, indirectly, that of deeper structures. Electrodes are attached to the scalp in an array known as the 10-20 system, and several different patterns of electrode pairing ("montages") are captured during each recording session. Reference electrodes are placed on the ear or mastoid process or an averaged reference is created electronically. Ideally, recordings capture the fully awake, drowsy, and sleeping states. To achieve the sleep state, the patient might require sleep deprivation on the night before the test.
	Stimulation procedures performed during the test include hyperventilation and photic stimulation, which are designed to elicit epileptiform patterns. If the referring question relates to a specific provocation (e.g., seizures when listening to music), the provocation should be simulated during testing. To capture epileptiform or ictal activity arising from temporal lobes (e.g., in partial seizures), anterior temporal (T1 and T2) and ear electrodes may be used; nasopharyngeal electrodes offer no advantage and are uncomfortable for the patient. If the referring question relates to encephalopathy, the patient may require specific alerting procedures; for example, they may be asked to count backward from 20, or the technician might provide a tapping stimulus to maintain wakefulness. Standard EEG frequencies recorded range from 0.5 Hz to ~35 Hz, with frequencies divided into bands as follows: delta=0.5–4 Hz theta=5–7.5 Hz alpha=8–12 Hz beta=13–35 Hz Higher frequencies often represent artifactual muscle activity.
Relevance to psychiatry and behavioral science	In psychiatric practice, the EEG finds greatest utility in the diagnosis and differential diagnosis of delirium. It is exquisitely sensitive to the changes in brain metabolism and activity accompanying the clinical signs and symptoms of delirium, showing generalized slow-wave activity in the delta and theta ranges, slowing of the posterior dominant frequency, disorganization of the background rhythm, and loss of reactivity to eye opening and closing. The EEG can be used to distinguish delirium from primary psychosis because it is usually normal in the latter condition. It can be used to detect the presence of delirium superimposed on dementia, in which case the amount of slow-wave activity may be greatly increased over the baseline tracing.

Electroencephalogram (EEG) *(continued)*

Relevance to psychiatry and behavioral science *(continued)*	Serial EEGs can be helpful in gauging response to treatment of delirium, with serial studies showing improvement in slowing and increase in mean frequency when treatment is successful.
	Another use of the EEG in psychiatry is to help distinguish seizures from pseudoseizures if the ictal event can be captured during the recording and neither spike nor spike-and-wave activity is seen. Caveats here relate to the fact that the interictal EEG may be completely normal, that patients who have pseudoseizures may also have true seizures, and that some patients who have convincing signs and symptoms but no EEG correlates may, in fact, have deep epileptogenic foci, with activity captured only by depth recording. When the EEG is used for the workup of "mental status changes" or confusional states, it may capture non-convulsive status epilepticus, a condition disproportionately affecting elderly females who present in an ongoing oneiric state or stupor. In these cases, the EEG shows sustained ictal activity.
	Characteristic EEG changes are also seen in sporadic CJD and in subacute sclerosing panencephalitis. In addition, the EEG may detect toxic effects of drugs such as lithium, in which case a disorganized rhythm, interspersed slow-wave activity, and triphasic waves may be seen.
Preparation of patient	Some patients need reassurance that the EEG only *records* electrical activity and does not deliver an electrical stimulus. The process of electrode application should be explained; this often includes use of collodion, an adhesive gel that requires vigorous cleansing for removal. Patients should avoid sedatives before testing. If a hypnotic is required to capture sleep during test, chloral hydrate is often used in preference to alternatives; other sedatives have been studied, but no consensus has been achieved as to superiority. Sleep deprivation may be needed to ensure an adequate sleep sample is obtained (e.g., in the case of suspected seizures). Sleep deprivation protocol is to awaken patient at 4:00 A.M. and then keep them awake without naps or stimulants until the time of testing.
Indications	• Confirming diagnosis of delirium
	• Distinguishing delirium from catatonia
	• Monitoring course of delirium (serial studies)
	• Detecting presence of epileptiform or ictal activity
	• Monitoring efficacy of antiepileptic drugs
	• Diagnosing non-convulsive status epilepticus
	• Diagnosing CJD
	• Diagnosing subacute sclerosing panencephalitis
	• Providing evidence for lithium toxicity

Electroencephalogram (EEG) *(continued)*

Indications *(continued)*	• Various indications in critical care: evaluating coma, confirming brain death • Aiding in the diagnosis of functional neurological symptom disorders (e.g., suspected pseudoseizures)
Normal patterns	• Posterior dominant (alpha) frequency 8–12 Hz • Presence of beta activity during wakefulness, prominent in frontal areas • Abundant theta and delta slow-wave activity only in drowsiness and sleep • Frontal intermittent rhythmic delta activity (FIRDA) only in transitions to and from sleep • In drowsiness and light sleep: vertex sharp waves • In stage 2 sleep: sleep spindles, K complexes • No epileptiform activity or focal slowing • No abnormalities elicited by hyperventilation or photic stimulation
Abnormal patterns	Spike, spike-and-slow-wave complexes, slow waves in the awake state, focal slowing, periodic patterns, triphasic waves; FIRDA outside of transitions. Abnormalities may only be seen with stimulation procedures.
Interfering factors	For intermittent EEG abnormalities, single EEG may be a low-yield procedure. This is particularly true for epileptiform or ictal (seizure) activity when clinical manifestations do not appear during EEG recording or when provoking stimulus cannot be simulated in the laboratory. For seizure activity, yield increases with sleep deprivation, greater number of EEG recordings, and longer times of recording. For this purpose, ambulatory (24-hour) EEG or EEG telemetry may be used for monitoring. EEG study that does not include wakefulness, drowsiness, and at least stage 2 sleep along with hyperventilation and photic stimulation is considered incomplete for detection of epileptiform activity. EEG study that does not explicitly produce and document alerting stimuli is considered incomplete for patients with a depressed level of consciousness (e.g., suspected delirium). Many psychotropic drugs affect EEG, usually introducing either slow-wave activity (e.g., antipsychotics and mood stabilizers) or beta activity (e.g., sedative-hypnotics and alcohol).
Cross-references	**Creutzfeldt-Jakob Disease** **Delirium** **Quantitative Electroencephalogram** **Seizures**

Electroencephalogram (EEG) *(continued)*

Fauci AS, Braunwald E, Kasper DL, et al (eds): Harrison's Principles of Internal Medicine, 17th Edition. New York, McGraw-Hill, 2008

Fernandes ML, Oliveira WM, Santos MV, Gomez RS: Sedation for electroencephalography with dexmedetomidine or chloral hydrate: a comparative study on the qualitative and quantitative electroencephalogram pattern. J Neurosurg Anesthesiol 27(1):21–25, 2015

Jacobson S, Jerrier H: EEG in delirium. Semin Clin Neuropsychiatry 5:86–92, 2000

Electrolytes panel

Type of test	Blood
Background and explanation of test	This panel includes the following four tests: • Sodium • Potassium • Chloride • Carbon dioxide
Relevance to psychiatry and behavioral science	This panel is used to screen and monitor for basic electrolyte abnormalities in patients considering treatment with lithium and certain other psychotropic drugs.
Preparation of patient	None needed
Indications	• Detecting or ruling out a specific lab abnormality • Monitoring a known condition and its associated lab abnormality
Reference range	See entries for individual tests.
Critical value(s)	See entries for individual tests.
Increased levels	See entries for individual tests.
Decreased levels	See entries for individual tests.
Interfering factors	See entries for individual tests.
Cross-references	**Basic Metabolic Panel** **Comprehensive Metabolic Panel** See entries for individual tests.

Electromyography (EMG) and nerve conduction testing (NCT)

Type of test	Neurophysiology
Background and explanation of test	An EMG evaluates the electrical activity of muscles, and NCT evaluates the activity of nerves. In an EMG, needles are inserted into muscle tissue, and electrodes are attached to the skin. Recordings are made at rest and with voluntary muscle contraction. In NCT, electric current is applied to the nerve so the velocity of nerve transmission can be measured for either motor or sensory nerves. Neurological conditions with abnormal test results are listed below.
Relevance to psychiatry and behavioral science	The primary use of electromyography in psychiatric practice relates to the workup of functional neurological symptom disorders, for which normal test results aid in excluding muscle or nerve pathology as a cause of symptoms such as weakness or paralysis.
Preparation of patient	Patients should be instructed to bathe or shower, avoid application of deodorants and cosmetics (including powders and lotions), and avoid caffeine and tobacco prior to testing. An EMG takes 30–60 minutes.
Indications	• Neuromuscular disease • Primary myopathy • Neuropathy
Reference range	*EMG*: No electrical activity at rest *NCT*: Nerve conduction velocities range from 40 ms to 70 ms, varying with particular nerve studied.
Critical value(s)	None
Abnormal test	• Peripheral neuropathy • Carpal tunnel syndrome • Muscular dystrophy and other myopathies • Guillain-Barré syndrome • Myositis
Interfering factors	Drugs affecting neuromuscular conduction Poor patient cooperation
Cross-references	**Peripheral Neuropathy**

Chemali KR, Tsao B: Electrodiagnostic testing of nerves and muscles: when, why, and how to order. Cleve Clin J Med 72:37–48, 2005

Daube JR: Clinical Neurophysiology. Philadelphia, PA, FA Davis, 1996

Erythrocyte sedimentation rate (ESR)

Type of test	Blood
Background and explanation of test	The ESR is a measure of how rapidly RBCs settle out of anticoagulated blood. The sample is placed in a narrow vertical tube, and after 1 hour, the height of the clear supernatant is measured. The ESR of normal blood is low because RBCs do not normally aggregate. In the presence of infectious or inflammatory processes, blood proteins are altered such that RBCs become heavier and settle faster, so the measured supernatant value is larger. In general, the ESR is correlated with the plasma fibrinogen level.
	The ESR has been widely used in the diagnosis of inflammatory, infectious, and autoimmune diseases. It is sensitive and inexpensive and thus remains a screening test of choice. It is not specific to any particular disease process, so positive results are followed up with other tests. It should not be used to screen asymptomatic patients for disease.
	Several laboratory methods are used to measure ESR, the Westergren method being the standard. Automated methods are now common. In recent years, CRP has been increasingly used in preference to the ESR for many indications because the CRP more closely parallels the inflammatory state. At present, the cost difference between the two tests is minimal.
Relevance to psychiatry and behavioral science	The ESR has been used in the diagnostic workup for patients with unexplained mental status changes, including delirium. In geriatrics, it has been the blood test of choice when temporal arteritis is among the diagnostic considerations. The ESR is elevated in SLE and heavy metal poisoning and in response to several psychotropic drugs as noted below.
Preparation of patient	None needed
Indications	• Diagnosing temporal arteritis and polymyalgia rheumatica • Monitoring the course and treatment of temporal arteritis, polymyalgia rheumatica, and rheumatoid arthritis • Evaluating patients with suspected inflammatory, infectious, or neoplastic disease when the diagnosis cannot be made by other means • Monitoring the course of chronic inflammatory diseases • Assessing elderly patients who have vague symptoms and nonspecific exam findings *Note:* ESR may be normal in patients with cancer, infection, or connective tissue disease.
Reference range	Adult males: 0–15 mm/hour (>50 years, 0–20 mm/hour) Adult females: 0–20 mm/hour (>50 years, 0–30 mm/hour)

Erythrocyte sedimentation rate (ESR) *(continued)*

Critical value(s)	Extreme ESR elevations may be seen with malignant lymphocarcinoma of colon or breast, rheumatoid arthritis, or myeloma.
Increased levels	• Temporal arteritis • Polymyalgia rheumatica • SLE • Infection • Inflammatory disease • Acute heavy metal poisoning • Tissue destruction (e.g., MI) • Malignant neoplasm • Macroglobulinemia • Multiple myeloma • Anemia (acute or chronic disease) • Late pregnancy, eclampsia • Hypothyroidism or hyperthyroidism
Decreased levels	Certain medications, as noted below
Interfering factors	Some elderly females have ESR elevations up to 60 mm/hour in the absence of disease. In younger females, menstruation and pregnancy can cause ESR elevations. Other factors associated with increased ESR include anemia, macrocytosis, and elevated blood levels of cholesterol, fibrinogen, or globulins. Certain drugs tend to increase ESR, including carbamazepine and other anticonvulsants, clozapine, isotretinoin, oral contraceptives, misoprostol, sulfamethoxazole, and zolpidem. Other drugs tend to decrease ESR, including corticotropin, cortisone, prednisone, hydroxychloroquine, methotrexate, NSAIDs, quinine, sulfasalazine, and trimethoprim.
Cross-references	**C-Reactive Protein** **Systemic Lupus Erythematosus**

American Association for Clinical Chemistry: Testing.com. Available at: https://www.testing.com. Accessed June 2021.

Fischbach FT, Fischbach MA: A Manual of Laboratory and Diagnostic Tests, 10th Edition. Philadelphia, PA, Wolters Kluwer Health/Lippincott Williams and Wilkins, 2018

Estrogens

Type of test	Blood
Background and explanation of test	The estrogens are hormones that regulate the development of female sex organs and secondary sex characteristics. Total estrogen measurement has largely been replaced by specific hormone assays. The three most important estrogen fractions are estrone (E1), estradiol (E2), and estriol (E3). Estradiol is the most active of the estrogens and the most often tested. In females, estradiol is produced mainly in the ovaries and is responsible for ovulation, conception, and pregnancy. It also regulates cholesterol levels and promotes bone health. Estriol is the estrogen of pregnancy, produced in the placenta. Estrone is the major estrogen present after menopause, derived from adrenal gland metabolites and produced in adipose tissue.
Relevance to psychiatry and behavioral science	Reduced estradiol levels with menopause may be associated with low energy, fatigue, insomnia, and depression. When these symptoms are present in a female age 45 years or older with a history of typical symptoms of menopause, it is not necessary to measure estradiol levels. Specific indications for hormone measurement are listed below. In psychiatry, estradiol may be measured in cases of precocious puberty, female characteristics developing in a male, individuals undergoing male-to-female transition, or amenorrhea in the context of anorexia nervosa.
Preparation of patient	None needed
Indications	*Estradiol* • Abnormal or heavy menstrual bleeding • Unexplained abnormal menstrual cycles (e.g., amenorrhea) • Symptoms of menopause in female <45 years of age • Infertility workup • Early development of sex organs in a female • Female characteristics in a male (e.g., gynecomastia) • Evaluating ovarian estrogen-producing tumors in non-menstruating females • Monitoring hormone replacement therapy after menopause • Monitoring feminizing hormone therapy *Estriol:* Evaluating fetal-placental status in early pregnancy
Reference range	*Estradiol* For menstruating females, dependent on menstrual phase: • Midfollicular: 24–114 pg/mL • Midluteal: 80–273 pg/mL • Periovulatory: 62–534 pg/mL

Estrogens *(continued)*

Reference range *(continued)*	Postmenopausal females: 20–88 pg/mL
	Females taking oral contraceptives: 12–50 pg/mL
	Adult males: 20–75 pg/mL
	Feminizing hormone therapy: maintain estradiol level <200 pg/mL (and testosterone level <50 ng/dL)
	Estriol: dependent on duration of pregnancy, time of day (diurnal variation)
Critical value(s)	None
Increased levels	*Estradiol:* precocious puberty, cirrhosis, gynecomastia in males, hyperthyroidism, Klinefelter's syndrome, polycystic ovary syndrome, and tumors of the adrenal glands, ovary, or testes
	Estriol: precocious puberty, cirrhosis, multiple pregnancy, feminizing tumors
Decreased levels	*Estradiol:* amenorrhea, anorexia nervosa, extreme exercise, hypopituitarism, menopause, infertility, osteoporosis, hypogonadism, Turner syndrome
	Estriol: failing pregnancy, increased risk of various fetal abnormalities
Interfering factors	Diurnal variation, menstrual cycle variation, hypertension, anemia, and liver or kidney dysfunction
	Certain drugs tend to increase estrogen levels: steroids, ampicillin, phenothiazines, tetracyclines, hydrochlorothiazide, prochlorperazine, cascara sagrada (stimulant laxative), and estrogen-containing drugs.
	Clomiphene may decrease estrogen levels.
Cross-references	**Anorexia Nervosa**
	Cirrhosis
	Klinefelter's Syndrome
	Thyrotoxicosis

American Association for Clinical Chemistry: Testing.com. Available at: https://www.testing.com. Accessed June 2021.

Fauci AS, Braunwald E, Kasper DL, et al (eds): Harrison's Principles of Internal Medicine, 17th Edition. New York, McGraw-Hill, 2008

Fischbach FT, Fischbach MA: A Manual of Laboratory and Diagnostic Tests, 10th Edition. Philadelphia, PA, Wolters Kluwer Health/Lippincott Williams and Wilkins, 2018

Klein DA, Paradise SL, Goodwin ET: Caring for transgender and gender-diverse persons: what clinicians should know. Am Fam Physician 98(11):645–653, 2018

Wu AHB: Tietz Clinical Guide to Laboratory Tests, 4th Edition. St. Louis, MO, WB Saunders, 2006

Ethylene glycol level

Type of test	Blood
Background and explanation of test	Ethylene glycol is an odorless, sweet-tasting substance found in certain detergents, paints, de-icing products, brake fluid, and antifreeze. Ingestion of as little as 4 fl oz of ethylene glycol can be fatal for an average-sized adult. Ethylene glycol can be accidentally ingested by children, intentionally taken in overdose, or abused as a substance in place of ethanol. Symptoms of toxicity include drunkenness, CNS depression, metabolic acidosis, hypocalcemia, and kidney injury. An elevated osmolal gap may be seen.

The diagnosis of ethylene glycol poisoning can be confirmed by the ethylene glycol level, although this test is not available in all settings. |
Relevance to psychiatry and behavioral science	Alcoholic patients without access to ethanol sometimes abuse ethylene glycol. Initial symptoms of ethylene glycol poisoning resemble those of alcohol intoxication, except that the patient's breath does not smell like alcohol.
Preparation of patient	None needed
Indications	Clinical suspicion of ethylene glycol ingestion
Reference range	Assay will not detect level <5 mg/dL.
Critical value(s)	Toxicity common at levels >20 mg/dL.

In susceptible individuals, any amount in plasma may be associated with toxicity. |
| Increased levels | • Accidental ingestion (e.g., by a child)

• Intentional overdose

• Abuse in place of ethanol |
| Decreased levels | Not applicable |
| Interfering factors | Plasma level may be below assay's limit of detection even though patient shows signs of toxicity. |
| Cross-references | **Ethylene Glycol Poisoning**

Osmolality |

ARUP Laboratories: Ethylene glycol, in Lab Test Directory. Salt Lake City, UT, ARUP Laboratories, 2021. Available at: https://ltd.aruplab.com/Tests/Pub/0090110. Accessed June 2021.

Barceloux DG, Krenzelok EP, Olson K, Watson W: American Academy of Clinical Toxicology practice guidelines on the treatment of ethylene glycol poisoning. Ad Hoc Committee. J Toxicol Clin Toxicol 37:537–560, 1999

Bobbitt WH, Williams RM, Freed CR: Severe ethylene glycol intoxication with multisystem failure. West J Med 144:225–228, 1986

Brent J: Current management of ethylene glycol poisoning. Drugs 61:979–988, 2001

Event-related potential (ERP) testing

Type of test	Neurophysiology
Background and explanation of test	Whereas evoked potential testing involves stimuli introduced to test the integrity of primary sensory pathways, ERP testing introduces an anomaly into the stimulus set so that the brain's processing of that anomaly can be examined. The anomaly can be as simple as a rare or unexpected tone, and in response to the tone, a late-appearing wave known as the P300 (or P3) is generated. The stimulus set is repeated many times, and the responses are averaged so that the target waveform can be distinguished from background EEG activity, which varies from sample to sample. The P300 and other late-appearing waves reflect higher-order cognitive processes such as selective attention, language processing, and decision-making.
Relevance to psychiatry and behavioral science	ERP testing has been used clinically to assist in the evaluation of patients who are unable to undergo cognitive testing to determine whether problems reside in language only, involve more global cognitive deficits, or involve a primary psychiatric disorder such as depression or psychosis.
Preparation of patient	Hair should be washed and rinsed before testing, but hair products other than shampoo should not be used.
Indications	Suspected dementia in absence of confirmatory cognitive testing
Reference range	Depends on testing protocol
Critical value(s)	None
Abnormal test	Abnormal ERP latencies have been identified in conditions such as the following: • Alzheimer's disease • Schizophrenia • Metabolic encephalopathy (delirium) • Brain tumor • Hydrocephalus • Epilepsy
Interfering factors	None
Cross-references	**Evoked Potential Testing**

Bennys K, Portet F, Touchon J, et al: Diagnostic value of event-related evoked potentials N200 and P300 subcomponents in early diagnosis of Alzheimer's disease and mild cognitive impairment. J Clin Neurophysiol 24:405–412, 2007

Daube JR: Clinical Neurophysiology. Philadelphia, PA, FA Davis, 1996

Evoked potential (EP) testing

Type of test	Neurophysiology
Background and explanation of test	In EP testing, electroencephalographic electrodes are placed at specific sites on the scalp, and the brain's electrical response to stimuli such as clicks, checkerboard pattern flashes, or electrical stimulation is captured digitally for computerized analysis. The latency of the response yields information about the integrity of the tested sensory circuit. Three circuits are commonly tested: brainstem auditory, somatosensory, and visual. Indications are listed below.
Relevance to psychiatry and behavioral science	Evoked responses are usually ordered in consultation with a neurologist or neurosurgeon. These tests may be useful in the evaluation of children with hearing impairment or developmental language problems. Less commonly, the tests are used in the evaluation of patients with disorders manifesting as sensorimotor symptoms in the extremities, to exclude functional neurological symptom disorders.
Preparation of patient	Hair should be washed and rinsed before testing, but hair products other than shampoo should not be used.
Indications	*Brainstem auditory evoked response* • Evaluation of coma and coma-like states (brain death vs. reversible coma) • Suspected neurological hearing impairment • Evaluation of children with language impairment • Evaluation of mass lesions of cerebellopontine angle or brainstem • Multiple sclerosis • Brainstem stroke • Migraine headaches • Evaluation of acoustic neuroma *Somatosensory evoked response* • Spinal cord lesions • Spinal cord stroke • Weakness or numbness of extremities *Visual evoked response* • Diagnosis of lesions involving optic nerve and tracts • Multiple sclerosis
Reference range	Normal values for each wave in complex waveform responses included in lab report
Critical value(s)	None
Abnormal test	See *Indications* section above.
Interfering factors	None

Evoked potential (EP) testing *(continued)*

Cross-references	Event-Related Potential Testing
	Multiple Sclerosis

Daube JR: Clinical Neurophysiology. Philadelphia, PA, FA Davis, 1996

Fischbach FT, Fischbach MA: A Manual of Laboratory and Diagnostic Tests, 10th Edition. Philadelphia, PA, Wolters Kluwer Health/Lippincott Williams and Wilkins, 2018

Fecal blood testing

Type of test	Stool
Background and explanation of test	Blood from the upper GI tract may appear as black tarry stool, whereas blood from the lower GI tract may appear as frank blood in stool. In the early stages of GI diseases such as cancer, no visible signs of bleeding may be seen, but occult blood may be present. This can be detected using a fecal occult blood test (FOBT). A positive test may suggest the presence of gastric ulcer or early localized colon cancer.
	There has been considerable controversy about the validity of the FOBT, even for office-based sampling. Multiple samples collected at home according to package instructions are in fact superior to a single sample collected in the physician's office.
	The fecal immunochemical test (FIT) is a newer test that uses an antibody to detect human hemoglobin in stool. Only two samples are needed for this test, and fecal material is collected with a brush, so the test has higher patient acceptance in addition to having improved reliability. FIT testing is often combined with stool DNA testing (Cologuard) to improve sensitivity.
Relevance to psychiatry and behavioral science	Upper GI bleeding can occur during treatment with SSRIs or SNRIs. The risk is increased when medications such as NSAIDs are used concomitantly.
Preparation of patient	Package instructions are provided for sample collection. For the FOBT, patients should be instructed to avoid aspirin and dental procedures before testing. Foods that should be avoided for 2–3 days before testing are listed in the *Interfering Factors* section below. For FIT and FIT-DNA, no dietary or other restrictions are needed.
Indications	• Routine health screening (yearly, starting at age 50 years) • Change in stool pattern or appearance • Workup for anemia
Reference range	Negative for blood
Positive test	• Ulcer • Cancer • Trauma from swallowed objects • Diverticular disease • Colon polyps • Inflammatory bowel disease • Hemorrhoids

Fecal blood testing *(continued)*

Interfering factors	False-positive FOBT results are seen when certain foods or drugs have been ingested, including beets, broccoli, radishes, grapefruit, carrots, turnips, horseradish, red meat, fish, poultry, iron, colchicine, iodine, or boric acid.
	False-negative FOBT results are seen when vitamin C has been ingested.
	For all tests, intermittent bleeding may not be detected.
Cross-references	**Anemia**

Collins JF, Lieberman DA, Durbin TE, et al: Accuracy of screening for fecal occult blood on a single stool sample obtained by digital rectal examination: a comparison with recommended sampling practice. Ann Intern Med 142:81–85, 2005

Fischbach FT, Fischbach MA: A Manual of Laboratory and Diagnostic Tests, 10th Edition. Philadelphia, PA, Wolters Kluwer Health/Lippincott Williams and Wilkins, 2018

Imperiale TF, Ransohoff DF, Itzkowitz SH, et al: Fecal DNA versus fecal occult blood for colorectal-cancer screening in an average-risk population. N Engl J Med 351:2704–2714, 2004

Ferritin

Type of test	Blood
Background and explanation of test	In healthy individuals, most iron is stored as ferritin, an intracellular protein found mainly in the liver but also in the bone marrow, spleen, and skeletal muscle. When iron is depleted from the body, iron stores are used first, then the ferritin level falls, and then iron deficiency develops. Several weeks may elapse before anemia can be detected. The ferritin level serves as an early indicator of iron deficiency.
	In iron overload, serum ferritin is less useful. Serum iron, total iron-binding capacity, and percent transferrin saturation are more sensitive tests.
Relevance to psychiatry and behavioral science	Patients with either iron deficiency anemia or hemochromatosis may present with fatigue, lethargy, and weakness that could be mistaken for depression.
Preparation of patient	None needed
Indications	Diagnosing iron deficiency
Reference range	Adult males: 20–250 ng/mL
	Adult females: 10–120 ng/mL
Critical value(s)	Iron deficiency: <10 ng/mL (<10 µg/L)
Increased levels	• Hemochromatosis • Alcoholic liver disease (acute or chronic) • Inflammation • Certain cancers • History of multiple transfusions • Other anemias (hemolytic, megaloblastic, thalassemia) • Iron administration (oral or parenteral) • End-stage renal disease
Decreased levels	Iron deficiency anemia
Interfering factors	Spurious results seen with hemolyzed blood or with recent intake of oral contraceptives or antithyroid drugs.
	Ferritin levels generally increase with age and are higher in those who consume red meat compared with vegetarians.
	Injury to ferritin-containing organs such as the liver may cause ferritin elevation.
	Ferritin cannot be used to evaluate iron status in patients with alcoholic liver disease, autoimmune disease, cancer, or chronic infection.
Cross-references	**Anemia** **Hemochromatosis** **Iron Level**

Ferritin *(continued)*

Cross-references *(continued)*	Total Iron-Binding Capacity
	Transferrin; Transferrin Saturation

American Association for Clinical Chemistry: Testing.com. Available at: https://www.testing.com. Accessed June 2021.

ARUP Laboratories: Ferritin, in Lab Test Directory. Salt Lake City, UT, ARUP Laboratories, 2021. Available at: https://ltd.aruplab.com/Tests/Pub/0070065. Accessed June 2021.

Fauci AS, Braunwald E, Kasper DL, et al (eds): Harrison's Principles of Internal Medicine, 17th Edition. New York, McGraw-Hill, 2008

Flurazepam level

Type of test	Blood
Background and explanation of test	Benzodiazepines are Schedule IV sedative-hypnotic drugs used to treat anxiety and insomnia. Flurazepam is a fast acting drug with a negligible half-life for the parent compound and a long half-life for the metabolite *N*-desalkylflurazepam. In general, metabolite level could be checked when overdose, noncompliance, or nonprescription use is suspected. Commonly used urine drug screens are not designed to detect flurazepam or its metabolites, and blood tests are not often ordered because this drug is rarely used today.
Relevance to psychiatry and behavioral science	Toxicity with chronic benzodiazepine ingestion may manifest as confusion, disorientation, memory impairment, ataxia, decreased reflexes, and dysarthria. With acute overdose, patients may exhibit somnolence, confusion, ataxia, decreased reflexes, vertigo, dysarthria, respiratory depression, and coma. More serious consequences usually involve co-ingestion of alcohol or other sedatives. Administration of flumazenil does not affect flurazepam level. Activated charcoal is no longer recommended as a treatment because of the high risk of aspiration. Supportive care, including intubation as indicated, is the mainstay of treatment.
Preparation of patient	None needed
Indications	• Screening for drug use • Suspicion of overdose • Signs of toxicity in treated patient • Suspected noncompliance with prescribed therapy
Reference range	*N*-desalkylflurazepam: 0.01–0.24 µg/mL
Critical value(s)	*N*-desalkylflurazepam: • Toxic >0.30 µg/mL • Lethal >0.50 µg/mL
Increased levels	• Overdose • Overuse • Poor metabolism
Decreased levels	Noncompliance
Interfering factors	None
Cross-references	**Benzodiazepines** **Urine Drug Screen**

Chernecky CC, Berger BJ: Laboratory Tests and Diagnostic Procedures, 5th Edition. St. Louis, MO, WB Saunders, 2008

Galanter M, Kleber HD (eds): The American Psychiatric Publishing Textbook of Substance Abuse Treatment, 4th Edition. Washington, DC, American Psychiatric Publishing, 2008

Wu AHB: Tietz Clinical Guide to Laboratory Tests, 4th Edition. St. Louis, MO, WB Saunders, 2006

Folate level

Type of test	Blood
Background and explanation of test	Folate is a water-soluble vitamin with several important cellular and metabolic functions. Regular intake of folate is required and is particularly crucial during the first trimester of pregnancy to avoid neural tube defects in the developing fetus.
	Four stages of folate deficiency are recognized. In Stage 1, the plasma or serum folate level drops. If folate is not replaced, then the RBC folate level falls. In Stage 2, RBC folate level falls. In Stage 3, hypersegmented granulocytes are seen. In Stage 4, a frank anemia develops, with hemoglobin <10 g/dL and macrocytic RBCs seen.
	In the general North American population, folate deficiency is now less common because cereals, breads, and grain products are folate-enriched, but the deficiency can still be seen in those with low intake of these foods as well as inadequate intake of fresh green vegetables and beans. Folate deficiency is still common in developing countries. This deficiency is also seen in specific patient populations. Malabsorption of folate (along with vitamin B_{12}) can affect individuals with disease or surgical conditions involving the small intestine, such as celiac disease or gastric bypass surgery. Accelerated loss of folate can occur in patients with liver disease, alcoholism, or kidney disease. Medications that can decrease folate levels include phenytoin, metformin, carbamazepine, oral contraceptives, trimethoprim, triamterene, and methotrexate.
	Folate can be measured in serum/plasma or in RBCs. Serum/Plasma measurements are cheaper and more widely available. It was once thought that RBC folate was superior because it was more closely correlated with tissue stores, but more recent studies suggest that the two measures are clinically comparable. When folate is checked, vitamin B_{12} should also be checked because the two deficiencies can occur together. When folate and vitamin B_{12} are both low, B_{12} should be replaced first to avoid the serious neurological complication of subacute combined degeneration of the spinal cord.
Relevance to psychiatry and behavioral science	Low folate levels are often found in community-dwelling individuals with an unhealthy diet and are correlated with depression and a poor response to antidepressant medication. Some patients with depression respond to folate augmentation of antidepressant medication even when their folate levels are in the normal or low-normal range. Folate levels are also correlated with dementia in certain patient populations, so folate is one of the laboratory tests routinely ordered in the evaluation of cognitive impairment. Newly admitted psychiatric patients with a variety of diagnoses are more likely than the general population to have low folate levels.

Folate level *(continued)*

Preparation of patient	Patients should fast for 6–8 hours before test.
Indications	• Physical symptoms of folate deficiency • Mental or behavioral changes, especially in elderly patients • Suspected malnutrition or malabsorption in patients with conditions such as alcoholism, celiac disease, Crohn's disease, or cystic fibrosis • Evaluation of megaloblastic anemia
Reference range	Serum folate: ≥5.9 ng/mL RBC folate: ≥366 ng/mL
Critical value(s)	Serum folate ≤3.9 ng/mL indicates deficiency.
Increased levels	• Supplementation • Acute renal failure • Active liver disease
Decreased levels	• Malabsorption: liver disease, alcoholism, gastric bypass, celiac disease • Use of certain medications noted in *Background* section above • Inadequate dietary intake • Increased metabolism • Increased requirements (e.g., pregnancy) • Renal dialysis • Malignancy (e.g., lymphoproliferative disease) • Increased hematopoiesis (e.g., thalassemia major)
Interfering factors	RBC hemolysis Radioactive scan within 48 hours of testing Specimen handling (must be protected from light) Ethnicity (values higher in Whites than in other ethnic groups)
Cross-references	**Alcohol Use Disorder** **Anemia** **Depressive Disorder Due to Another Medical Condition** **Folate Deficiency** **Vitamin B$_{12}$ Deficiency** **Vitamin B$_{12}$ Level**

ARUP Laboratories: Folate, RBC, in Lab Test Directory. Salt Lake City, UT, ARUP Laboratories, 2021. Available at: https://ltd.aruplab.com/Tests/Pub/0070385. Accessed June 2021.
ARUP Laboratories: Folate, serum, in Lab Test Directory. Salt Lake City, UT, ARUP Laboratories, 2021. Available at: https://ltd.aruplab.com/Tests/Pub/0070070. Accessed June 2021.

Folate level *(continued)*

Bender A, Hagan KE, Kingston N: The association of folate and depression: a meta-analysis. J Psychiatr Res 95:9–18, 2017

Khosravi M, Sotoudeh G, Amini M, et al: The relationship between dietary patterns and depression mediated by serum levels of folate and vitamin B_{12}. BMC Psychiatr 20(1):63, 2020

Kim JM, Stewart R, Kim SW, et al: Predictive value of folate, vitamin B_{12} and homocysteine levels in late-life depression. Br J Psychiatry 192:268–274, 2008

Lerner V, Kanevsky M, Dwolatzky T, et al: Vitamin B_{12} and folate serum levels in newly admitted psychiatric patients. Clin Nutr 25:60–67, 2006

Morris DW, Trivedi MH, Rush AJ: Folate and unipolar depression. J Altern Complement Med 14:277–285, 2008

Follicle-stimulating hormone (FSH)

Type of test	Blood
Background and explanation of test	FSH is an anterior pituitary hormone that acts on the ovaries to stimulate follicle maturation and on the testes to stimulate sperm development. FSH is regulated by gonadotropin-releasing hormone (GnRH) from the hypothalamus as well as estrogen and progesterone in females and testosterone in males.
	The menstrual cycle is divided into two phases—follicular and luteal—by a midcycle surge of FSH and LH, which is followed by ovulation. In the follicular phase, FSH stimulates estradiol production by the egg follicle, and these two hormones promote follicle maturation. In the luteal phase, FSH stimulates progesterone production. FSH also facilitates the ovaries' response to LH. At menopause, when the ovaries cease to function, FSH levels rise.
	FSH is used in combination with LH to diagnose primary ovarian failure, in which both hormone levels are elevated. Hormone levels are not needed to confirm ovarian failure in females 45 years or older who have typical symptoms of menopause; in these cases, a clinical diagnosis is the standard. The FSH assay can be useful in females <45 years with possible early menopause and females <40 years with suspected premature ovarian failure. In these cases, two separate FSH values >40 IU/L obtained 4–8 weeks apart would be consistent with ovarian failure.
	Fertility declines with FSH values >25 IU/L, but the assay provides no guarantee of infertility. Advice about discontinuation of contraception should be based on the duration of amenorrhea.
	In males, FSH promotes production of androgen-binding proteins in addition to promoting sperm development. Once puberty is reached, FSH levels in males are stable.
Relevance to psychiatry and behavioral science	FSH levels are influenced by various conditions encountered in psychiatric practice, including alcohol use disorder, anorexia nervosa, Klinefelter's syndrome, precocious or delayed puberty, and pituitary or hypothalamic disease. In addition, medications such as phenothiazines and megestrol act to lower FSH levels.
Preparation of patient	None needed
Indications	• Component of infertility workup in both males and females • Determining cause of a low sperm count in males • Workup of menstrual irregularities • Confirming onset of menopause (not recommended for routine use; duration of amenorrhea is more reliable) • Confirming onset of menopause in females taking oral contraceptives and those who have undergone hysterectomy (if oligomenorrhea or amenorrhea do not apply)

Follicle-stimulating hormone (FSH) *(continued)*

Indications *(continued)*	• Aiding in the diagnosis of pituitary disorders and diseases of the ovaries or testes
	• Used with other tests to determine cause of hypothyroidism in females and endocrine dysfunction in males
	• In children, used with LH to diagnose precocious or delayed puberty
Reference range	See ranges published by individual laboratories. Values differ by stage of puberty, sex, and phase of menstrual cycle. FSH values increased in pregnancy, with degree of increase dependent on trimester. Reference range units differ according to laboratory methods.
Critical value(s)	None
Increased levels	• Primary gonadal failure (ovarian or testicular)
	• Ovarian or testicular agenesis
	• Klinefelter's syndrome
	• Reifenstein syndrome
	• Menopause
	• Castration
	• Alcohol use disorder
	• Gonadotropin-secreting pituitary tumor
	• Orchitis or other testicular injury (from radiation, chemotherapy, tumor, autoimmune disease, trauma, or viral infection such as mumps)
Decreased levels	• Secondary ovarian failure due to pituitary or hypothalamic lesion
	• Pregnancy
	• Anorexia nervosa
	• Polycystic ovary syndrome
	• Hemochromatosis
	• Sickle cell anemia
	• Severe illness
	• Hyperprolactinemia
	• Delayed puberty
Interfering factors	FSH levels can be increased with use of low-dose estrogens, cimetidine, clomiphene, digitalis, and levodopa.
	FSH levels can be decreased with use of high-dose estrogens, oral contraceptives, megestrol, phenothiazines, and GnRH analogues.
Cross-references	**Alcohol Use Disorder**
	Anorexia Nervosa
	Klinefelter's Syndrome

Follicle-stimulating hormone (FSH) *(continued)*

American Association for Clinical Chemistry: Testing.com. Available at: https://www.testing.com. Accessed July 2021.

ARUP Laboratories: Luteinizing hormone and follicle stimulating hormone, Lab Test Directory. Salt Lake City, UT, ARUP Laboratories, 2021. Available at: https://ltd.aruplab.com/Tests/Pub/0070193. Accessed July 2021.

Fauci AS, Braunwald E, Kasper DL, et al (eds): Harrison's Principles of Internal Medicine, 17th Edition. New York, McGraw-Hill, 2008

Fischbach FT, Fischbach MA: A Manual of Laboratory and Diagnostic Tests, 10th Edition. Philadelphia, PA, Wolters Kluwer Health/Lippincott Williams and Wilkins, 2018

Fragile X DNA testing

Type of test	Genetic
Background and explanation of test	The expansion of a segment of DNA known as a CGG (cytosine-guanine-guanine) trinucleotide repeat in the non-coding region of the fragile X mental retardation 1 gene (*FMR1*) underlies the development of several fragile X–associated disorders.
	FXS develops in those with >200 CGG repeats (a full mutation). This is a neurodevelopmental disorder involving intellectual disability and autism spectrum disorder (ASD) in more than half of affected individuals.
	A premutation involving 55–200 CGG repeats is associated with fragile X tremor/ataxia syndrome (FXTAS), fragile X primary ovarian insufficiency (FXPOI), and fragile X–associated neuropsychiatric disorders (FXAND).
	This test uses PCR methods for the analysis.
Relevance to psychiatry and behavioral science	FXS involves a constellation of symptoms related to silencing of *FMR1*: intellectual disability, ASD, generalized anxiety, social avoidance, and hyperactive behaviors. Other associated childhood conditions include seizures, recurrent otitis media, strabismus, and obesity. In adults with FXS, there is increased risk of hypertension, obesity, GI disorders, parkinsonism, mood disorders, and anxiety. Structural MRI shows enlargement of the caudate nucleus and lateral ventricles and reduction of the cerebellar vermis volume.
	A subset of premutation carriers will go on to develop FXTAS, a neurodegenerative disease with an incidence that increases with age. Symptoms include kinetic tremor, cerebellar ataxia, neuropathy, impaired executive function, memory problems, and personality changes. MRI findings that occur long before clinical symptoms include loss of cerebellar and brainstem volume and white matter changes.
	FXAND that occur in premutation carriers are not as well characterized but include anxiety disorders (generalized anxiety disorder, specific phobia, social phobia) and OCD. These conditions affect both adults and children.
Preparation of patient	Genetic counseling, both before and after testing
Indications	• Individuals with intellectual disability, developmental delay, speech and language delay, ASD, or learning disabilities of unknown cause
	• Females with infertility, elevated FSH levels, premature ovarian failure, primary ovarian insufficiency, or irregular menstrual periods
	• Adults older than 50 years with features of FXTAS
	• Females who are pregnant or considering pregnancy who request fragile X carrier testing

Fragile X DNA testing *(continued)*

Positive test	• >200–1,000 repeats—full mutation
	• 55–200 repeats—premutation (risk of FXTAS, FXPOI, and FXAND)
Negative test	A normal result is 5–40 CGG repeats.
Interfering factors	None known
Cross-references	**Fragile X Syndrome**

Grigsby J, Brega AG, Bennett RE, et al: Clinically significant psychiatric symptoms among male carriers of the fragile X premutation, with and without FXTAS, and the mediating influence of executive functioning. Clin Neuropsychol 30(6):944–959, 2016

Hagerman RJ, Hagerman P: Fragile X-associated tremor/ataxia syndrome: features, mechanisms and management. Nat Rev Neurol 12(7):403–412, 2016

Hall DA, Berry-Kravis E: Fragile X syndrome and fragile X-associated tremor ataxia syndrome. Handb Clin Neurol 147:377–391, 2018

Salcedo-Arellano MJ, Dufour B, McLennan Y, et al: Fragile X syndrome and associated disorders: clinical aspects and pathology. Neurobiol Dis 136:104740, 2020

Santos E, Emeka-Nwonovo C, Wang JY, et al: Developmental aspects of FXAND in a man with the FMR1 premutation. Mol Genet Genomic Med 8(2):e1050, 2020

Functional magnetic resonance imaging (fMRI)

Type of test	Imaging
Background and explanation of test	fMRI of the brain is an enhancement of MRI in which images are taken in rapid succession while the patient performs a task. Change in signal intensity and blood flow from image to image facilitates understanding of brain function in the context of neurological or psychiatric disease. The test does not involve any radiation exposure. It is at present used only for presurgical planning and in research.
Relevance to psychiatry and behavioral science	In patients with schizophrenia, studies of prefrontal cortex activation have yielded conflicting findings, some with hypoactivation and others with hyperactivation. The discrepancies may be explained by the differing baseline cognitive efficiency of subjects and the memory load of the tasks presented, among other factors. In patients with mood disorders, state-dependent (manic vs. depressed) alterations are seen in frontolimbic activity. In addition, prefrontal cortex hypoactivity may underlie observed cognitive deficits. Patients with anxiety disorders (PTSD, social anxiety disorder, and specific phobias) show hyperactivation of the amygdala and insula on fMRI study.
Preparation of patient	Patients must be carefully screened to ensure that no loose metal objects enter the room where the scanner resides.
	This test takes about 1 hour, depending on the experimental protocol. During that time, the patient lies supine in the scanner wearing headphones and viewing a screen reflected in a mirror above their head. Patients must lie still during testing.
Indications	• Presurgical planning
	• Research protocols
Interfering factors	Metal produces artifacts and may endanger the patient and the magnet.
	Image may be distorted by patient movement.
Cross-references	**Magnetic Resonance Imaging**
	Magnetic Resonance Spectroscopy

Agarwal N, Port JD, Bazzocchi M, et al: Update on the use of MR for assessment and diagnosis of psychiatric diseases. Radiology 255:23–41, 2010

O'Connor EE, Zeffiro TA: Why is clinical fMRI in a resting state? Front Neurol 10:420, 2019

Gamma-glutamyltransferase (GGT)

Type of test	Blood
Background and explanation of test	The primary source of serum GGT is the liver, and elevated GGT can be used as a marker of recent heavy drinking. Mounting evidence suggests that GGT elevation is also linked to fatty liver disease, atherosclerosis, diabetes, cardiovascular disease, heart failure, lung inflammation, metabolic syndrome, neuroinflammation, cognitive decline, and vascular dementia. GGT is an independent risk factor for all-cause mortality.
	GGT elevation due to excessive alcohol use usually normalizes with abstinence within 2–3 weeks. If GGT remains elevated, further diagnostic evaluation may be warranted to exclude conditions such as fatty liver, biliary obstruction, cholangitis, or cholecystitis. Other laboratory measures can inform this workup; for example, elevation of GGT in combination with elevation of ALP suggests hepatobiliary disease.
Relevance to psychiatry and behavioral science	Elevation of GGT has high sensitivity for liver disease but low specificity in the evaluation of etiology. Specificity improves through patient selection; although the GGT assay would have little use in screening for alcoholic liver disease, it would be highly useful in confirming recent drinking in a chronic drinker in treatment who is supposedly abstinent. In males, GGT is used alone for this indication. In females, it is best used in tandem with CDT. Specificity also improves when elevated GGT is found in combination with an AST-to-ALT ratio >2, which is consistent with alcoholic liver disease. As noted above, elevated GGT may have a role in the pathogenesis of several other neuropsychiatric conditions.
Preparation of patient	Patients should fast for 8 hours and should abstain from alcohol for 24 hours before testing.
Indications	• Detecting covert alcohol ingestion (recent drinking) • Detecting hepatobiliary disease • Monitoring progression of liver disease or liver metastases
Reference range	Adult males: 7–47 U/L Adult females: 5–25 U/L Elderly individuals may have slightly higher levels. Values may vary with method used; consult lab reference values.
Critical value(s)	None
Increased levels	• Recent heavy drinking • Hepatic necrosis • Pancreatitis • Hepatic tumor or metastasis

Gamma-glutamyltransferase (GGT) *(continued)*

Increased levels *(continued)*	• Diabetes, metabolic syndrome • Pancreatic cancer • Hepatotoxic drugs • Epstein-Barr virus • Cholestasis • Cytomegalovirus • Renal failure • Reye's syndrome
Decreased levels	Late pregnancy
Interfering factors	Increased levels may be seen with phenytoin, phenobarbital, and anticoagulants because of enzyme induction, and with excessive meat consumption. Decreased levels seen with oral contraceptives or clofibrate.
Cross-references	**Alanine Transaminase** **Alcohol Use Disorder** **Aspartate Transaminase** **Carbohydrate-Deficient Transferrin** **Cirrhosis** **Liver Function Tests**

Bradley R, Fitzpatrick AL, Jenny NS, et al: Associations between total serum GGT activity and metabolic risk: MESA. Biomark Med 7(5):709–721, 2013

Corti A, Belcastro E, Dominici S, et al: The dark side of gamma-glutamyltransferase (GGT): pathogenic effects of an "antioxidant" enzyme. Free Radic Biol Med 160:807–819, 2020

Fujii H, Doi H, Ko T, et al: Frequently abnormal serum gamma-glutamyl transferase activity is associated with future development of fatty liver: a retrospective cohort study. BMC Gastroenterol 20(1):217, 2020

Hong SH, Lee JS, Kim JA, et al: Gamma-glutamyl transferase variability and the risk of hospitalisation for heart failure. Heart 106(14):1080–1086, 2020

Koenig G, Seneff S: Gamma-glutamyltransferase: a predictive biomarker of cellular antioxidant inadequacy and disease risk. Dis Markers 818570, 2015

Lee YB, Han K, Park S, et al: Gamma-glutamyl transferase variability and risk of dementia: a nationwide study. Int J Geriatr Psychiatry 35(10):1105–1114, 2020

Praetorius Björk M, Johansson B: Gamma-glutamyltransferase (GGT) as a biomarker of cognitive decline at the end of life: contrasting age and time to death trajectories. Int Psychogeriatr 30(7):981–990, 2018

Glucose

Type of test	Blood
Background and explanation of test	Glucose is the body's primary source of cellular energy, obtained from carbohydrates in the diet and conversion of glycogen stored in the liver and muscles. A constant supply of glucose is required for normal brain function. A variety of hormones regulate glucose levels, the most important of which are insulin and glucagon. Glucagon is secreted when glucose levels are low, and this results in a cascade of events that drive glucose levels up. Insulin is secreted when glucose levels are high, driving glucose into cells and lowering serum glucose levels.
	It is important to interpret serum levels with respect to the time of the last meal. Hyperglycemia in the fasting state suggests a diagnosis of diabetes mellitus. This can be confirmed with a glycosylated hemoglobin test or a glucose tolerance test. Hypoglycemia is most common in patients with "brittle" diabetes who have taken too much insulin. Very low blood sugar values as shown in the *Critical Values* section below may be injurious to the brain.
Relevance to psychiatry and behavioral science	High blood glucose levels can be associated with delirium, the metabolic syndrome, acute stress response, and acute pancreatitis and found in patients treated with atypical antipsychotics, phenothiazines, TCAs, lithium, or β-blockers (other than propranolol). Low blood glucose levels can be associated with alcohol use disorder, anorexia nervosa, panic attacks or other anxiety syndromes, depression, and agitation and may be seen in patients treated with propranolol or MAOIs.
Preparation of patient	Patients should fast for 8 hours before testing, with water allowed. They should not fast for >16 hours, because feedback processes can raise glucose levels. Insulin and oral hypoglycemic medications should be held until blood is drawn.
Indications	• Routine health screening • Suspicion of diabetes based on clinical signs and symptoms • Suspicion of hypoglycemia based on clinical signs and symptoms • Acute change in mental status • Workup for patients with panic attacks or unexplained anxiety • Monitoring patients taking atypical antipsychotics
Reference range	*Fasting plasma glucose in adults* • <60 years: 74–106 mg/dL • 60–90 years: 82–115 mg/dL • >90 years: 75–121 mg/dL Whole-blood glucose levels are 90% of plasma glucose levels.

Glucose *(continued)*

Critical value(s)	*Diagnosis of diabetes mellitus* (World Health Organization/American Diabetes Association criteria) • Fasting glucose ≥126 mg/dL, or • 2-hour level after 75-g oral glucose load ≥200 mg/dL, or • HbA1C ≥6.5% or • Random glucose ≥200 mg/dL plus symptoms of hyperglycemia *Panic values* • Males: <50 mg/dL or >400 mg/dL • Females: <40 mg/dL or >400 mg/dL
Increased levels	• Diabetes mellitus • Acute stress response • Cushing's syndrome • Pheochromocytoma • Chronic renal failure • Glucagonoma • Acute pancreatitis • Diuretic therapy • Acromegaly • Pregnancy • *Drugs:* TCAs, β-blockers, corticosteroids, dextrothyroxine, diazoxide, diuretics, epinephrine, estrogens, glucagon, isoniazid, lithium, phenothiazines, phenytoin, salicylate toxicity, triamterene
Decreased levels	• Insulinoma • Hypothyroidism • Hypopituitarism • Addison's disease • Severe liver disease • Insulin overdose • Starvation, anorexia nervosa • *Drugs:* acetaminophen, alcohol, anabolic steroids, clofibrate, disopyramide, gemfibrozil, insulin, MAOIs, pentamidine, propranolol, thiazolidinediones, sulfonylureas, biguanides, meglitinides, α-glucosidase inhibitors, incretin mimetics
Interfering factors	Dextrose-containing IV fluids
Cross-references	**Diabetes Mellitus** **Hyperglycemia** **Hypoglycemia**

Glucose *(continued)*

Chernecky CC, Berger BJ: Laboratory Tests and Diagnostic Procedures, 5th Edition. St. Louis, MO, WB Saunders, 2008

Fischbach FT, Fischbach MA: A Manual of Laboratory and Diagnostic Tests, 10th Edition. Philadelphia, PA, Wolters Kluwer Health/Lippincott Williams and Wilkins, 2018

Wu AHB: Tietz Clinical Guide to Laboratory Tests, 4th Edition. St. Louis, MO, WB Saunders, 2006

Heavy metal screening

Type of test	Blood, 24-hour urine
Background and explanation of test	Potentially toxic metals are found naturally in the environment and are used in various industrial processes. Toxic human exposure may occur due to accident, intentional overdose, or the cumulative effects of chronic, low-level exposure. In the latter case, exposure is usually occupational or occurs within the context of certain hobbies. Heavy metals can contaminate air, water, soil, or food. One well-known example of exposure from food is mercury poisoning from fish caught in polluted waters.
	The term *heavy metal* refers to a range of metals, from aluminum to lead, with relatively high atomic weights. Different laboratories offer different combinations of tests as heavy metal screening panels. One commonly offered panel is a blood screen for lead, mercury, and arsenic. Other metals tested include aluminum, beryllium, bismuth, cadmium, chromium, cobalt, copper, iron, manganese, molybdenum, nickel, platinum, selenium, silicon, silver, thallium, and zinc. Those metals with psychiatric or neurological toxic sequelae—lead, manganese, and mercury—are discussed in the **Diseases and Conditions** chapter.
	It should be noted that a panel of tests is not required for screening; any one metal can be ordered separately. Heavy metal testing is usually done on blood or a 24-hour urine sample, although for some indications, other samples such as hair or nails are used. Special containers are used to collect samples to minimize extraneous metal contamination.
	Interpretation of heavy metal screening results for acute toxic exposures is complicated by the fact that these metals are in the circulation for only a short time and are not present in urine for an extended period. In addition, apparently healthy people may have low levels of heavy metals present in blood and urine that reflect environmental levels.
Relevance to psychiatry and behavioral science	Heavy metals associated with neuropsychiatric signs and symptoms include lead, manganese, and mercury. Lead poisoning is well known to produce behavioral and cognitive problems in children and is associated with delirium, dementia, motor deficits, mood and personality changes, fatigue, weakness, and constitutional signs in patients of all ages.
	Manganese poisoning is associated with parkinsonism coupled with mood changes, psychosis, behavioral changes, dementia, sleep disturbances, sexual dysfunction, headaches, and speech problems.
	Mercury poisoning can produce vague symptoms such as fatigue, apathy, emotional instability, memory problems, headache, ataxia, and paresthesias or can be associated with specific deficits, including deafness, dysarthria, dysphagia, and visual disturbances.
Preparation of patient	None needed

Heavy metal screening *(continued)*

Indications	• Confirming suspected toxic metal exposure
	• Evaluating a patient with signs and symptoms of toxic exposure
	• Monitoring metal levels in a patient with known occupational exposure
Reference range	See **Lead Poisoning**, **Manganese Poisoning**, and **Mercury Poisoning** entries in the *Diseases and Conditions* chapter.
Critical value(s)	
Increased levels	
Decreased levels	
Interfering factors	
Cross-references	**Lead Poisoning**
	Manganese Poisoning
	Mercury Poisoning

American Association for Clinical Chemistry: Testing.com. Available at: https://www.testing.com. Accessed May 2010.

Brown JS: Environmental and Chemical Toxins and Psychiatric Illness. Washington, DC, American Psychiatric Publishing, 2002

Hales RE, Yudofsky SC, Gabbard GO (eds): The American Psychiatric Publishing Textbook of Psychiatry. Washington, DC, American Psychiatric Publishing, 2008

Kim JJ, Kim YS, Kumar V: Heavy metal toxicity: an update of chelating therapeutic strategies. J Trace Elem Med Biol 54:226–231, 2019

Sadock BJ, Sadock VA, Ruiz P (eds): Kaplan and Sadock's Comprehensive Textbook of Psychiatry. Philadelphia, PA, Lippincott Williams and Wilkins, 2009

Hematocrit

Type of test	Blood
Background and explanation of test	Hematocrit is a measure of the oxygen-carrying capacity of the blood and the primary determinant of blood viscosity. When the hematocrit is too low, oxygenation of tissues is compromised; when hematocrit is too high, thrombotic risk increases. For this test, RBCs are separated from plasma by centrifugation, and the resulting RBC mass is measured. Alternatively, the hematocrit can be calculated from the measured hemoglobin and MCV. As a rule, the hematocrit value is 3 times the hemoglobin value.
Relevance to psychiatry and behavioral science	A low hematocrit is associated with symptoms of fatigue, weakness, somnolence, anhedonia, and depression. Patients with restless legs syndrome may have a low hematocrit, and symptoms of this condition may improve with interventions to raise the hematocrit. Heavy smoking and lung disease often cause secondary elevation of the hematocrit, and modification of these health risks may lower it. High hematocrit in the third trimester of pregnancy has been suggested as a biomarker for postpartum depression and anxiety symptoms.
Preparation of patient	None needed
Indications	• Component of routine blood count • Determining anemia (low hematocrit) or polycythemia (high hematocrit)
Reference range	Normal hematocrit is ~45%, with the following normal ranges: • Adult females: 36%–48% • Adult males: 42%–52%
Critical value(s)	Hematocrit <20% associated with cardiac failure and death Hematocrit >60% associated with spontaneous blood clotting Persistent elevation above the upper limit of normal for >2 months should prompt referral to a hematologist for evaluation. The risk of events such as large-vessel occlusion increases with a hematocrit >45%.
Increased levels	• Erythrocytosis • Polycythemia vera • Shock, with hemoconcentration • Heavy smoking and lung disease • High altitude
Decreased levels	• Anemia • Leukemia, lymphoma, Hodgkin's disease, myeloproliferative disorders • Adrenal insufficiency

Hematocrit *(continued)*

Decreased levels *(continued)*	• Chronic disease • Acute and chronic blood loss • Hemolytic reaction (from incompatible blood transfusion, drug reactions, or reactions to chemicals, infections, or physical agents) • Old age, female sex, pregnancy
Interfering factors	Age affects the hematocrit, with differing normal ranges from birth to adulthood. Patients older than 60 years tend to have lower hematocrits. Females generally have lower hematocrit values than males. Pregnancy is associated with decreased hematocrit values. At high altitudes, hematocrit values are increased. Values tend to be unreliable immediately after acute blood loss or transfusion.
Cross-references	**Anemia** **Complete Blood Count** **Restless Legs Syndrome**

Brun JF, Varlet-Marie E, Richou M, et al: Seeking the optimal hematocrit: may hemorheological modelling provide a solution? Clin Hemorheol Microcirc 69(4):493–501, 2018

Chernecky CC, Berger BJ: Laboratory Tests and Diagnostic Procedures, 5th Edition. St. Louis, MO, WB Saunders, 2008

Fischbach FT, Fischbach MA: A Manual of Laboratory and Diagnostic Tests, 10th Edition. Philadelphia, PA, Wolters Kluwer Health/Lippincott Williams and Wilkins, 2018

Roomruangwong C, Kanchanatawan B, Sirivichayakul S, Maes M: Antenatal depression and hematocrit levels as predictors of postpartum depression and anxiety symptoms. Psychiatry Res 238:211–217, 2016

Hemoglobin

Type of test	Blood
Background and explanation of test	Hemoglobin binds and carries oxygen and carbon dioxide in RBCs. The oxygen-carrying capacity of the blood is thus directly related to the hemoglobin concentration. Hemoglobin also serves as a buffer for extracellular fluid to maintain physiological pH. The hemoglobin value is generally one-third that of the hematocrit. Several heritable hemoglobin variants exist, affecting almost 7% of the world population. Hemoglobin S, C, and E are the most common. Hemoglobin S is associated with sickle cell disease. Hemoglobin C and E are known to cause anemia.
Relevance to psychiatry and behavioral science	See **Hematocrit**.
Preparation of patient	None needed
Indications	• Component of routine CBC • Screening for anemia • Determining severity of anemia • Monitoring response to treatment for anemia • Evaluating polycythemia
Reference range	Adult females: 12.1–15.1 g/dL Adult males: 13.8–17.2 g/dL
Critical value(s)	<5.0 g/dL associated with heart failure and death >20.0 g/dL associated with capillary clogging
Increased levels	• Polycythemia vera • Congestive heart failure • Chronic obstructive pulmonary disease
Decreased levels	• Iron deficiency anemia • Thalassemia • Pernicious anemia • Hemoglobinopathies • Liver disease • Hypothyroidism • Hemorrhage • Hemolytic anemia (e.g., due to drug reactions, transfusion of incompatible blood, infectious disease, chemical exposure, burns, or artificial heart valves) • Systemic diseases (e.g., Hodgkin's disease, leukemia, lymphoma, lupus, sarcoidosis, carcinomatosis)
Interfering factors	Increased hemoglobin seen with extreme exercise and in those living at high altitude.

Hemoglobin *(continued)*

Interfering factors *(continued)*	Decreased hemoglobin seen in pregnancy and with excessive fluid intake.
	Hemoglobin variants may confound hemoglobin measurement.
Cross-references	**Anemia**
	Complete Blood Count

Chernecky CC, Berger BJ: Laboratory Tests and Diagnostic Procedures, 5th Edition. St. Louis, MO, WB Saunders, 2008

Fischbach FT, Fischbach MA: A Manual of Laboratory and Diagnostic Tests, 10th Edition. Philadelphia, PA, Wolters Kluwer Health/Lippincott Williams and Wilkins, 2018

Hasan MN, Fraiwan A, An R, et al: Paper-based microchip electrophoresis for point-of-care hemoglobin testing. Analyst 145(7):2525–2542, 2020

Hemoglobin A1C (HbA1C)

Type of test	Blood
Background and explanation of test	HbA1C is a form of glycosylated hemoglobin—glucose bound to hemoglobin—produced slowly over the 120-day life span of the RBC, with the amount formed proportional to the amount of glucose present in the blood. The measured HbA1C value reflects the average blood sugar level in the 2–3 months before the test, thus providing a longer-term view of blood sugar control for patients with diabetes. HbA1C is reported as a percentage of total hemoglobin. This test does not replace fasting blood sugar checks by blood draw or home glucose monitoring, which are required to determine whether dietary changes or immediate intervention is needed. To facilitate comparison of these numbers, the American Diabetes Association recommends that HbA1C values be converted to estimated average glucose (eAG) values, which correspond more closely to glucose meter results. The conversion can be made using published tables or the following formula: $28.7 \times \text{HbA1C} - 46.7 = \text{eAG}$.
Relevance to psychiatry and behavioral science	For patients with diabetes, this test can be ordered routinely with admission lab tests. It is useful in the detection of poor compliance with diabetic regimens. Patients with symptoms of the metabolic syndrome should be considered for HbA1C testing.
Preparation of patient	No fasting necessary
Indications	• Baseline HbA1C testing for adults ≥45 years. If normal, repeat every 3 years. • Baseline HbA1C testing for patients <45 years who are overweight and have risk factors for diabetes. • Routine health maintenance for patients with diabetes (type 1 or type 2): every 6 months for those meeting treatment goals, with stable glycemic control; every 3 months for those whose treatment has been changed or who are not meeting treatment goals.
Reference range	Normal: <5.7% Prediabetes: 5.7%–6.4% Diabetes: ≥6.5%
Critical value(s)	<4% is associated with increased all-cause mortality ≥8% indicates increased risk of diabetic complications >15% signifies uncontrolled diabetes 14.3%–20% corresponds to ketoacidosis
Increased levels	• Diabetes • Prediabetes
Decreased levels	Associated with increased all-cause mortality

Hemoglobin A1C (HbA1C) *(continued)*

Interfering factors	Numerous conditions are associated with falsely increased HbA1C levels, including anemia with reduced RBC turnover, uremia, asplenia, severe hypertriglyceridemia, severe hyperbilirubinemia, chronic alcohol ingestion, chronic salicylate ingestion, and chronic opioid ingestion.
	Conditions associated with falsely decreased HbA1C levels include anemia from blood loss, pregnancy, splenomegaly, vitamin E ingestion, monoclonal antibodies, and the drugs ribavirin and interferon-α.
	Falsely increased or decreased HbA1C levels can result from RBC transfusions, hemoglobin variants, and vitamin C ingestion.
Cross-references	**Diabetes Mellitus**
	Glucose
	Hyperglycemia
	Metabolic Syndrome

Carson AP, Fox CS, McGuire DK, et al: Low hemoglobin A1c and risk of all-cause mortality among US adults without diabetes. Circ Cardiovasc Qual Outcomes 3(6):661–667, 2010

Guo W, Zhou Q, Jia Y, Xu J: Increased levels of glycated hemoglobin A1c and iron deficiency anemia: a review. Med Sci Monit 25:8371–8378, 2019

Hasan MN, Fraiwan A, An R, et al: Paper-based microchip electrophoresis for point-of-care hemoglobin testing. Analyst 145(7):2525–2542, 2020

Nathan DM, Griffin A, Perez FM, et al: Accuracy of a point-of-care hemoglobin A1c assay. J Diabetes Sci Technol 13(6):1149–1153, 2019

Radin MS: Pitfalls in hemoglobin A1c measurement: when results may be misleading. J Gen Intern Med 29(2):388–394, 2014

Wright LA, Hirsch IB: Metrics beyond hemoglobin A1C in diabetes management: time in range, hypoglycemia, and other parameters. Diabetes Technol Ther 19(S2):S16–S26, 2017

Hepatitis panel

Type of test	Blood
Background and explanation of test	When a patient with no prior history of hepatitis presents with signs and symptoms suggestive of acute infectious hepatitis, a screening panel is ordered. In the United States, screening is carried out for hepatitis A, B, and C infection simultaneously, except in the case of a known exposure to a specific type. The panel includes the following tests: • Hepatitis A virus antibody, IgM • Hepatitis B virus core antibody, IgM • Hepatitis B virus surface antigen with reflex to confirmation • Hepatitis C virus antibody If the patient presents with signs and symptoms suggestive of acute hepatitis and has a known history of hepatitis B infection, the patient is tested for co-infection with delta hepatitis (hepatitis D). If the patient presents with signs and symptoms like those of hepatitis A but is seronegative, testing for hepatitis E by hepatitis E IgM antibody may be indicated.
Relevance to psychiatry and behavioral science	Hepatitis is highly prevalent among patients in psychiatric care. Hepatitis A and E are usually mild, self-limited diseases with complete recovery, whereas hepatitis B, C, and D can cause acute liver failure. Hepatitis B and C often result in chronic infection leading to cirrhosis or hepatocellular carcinoma. Hepatitis C infection is often associated with neuropsychiatric disorders, including cognitive impairment, stroke, and peripheral neuropathy. Hepatitis E infection is associated with Guillain-Barré syndrome, meningoencephalitis, and brachial plexus neuritis. Hepatitis A and E are transmitted by the fecal-oral route, involving contaminated food or water. Hepatitis B, C, and D are transmitted through body fluid exposure, most commonly from sexual contact or needle sharing.
Preparation of patient	None needed
Indications	• New-onset jaundice, dark urine, nausea, and/or anorexia • Exposure to hepatitis • Elevated liver enzymes • Suspicion of chronic hepatitis
Reference range	Negative testing for hepatitis A antibody, hepatitis B core antibody and surface antigen, and hepatitis C antibody
Critical value(s)	None

Hepatitis panel *(continued)*

Positive test	*Hepatitis A antibody positive*: acute hepatitis A
	Hepatitis B antibody positive and surface antigen positive: acute hepatitis B or chronic hepatitis (further testing indicated)
	Hepatitis C antibody positive: acute hepatitis C or chronic hepatitis (further testing indicated)
Negative test	Negative testing for hepatitis A antibody, hepatitis B core antibody and surface antigen, and hepatitis C antibody
Interfering factors	Individuals vaccinated for hepatitis B but never exposed will show only surface antibody positivity.
	False-negative results for hepatitis C may occur in hemodialysis patients and those who are immunocompromised.
	Hemolyzed or lipemic specimens, those containing particulate material, or heat-inactivated specimens invalidate results.
Cross-references	**Hepatitis, Viral**

Almeida PH, Matielo CEL, Curvelo LA, et al: Update on the management and treatment of viral hepatitis. World J Gastroenterol 27(23):3249–3261, 2021

American Association for Clinical Chemistry: Testing.com. Available at: https://www.testing.com. Accessed July 2021.

Bart G, Piccolo P, Zhang L, et al: Markers for hepatitis A, B and C in methadone-maintained patients: an unexpectedly high co-infection with silent hepatitis B. Addiction 103:681–686, 2008

Castaneda D, Gonzalez AJ, Alomari M, et al: From hepatitis A to E: a critical review of viral hepatitis. World J Gastroenterol 27(16):1691–1715, 2021

Fontana RJ, Engle RE, Gottfried M, et al: Role of hepatitis E virus infection in North American patients with severe acute liver injury. Clin Transl Gastroenterol 11(11):e00273, 2020

Jha AK, Kumar G, Dayal VM, et al: Neurological manifestations of hepatitis E virus infection: an overview. World J Gastroenterol 27(18):2090–2104, 2021

High-sensitivity C-reactive protein (hsCRP)

Type of test	Blood
Background and explanation of test	CRP is an acute-phase reactant secreted by the liver in response to inflammation or tissue injury when cytokines such as interleukin-6 are present in the circulation. CRP levels are very low or undetectable in the serum of healthy individuals. CRP levels rise within hours when the inflammatory response is stimulated and fall rapidly when inflammation subsides.
	Two separate CRP assays are available, both measuring the same molecule in blood, although using different assays:
	• CRP measures the molecule in the range 10–1,000 mg/L
	• hsCRP measures the molecule in the range 0.5–10 mg/L
	Because persistent, low-level inflammation is known to promote atherosclerosis, hsCRP testing is used to assess the risk of heart attack or stroke. Moreover, drugs used to prevent these outcomes also affect the hsCRP level. In fact, aspirin reduces the risk only in patients with elevated hsCRP levels. Statin drugs lower not only lipid levels but also hsCRP. Weight loss lowers hsCRP (and CRP) levels; for each kilogram of weight lost, CRP is reduced by 0.13 mg/L.
Relevance to psychiatry and behavioral science	hsCRP may be of use to behavioral health specialists working in cardiac or neurological rehabilitation settings, particularly in relation to risk reduction efforts such as weight management programs.
Preparation of patient	Patients should fast (no food or fluids) for 4 hours before test.
Indications	• Assessing cardiovascular risk
	• Assessing stroke risk
	• Assessing degree of vascular inflammation
Reference range	In general, hsCRP ≥1 mg/L constitutes a positive test; exact reference values depend on testing methods.
	In the absence of inflammation, hsCRP is <0.2 mg/L.
	hsCRP cardiovascular risk stratification:
	• Low risk: <1.0 mg/L
	• Average risk: 1.0–3.0 mg/L
	• High risk: 3.1–9.9 mg/L
	• Very high risk: >9.9 mg/L
Critical value(s)	Values >10 mg/L on repeated measurement indicate a non-cardiovascular cause of inflammation.
Increased levels	• Elevated risk of stroke
	• Elevated risk of MI
	• Postoperative state
Decreased levels	Not applicable

High-sensitivity C-reactive protein (hsCRP) *(continued)*

Interfering factors	Obesity and late-stage pregnancy affect results.
	Chronic inflammatory conditions such as arthritis may interfere with risk assessment.
	Use of NSAIDs dampens CRP response.
Cross-references	**Cardiovascular Risk Assessment** (Appendix C)
	C-Reactive Protein
	Metabolic Syndrome

Abi-Saleh B, Iskandar SB, Elgharib N, et al: C-reactive protein: the harbinger of cardiovascular diseases. South Med J 101:525–533, 2008

American Association for Clinical Chemistry: Testing.com. Available at: https://www.testing.com. Accessed July 2021.

Ben-Yehuda O: High-sensitivity C-reactive protein in every chart? The use of biomarkers in individual patients. J Am Coll Cardiol 49:2139–2141, 2007

Lin MS, Shih SR, Li HY, et al: Serum C-reactive protein levels correlates better to metabolic syndrome defined by International Diabetes Federation than by NCEP ATP III in men. Diabetes Res Clin Pract 77:286–292, 2007

Patel AA, Budoff MJ: Screening for heart disease: C-reactive protein versus coronary artery calcium. Expert Rev Cardiovasc Ther 8:125–131, 2010

Selvin E, Paynter NP, Erlinger TP: The effect of weight loss on C-reactive protein: a systematic review. Arch Intern Med 167:31–39, 2007

HIV testing

Type of test	Blood or oral fluid
Background and explanation of test	HIV infection continues to be a global public health problem with no cure but now with effective prevention, diagnosis, and treatment that enables affected people to lead long and healthy lives. In the United States, ~1.2 million people live with HIV, and ~13% of them are not aware of this fact and need testing. New cases disproportionately affect racial and ethnic minorities and gay, bisexual, and other men who have sex with men. Three types of tests are used to diagnose HIV: • Antibody tests—use blood or oral fluid. Most rapid tests and home-use tests are of this type. • Antigen/antibody tests—detect parts of the virus itself as well as the body's response to it. • Nucleic acid tests—detect HIV virus in blood. Initial testing is with either an antibody test or an antigen/antibody test. Nucleic acid tests are costly and are not used for screening except for high-risk exposure or possible exposure with early HIV symptoms. If the initial test is positive, a follow-up test is conducted. A second positive test confirms HIV.
Relevance to psychiatry and behavioral science	Psychiatrists should be aware of the rate of HIV infection in their catchment areas and that homeless and drug-abusing populations have greatly increased risk. Where patients with chronic mental illness use their mental health professional as a primary care provider, knowledge about testing and follow-up is essential.
Preparation of patient	Patient counseling is mandatory for HIV testing. The following information should be provided to the patient, whether for an office-based or a laboratory-based test: information about the HIV test, its benefits and consequences, ways HIV is transmitted and how it can be prevented, the meaning of the test results, and where to obtain further information and other services, including treatment. Those tested with rapid tests should be informed that results will be available during the visit and that confirmatory testing will be needed if the rapid test is positive. In this case, a return visit should be scheduled to discuss the confirmatory test results.
Indications	HIV testing should be performed: • At least once for all patients ages 13–64 years as part of routine medical care • Yearly for those at higher risk • Every 3–6 months for sexually active gay and bisexual men

HIV testing *(continued)*

Indications *(continued)*	Factors that increase risk include the following: • Having vaginal or anal sex with someone who is HIV positive or whose HIV status is unknown • Injecting drugs and sharing needles, syringes, or other drug equipment with others • Exchanging sex for money or drugs • Having a sexually transmitted disease, such as syphilis • Having hepatitis or tuberculosis • Having sex with anyone who has any of the above risk factors
Negative test	Either no HIV infection is present or the test was performed outside window of detection. No test can detect HIV immediately after infection. Antibody tests can take 23–90 days to detect infection, with oral fluid or finger-prick samples taking longer than venous blood. Antigen/antibody tests can take 18–45 days, with finger-prick samples taking longer (up to 90 days). Nucleic acid testing can detect infection 10–33 days after exposure.
Positive test	A positive test is followed up by a confirmatory test. If the second test is positive, HIV infection is presumed present.
Indeterminate test	Usually caused by cross-reacting antibodies in an uninfected patient. The patient should be retested in 4–8 weeks and then again in 6 months.
Interfering factors	As noted above, if the patient tested too soon after exposure, the test may be falsely negative. Cross-reacting antibodies may cause a false-positive result.
Cross-references	**HIV and AIDS**

Centers for Disease Control and Prevention: Types of HIV tests. Atlanta, GA, Centers for Disease Control and Prevention, 2021. Available at: https://www.cdc.gov/hiv/basics/hiv-testing/test-types.html. Accessed July 2021.

HIV.gov: U.S. Statistics. Washington, DC, U.S. Department of Health and Human Services, 2021. Available at: https://www.hiv.gov/hiv-basics/overview/data-and-trends/statistics. Accessed July 2021.

National Institutes of Health: HIV overview. HIVinfo, 2021. Available at: https://hivinfo.nih.gov/understanding-hiv/fact-sheets/hiv-testing. Accessed July 2021.

Price RW, Epstein LG, Becker JT, et al: Biomarkers of HIV-1 CNS infection and injury. Neurology 69:1781–1788, 2007

Syed Iqbal H, Balakrishnan P, Murugavel KG, et al: Performance characteristics of a new rapid immunochromatographic test for the detection of antibodies to human immunodeficiency virus (HIV) types 1 and 2. J Clin Lab Anal 22:178–185, 2008

Taylor MM, Hawkins K, Gonzalez A, et al: Use of the serologic testing algorithm for recent HIV seroconversion (STARHS) to identify recently acquired HIV infections in men with early syphilis in Los Angeles County. J Acquir Immune Defic Syndr 38:505–508, 2005

Homocysteine level

Type of test	Blood
Background and explanation of test	Homocysteine is an intermediate product of methionine metabolism that can be elevated with certain nutritional deficiencies, including vitamin B_{12}, vitamin B_6, and folate. Serum homocysteine is toxic to vascular endothelial cells, and elevations have been found to be associated with a range of diseases: cardiovascular disease, hypertension, stroke, cognitive dysfunction, dementia (Alzheimer's disease [AD] and vascular dementia), chronic kidney disease, cancer, and bone tissue damage. A recent prospective study found that an increment in the homocysteine level of 5 µmol/L increased the risk of developing AD by 40%. Serum homocysteine levels can also be used to detect vitamin B_{12} and/or folate deficiency. Supplementation with these vitamins can lower the homocysteine level.
Relevance to psychiatry and behavioral science	As noted above, elevation of the serum homocysteine level increases the risk of various diseases of interest to psychiatrists. In addition to the established use of serum homocysteine to detect folate or early vitamin B_{12} deficiency, compelling evidence suggests that serum total homocysteine should be checked as part of the evaluation for dementia or cognitive impairment and that, for this patient population, supplementation should be considered for homocysteine levels ≤10 µmol/L. These vitamins are not stored by the body; any excess is excreted in urine. Although understudied in psychiatry generally, serum homocysteine is thought to be elevated in alcohol use disorder, schizophrenia, epilepsy, and hypothyroidism.
Preparation of patient	Patients should fast for ≥8 hours before testing.
Indications	• Patients with poor nutritional status, in whom vitamin deficiency is suspected: elderly patients, patients with alcohol use disorder and/or substance abuse/dependence • Patients with peripheral neuropathy or myelopathy • Vegetarians not taking vitamin B_{12} supplements • Patients using medications known to interfere with folate metabolism (e.g., antiepileptic drugs, methotrexate)
Reference range	0–15 µmol/L A slightly lower upper limit of normal (8–10 µmol/L) may be appropriate for prevention of cognitive impairment in elderly patients.
Critical value(s)	>15 µmol/L
Increased levels	• Vitamin B_{12} deficiency • Folate deficiency • Vitamin B_6 deficiency • Inherited disorders of methionine metabolism • Chronic kidney disease

Homocysteine level *(continued)*

Decreased levels	Not applicable
Interfering factors	False elevation may be seen if serum is not promptly separated from cells when specimen is collected.
	Medications that affect homocysteine levels include azaribine, carbamazepine, methotrexate, nitrous oxide, and phenytoin.
Cross-references	**Folate Deficiency**
	Folate Level
	Methylmalonic Acid Level
	Vitamin B$_{12}$ Deficiency
	Vitamin B$_{12}$ Level

ARUP Laboratories: Homocysteine, total, in Lab Test Directory. Salt Lake City, UT, ARUP Laboratories, 2021. Available at: https://ltd.aruplab.com/Tests/Pub/0099869. Accessed July 2021.

Chen S, Honda T, Ohara T, et al: Serum homocysteine and risk of dementia in Japan. J Neurol Neurosurg Psychiatry 91(5):540–546, 2020

Fischbach FT, Fischbach MA: A Manual of Laboratory and Diagnostic Tests, 10th Edition. Philadelphia, PA, Wolters Kluwer Health/Lippincott Williams and Wilkins, 2018

Jiang B, Yao G, Yao C, Zheng N: The effect of folate and VitB12 in the treatment of MCI patients with hyperhomocysteinemia. J Clin Neurosci 81:65–69, 2020

Li S, Guo Y, Men J, et al: The preventive efficacy of vitamin B supplements on the cognitive decline of elderly adults: a systematic review and meta-analysis. BMC Geriatr 21(1):367, 2021

Mielech A, Puscion-Jakubik A, Markiewicz-Zukowska R, Socha K: Vitamins in Alzheimer's disease: review of the latest reports. Nutrients 12(11):3458, 2020

Seshadri S, Beiser A, Selhub J, et al: Plasma homocysteine as a risk factor for dementia and Alzheimer's disease. N Engl J Med 346(7):476–483, 2002

Smith AD, Refsum H, Bottiglieri T, et al: Homocysteine and dementia: an international consensus statement. J Alzheimers Dis 62(2):561–570, 2018

Sun J, Han W, Wu S, et al: Associations between hyperhomocysteinemia and the presence and severity of acute coronary syndrome in young adults≤35 years of age. BMC Cardiovasc Disord 21(1):47, 2021

Yang Q, Lu Y, Deng Y, et al: Homocysteine level is positively and independently associated with serum creatinine and urea nitrogen levels in old male patients with hypertension. Sci Rep 10(1):18050, 2020

Human chorionic gonadotropin (hCG)

Type of test	Urine (hCG), blood (β-hCG)
Background and explanation of test	hCG is a hormone produced by the developing placenta that is excreted in urine. Its level is elevated in pregnancy and in the presence of trophoblastic or germ cell tumors. An elevation at menopause also occurs in which the hCG is of pituitary origin. Of the two subunits of hCG (α and β), the β subunit is the more sensitive and specific for early pregnancy. For routine pregnancy testing, a qualitative test is performed on a urine specimen. The test becomes positive within 3 days of egg implantation, just after the first missed period. A urine home pregnancy test can be used for this purpose; these tests are accurate if used according to package instructions. For nonroutine pregnancy testing and for testing of conditions other than pregnancy, quantitative testing of β-hCG in blood is performed. This is the most sensitive and specific test to detect early pregnancy, estimate gestational age, and diagnose ectopic pregnancy or threatened abortion. This test is also used to diagnose and monitor various hormone-producing tumors.
Relevance to psychiatry and behavioral science	Pregnancy tests are performed in females of reproductive age being considered for procedures such as ECT or before initiation of potentially teratogenic medications (including psychotropics such as valproate, carbamazepine, and lithium). Pregnancy itself can precipitate psychiatric symptoms in some patients, and when this is suspected, pregnancy testing is part of the diagnostic workup.
Preparation of patient	For urine testing, instruct patient to collect their first morning urine specimen, which contains the highest concentration of β-hCG. If a random specimen is used, the specific gravity must be >1.005 for the result to be valid. Specimens containing gross blood should not be used.
Indications	• Confirming or ruling out pregnancy • Diagnosing ectopic pregnancy • Diagnosing and monitoring gestational trophoblastic tumors • Ruling out pregnancy before initiating ECT • Ruling out pregnancy before initiating that is potentially teratogenic medications • Ruling out pregnancy before procedures involving ionizing radiation or contrast media potentially harmful to fetus
Reference range	*Urine* • Positive: pregnant • Negative: not pregnant

Human chorionic gonadotropin (hCG) *(continued)*

Reference range *(continued)*	*Blood, quantitative*
	• Males and nonpregnant females: <5.0 IU/L
	• Pregnant females: wide variation, dependent on gestational age
Critical value(s)	None
Increased levels	Positive urine results also occur in choriocarcinoma, hydatidiform mole, testicular and trophoblastic tumors in males, *chorioadenoma destruens*, or ectopic pregnancy.
	Increased blood values also occur in hydatidiform mole, choriocarcinoma, seminoma, ovarian and testicular teratomas, ectopic pregnancy, certain cancers (lung, stomach, pancreas), or Down syndrome.
Decreased levels	Negative urine results also occur in fetal demise, abortion, or threatened abortion.
	Decreased blood values also occur in ectopic pregnancy, trisomy 18.
Interfering factors	*Urine false-positive:* proteinuria, hematuria, excess pituitary gonadotropin, certain drugs (including phenothiazines and methadone)
	Urine false-negative: specimen obtained too early in pregnancy or urine too dilute
	Blood factors: lipemia, hemolysis, radioisotope administration within 1 week. Positive result persists for 1 week after completed abortion. Presence of heterophile antibodies may increase or decrease quantitative results.
Cross-references	**Medical Evaluation for Electroconvulsive Therapy** (Appendix C)

Fischbach FT, Fischbach MA: A Manual of Laboratory and Diagnostic Tests, 10th Edition. Philadelphia, PA, Wolters Kluwer Health/Lippincott Williams and Wilkins, 2018

Wu AHB: Tietz Clinical Guide to Laboratory Tests, 4th Edition. St. Louis, MO, WB Saunders, 2006

Human growth hormone level

Type of test	Blood
Background and explanation of test	Growth hormone (GH) released by the anterior pituitary gland is critical for normal growth in children. During the growth years, if too little GH is secreted, children grow more slowly and are small for their age. In extreme cases, dwarfism results. If too much is secreted, children may develop gigantism, with long bones growing beyond puberty, thickened facial features, weakness, headaches, and delayed puberty.
	In adults, GH subserves metabolic functions such as muscle protein synthesis and lipolysis (especially of visceral fat) and has beneficial effects on the lipid profile. GH deficiency—associated with TBI, pituitary disease, vascular compromise, or cranial irradiation—is associated with central obesity, decreased bone density and muscle mass, and elevated lipid levels in addition to the psychiatric symptoms noted below. GH excess in adults, which can result from pituitary tumors, is associated with acromegaly.
	GH is released in pulses, primarily at night, and daytime levels may be undetectable, especially in elderly or obese individuals. In determining deficiency, random GH levels are not useful, so biomarkers such as insulin-like growth factor (IGF)-1 (a downstream product of GH) are used. Definitive diagnosis is made by a blunted GH response to two or more validated provocative tests that induce GH release. Insulin-induced hypoglycemia is the gold standard for diagnosis.
	A separate issue relating to GH is that its effects on muscle strength and endurance have made this hormone popular as a performance-enhancing supplement for athletes. This is a different situation from GH replacement in patients with GH deficiency. In general, this practice of supplementing GH is not safe because of myriad adverse effects, including diabetes, osteoporosis, and increased risk of cancer. Use of GH is prohibited by the World Anti-Doping Agency, and testing for GH ingestion is now routine. Use of GH to increase energy and drive in elderly patients, whose GH levels are naturally low, is similarly ill-advised.
Relevance to psychiatry and behavioral science	Children with GH abnormalities may come to clinical attention because of concerns about stature or physical anomalies. These patients should be referred promptly for endocrinological evaluation. In adults, GH deficiency is associated with social isolation, reduced quality of life, low self-esteem, low energy, and reduced drive, symptoms that could be mistaken for depression. Adults and children with Prader-Willi syndrome have reduced GH secretion and have signs and symptoms like those of other causes of GH deficiency, such as TBI. In these cases, GH replacement may be indicated.
Preparation of patient	Patients should fast and limit physical activity for 10–12 hours before testing.

Human growth hormone level *(continued)*

Indications	• Evidence of pituitary or parasellar mass • Characteristic symptoms in patients with a history of hypothalamic-pituitary insult (surgery, radiation therapy, TBI, brain tumor, stroke) • Slow growth in children • Gigantism in children • Acromegaly in adults
Reference range	See laboratory reference ranges for various test protocols.
Critical value(s)	None
Increased levels	• Pituitary tumor/hyperpituitarism • Acromegaly • Gigantism • Anorexia nervosa • Diabetes in adolescents • Hypoglycemia, starvation • Surgery • Deep sleep states • *Drugs*: gamma-hydroxybutyrate (GHB), gamma-butyrolactone (GBL), amphetamines, β-blockers, estrogens, oral contraceptives, histamine, insulin, niacin, levodopa, arginine, glucagon, St. John's wort
Decreased levels	• Congenital hypoplasia; lesions of hypothalamus or pituitary • Congenital GH deficiency • Prader-Willi syndrome • Dwarfism • Failure to thrive • Acute lymphoblastic leukemia • Chronic atrophic gastritis • Hyperglycemia • Urban pollutants • *Drugs:* corticosteroids, phenothiazines, SSRIs
Interfering factors	Stress and exercise affect GH levels. Use of radioactive contrast material in the week before testing may affect the results. Obesity and advanced age may cause a blunted GH response to provocation.
Cross-references	**Anorexia Nervosa**

Human growth hormone level *(continued)*

American Association for Clinical Chemistry: Testing.com. Available at: https://www.testing.com. Accessed July 2021.

Deal CL, Tony M, Höybye C, et al: Growth Hormone Research Society workshop summary: consensus guidelines for recombinant human growth hormone therapy in Prader-Willi syndrome. J Clin Endocrinol Metab 98(6):E1072–E1087, 2013

Fischbach FT, Fischbach MA: A Manual of Laboratory and Diagnostic Tests, 10th Edition. Philadelphia, PA, Wolters Kluwer Health/Lippincott Williams and Wilkins, 2018

Melmed S: Pathogenesis and diagnosis of growth hormone deficiency in adults. N Engl J Med 380(26):2551–2562, 2019

Siebert DM, Rao AL: The use and abuse of human growth hormone in sports. Sports Health 10(5):419–426, 2018

Huntingtin gene mutation

Type of test	Genetic
Background and explanation of test	The huntingtin gene (*HTT*) codes for a protein with a critical role in prenatal brain development. One area of the gene contains a segment of DNA known as a CAG (cytosine-adenine-guanine) trinucleotide repeat that appears several times in a row. A normal number of CAG repeats is 10–26. When more repeats are present, the CAG segment becomes unusually long. This elongated protein is processed into smaller fragments that are neurotoxic, resulting in dysfunction and death of neurons. The more repeats, the earlier the onset of clinical Huntington's disease (HD), although age at onset is modified by environmental factors and variants elsewhere in the genome.
	As the mutation is passed to the next generation, the size of the CAG repeat segment often increases, a phenomenon known as "anticipation."
	Early presentations of HD (age <20 years) are associated with a wide range of cognitive, psychiatric, and motor symptoms, whereas late presentations (age ≥60 years) are marked by motor symptoms. This progression is mirrored by neocortical atrophy, which occurs early in anterior areas and late in occipital and parietal areas.
	More sensitive testing methods as well as treatments that partially reduce variant *HTT* are under active investigation.
Relevance to psychiatry and behavioral science	Psychiatric symptoms of HD include irritability, depression, psychosis, personality changes, apathy, and cognitive impairment. Depression and irritability can precede motor symptoms by many years, whereas apathy and cognitive impairment tend to occur after motor symptoms. Suicidal ideation, suicide attempt, and completed suicide are more common in HD patients than in the general population. Involuntary movements such as chorea—the hallmark of HD—may be subtle until later stages of the disease. Motor abnormalities also include dystonia, ataxia, parkinsonism, oculomotor problems, dysarthria, dysphagia, incoordination, clumsiness, and seizures.
Preparation of patient	All patients require genetic counseling, both before and after testing.
Indications	• Positive family history of HD confirmed by genetic testing • Presence of mood, motor, and/or cognitive symptoms suggestive of HD • Presence of FTD/amyotrophic lateral sclerosis, with concern for variant *HTT*
Positive test	• *27–35 repeats*: Patients will not develop HD, but children are at risk because CAG repeat size may increase into HD range as the gene is transmitted from parent to child. • *36–39 repeats*: Patients may or may not develop HD.

Huntingtin gene mutation *(continued)*

Positive test *(continued)*	• ≥ 40 *repeats*: HD will develop. • ≥ 60 *repeats*: Early onset HD will develop.
Negative test	A normal result is 10–26 CAG repeats.
Interfering factors	None known
Cross-references	**Huntington's Disease**

De Luca A, Morella A, Consoli F, et al: A novel triplet-primed PCR assay to detect the full range of trinucleotide CAG repeats in the huntingtin gene (HTT). Int J Mol Sci 22(4):1689, 2021

Dewan R, Chia R, Ding J, et al: Pathogenic huntingtin repeat expansions in patients with frontotemporal dementia and amyotrophic lateral sclerosis. Neuron 109(3):448–460, 2021

Fischbach FT, Fischbach MA: A Manual of Laboratory and Diagnostic Tests, 10th Edition. Philadelphia, PA, Wolters Kluwer Health/Lippincott Williams and Wilkins, 2018

Johnson EB, Ziegler G, Penny W, et al: Dynamics of cortical degeneration over a decade in Huntington's disease. Biol Psychiatry 89(8):807–816, 2021 [published correction appears in Biol Psychiatry 90(7):505, 2021].

Kachian ZR, Cohen-Zimerman S, Bega D, et al: Suicidal ideation and behavior in Huntington's disease: systematic review and recommendations. J Affect Disord 250:319–329, 2019

Leavitt BR, Kordasiewicz HB, Schobel SA: Huntingtin-lowering therapies for Huntington disease: a review of the evidence of potential benefits and risks. JAMA Neurol 77(6):764–772, 2020 [published correction appears in JAMA Neurol 2020 77(8):1040]

McAllister B, Gusella JF, Landwehrmeyer GB, et al: Timing and impact of psychiatric, cognitive, and motor abnormalities in Huntington disease. Neurology 96(19):e2395–e2406, 2021

van der Plas E, Langbehn DR, Conrad AL, et al: Abnormal brain development in child and adolescent carriers of mutant huntingtin. Neurology 93(10):e1021–e1030, 2019

Iron level

Type of test	Blood
Background and explanation of test	Iron is an essential nutrient required for the production of healthy RBCs. When iron is taken in from dietary sources, very small amounts are absorbed. Iron is transported in the body by the protein transferrin. Most of the iron in the blood is incorporated into hemoglobin, which carries oxygen from the lungs to tissue and helps to carry carbon dioxide back to the lungs. Iron is stored in the liver and reticuloendothelial tissues in the form of ferritin and hemosiderin and is released from these stores as needed by the body.
	Iron deficiency refers to the depletion of storage iron, whereas *anemia* refers to a decrease in the amount of hemoglobin in the blood. When iron stores are depleted, anemia does not develop immediately, so early iron deficiency is often asymptomatic. When the hemoglobin level drops to ≤10 g/dL, however, patients may begin to experience palpitations and fatigue. Then, with further lowering of hemoglobin, shortness of breath, dizziness, headache, and even angina may develop.
	Chronic iron deficiency can be associated with pica (craving for dirt, clay, or chalk), burning or smooth tongue, sores at the corners of the mouth, and spoon-shaped nails.
	When the serum iron level is checked in the workup of iron deficiency or iron overload, serum ferritin, transferrin, and total iron-binding capacity are also checked.
Relevance to psychiatry and behavioral science	Both iron deficiency and iron overload (hemochromatosis) are associated with psychiatric and behavioral symptoms. Furthermore, an association between low iron levels and schizophrenia has been discovered that is particularly marked in patients with akathisia. The explanation for this relationship is not known.
	There is some evidence that iron overload underlies liver injury observed in COVID-19 patients.
Preparation of patient	Some sources suggest that patients fast overnight and have their blood drawn in the morning for iron testing. Patients should not take iron supplements for 24 hours before testing. If the patient has had a transfusion, several days should elapse before testing.
Indications	• Determining cause of anemia • Monitoring treatment of iron deficiency • Workup of suspected hemochromatosis • Suspected iron poisoning
Reference range	Adult males: 50–160 µg/dL Adult females: 40–150 µg/dL

Iron level *(continued)*

Critical value(s)	>300 µg/dL
Increased levels	• Multiple blood transfusions • Accidental overdose • Iron injections • Lead poisoning • Hemochromatosis • Acute hepatitis • Aplastic anemia • Hemolytic anemia • Polycythemia • Thalassemia • Vitamin B_6 deficiency • Nephritis
Decreased levels	• Bleeding • Pregnancy • Burns • Carcinoma • Postoperative state • Postgastrectomy • Malnutrition • Malabsorption • Rheumatoid arthritis • Schizophrenia • Uremia
Interfering factors	Specimen hemolysis invalidates test result. Vitamin B_{12} taken within 48 hours of testing may increase iron level.
Cross-references	**Anemia** **Hemochromatosis** **Pica**

American Association for Clinical Chemistry: Testing.com. Available at https://www.testing.com. Accessed July 2021.

Del Nonno F, Nardacci R, Colombo D, et al: Hepatic failure in COVID-19: is iron overload the dangerous trigger? Cells 10(5):1103, 2021

Fischbach FT, Fischbach MA: A Manual of Laboratory and Diagnostic Tests, 10th Edition. Philadelphia, PA, Wolters Kluwer Health/Lippincott Williams and Wilkins, 2018

Kuloglu M, Atmaca M, Ustundag B, et al: Serum iron levels in schizophrenic patients with or without akathisia. Eur Neuropsychopharmacol 13:67–71, 2003

Tojo K, Sugawara Y, Oi Y, et al: The U-shaped association of serum iron level with disease severity in adult hospitalized patients with COVID-19. Sci Rep 11(1):13431, 2021

Lipase

Type of test	Blood
Background and explanation of test	Lipase is a pancreatic enzyme involved in the metabolism of long-chain fatty acids. With pancreatic injury, the lipase level in the circulation rises. When the level is ≥3 times the upper limit of normal (ULN), acute pancreatitis may be diagnosed in the presence of typical symptoms such as epigastric pain, nausea, and vomiting. The lipase level in this condition rises within 4–8 hours, peaks at 24 hours, and normalizes over the following 8–14 days. Because the duration of the lipase elevation is longer than that of amylase, lipase is the preferred test for pancreatitis. Past practice has been to check both amylase and lipase simultaneously, but this has been found to be unnecessary. Rechecking lipase (or amylase) in the course of illness is also unnecessary.
Relevance to psychiatry and behavioral science	Patients at risk for pancreatitis include those with alcohol use disorder (especially males), gallstones (especially females), and hyperlipidemia and those treated with medications such as valproate, corticosteroids, or isoniazid.
	A false-positive report of pancreatitis can occur with other serious conditions such as bowel obstruction or peritonitis, so it is important to consider the differential diagnosis. On the other hand, a false-negative report could delay critical treatment for pancreatitis, so the standard of care is to admit and treat patients who demonstrate typical symptoms, even if their lipase level does not meet the criterion.
	In patients admitted to the hospital with COVID-19 infection, elevated lipase levels predict a more severe course of illness, often with ICU admission and intubation.
Preparation of patient	None needed
Indications	Clinical suspicion of pancreatitis
Reference range	Normal values vary according to testing method and age of patient; consult lab report for normal range.
	≥3 times the ULN is consistent with acute pancreatitis.
Critical value(s)	>600 IU/L
Increased levels	• Pancreatitis • Chronic renal failure • Pancreatic carcinoma • Cholecystitis • Hemodialysis • Bowel obstruction or infarction • Peritonitis • Primary biliary cirrhosis
Decreased levels	Not applicable

Lipase *(continued)*

Interfering factors	EDTA anticoagulant interferes with test.
	Drugs associated with increased lipase levels include clozapine, desipramine, donepezil, mirtazapine, risperidone, valproate, many opioids, and numerous non-psychotropics, including acetaminophen, NSAIDs, and steroids.
	Drugs associated with decreased lipase levels include calcium, hydroxyurea, mesalamine, protamine, and somatostatin.
Cross-references	**Amylase**
	Pancreatitis, Acute

Aljomah AS, Hammami MM: Superfluous amylase/lipase testing at a tertiary care hospital: a retrospective study. Ann Saudi Med 39(5):354–358, 2019

Barlass U, Wiliams B, Dhana K, et al: Marked elevation of lipase in COVID-19 disease: a cohort study. Clin Transl Gastroenterol 11(7):e00215, 2020

Cappell MS: Acute pancreatitis: etiology, clinical presentation, diagnosis, and therapy. Med Clin North Am 92:889–923, 2008

Fischbach FT, Fischbach MA: A Manual of Laboratory and Diagnostic Tests, 10th Edition. Philadelphia, PA, Wolters Kluwer Health/Lippincott Williams and Wilkins, 2018

Hameed AM, Lam VW, Pless HC: Significant elevations of serum lipase not caused by pancreatitis: a systematic review. HPB (Oxford) 17(2):99–112, 2015

Matull WR, Pereira SP, O'Donohue JW: Biochemical markers of acute pancreatitis. J Clin Pathol 59:340–344, 2006

Ritter JP, Ghirimoldi FM, Manuel LSM, et al: Cost of unnecessary amylase and lipase testing at multiple academic health systems. Am J Clin Pathol 153(3):346–352, 2020

Rompianesi G, Hann A, Komolafe O, et al: Serum amylase and lipase and urinary trypsinogen and amylase for diagnosis of acute pancreatitis. Cochrane Database Syst Rev 4(4):CD012010, 2017

Lipid panel

Type of test	Blood
Background and explanation of test	A standard lipid panel includes total cholesterol, low-density lipoprotein cholesterol (LDL-C), high-density lipoprotein cholesterol (HDL-C), and triglycerides (TG). LDL-C—the primary target for lowering the risk of coronary heart disease and stroke—can be calculated or measured directly. The calculated value for LDL-C is valid only if the TG content is <400 mg/dL. With higher TG values, LDL-C is measured directly. LDL-C is highly correlated with the risk of atherosclerotic cardiovascular disease. The lower the LDL-C level, the better, at least down to ~40 mg/dL. Guidelines emphasize the importance of treating to get LDL-C levels as low as possible. U.S. guidelines suggest a target LDL-C level for very-high-risk patients of <70 mg/dL, whereas European guidelines suggest a target of <55 mg/dL. Both guidelines recommend at least a 50% reduction in LDL-C. In addition to dietary and other lifestyle interventions, LDL-C-lowering drugs such as PCSK9 inhibitors are now available to help achieve these endpoints. Hypertriglyceridemia identified from non-fasting blood samples is also associated with increased cardiovascular and stroke risk, with the risk of an adverse event doubled for those with TG ≥171 mg/dL. Fasting TG levels are less predictive. Very elevated non-fasting TG levels (≥500 mg/dL) also increase the risk of pancreatitis. HDL-C level is inversely related to coronary risk; intervention may be indicated when this value is low. Healthy adults should have their lipid profile checked every 4–6 years. After age 40, a 10-year cardiac risk assessment should be performed that can guide further testing and treatment.
Relevance to psychiatry and behavioral science	Many psychotropic medications—particularly atypical antipsychotics and antidepressants—have adverse effects on cholesterol levels. In addition, certain psychiatric patient populations are at high risk of lipid abnormalities, obesity, and the metabolic syndrome.
Preparation of patient	Fasting is no longer recommended before lipid testing
Indications	• Routine health screening for all adults ≥20 years of age, obtained every 4–6 years; more often for those at higher risk (e.g., with diabetes, known heart disease, or family history of high cholesterol) • Lipid panel 1–3 months after intervention to lower lipid levels
Reference range	Total cholesterol: <200 mg/dL LDL-C: <100 mg/dL HDL-CL ≥60 mg/dL TG: <150 mg/dL

Lipid panel *(continued)*

Critical value(s)	Total cholesterol: ≥240 mg/dL
	LDL-C: ≥160 mg/dL
	HDL-C: ≤39 mg/dL
	TG: ≥200 mg/dL
Increased levels	• Familial hyperlipidemias
	• Glycogen storage disease
	• Coronary heart disease
	• Obstructive liver disease
	• Primary biliary cirrhosis
	• Nephrotic syndrome
	• Chronic renal failure
	• Cushing's syndrome
	• Diabetes, type 2
	• Anorexia nervosa
	• Hypothyroidism
	• Obesity
	• Pregnancy
	• *Drugs:* levodopa, phenytoin
Decreased levels	• Tangier disease
	• Abetalipoproteinemia, hypobetalipoproteinemia
	• Hepatocellular necrosis
	• Hepatitis
	• Porphyria
	• Tuberculosis
	• Malignancy
	• Hyperthyroidism
	• Malabsorption
	• Malnutrition
	• Severe acute illness
	• Cirrhosis
	• Depression, suicidal behavior
	• Epilepsy
	• Pernicious anemia
	• Inflammation
	• Infection
	• *Drugs:* haloperidol, MAOIs

Lipid panel *(continued)*

Interfering factors	High TG concentrations the affect accuracy of methods used by many laboratories to calculate LDL-C.
	Drugs associated with reduced cholesterol levels include thyroid hormone and all cholesterol-lowering treatments.
	Drugs associated with increased cholesterol levels include carbamazepine, steroids, levodopa, phenothiazines, and HIV protease inhibitors.
Cross-references	**Cardiovascular Risk Assessment** (Appendix C)
	Metabolic Syndrome
	Triglycerides

Atar D, Jukema JW, Molemans B, et al: New cardiovascular prevention guidelines: how to optimally manage dyslipidaemia and cardiovascular risk in 2021 in patients needing secondary prevention? Atherosclerosis 319:51–61, 2021

Doran B, Guo Y, Xu J, et al: Prognostic value of fasting versus nonfasting low-density lipoprotein cholesterol levels on long-term mortality: insight from the National Health and Nutrition Examination Survey III (NHANES-III). Circulation 130(7):546–553, 2014

Fischbach FT, Fischbach MA: A Manual of Laboratory and Diagnostic Tests, 10th Edition. Philadelphia, PA, Wolters Kluwer Health/Lippincott Williams and Wilkins, 2018

Oh RC, Trivette ET, Westerfield KL: Management of hypertriglyceridemia: common questions and answers. Am Fam Physician 102(6):347–354, 2020

Lithium level

Type of test	Blood
Background and explanation of test	Lithium is an alkali metal salt used to treat bipolar disorder and mood instability in the context of dementia and other neuropsychiatric conditions. Mounting evidence has demonstrated that lithium has neuroprotective effects by virtue of molecular actions that include the inhibition of glycogen synthase kinase-3β (GSK-3β) and inositol monophosphatase (IMP) as well as increased secretion of brain-derived neurotrophic factor (BDNF). When used chronically for bipolar disorder, lithium appears to counteract the cortical thinning and reduced hippocampal volumes seen in the normal course of the disease. There is now interest in the potential of lithium to prevent or slow degenerative processes in mild cognitive impairment, Alzheimer's disease, Parkinson's disease, and amyotrophic lateral sclerosis.

These beneficial effects of lithium are contingent on maintaining the lithium level within a narrow therapeutic range and monitoring potential adverse effects on the kidneys, heart, and thyroid gland. Over the years, the suggested upper limit of the therapeutic range has been progressively lowered, particularly for elderly patients. Once-daily dosing is recommended, with the target level kept as low as possible to minimize effects on the kidney.

When the lithium level is checked, blood should be drawn 12 hours after the last dose (a trough level) for proper interpretation of results. When lithium is initiated or a change is made in the dosage, levels should be checked in 1 week and then every 2–3 months for the first 6 months of treatment. After 6 months, levels should be checked every 6–12 months. Other lab tests needed for screening and monitoring of lithium therapy are noted in the **Psychotropic Medications** chapter. |
| Relevance to psychiatry and behavioral science | Lithium toxicity can be acute, chronic, or acute-on-chronic. In patients on high-dosage maintenance treatment, lithium can accumulate in the CNS to toxic levels. If the patient then stops lithium because of symptoms, the measured serum level may be normal even though the CNS level remains toxic, so the level must be interpreted in relation to the time since the last dose.

With acute toxicity, GI symptoms are prominent, the correlation of lithium level with signs and symptoms is poor, and rapid recovery on holding the drug is the rule. With chronic toxicity, CNS symptoms are more evident, and renal, cardiac, and thyroid effects may be seen. Also with chronic toxicity, the correlation of lithium level with signs and symptoms is relatively good. |
| Preparation of patient | Patients should be instructed to hold lithium until after blood is drawn, and the phlebotomy appointment should be scheduled as closely as possible to the 12-hour mark described in the *Background* section above. |

Lithium level *(continued)*

Indications	• Routine monitoring of lithium therapy • Signs/symptoms of lithium toxicity
Reference range	*Adults: standard range 0.60–0.80 mEq/L* • If poorly tolerated, but with good response, range could be lowered to 0.40–0.60 mEq/L. • If well tolerated, but with inadequate response, range could be raised to 0.80–1.00 mEq/L. *Elderly patients: standard range 0.40–0.60 mEq/L* • If tolerated but response is inadequate, range could be raised to a maximum of 0.70 or 0.80 mEq/L in patients ages 65–79 years or a maximum of 0.70 mEq/L in those ≥80 years.
Critical value(s)	≥1.5 mEq/L indicates toxicity.
Increased levels	• Overdose • Sodium restriction • Coadministration of NSAIDs, ACE inhibitors, angiotensin receptor blockers, thiazide diuretics, spironolactone, diltiazem, verapamil, or fluoxetine
Decreased levels	Coadministration of sodium chloride, sodium bicarbonate, psyllium, fleawort or fleabane (herbals), acetazolamide, aminophylline, or theophylline
Interfering factors	Collection of blood into a lithium heparin tube will cause a spurious elevation in level.
Cross-references	**Bipolar and Related Disorder Due to Another Medical Condition** **Lithium**

Czarnywojtek A, Zgorzalewicz-Stachowiak M, Czarnocka B, et al: Effect of lithium carbonate on the function of the thyroid gland: mechanism of action and clinical implications. J Physiol Pharmacol 71(2), 2020

Davis J, Desmond M, Berk M: Lithium and nephrotoxicity: a literature review of approaches to clinical management and risk stratification. BMC Nephrol 19(1):305, 2018

Forlenza OV, De-Paula VJ, Diniz BS: Neuroprotective effects of lithium: implications for the treatment of Alzheimer's disease and related neurodegenerative disorders. ACS Chem Neurosci 5(6):443–450, 2014

Foulser P, Abbasi Y, Mathilakath A, Nilforooshan R: Do not treat the numbers: lithium toxicity. BMJ Case Rep 2017:bcr-2017-220079, 2017

Giakoumatos CI, Nanda P, Mathew IT, et al: Effects of lithium on cortical thickness and hippocampal subfield volumes in psychotic bipolar disorder. J Psychiatr Res 61:180–187, 2015

Gong R, Wang P, Dworkin L: What we need to know about the effect of lithium on the kidney. Am J Physiol Renal Physiol 311(6):F1168–F1171, 2016

Mehta N, Vannozzi R: Lithium-induced electrocardiographic changes: a complete review. Clin Cardiol 40(12):1363–1367, 2017

Nolen WA, Licht RW, Young AH, et al: What is the optimal serum level for lithium in the maintenance treatment of bipolar disorder? A systematic review and recommendations from the ISBD/IGSLI Task Force on Treatment With Lithium. Bipolar Disord 21(5):394–409, 2019

Lithium level *(continued)*

Schoot TS, Molmans THJ, Grootens KP, Kerckhoffs APM: Systematic review and practical guideline for the prevention and management of the renal side effects of lithium therapy. Eur Neuropsychopharmacol 31:16–32, 2020

Wen J, Sawmiller D, Wheeldon B, Tan J: A review for lithium: pharmacokinetics, drug design, and toxicity. CNS Neurol Disord Drug Targets 18(10):769–778, 2019

Liver function tests (LFTs)

Type of test	Blood
Background and explanation of test	LFTs usually include ALT, AST, ALP, direct and total serum bilirubin, albumin, and PT. The tests can be grouped conceptually as follows: • Tests of hepatocellular injury—ALT and AST • Tests of cholestasis—ALP • Tests of excretory function—bilirubin (direct and total) • Tests of biosynthetic function—albumin and PT The first two categories do not measure liver function per se, but instead indicate whether the pattern of liver injury is primarily hepatocellular or cholestatic. Disproportionate elevations of ALT and AST compared to ALP are associated with acute or chronic injury to the liver itself. A disproportionate elevation of ALP compared to ALT and AST is associated with bile duct obstruction. Isolated bilirubin elevation may reflect a disorder of bilirubin processing. The inclusion of biosynthetic tests helps to minimize false-negative results in patients with advanced hepatocellular injury (e.g., alcoholic cirrhosis), in whom AST and ALT values may be normal or low. It should be noted, however, that albumin can be low and PT prolonged for reasons other than liver disease. Tests used to follow up on screening abnormalities include GGT to determine whether ALP elevations are due to liver disease or bone disease, hepatitis serology to detect viral hepatitis, and autoimmune disease markers. If non-alcoholic fatty liver disease is suspected, imaging studies (ultrasound, CT, or MRI) are used to visualize the liver, and transient elastography using ultrasound may be used to measure liver stiffness.
Relevance to psychiatry and behavioral science	LFTs may be abnormal in several conditions encountered in psychiatry, including alcohol use disorder, hepatitis B and C viral infections, the metabolic syndrome, Wilson's disease, and during refeeding in severe anorexia nervosa. Drugs of abuse that can cause abnormal LFTs include cocaine, ecstasy, phencyclidine (PCP), toluene inhalants, and anabolic steroids. Many herbal and alternative medical remedies affect the liver, and these substances are often overlooked as potential culprits. Especially problematic from a liver function standpoint are the herbs chaparral, gentian, skullcap, germander, alchemilla, and senna. A variety of Chinese herbs are implicated as well, as is shark cartilage. Numerous prescribed medications are known to affect LFTs, including all classes of psychotropic drugs. Antipsychotic drugs have in rare cases been reported to cause fatal hepatic injury, with chlorpromazine possibly the worst offender.

Liver function tests (LFTs) *(continued)*

Relevance to psychiatry and behavioral science *(continued)*	AST and ALT often increase when a drug is initiated or with a dosage increase, but this is not necessarily an indication for drug discontinuation. If AST and ALT values are <3 times the baseline value and the ALP and bilirubin are normal, LFTs can simply be checked weekly. When values plateau, testing intervals can be lengthened. If AST and/or ALT rises >3 times the baseline or >2 times the upper limit of normal (ULN), the drug should be stopped and/or GI consultation obtained. Other indications for drug discontinuation include elevation of ALP or bilirubin, PT prolongation, and clinical signs or symptoms of hepatotoxicity.
Preparation of patient	None needed
Indications	• Routine health screening (part of CMP) • Signs/symptoms of liver dysfunction • History of alcohol overuse • Exposure to hepatitis • Exposure to hepatotoxic drug(s) or chemicals • Monitoring liver dysfunction
Reference range	See entries for individual LFTs.
Critical value(s)	See entries for individual LFTs.
Abnormal test	• Non-alcoholic fatty liver disease—now the most common cause of chronic liver disease—is associated with mild elevations of ALT and AST. Other common causes are alcohol-related liver injury and chronic viral hepatitis. • An AST-to-ALT ratio ≥3:1 suggests alcoholic liver disease. • If ALP is elevated, GGT should be checked. If GGT is elevated and ALP is ≥2 times the ULN or the symptoms or elevations persist, a liver ultrasound should be obtained to evaluate possible biliary obstruction. • Bilirubin levels are a reliable marker of severity of liver disease. • Low serum albumin indicates advanced disease in cirrhosis but is not a reliable marker of acute liver injury. • Prolonged PT is a reliable marker of acute liver injury affecting synthetic capacity and consistent with liver failure. • Abnormal LFTs are highly prevalent in patients with COVID-19 infection, but the significance of this finding is not yet clear.
Interfering factors	See entries for individual LFTs.
Cross-references	**Alanine Transaminase** **Albumin** **Alcohol Use Disorder** **Alkaline Phosphatase**

Liver function tests (LFTs) *(continued)*

Cross-references *(continued)*	Aspartate Transaminase
	Bilirubin
	Hepatitis, Viral
	Metabolic Syndrome
	Wilson's Disease

Bertolini A, van de Peppel IP, Bodewes FAJA, et al: Abnormal liver function tests in patients with COVID-19: relevance and potential pathogenesis. Hepatology 72(5):1864–1872, 2020

Fischbach FT, Fischbach MA: A Manual of Laboratory and Diagnostic Tests, 10th Edition. Philadelphia, PA, Wolters Kluwer Health/Lippincott Williams and Wilkins, 2018

Gopal DV, Rosen HR: Abnormal findings on liver function tests: interpreting results to narrow the diagnosis and establish a prognosis. Postgrad Med 107:100–114, 2000

Harris RH, Sasson G, Mehler PS: Elevation of liver function tests in severe anorexia nervosa. Int J Eat Disord 46(4):369–374, 2013

Johnston DE: Special considerations in interpreting liver function tests. Am Fam Physician 59:2223–2230, 1999

Marwick KF, Taylor M, Walker SW: Antipsychotics and abnormal liver function tests: systematic review. Clin Neuropharmacol 35(5):244–253, 2012

Piano S, Dalbeni A, Vettore E, et al: Abnormal liver function tests predict transfer to intensive care unit and death in COVID-19. Liver Int 40(10):2394–2406, 2020

Woreta TA, Alqahtani SA: Evaluation of abnormal liver tests. Med Clin North Am 98(1):1–16, 2014

Lorazepam level

Type of test	Blood
Background and explanation of test	Benzodiazepines are Schedule IV sedative-hypnotic drugs used to treat anxiety and insomnia. Lorazepam is an intermediate-acting drug with a half-life of 9–16 hours with no active metabolites. It is not extensively metabolized in the liver. Levels are rarely checked except to confirm overdose, noncompliance, or use without a prescription. In the latter case, a urine drug screen is more likely to be used than a blood level.
Relevance to psychiatry and behavioral science	Lorazepam is often a drug of choice among sedatives for a variety of psychiatric indications. Toxicity with chronic benzodiazepine ingestion may manifest as confusion, disorientation, memory impairment, ataxia, decreased reflexes, and dysarthria. Past practice using prolonged dosing of IV lorazepam to control agitation in the ICU resulted in numerous cases of propylene glycol toxicity associated with the diluent, so that practice has been discontinued. With acute overdose, patients may exhibit somnolence, confusion, ataxia, decreased reflexes, vertigo, dysarthria, respiratory depression, and coma. More serious consequences usually involve co-ingestion of alcohol or other sedatives. Activated charcoal is no longer recommended as a treatment because of the high risk of aspiration. Supportive care, including intubation as indicated, is the mainstay of treatment.
Preparation of patient	None needed
Indications	• Screening for drug use • Suspected overdose • Signs of toxicity in a treated patient • Suspected noncompliance with prescribed therapy
Reference range	50–240 ng/mL (with dosage of 1–10 mg/day)
Critical value(s)	Toxicity >300 ng/mL *Note:* Administration of flumazenil does not affect drug level.
Increased levels	• Overdose • Overuse
Decreased levels	Noncompliance
Interfering factors	None
Cross-references	**Urine Drug Screen**

ARUP Laboratories: Lorazepam, in Lab Test Directory. Salt Lake City, UT, ARUP Laboratories, 2021. Available at: https://ltd.aruplab.com/Tests/Pub/0090181. Accessed August 2021.

Chernecky CC, Berger BJ: Laboratory Tests and Diagnostic Procedures, 5th Edition. St. Louis, MO, WB Saunders, 2008

Wu AHB: Tietz Clinical Guide to Laboratory Tests, 4th Edition. St. Louis, MO, WB Saunders, 2006

Lyme antibodies

Type of test	Blood
	CSF in suspected Lyme meningitis
	Synovial fluid in suspected Lyme arthritis
Background and explanation of test	Lyme disease, caused by the spirochete *Borrelia burgdorferi*, is the most common tick-borne illness in the United States and Europe. It often begins with the characteristic skin lesion known as *erythema migrans* at the site of the tick bite. Within days to weeks, the spirochete may disseminate so that patients develop cardiac, neurological, and/or rheumatological symptoms. Treatment with an antibiotic accelerates resolution of the disease. If no treatment is given, the disease may resolve spontaneously but can then recur.
	In the United States, laboratory testing for Lyme disease has been greatly overused. Guidelines for testing are as follows:
	• The tick should be saved for species identification, but the tick itself should not be tested.
	• Asymptomatic patients with a tick-bite history do not require testing.
	• Patients presenting with an erythema migrans rash should be treated immediately; confirmatory testing is not needed.
	• Testing methods for the diagnosis of Lyme disease are of two types: antigen testing for *B. burgdorferi* and antibody testing to detect the immune response. Antigen testing is not recommended at this time, in part because of the low sensitivity of existing assays.
	• Antibody testing uses a two-tiered approach, with an initial enzyme immunoassay (EIA) followed by either a second EIA or Western blots if the first EIA test is positive or borderline. This approach works well for later stages of infection but has low sensitivity for early infection. These assays do not distinguish active from inactive infection, and seropositivity may persist for years, even after treatment and resolution of the clinical disease.
	• A culture of *B. burgdorferi* has low sensitivity, requires a lengthy incubation, and dictates special media and expertise. It is not routinely used.
	• PCR assay for *B. burgdorferi* is used for evaluation of synovial fluid samples in patients with suspected Lyme arthritis and in cases of reinfection in which persistent antibodies make the usual serological tests unreliable.
	• To test for Lyme neuroborreliosis, simultaneous sampling of serum and CSF for antibodies is recommended, because sampling only CSF could yield spurious results due to passive transfer of antibodies from blood to CSF. The two-tiered approach is used.

Lyme antibodies *(continued)*

Background and explanation of test *(continued)*	• ECG should be performed in patients evaluated for Lyme disease who have signs or symptoms of carditis: dyspnea, edema, palpitations, lightheadedness, chest pain, and/or syncope.
Relevance to psychiatry and behavioral science	Lyme disease affects the nervous system in 10%–15% of cases, with manifestations including lymphocytic meningitis, cranial neuritis, painful radiculoneuritis, and mononeuropathy multiplex. During active systemic infection, encephalopathy can be seen.
	Individuals diagnosed with Lyme disease have a greatly increased risk of psychiatric disorders, including mood disorders, suicidality, and completed suicide, that is highest in the first 1–3 years after diagnosis. Recurrence of Lyme disease symptoms further elevates this risk. It should be noted that the converse is not true; individuals diagnosed with psychiatric disorders do not necessarily have an increased risk of Lyme disease, and testing in the general psychiatric population has given rise to a great deal of controversy.
	Symptoms that have been attributed to "chronic Lyme disease" may in some cases be due to "posttreatment Lyme disease," a syndrome characterized by symptoms seen within 6 months of treatment that persist for 6 months or longer. This posttreatment syndrome is thought to arise from persistent immune activation, a hypothesis bolstered by recent [^{11}C]DPA-713 PET studies of the TSPO in affected patients vs. healthy control subjects.
Preparation of patient	None needed
Indications	Suspected Lyme disease in a symptomatic patient
Reference range	Negative EIA test Negative Western blot analysis
Critical value(s)	None
Positive test	• Recent infection with *B. burgdorferi* • Past exposure to *B. burgdorferi* • Exposure to another spirochete
Negative test	No exposure Blood drawn too early for antibodies to have formed
Interfering factors	False-positive results can be seen with other spirochetes, including the organisms that cause syphilis and leptospirosis. Other diseases can also cause false-positive results, including HIV infection, malaria, Epstein-Barr virus, and autoimmune disorders such as SLE and rheumatoid arthritis. IgG antibodies may be present from Lyme infection in the distant past. Antibiotics can change test results in some cases.
Cross-references	**Lyme Disease**

Lyme antibodies *(continued)*

Chaconas G, Castellanos M, Verhey TB: Changing of the guard: how the Lyme disease spirochete subverts the host immune response. J Biol Chem 295(2):301–313, 2020

Coughlin JM, Yang T, Rebman AW, et al: Imaging glial activation in patients with post-treatment Lyme disease symptoms: a pilot study using [11C]DPA-713 PET. J Neuroinflammation 15(1):346, 2018

Dumes AA: Lyme disease and the epistemic tensions of "medically unexplained illnesses." Med Anthropol 39(6):441–456, 2020

Hinds K, Sutcliffe K: Heterodox and orthodox discourses in the case of Lyme disease: a synthesis of arguments. Qual Health Res 29(11):1661–1673, 2019

John TM, Taege AJ: Appropriate laboratory testing in Lyme disease. Cleve Clin J Med 86(11):751–759, 2019

Lantos PM: Chronic Lyme disease. Infect Dis Clin North Am 29(2):325–340, 2015

Lantos PM, Rumbaugh J, Bockenstedt LK, et al: Clinical practice guidelines by the Infectious Diseases Society of America (IDSA), American Academy of Neurology (AAN), and American College of Rheumatology (ACR): 2020 Guidelines for the Prevention, Diagnosis, and Treatment of Lyme Disease. Arthritis Care Res (Hoboken) 73(1):1–9, 2021

Marques AR: Laboratory diagnosis of Lyme disease: advances and challenges. Infect Dis Clin North Am 29(2):295–307, 2015

Mead P, Petersen J, Hinckley A: Updated CDC recommendation for serologic diagnosis of Lyme disease. MMWR Morb Mortal Wkly Rep 68(32):703, 2019

Moore A, Nelson C, Molins C, et al: Current guidelines, common clinical pitfalls, and future directions for laboratory diagnosis of Lyme disease, United States. Emerg Infect Dis 22(7):1169–1177, 2016

Nigrovic LE, Lewander DP, Balamuth F, et al: The Lyme disease polymerase chain reaction test has low sensitivity. Vector Borne Zoonotic Dis 20(4):310–313, 2020

Schriefer ME: Lyme disease diagnosis: serology. Clin Lab Med 35(4):797–814, 2015

Schutzer SE, Body BA, Boyle J, et al: Direct diagnostic tests for Lyme disease. Clin Infect Dis 68(6):1052–1057, 2019

Shapiro ED. Clinical practice: Lyme disease. N Engl J Med 370(18):1724–1731, 2014

Waddell LA, Greig J, Mascarenhas M, et al: The accuracy of diagnostic tests for Lyme disease in humans, a systematic review and meta-analysis of North American research. PLoS One 11(12):e0168613, 2016

Magnesium

Type of test	Blood
Background and explanation of test	Magnesium is a micronutrient required for the regulation of blood pressure, muscle and nerve function, blood clotting, carbohydrate metabolism, and protein and nucleic acid synthesis. Magnesium and calcium are functionally linked, with magnesium required for calcium absorption by the intestine and involved in calcium metabolism. With magnesium deficiency, calcium is removed from the bones and can cause calcification of the aorta and kidney. In addition, a low calcium level may be difficult to correct unless low magnesium is also corrected. Under normal conditions, only about 1% of total body magnesium is present in serum. Decreased renal function can be associated with increased serum levels. Magnesium comes from the diet, with levels in the body regulated by control of excretion through the kidneys and absorption from the GI tract. Abnormal levels may be seen when either of these controls is compromised. When magnesium levels are low, potassium levels are often also low.
Relevance to psychiatry and behavioral science	Alcohol use disorder (AUD) and anorexia nervosa are both associated with low magnesium levels, which can manifest as agitation, delirium, or seizures. Lithium use, abuse of laxatives, and overuse of antacids are associated with high magnesium levels, which can manifest as a delirium of subacute onset. Patients with depression who are deficient in magnesium may show improvement in mood with magnesium supplementation.
Preparation of patient	Patients should fast for 4 hours before testing.
Indications	• Component of admission lab workup to evaluate electrolyte status • Symptoms of abnormally low magnesium level, such as muscle weakness, twitching, cramping, confusion, cardiac arrhythmia, or seizures • Workup for malnutrition, diarrhea, or suspected malabsorption • Evaluating acute illness in patients with AUD • Workup for patients with chronically low calcium and potassium levels
Reference range	*Fasting serum levels* • <60 years: 1.6–2.6 mg/dL • 60–90 years: 1.6–2.4 mg/dL • >90 years: 1.7–2.3 mg/dL
Critical value(s)	Hypomagnesemia: <1 mg/dL Hypermagnesemia: >9 mg/dL

Magnesium *(continued)*

Increased levels	• Oversupplementation or overuse of medications containing magnesium, including antacids and laxatives • Prolonged lithium or salicylate therapy • Renal failure or insufficiency (acute or chronic) • Low urine output • Dehydration • Hypothyroidism • Addison's disease or adrenalectomy • Severe diabetic ketoacidosis
Decreased levels	• Low dietary intake • Malabsorption due to GI disorders (e.g., Crohn's disease) • Excessive body fluid loss (e.g., diuretic abuse, diarrhea) • AUD with cirrhosis • Chronic kidney disease • Preeclampsia • Uncontrolled diabetes, diabetic ketoacidosis • Hemodialysis • Tissue trauma (surgery or burns)
Interfering factors	Sample hemolysis invalidates results. Upright posture increases level by 4%. Calcium gluconate and other drugs can falsely decrease levels. Levels are normally low in pregnancy after the first trimester.
Cross-references	**Alcohol Use Disorder** **Anorexia Nervosa** **Hypermagnesemia** **Hypomagnesemia**

American Association for Clinical Chemistry: Testing.com. Available at: https://www.testing.com. Accessed August 2021.

ARUP Laboratories: Critical Values List. Salt Lake City, UT, ARUP Laboratories, 2019. Available at: https://www.aruplab.com/Testing-Information/resources/PDF_Brochures/ARUP_Critical_Values.pdf. Accessed December 2021.

Fischbach FT, Fischbach MA: A Manual of Laboratory and Diagnostic Tests, 10th Edition. Philadelphia, PA, Wolters Kluwer Health/Lippincott Williams and Wilkins, 2018

Li J, Hovey KM, Andrews CA, et al: Association of dietary magnesium intake with fatal coronary heart disease and sudden cardiac death. J Womens Health (Larchmt) 29(1):7–12, 2020

Peeri NC, Egan KM, Chai W, Tao MH: Association of magnesium intake and vitamin D status with cognitive function in older adults: an analysis of US National Health and Nutrition Examination Survey (NHANES) 2011 to 2014. Eur J Nutr 60(1):465–474, 2021

Rajizadeh A, Mozaffari-Khosravi H, Yassini-Ardakani M, Dehghani A: Effect of magnesium supplementation on depression status in depressed patients with magnesium deficiency: a randomized, double-blind, placebo-controlled trial. Nutrition 35:56–60, 2017

Magnesium *(continued)*

Reddy P, Edwards LR: Magnesium supplementation in vitamin D deficiency. Am J Ther 26(1):e124–e132, 2019

Tarleton EK, Littenberg B: Magnesium intake and depression in adults. J Am Board Fam Med 28(2):249–256, 2015

Magnetic resonance imaging

Type of test	Imaging
Background and explanation of test	MRI uses a superconducting magnet and radiofrequency signals to form high-resolution images of soft tissue, including white matter tracts, arteries, and lesions in the brain and other CNS structures. The development of techniques over the past few decades has made it possible to visualize tissue architecture at a microscopic level, making MRI the tool of choice in the investigation of stroke, white matter disease, and other pathologies. Diffusion techniques have made it possible to visualize the area of tissue ischemia in stroke before that tissue has been infarcted, facilitating time-sensitive interventions such as tissue plasminogen activator (tPA).
	MRI studies usually include a series of pulse sequences such as sagittal T1, axial T1, T2, diffusion-weighted, and FLAIR images throughout the brain, without contrast. The contrast agent gadolinium can be used to enhance visualization of lesions such as stroke, tumor, or abscess. With contrast, sequences such as T1 spoiled gradient recalled echo and axial T1 spin echo are used. In general, T1-weighted images are used to identify anatomy, and T2-weighted images are used to identify white matter disease. Brain MRI is superior to head CT in the detection of ischemia and demyelination. It is also better for viewing the brainstem and posterior fossa structures. MRI is preferred to CT in identifying lesions representing seizure focus, nonmeningeal tumors, and vascular malformations. On the other hand, MRI is about twice as expensive as CT and is not universally available for clinical use 24 hours a day.
	For the MRI procedure, which takes about 45 minutes, patients are positioned supine on a flat table. During the test, a loud tapping noise is heard that may be mitigated somewhat by headphones. In a standard MRI, the patient's head and upper body are inside a narrow tube, and this can cause problems for those who are claustrophobic. An open MRI is available in which the sides of the tube do not obstruct the view, so patients feel less confined. The open MRI is also more suitable for obese patients. The problem with open MRI is low magnet strengths; magnets used in clinical settings range from 1.5 T to 3.0 T for closed systems and 0.2 T to 0.35 T for open systems. In general, the stronger the magnet, the better the image resolution. Research studies are now done with extremely strong magnets of ≥ 7.0 T, and 7.0 T magnets have now been approved for clinical use in the United States.
Relevance to psychiatry and behavioral science	Characteristic MRI findings in schizophrenia include reduced total cerebral volume and atrophy of temporal lobe(s); subcortical and limbic structures may or may not show abnormalities. Characteristic MRI findings in affective disorders include areas of high signal intensity in white matter, volume loss in the prefrontal cortex, and alterations in the subcortical and limbic structures.

Magnetic resonance imaging *(continued)*

Relevance to psychiatry and behavioral science *(continued)*	In ADHD, a 3%–4% reduction in total cerebral and cerebellar volumes, thinning of the medial prefrontal cortex, and volume reduction in the dorsal anterior cingulate cortex are characteristic. In autism spectrum disorder, gray matter abnormalities have been found in the social brain network that includes the amygdala and superior temporal sulcus.
Preparation of patient	No pretest preparation is needed. Patients should be informed that gadolinium contrast material can deposit itself in the brain, mostly in the dentate nuclei and globus pallidus, and current recommendations are to use contrast agents with caution. MRI should not be performed on patients with implanted metal devices including pacemakers, defibrillators, cochlear implants, metal heart valves, pumps, neurostimulators, certain prostheses, and certain intrauterine devices. For surgical implants that are MRI compatible, the brand, style, and serial number should be requested to confirm compatibility. Guidelines for MRI in pregnancy have been updated to reflect the safety of this modality, with the understanding that gadolinium contrast should be used only if it significantly improves diagnostic yield.
Indications (selected)	• Evaluating for dementia • Suspected NPH • Suspected Huntington's disease • Suspected neurodegenerative disease with brain iron accumulation • Parkinsonian syndrome with atypical features • New focal neurological deficit • TIA involving carotid or vertebrobasilar arteries • Ataxia, acute or slowly progressive • Sudden-onset unilateral headache • New headache: patients older than 60 years with suspected temporal arteritis, patients with suspected meningitis/encephalitis, HIV-positive patients, pregnant patients
Normal test	• Normal structures (pituitary gland and corpus callosum) • No herniation of cerebellar tonsils • No evidence of mass lesion, hemorrhage, or acute ischemic injury • No abnormality of gray or white matter on FLAIR images • No abnormal fluid collections or displacement of midline structures • No areas of abnormal enhancement with contrast • Normal flow voids in major arteries

Magnetic resonance imaging *(continued)*

Normal test *(continued)*	• Normal visualized portions of the paranasal sinus, orbits, and mastoids • No abnormality of the calvarium
Abnormal test	• Periventricular or subcortical white matter changes (ischemia) • Stroke, acute or old • Hemorrhage • Atrophy, focal or regional • Generalized atrophy (graded as mild, moderate, or severe) • Ventricular dilatation (hydrocephalus) • Vascular abnormalities (aneurysms, arteriovenous malformations) • Vasculitis • Neoplasm, abscess, or other mass lesion • Infectious disease: toxoplasmosis, tuberculosis, or herpes encephalitis
Interfering factors	Perivascular spaces (Virchow-Robin spaces) can be mistaken for lacunar infarcts. These spaces are filled with interstitial fluid and are isointense with ventricles. Virchow-Robin spaces appear as round, oval, or linear (depending on plane of section) and are usually ≤5 mm, although they can be larger. Usually, Virchow-Robin spaces are suppressed completely on FLAIR images.
Cross-references	**Angiography, Magnetic Resonance (Cerebrovascular)** **Computed Tomography Scan, Head** **Neuroimaging Signal Appearance** (Appendix B)

Agarwal N, Port JD, Bazzocchi M, et al: Update on the use of MR for assessment and diagnosis of psychiatric diseases. Radiology 255:23–41, 2010

Gulani V, Calamante F, Shellock FG, et al: Gadolinium deposition in the brain: summary of evidence and recommendations. Lancet Neurol 16(7):564–570, 2017

Le Bihan D: Diffusion MRI: what water tells us about the brain. EMBO Mol Med 6(5):569–573, 2014

Le Bihan D, Johansen-Berg H: Diffusion MRI at 25: exploring brain tissue structure and function. Neuroimage 61(2):324–341, 2012

Mitelman SA: Transdiagnostic neuroimaging in psychiatry: a review. Psychiatry Res 277:23–38, 2019

Magnetic resonance spectroscopy (MRS)

Type of test	Neuroimaging
Background and explanation of test	Brain MRS uses the same basic technology and scanning equipment as MRI, with software programmed to acquire data regarding tissue metabolite levels. Three methods in common use include ^{1}H MRS, ^{31}P MRS, and ^{23}Na MRS. ^{1}H MRS is the fastest to perform and has the best signal-to-noise ratio of the three. Results of scanning are reported as a spectrum, with peaks representing signal intensities as a function of frequency (expressed as ppm). Data are obtained either from one area of interest (single-voxel spectroscopy) or from multiple regions (magnetic resonance spectroscopic imaging).
	With ^{1}H MRS, the following metabolites can be detected:
	• Lipids—products of brain destruction at 0.9–1.4 ppm
	• Lactate—product of anaerobic metabolism at 1.3 ppm
	• *N*-acetylaspartate (NAA)—neuronal density at 2.0 ppm
	• Glutamine and GABA—neurotransmitters at 2.2–2.4 ppm
	• Creatine—reflecting energy stores at 3.0 ppm
	• Choline—marker of cellular turnover at 3.2 ppm
	• Myoinositol—glial cell marker, osmolyte at 3.5 ppm
	• Other detectable substances include ethanol, glucose, mannitol, and alanine.
	Other neurotransmitters (dopamine, serotonin, acetylcholine) are invisible to MRS, as are DNA, RNA, and most proteins and enzymes.
Relevance to psychiatry and behavioral science	MRS can probe pathological processes occurring at the cellular level before morphological changes appear on structural study. Unlike existing imaging modalities that detect only coarse brain disease, MRS has the potential to investigate chemical abnormalities underlying various psychiatric disorders. In bipolar disorder, ^{1}H MRS shows reduced NAA in the prefrontal cortex and hippocampus in adults, adolescents, and at-risk patients. Alterations in the myoinositol-to-creatine ratio generally parallel mood state, with increased ratios in mania and euthymia and decreased ratios in bipolar depression. ^{31}P MRS in bipolar disorder shows altered phospholipid metabolism. Disorders such as PTSD, OCD, and generalized anxiety disorder show reduced NAA in the striatum and anterior cingulate cortex. The ratio of NAA to creatine tends to be lower in subjects with mild cognitive impairment who convert to dementia compared with those who do not.
Preparation of patient	See **Magnetic Resonance Imaging**. Use of ^{1}H MRS adds ~15 minutes to the MRI study.

Magnetic resonance spectroscopy (MRS) *(continued)*

Indications	MRS is used clinically to investigate the following: • Brain tumors • Hypoxic/ischemic insults • Cases of near drowning • TBI • Brain infections, such as abscess • Demyelinating disorders Clinical use is emerging for application of MRS to neurodegenerative diseases, stroke, and epilepsy.
Normal result	Principal metabolite peaks are those of NAA, creatine, choline, and myoinositol. *Normal ratios* • NAA-to-creatine: 2.0 • NAA-to-choline: 1.6 • Choline-to-creatine: 1.2
Abnormal result	Examples of abnormal findings: • With malignancy, NAA and creatine decrease and choline, lactate, and lipids increase. • Marked elevation of lactate is consistent with ischemia. • Increase in lipids occurs with stroke. • In AIDS dementia, NAA is reduced and choline elevated. • In hepatic encephalopathy, marked reduction in myoinositol is seen, along with reduced choline and increased glutamine. • In advanced Alzheimer's disease, NAA is reduced and myoinositol elevated. Myoinositol elevation is not seen in other dementias. *Abnormal ratios* • NAA-to-creatine: <1.6 • NAA-to-choline: <1.2 • Choline-to-creatine: >1.5
Interfering factors	MRS is a technically complex imaging modality. Factors that affect results include nonuniformity of magnetic fields and variability among subjects, age groups, and developmental stages in infants. Over the past decade, concerted efforts have been made to standardize acquisition protocols across laboratories.
Cross-references	**Magnetic Resonance Imaging**

Magnetic resonance spectroscopy (MRS) *(continued)*

Agarwal N, Port JD, Bazzocchi M, et al: Update on the use of MR for assessment and diagnosis of psychiatric diseases. Radiology 255:23–41, 2010

Currie S, Hadjivassiliou M, Craven IJ, et al: Magnetic resonance spectroscopy of the brain. Postgrad Med J 89(1048):94–106, 2013

Gharzeddine K, Hatzoglou V, Holodny AI, Young RJ: MR Perfusion and MR spectroscopy of brain neoplasms. Radiol Clin North Am 57(6):1177–1188, 2019

Gupta RK, Jobanputra KJ, Yadav A: MR spectroscopy in brain infections. Neuroimaging Clin N Am 23(3):475–498, 2013

Oz G, Alger JR, Barker PB, et al: Clinical proton MR spectroscopy in central nervous system disorders. Radiology 270(3):658–679, 2014

Schmitz B, Wang X, Barker PB, et al: Effects of aging on the human brain: a proton and phosphorus MR spectroscopy study at 3T. J Neuroimaging 28(4):416–421, 2018

Mammography

Type of test	Imaging
Background and explanation of test	Mammography is an X-ray examination of the breast and surrounding soft tissue used to detect masses too small to be palpable by clinical breast exam. Screening mammography has been the subject of a great deal of controversy in medicine because of concerns that the harms of false-positive results outweigh the benefits. In females of average breast cancer risk, however, screening is known to reduce breast cancer mortality.
	For patients who have symptoms, palpable masses, or a history of breast cancer or abnormal mammogram, a diagnostic mammogram is performed instead of a screening exam.
	A relatively new enhancement to the standard mammogram—three-dimensional (3D) mammography, or breast tomosynthesis—involves capture of multiple breast images in different planes that are then reconstructed digitally into 3D images that improve the accuracy of detection and reduce false-positive rates, particularly in patients with dense breast tissue. Another enhancement is contrast-enhanced digital mammography, which is utilized to stage newly diagnosed breast cancer and to evaluate response to chemotherapy.
Relevance to psychiatry and behavioral science	The incidence of brain metastases among females with metastatic breast cancer ranges from 10% to 30%. Breast cancer that metastasizes to the brain is more likely to involve triple-negative tumors and/or tumors overexpressing *HER2*. Clinical symptoms of brain metastases include headaches, memory problems, mood or personality changes, seizures, stroke or TIA, and impaired sensation and motor function.
Preparation of patient	Radiation exposure for mammography is minimal. The test involves compression of each breast between plates for several seconds while each image is acquired, which is uncomfortable for most females. Patients should be instructed not to apply deodorant, powder, perfume, or lotion to the underarm area on the day of the test because these may obscure the images obtained. Patients with painful breasts due to fibrocystic breast disease may benefit from abstaining from caffeinated beverages in the week before the test to reduce breast tenderness.
Indications	Testing recommendations of the American Cancer Society are as follows: • Females at average risk of breast cancer* have the option of starting annual screening mammography between ages 40 and 44. • Females ages 45–54 should undergo annual screening mammography. • Females age 55+ may switch to every-other-year mammography or continue annual mammography.

Mammography *(continued)*

Indications *(continued)*	• Mammography exams should continue as long as the patient is in good health and expected to live another 10 years. • Patients at high risk of breast cancer* should undergo mammography and breast MRI annually starting at age 30 years.
Normal findings	Normal breast tissue is imaged. Any calcifications are evenly distributed. Normal duct contrast and architecture.
Abnormal findings	• Mass in breast tissue or nipple • Signs of breast cancer: asymmetric density; poorly defined, spiculated mass; fine, stippled, clustered calcifications; thickening of overlying skin • Signs of malignant breast cancer: irregular, poorly defined, unilateral mass
Interfering factors	False-positive findings may result from fibrocystic breast disease, postoperative changes, post–radiation therapy changes, tattoos on overlying skin, sebaceous gland secretions, or talcum powder. Dense breast tissue or breast implants may yield false-negative findings.
Cross-references	**Brain Tumor**

*See the American Cancer Society guidelines referenced below for definitions of average and high risk.

American Cancer Society: Recommendations for the Early Detection of Breast Cancer. Atlanta, GA, American Cancer Society, 2021. Available at: https://www.cancer.org/cancer/breast-cancer/screening-tests-and-early-detection/american-cancer-society-recommendations-for-the-early-detection-of-breast-cancer.html. Accessed November 2021.

Brosnan EM, Anders CK: Understanding patterns of brain metastasis in breast cancer and designing rational therapeutic strategies. Ann Transl Med 6(9):163, 2018

Løberg M, Lousdal ML, Bretthauer M, Kalager M: Benefits and harms of mammography screening. Breast Cancer Res 17(1):63, 2015

Narayan AK, Lee CI, Lehman CD: Screening for breast cancer. Med Clin North Am 104(6):1007–1021, 2020

Polat DS, Evans WP, Dogan BE: Contrast-enhanced digital mammography: technique, clinical applications, and pitfalls. Am J Roentgenol 215(5):1267–1278, 2020

Schattner E: Correcting a decade of negative news about mammography. Clin Imaging 60(2):265–270, 2020

Mean corpuscular volume (MCV)

Type of test	Blood
Background and explanation of test	The MCV is the average volume (size) of RBCs in circulation, either measured directly or calculated from the hematocrit and RBC count. Included as a component of the CBC, the MCV is primarily used in the differential diagnosis of anemia.
	A mildly abnormal MCV can be an incidental finding on the CBC in the absence of anemia or other pathology. Very elevated MCV values may be found in association with vitamin B_{12} or folate deficiency and in disease states involving release of cold agglutinins (e.g., viral infections).
	Recent studies have shown increased mortality in patients with elevated MCV in the context of medical conditions such as esophageal cancer and chronic kidney disease, but the pathophysiology of this association is not yet understood. At the other end of the spectrum, benign elevation of MCV that is relatively mild (<115 fL) in the absence of anemia and other abnormalities on history, physical exam, and other laboratory tests does not require treatment.
Relevance to psychiatry and behavioral science	Several conditions relevant to clinical psychiatry are associated with an elevated MCV. These include alcohol use disorder, liver disease/cirrhosis, vitamin B_{12} or folate deficiency, smoking, and hypothyroidism. The greater the MCV elevation, the more likely it is due to vitamin B_{12} or folate deficiency.
Preparation of patient	None needed
Indications	Component of CBC
Reference range	*Adults 18–44 years* • Males: 80–99 fL • Females: 81–100 fL *Adults 45–64 years* • Males: 81–101 fL • Females: 81–101 fL *Adults 65–74 years* • Males: 81–103 fL • Females: 81–102 fL
Increased levels	• Excessive alcohol intake • Vitamin B_{12} deficiency • Folate deficiency • Increased RBC production (acute blood loss, hemolysis, liver disease, or disseminated malignancy) • Myelodysplastic syndrome • Multiple myeloma • Hypothyroidism

Mean corpuscular volume (MCV) *(continued)*

Increased levels *(continued)*	• Smoking • Advanced age • Pregnancy • *Drugs:* antihistamines, proton pump inhibitors, anticonvulsants, aspirin, acyclovir, isoniazid, metformin, chemotherapeutic agents, neomycin, colchicine, allopurinol, triamterene, nitrofurantoin, oral contraceptives, trimethoprim, valproic acid, and reverse transcriptase inhibitors, among others
Decreased levels	• Iron deficiency anemia • Anemia of chronic disease • Thalassemia • Certain hemoglobinopathies • Hypothyroidism (uncommon presentation)
Interfering factors	The MCV value is not reliable in the presence of large numbers of reticulocytes, abnormal erythrocytes (e.g., sickle cells), or a dimorphic population of erythrocytes. A common cause of falsely elevated MCV is RBC clumping in the test tube, which occurs in the presence of inflammatory or neoplastic disorders, cold agglutinins, or anticoagulant malfunction in the blood drawing tube. Severe hyperglycemia or leukocytosis may also falsely elevate MCV.
Cross-references	**Alcohol Use Disorder** **Anemia** **Cirrhosis** **Complete Blood Count** **Folate Deficiency** **Vitamin B$_{12}$ Deficiency**

Fischbach FT, Fischbach MA: A Manual of Laboratory and Diagnostic Tests, 10th Edition. Philadelphia, PA, Wolters Kluwer Health/Lippincott Williams and Wilkins, 2018

Hsieh YP, Chang CC, Kor CT, et al: Mean corpuscular volume and mortality in patients with CKD. Clin J Am Soc Nephrol 12(2):237–244, 2017

Veda P: Evaluation of macrocytosis in routine hemograms. Indian J Hematol Blood Transfus 29(1):26–30, 2013

Wu AHB: Tietz Clinical Guide to Laboratory Tests, 4th Edition. St. Louis, MO, WB Saunders, 2006

Metanephrines

Type of test	Blood, urine
Background and explanation of test	Metanephrines are breakdown products of epinephrine found in blood and urine that aid in the diagnosis of the chromaffin cell tumors *pheochromocytoma* and *paraganglioma*. Patients with these tumors have variable clinical presentations, the classic triad being episodic headache, sweating, and tachycardia. The predominant symptom for many patients is severe, variable hypertension that is associated with end-organ damage. Anxiety and panic attacks often bring patients to the attention of psychiatrists. Other symptoms are discussed in the **Pheochromocytoma** entry in the ***Diseases and Conditions*** chapter. Pheochromocytoma and paraganglioma are diagnosed by plasma free metanephrines or urine metanephrines, with plasma metanephrine testing preferred because of convenience and factors interfering with urine testing. Because metanephrines are secreted continuously by the tumor, blood can be drawn at any time; it is not necessary to draw samples *during* a panic attack or hypertensive episode.
Relevance to psychiatry and behavioral science	Pheochromocytoma and paraganglioma can cause episodic panic attacks that closely resemble primary panic disorder. Attacks are associated with somatic signs and symptoms noted in the **Pheochromocytoma** entry referenced above. Attacks may be spontaneous or induced by a range of stimuli, including abdominal compression, urination, trauma, anesthesia, surgery, biopsy or other invasive procedures, medications, or foods with high tyramine content.
Preparation of patient	Strict preparation requires a 3-day diet without caffeine, black tea, nicotine, alcohol, bananas, cheese, almonds, nuts, chocolate, eggs, or vanilla. Drugs listed below that may cause spurious results should be avoided if possible.
Indications	Clinical suspicion of pheochromocytoma or paraganglioma
Reference range	Free normetanephrine: 0.0–0.89 nmol/L Free metanephrine: 0.0–0.49 nmol/L
Critical value(s)	Plasma levels >2 times the upper limit of normal for the laboratory reference range are consistent with pheochromocytoma. Most patients with one of these tumors have a plasma free normetanephrine level >2.2 nmol/L and/or a metanephrine level >1.1 nmol/L.
Increased levels	Pheochromocytoma, paraganglioma
Decreased levels	Not applicable
Interfering factors	Patient positioning affects the results; blood should be drawn after 15 minutes of rest, with the patient in the supine position. Drugs and some foods (see *Preparation of Patient* section above) affect the results.

Metanephrines *(continued)*

Interfering factors *(continued)*	Spurious results can be obtained with the following: acetaminophen, alcohol (withdrawal), aminophylline, amphetamines, benzodiazepines (withdrawal), buspirone, caffeine, chloral hydrate, chlorpromazine, clonidine, dexamethasone, epinephrine, imipramine, lithium, MAOIs, opioids, salicylates, TCAs, and tobacco, among other drugs. Vigorous exercise can affect results.
Cross-references	**Pheochromocytoma**

ARUP Laboratories: Metanephrines, plasma (free), in Lab Test Directory. Salt Lake City, UT, ARUP Laboratories, 2021. Available at: https://ltd.aruplab.com/Tests/Pub/0050184. Accessed August 2021.

Därr R, Kuhn M, Bode C, et al: Accuracy of recommended sampling and assay methods for the determination of plasma-free and urinary fractionated metanephrines in the diagnosis of pheochromocytoma and paraganglioma: a systematic review. Endocrine 56(3):495–503, 2017

Farrugia FA, Martikos G, Tzanetis P, et al: Pheochromocytoma, diagnosis and treatment: review of the literature. Endocr Regul 51(3):168–181, 2017

Garcia-Carbonero R, Matute Teresa F, Mercader-Cidoncha E, et al: Multidisciplinary practice guidelines for the diagnosis, genetic counseling and treatment of pheochromocytomas and paragangliomas. Clin Transl Oncol 23(10):1995–2019, 2021

Peaston RT, Graham KS, Chambers E, et al: Performance of plasma free metanephrines measured by liquid chromatography–tandem mass spectrometry in the diagnosis of pheochromocytoma. Clin Chim Acta 411:546–552, 2010

Methanol level

Type of test	Blood
Background and explanation of test	Methanol, also known as methyl alcohol or wood alcohol, is a highly toxic substance found in windshield washer fluid, gas line antifreeze, carburetor cleaner, copy machine fluid, perfumes, food warming fuel, and other types of fuels. In the past, exposure to methanol occurred accidentally, because of contaminated home-distilled and fermented beverages, or intentionally, with ingestion of products such as windshield washer fluid as a means of suicide, use of food-warming fuel as a substitute for ethanol when the latter was unavailable, and abuse of carburetor cleaner via inhalation ("huffing"). More recently, worldwide exposures occurred starting in 2020 with the COVID-19 pandemic, when false rumors appeared on social media that the virus could be prevented or treated by drinking or gargling hand sanitizer. A significant number of those hand sanitizers, notably those from Mexico, contained methanol rather than ethyl alcohol or isopropanol. As little as 2 tbsp of methanol can be lethal for a child, and 2 fl oz for an adult. The prognosis with poisoning depends on the amount ingested and how soon treatment is administered. Once ingested, methanol is rapidly absorbed and oxidized by alcohol dehydrogenase to formaldehyde, and then by aldehyde dehydrogenase to formic acid. As metabolism proceeds, an initial high osmolal gap decreases and an anion gap increases. Formic acid is the primary toxic metabolite, causing retinal toxicity and later parkinsonism. Treatment consists of supportive care, correction of acidosis, use of an alcohol dehydrogenase inhibitor (fomepizole, or ethanol orally or intravenously if fomepizole is not available), and hemodialysis. Left untreated, methanol poisoning can be fatal.
Relevance to psychiatry and behavioral science	Psychiatrists may encounter methanol poisoning in patients who are suicidal, in those with alcohol use disorder who lack access to ethanol, in patients using solvents for "huffing," and in misguided patients ingesting hand sanitizer. On presentation, patients might initially appear normal or inebriated. Onset of clinical and laboratory features can be delayed for days with co-ingestion of ethanol. Initial symptoms are GI related, followed by CNS depression and hyperventilation. Visual changes such as blurred vision, decreased acuity, photophobia, and "halo vision" are associated with an abnormal funduscopic exam. Seizures can occur. Several weeks after exposure, parkinsonian signs can be seen, with tremor, cogwheel rigidity, hypokinesia, stooped posture, and shuffling gait. Necrosis of the putamen and globus pallidus are associated with these findings.
Preparation of patient	None needed
Indications	Clinical suspicion of methanol ingestion
Reference range	Not applicable. Methanol is not detectable at levels <5 mg/dL.
Critical values	Toxicity at levels >20 mg/dL

Methanol level *(continued)*

Increased levels	<ul><li>Ingestion of hand sanitizer containing methanol</li><li>Accidental ingestion</li><li>Intentional overdose</li><li>Abuse in place of ethanol</li></ul>
Decreased levels	Not applicable
Interfering factors	Plasma level may be below the assay's limit of detection even though the patient shows signs of toxicity. Laboratory findings may be delayed up to 3–4 days when ethanol is co-ingested.
Cross-references	**Methanol Poisoning** **Osmolality**

ARUP Laboratories Test Directory: Methanol, in Lab Test Directory. Salt Lake City, UT, ARUP Laboratories, 2021. Available at: https://ltd.aruplab.com/Tests/Pub/0090165. Accessed August 2021.

Liu YS, Lin KY, Masur J, et al: Outcomes after recurrent intentional methanol exposures not treated with alcohol dehydrogenase inhibitors or hemodialysis. J Emerg Med 58(6):910–916, 2020

Mehrpour O, Sadeghi M: Toll of acute methanol poisoning for preventing COVID-19. Arch Toxicol 94(6):2259–2260, 2020

Sefidbakht S, Lotfi M, Jalli R, et al: Methanol toxicity outbreak: when fear of COVID-19 goes viral. Emerg Med J 37(7):416, 2020

Yip L, Bixler D, Brooks DE, et al: Serious adverse health events, including death, associated with ingesting alcohol-based hand sanitizers containing methanol: Arizona and New Mexico, May–June 2020. MMWR Morb Mortal Wkly Rep 69(32):1070–1073, 2020

Zakharov S, Pelclova D, Navratil T, et al: Fomepizole versus ethanol in the treatment of acute methanol poisoning: comparison of clinical effectiveness in a mass poisoning outbreak. Clin Toxicol (Phila) 53(8):797–806, 2015

Methylmalonic acid (MMA) level

Type of test	Blood
Background and explanation of test	In past practice, the serum MMA level was often used (along with serum total homocysteine) to determine the significance of a low-normal vitamin B_{12} level. In normal metabolism, vitamin B_{12} is a necessary cofactor for the conversion of methylmalonyl coenzyme A (CoA) to succinyl CoA; when B_{12} is deficient, methylmalonyl CoA is converted to MMA instead, and levels rise in the blood and urine. Research has demonstrated that a substantial proportion of individuals with low B_{12} levels have normal MMA levels, and clinical opinion now differs as to the utility of MMA in determining B_{12} status. Serum holotranscobalamin is a more sensitive indicator of B_{12} deficiency, although that test is not available in all laboratories. Serum MMA is still used in some centers for the workup of suspected B_{12} deficiency.
Relevance to psychiatry and behavioral science	Vitamin B_{12} deficiency is associated with numerous psychiatric signs and symptoms, as noted in the **Diseases and Conditions** chapter.
Preparation of patient	Ideally, patients should fast overnight before the test.
Indications	• Detecting early or mild vitamin B_{12} deficiency • Follow-up to B_{12} levels at lower end of the normal range • Diagnosing methylmalonic acidemia (plasma and urine) • Detecting cobalamin genetic defects (plasma and urine)
Reference range	Adults: <0.2 µmol/L *Note*: Degree of elevation above this cutoff correlates poorly with severity of deficiency as well as prognosis.
Critical value(s)	≥0.3 µmol/L associated with poor functional status
Increased levels	• Vitamin B_{12} deficiency • Impaired kidney function • Cobalamin genetic defects • Methylmalonic acidemia (in infants)
Decreased levels	Not known to have clinical significance
Interfering factors	Results invalidated by renal failure and volume depletion (dehydration). Broad-spectrum antibiotic therapy at time of testing may lead to false-negative results.
Cross-references	**Folate Deficiency** **Folate Level** **Homocysteine Level** **Vitamin B_{12} Deficiency** **Vitamin B_{12} Level**

Methylmalonic acid (MMA) level *(continued)*

American Association for Clinical Chemistry: Testing.com. Available at: https://www.testing.com. Accessed August 2021.

ARUP Laboratories: Methylmalonic acid, serum or plasma (vitamin B_{12} status), in Lab Test Directory. Salt Lake City, UT, ARUP Laboratories, 2021. Available at: https://ltd.aruplab.com/Tests/Pub/0099431. Accessed August 2021.

Hill MH, Flatley JE, Barker ME, et al: A vitamin B-12 supplement of 500 µg/d for eight weeks does not normalize urinary methylmalonic acid or other biomarkers of vitamin B-12 status in elderly people with moderately poor vitamin B-12 status. J Nutr 143(2):142–147, 2013

Remacha AF, Sardà MP, Canals C, et al: Role of serum holotranscobalamin (holoTC) in the diagnosis of patients with low serum cobalamin: comparison with methylmalonic acid and homocysteine. Ann Hematol 93(4):565–569, 2014

Wolffenbuttel BHR, Wouters HJCM, de Jong WHA, et al: Association of vitamin B_{12}, methylmalonic acid, and functional parameters. Neth J Med 78(1):10–24, 2020

Multiple sleep latency test (MSLT) and maintenance of wakefulness test (MWT)

Type of test	Neurophysiology
Background and explanation of test	The MSLT provides an objective index of an individual's degree of daytime sleepiness and detects the inappropriate early appearance of REM sleep after sleep onset. The MSLT is an all-day test consisting of four or five scheduled naps separated by 2-hour breaks. It is performed the day after a PSG study in which sleep quality and duration are observed. The MSLT monitors EEG, eye and muscle movement, and ECG and identifies times of sleep onset and sleep stages, including REM sleep. The results are used to diagnose narcolepsy and idiopathic hypersomnia. The MWT provides an objective index of an individual's daytime alertness. In this test, patients are instructed to resist the urge to fall asleep during the test period of ≤40 minutes; otherwise, the protocol is much like that used for the MSLT. Results can be used to assess an individual's ability to stay awake when there is a question of individual or public safety and to evaluate response to treatment for excessive daytime sleepiness.
Relevance to psychiatry and behavioral science	Daytime somnolence is often reported by patients with Parkinson's disease, Alzheimer's disease, chronic fatigue syndrome, depression, and fibromyalgia and other chronic pain syndromes. It also plagues those treated with highly sedating medications such as anticonvulsants, antipsychotics, and certain antidepressants. Positive urine drug screens in a substantial minority of patients presenting for MSLT/MWT prompted the current recommendation that urine drug screening be performed on the morning of testing. Drugs detected included amphetamines, cannabinoids, opiates, and benzodiazepines, and use of these drugs was not self-reported. Drug and medication use must be known in order to correctly interpret MSLT/MWT results.
Preparation of patient	A sleep medicine consult should be performed before the test is scheduled. All wake-promoting and REM-suppressing drugs should be stopped ≥15 days before testing (≥5 half-lives of drug and metabolites). Cannabis (THC and cannabidiol [CBD]) cause REM rebound and sleep-onset REM when discontinued; 4 weeks of abstinence is recommended. Smoking should be stopped 30 minutes before each nap. As noted in the *Relevance* section above, urine drug screen should be performed on the morning of testing.
Indications	• Confirming clinical diagnoses of narcolepsy and idiopathic hypersomnia • Evaluating daytime hypersomnia • Determining effectiveness of treatment for hypersomnia

Multiple sleep latency test (MSLT) and maintenance of wakefulness test (MWT) *(continued)*

Reference range	MSLT: Normal mean sleep latency is 10–20 minutes.
	MWT: Mean sleep latency is 35 minutes on the 40-minute test; most individuals with normal sleep can resist falling asleep and stay awake for the duration.
Positive test	MSLT: Mean sleep latency is <8 minutes. Sleep-onset REM periods occur on more than two naps.
	MWT: Mean sleep latency is <8 minutes.
Critical value(s)	Mean sleep latency in patients with narcolepsy with cataplexy is usually 2–3 minutes.
	In this condition, three to five sleep-onset REM periods are often observed.
Interfering factors	Test-retest reliability for MSLT is good for narcolepsy with cataplexy but not for narcolepsy without cataplexy or for idiopathic hypersomnia.
	Sleep deprivation, which affects individuals attempting to sleep in artificial laboratory conditions, interferes with both MSLT and MWT. Anxiety may affect patients' ability to fall asleep.
	Environmental factors such as light, temperature, and noise affect test validity. Caffeine or other stimulants and sedative-hypnotic medications taken before testing may invalidate results.
	Drugs that cause REM sleep rebound when discontinued affect results.
Cross-references	**Narcolepsy**
	Polysomnography

Anniss AM, Young A, O'Driscoll DM: Importance of urinary drug screening in the multiple sleep latency test and maintenance of wakefulness test. J Clin Sleep Med 12(12):1633–1640, 2016

Kluge M, Himmerich H, Wehmeier PM, et al: Sleep propensity at daytime as assessed by multiple sleep latency tests (MSLT) in patients with schizophrenia increases with clozapine and olanzapine. Schizophr Res 135(1–3):123–127, 2012

Kolla BP, Jahani Kondori M, Silber MH, et al: Advance taper of antidepressants prior to multiple sleep latency testing increases the number of sleep-onset rapid eye movement periods and reduces mean sleep latency. J Clin Sleep Med 16(11):1921–1927, 2020

Plante DT: Sleep propensity in psychiatric hypersomnolence: a systematic review and meta-analysis of multiple sleep latency test findings. Sleep Med Rev 31:48–57, 2017

Rack M, Davis J, Roffwarg HP, et al: The multiple sleep latency test in the diagnosis of narcolepsy. Am J Psychiatry 162:2198–2199, 2005

Sullivan SS, Kushida CA: Multiple sleep latency test and maintenance of wakefulness test. Chest 134:854–861, 2008

Osmolality

Type of test	Blood, urine
Background and explanation of test	Osmolality refers to the number of solute particles in 1 kg of solvent. A related variable—osmolarity—is the number of solute particles in 1 L of solvent. (A simple mnemonic: osmolaRity refers to liteR.) Because measurements of osmolarity are temperature-dependent, *osmolality* is the preferred term for biological systems.
	Osmolality is used to evaluate fluid and electrolyte balance, determine the cause of increased or decreased urine output, investigate abnormal levels of sodium, and detect the presence of ingested toxins such as methanol or acetylsalicylic acid. Serum and urine osmolality are most often measured at the same time so that results can be correctly interpreted. Under normal conditions, the body maintains osmolality within a certain range through secretion of antidiuretic hormone (ADH) by the posterior pituitary.
	Serum osmolality is primarily a reflection of sodium concentration, whereas urine osmolality is primarily a measure of waste products (urea and creatinine). Under pathological conditions, serum osmolality can also reflect glucose levels (in hyperglycemia) or blood urea levels (in renal failure). Serum osmolality aids in the evaluation of hyponatremia, which can be secondary to urinary sodium losses or to increased fluid in the circulation (e.g., from polydipsia, water retention, inability of kidneys to produce a dilute urine, or high glucose levels).
	Another application of serum osmolality is to compare it with a calculation of predicted osmolality based on measurements of the major solutes (sodium, glucose, BUN), a difference termed the *osmolal gap*. Such a gap indicates the presence of additional osmotically active substances such as ethanol, methanol, or ethylene glycol in the blood.
Relevance to psychiatry and behavioral science	Acute osmolality changes can be associated with dehydration, hyperglycemia, alcohol withdrawal, TBI, and other conditions. Subacute or chronic changes can be seen in psychogenic polydipsia, tuberculosis, subdural hematoma, hydrocephalus, AIDS, or multiple sclerosis or be associated with medications (e.g., diabetes insipidus in patients treated with lithium, or SIAD in patients treated with antidepressants, antipsychotics, opioids, or carbamazepine). Acute changes in osmolality can cause delirium or—in extreme cases—coma.
Preparation of patient	None needed
Indications	• Determining cause of hyponatremia • Assessing fluid and electrolyte balance • Determining cause of abnormal urine output • Evaluating suspected SIAD, diabetes insipidus, or psychogenic polydipsia

Osmolality *(continued)*

Indications (*continued*)	• Detecting ingested toxins: methanol, ethylene glycol, or acetylsalicylic acid
Reference range	Serum osmolality in adults age ≥17 years: 280–303 mOsm/kg Urine osmolality in adults age ≥17 years: 50–800 mOsm/kg Normal ratio of urine to serum osmolality: 3:1
Critical value(s)	Serum osmolality <240 mOsm/kg or >320 mOsm/kg Respiratory arrest can occur at >360 mOsm/kg.
Increased levels	• *Serum osmolality*: dehydration, diabetes insipidus, hyperglycemia, hypercalcemia, cerebral lesions, hypernatremic ethanol intoxication, tube feeding, high-protein diet, hypovolemic shock, poisoning (e.g., methanol, ethylene glycol) • *Urine osmolality*: dehydration, prerenal azotemia, congestive heart failure, SIAD, Addison's disease, amyloidosis, hypernatremia, high-protein diet
Decreased levels	• *Serum osmolality*: overhydration, primary (psychogenic) polydipsia, Addison's disease, acute renal failure, panhypopituitarism, postoperative states, SIAD • *Urine osmolality*: acute renal failure, diabetes insipidus, primary (psychogenic) polydipsia, compulsive water drinking, electrolyte derangement (hypokalemia, hypernatremia, or hypercalcemia)
Interfering factors	IV fluids (dextrose and water; sodium) influence osmolality results. Specimen hemolysis or lipemic serum influences results. Several herbs and natural remedies increase osmolality, either through ADH antagonism or diuretic effects. Increased serum osmolality can result from ingestion of mineralocorticoids, osmotic diuretics, insulin, or mannitol. Abnormal urine osmolality can result from anesthetic agents, antibiotics, carbamazepine, diuretics, glucose, mannitol, or X-ray contrast agents. Urine osmolality is also affected by an aging-related inability to fully concentrate urine.
Cross-references	**Adrenal Insufficiency** **Diabetes Insipidus** **Hyperglycemia** **Hyponatremia** **Psychogenic Polydipsia** **Syndrome of Inappropriate Antidiuresis**

Osmolality *(continued)*

American Association for Clinical Chemistry: Testing.com. Available at: https://www.testing.com. Accessed August 2021.

ARUP Laboratories: Osmolality, urine, in Lab Test Directory. Salt Lake City, UT, ARUP Laboratories, 2021. Available at: https://ltd.aruplab.com/Tests/Pub/0020228. Accessed August 2021.

ARUP Laboratories: Osmolality, serum or plasma, in Lab Test Directory. Salt Lake City, UT, ARUP Laboratories, 2021. Available at: https://ltd.aruplab.com/Tests/Pub/0020046. Accessed August 2021.

Fischbach FT, Fischbach MA: A Manual of Laboratory and Diagnostic Tests, 10th Edition. Philadelphia, PA, Wolters Kluwer Health/Lippincott Williams and Wilkins, 2018

Oxazepam level

Type of test	Blood
Background and explanation of test	Benzodiazepines are Schedule IV sedative-hypnotic drugs used to treat anxiety and insomnia. Oxazepam is a drug with a slow onset of action and a short half-life. It is not extensively metabolized in the liver. In general, levels of the drug are checked when either overdose or noncompliance is suspected or to detect use without a prescription. In the latter case, a urine drug screen is more likely to be ordered than a blood level.
Relevance to psychiatry and behavioral science	Toxicity with chronic benzodiazepine ingestion may manifest as confusion, disorientation, memory impairment, ataxia, decreased reflexes, and dysarthria. With acute overdose, patients may exhibit somnolence, confusion, ataxia, decreased reflexes, vertigo, dysarthria, respiratory depression, and coma. Treatment is supportive. More serious consequences usually involve co-ingestion of alcohol or other sedatives, and in these cases, airway management is required. The decision to use flumazenil, an antagonist at the benzodiazepine receptor, is made on a case-by-case basis. Activated charcoal is no longer recommended, and neither dialysis nor bowel irrigation has a role in treatment.
Preparation of patient	None needed
Indications	• Screening for drug use • Suspicion of overdose • Signs of toxicity in a treated patient • Suspected noncompliance with prescribed therapy
Reference range	200–500 ng/mL
Critical value(s)	>2,000 ng/mL
Increased levels	• Overdose • Overuse
Decreased levels	Noncompliance
Interfering factors	None
Cross-references	**Benzodiazepines** **Urine Drug Screen**

Kang M, Galuska MA, Ghassemzadeh S: Benzodiazepine toxicity, in StatPearls. Treasure Island, FL, Stat-Pearls Publishing, 2021. Available at: https://www.statpearls.com/ArticleLibrary/viewarticle/30312. Accessed September 2021

Mayo Clinic Laboratories: Test Catalog: Oxazepam (Serax), Serum. Available at: https://www.mayocliniclabs.com/test-catalog/Overview/90108. Accessed August 2021.

Parathyroid hormone (PTH)

Type of test	Blood
Background and explanation of test	PTH, which is secreted from four small glands on the posterior aspect of the thyroid gland, regulates calcium levels in the blood and extracellular fluids. When circulating calcium levels are low, PTH causes calcium to be released from bones and increases the reabsorption of calcium in the proximal convoluted tubule of the kidney, bringing calcium levels back to the normal range. When circulating calcium levels are high, the glands stop producing PTH. The PTH test is used to diagnose hyperparathyroidism and hypoparathyroidism, to determine whether abnormal calcium levels are due to pathology in the parathyroid gland itself, and to monitor kidney disease. When the PTH level is drawn, calcium and creatinine are checked at the same time for proper test interpretation.
Relevance to psychiatry and behavioral science	Dysregulation of PTH is associated with altered mental status, including delirium. In hypoparathyroidism, secondary anxiety syndromes can be seen. In hyperparathyroidism, depression, fatigue, loss of appetite, and personality changes can be seen. Hypoparathyroidism is most often due to parathyroid injury or accidental removal during thyroid surgery. Several psychotropic drugs affect the PTH level, including lithium, steroids, anticonvulsants, and propranolol.
Preparation of patient	Fasting is no longer required for testing. The time at which the sample is drawn may be prescribed, because PTH levels fluctuate over a 24-hour period. Certain drugs may have to be discontinued prior to testing.
Indications	• Determining cause of calcium derangement • Evaluating parathyroid function • Diagnosing hyperparathyroidism • Diagnosing hypoparathyroidism • Confirming removal of pathological parathyroid tissue during surgery • Monitoring chronic kidney disease
Reference range	15–65 pg/mL
Critical value(s)	None
Increased levels	• Primary hyperparathyroidism • Secondary hyperparathyroidism • Zollinger-Ellison syndrome • Pseudogout • Spinal cord injury

Parathyroid hormone (PTH) *(continued)*

Increased levels *(continued)*	• Familial medullary thyroid carcinoma • Multiple endocrine neoplasia (MEN I, IIA, IIB)
Decreased levels	• Autoimmune hypoparathyroidism • Surgical hypoparathyroidism (after thyroidectomy) • Sarcoidosis • Hyperthyroidism • Nonparathyroid hypercalcemia • Magnesium deficiency • DiGeorge syndrome
Interfering factors	Elevated blood lipids and hemolysis interfere with the PTH test itself. The time of blood draw influences the results. Ingestion of milk before the test may falsely reduce the PTH result. Oversupplementation with vitamins A and D reduces PTH. Drugs that cause increased PTH include anticonvulsants, corticosteroids, isoniazid, lithium, phosphates (large effect), estrogen/progestin, ketoconazole, nifedipine, verapamil, phenytoin, prednisone, and rifampin. Drugs that cause decreased PTH include aluminum hydroxide, cimetidine, gentamicin, magnesium sulfate, pindolol, propranolol, and thiazides.
Cross-references	**Calcium** **Hypercalcemia** **Hypocalcemia**

American Association for Clinical Chemistry: Testing.com. Available at: https://www.testing.com. Accessed August 2021.

ARUP Laboratories: Parathyroid hormone, intact, in Lab Test Directory. Salt Lake City, UT, ARUP Laboratories, 2021. Available at: https://www.aruplab.com/Tests/Pub/0070346. Accessed August 2021.

Fischbach FT, Fischbach MA: A Manual of Laboratory and Diagnostic Tests, 10th Edition. Philadelphia, PA, Wolters Kluwer Health/Lippincott Williams and Wilkins, 2018

Peacock M: Calcium metabolism in health and disease. Clin J Am Soc Nephrol 5(Suppl):S23–S30, 2010

Verrotti A, Coppola G, Parisi P, et al: Bone and calcium metabolism and antiepileptic drugs. Clin Neurol Neurosurg 112:1–10, 2010

Phosphate

Type of test	Blood
Background and explanation of test	This test, also known as *phosphorus*, measures the level of a dietary nutrient ingested from meat, chicken, fish, eggs, dairy products, beans, nuts, and cereals. Its absorption in the small intestine is facilitated by vitamin D. In humans, ≤85% of phosphorus binds to calcium to form bones and teeth; of the remainder, 10% resides in muscle, 1% in nerve tissue, and 1% in the blood. Phosphate levels are regulated by changes in intestinal absorption or renal excretion. They are most often checked along with levels of calcium, PTH, and vitamin D to diagnose and monitor treatment of conditions that affect both phosphate and calcium levels.
	Phosphates have several important functions in the body, including acid-base balance, carbohydrate and lipid metabolism, and storage and transfer of energy. Patients with mild to moderate phosphate deficiency may be asymptomatic. Those with severe deficiency may exhibit muscle weakness, reduced cardiac contractility, reduced platelet function, paresthesias, and confusion. Patients who are on a ventilator may have difficulty weaning if phosphate deficiency is present. As the severity of phosphate deficiency worsens, muscle cramps, delirium, and seizures may be seen.
	Athletes are known to supplement phosphates to improve performance in high-intensity sports such as cycling and sprinting. This practice may prove to be dangerous because high phosphate levels are associated with osteoporosis, cardiovascular events, and all-cause mortality. Higher phosphate levels—even high-normal levels—contribute to microvascular dysfunction and may be a cause of aortic stenosis. Many prescription drugs are known to contain phosphates, and this can prove problematic for patients with kidney failure. Many soft drinks and prepackaged foods are high in phosphates, possibly contributing to overconsumption in the general population. Other sources include phosphate-containing laxatives and enemas, excessive vitamin D supplementation, and IV glucose administration.
Relevance to psychiatry and behavioral science	Alcohol use disorder is associated with decreased phosphate levels, whereas cirrhosis is associated with increased levels. Patients who ingest large volumes of soft drinks or large amounts of prepackaged foods can develop toxic levels of phosphate.
Preparation of patient	Patients should fast for 8–12 hours before testing.
Indications	• Abnormal calcium test result • Symptoms of an abnormal calcium level • Diagnosing and monitoring kidney disease • Diagnosing and monitoring bone disorders • Diagnosing and monitoring GI disease • Diagnosing parathyroid disease

Phosphate *(continued)*

Reference range	Adults: 2.7–4.5 mg/dL
Critical value(s)	<1.0 mg/dL
Increased levels	Kidney failure, excessive intake of phosphate supplements, hypoparathyroidism, hypocalcemia, excessive vitamin D intake, liver disease and cirrhosis, pulmonary embolism, Addison's disease, acromegaly, healing fractures, osteolytic bone tumors and metastases
Decreased levels	Hyperparathyroidism, hypercalcemia, malnutrition, malabsorption, vomiting and/or severe diarrhea, acid-base imbalance, serious burns, hypothyroidism, chronic use of antacids or laxatives, overuse of diuretics, alcohol use disorder, liver disease, vitamin D deficiency (rickets or osteomalacia), growth hormone deficiency, continuous IV glucose administration, salicylate poisoning, sepsis
Interfering factors	Phosphate levels show diurnal fluctuation, with highest levels in late morning and lowest in evening. Seasonal variations are also seen, with highest values in May and June and lowest values in winter.
	Falsely elevated phosphate levels may be measured if serum or plasma is not separated from erythrocytes within 1 hour after blood is drawn.
	Many prescription drugs affect phosphate levels; a complete drug history is needed for proper test interpretation.
Cross-references	**Anorexia Nervosa**
	Calcium
	Chronic Fatigue Syndrome
	Magnesium
	Parathyroid Hormone
	Renal Function Panel
	Vitamin D Level

American Association for Clinical Chemistry: Lab Tests Online. Available at: https://www.testing.com. Accessed August 2021

Brewer CP, Dawson B, Wallman KE, Guelfi K: Effect of sodium phosphate supplementation on repeated high-intensity cycling efforts. J Sports Sci 33(11):1109–1116, 2015

Ginsberg C, Houben AJHM, Malhotra R, et al: Serum phosphate and microvascular function in a population-based cohort. Clin J Am Soc Nephrol 14(11):1626–1633, 2019

Nelson SM, Sarabia SR, Christilaw E, et al: Phosphate-containing prescription medications contribute to the daily phosphate intake in a third of hemodialysis patients. J Ren Nutr 27(2):91–96, 2017

Wald DS, Bestwick JP: Association between serum calcium, serum phosphate and aortic stenosis with implications for prevention. Eur J Prev Cardiol 25(5):551–556, 2018

Platelet count

Type of test	Blood
Background and explanation of test	Platelets—also known as *thrombocytes*—are disc-shaped, non-nucleated cells that develop in the bone marrow and spend most of their 1-week lifespan in the circulation. They have a critical role in blood clotting, vasoconstriction, and maintenance of small blood vessels. Platelets link these hemostatic functions with inflammatory processes and are known to have altered function under pro-inflammatory conditions. Increased platelet activity heightens the risk of thrombotic events such as heart attack and stroke. Number and size (volume) of platelets are reported as part of the CBC. An insufficient number of platelets is associated with spontaneous bleeding and easy bruising. The mean platelet volume (MPV) is an indicator of the average age of platelets; newly formed platelets are larger than old platelets. *Thrombocytosis* refers to an increased number of platelets, whereas *thrombocytopenia* refers to a decreased number.
Relevance to psychiatry and behavioral science	Psychotropic drugs associated with thrombocytopenia include antidepressants (all classes), antipsychotics (conventional and atypical), anticonvulsants, prescribed stimulants, acetylcholinesterase inhibitors, β-blockers, and commonly used analgesics (aspirin, acetaminophen, codeine, ibuprofen, and others). Drugs associated with thrombocytosis include amoxapine, clozapine, danazol, donepezil, steroids, immune globulin, lithium, megestrol, metoprolol, paroxetine, propranolol, venlafaxine, and zidovudine, among others.
Preparation of patient	None needed
Indications	• Evaluating bleeding disorders • Monitoring bone marrow failure • Abnormal estimated platelet count on blood smear • Component of coagulation profile
Reference range	Adults: $140–400 \times 10^3/\text{mm}^3$ The lower limit of normal may be lower for those of Afro-Caribbean or African ancestry.
Critical values	$<20 \times 10^3/\text{mm}^3$ associated with spontaneous bleeding $>1,000 \times 10^3/\text{mm}^3$ associated with myeloproliferative disorders. Patients may have bleeding because of abnormal platelet function. Half of patients with unexpected increase in platelet count have malignancy.
Increased levels	Essential thrombocytosis, rapid blood regeneration (e.g., with acute bleeding), leukemia, myeloproliferative disease, Hodgkin's disease, lymphoma, other malignancies, polycythemia vera, splenectomy, iron deficiency anemia, acute infection, acute inflammation, rheumatoid arthritis, SLE, other collagen diseases, chronic pancreatitis, inflammatory bowel disease, tuberculosis, renal failure, recovery from bone marrow suppression, and numerous drugs, including psychotropics

Platelet count *(continued)*

Decreased levels	Idiopathic thrombocytopenic purpura, various heritable syndromes, anemia (pernicious, hemolytic, aplastic), thrombopoietin deficiency, dilutional effect of a large blood transfusion, infection (viral, bacterial, or rickettsial), congestive heart failure, congenital heart disease, chemotherapy or radiation therapy, exposure to DDT and other chemicals, HIV infection, bone marrow disease (leukemia, carcinoma, myelofibrosis), disseminated intravascular coagulation, thrombotic thrombocytopenic purpura, preeclampsia, eclampsia, alcohol use disorder, excessive alcohol ingestion, hypersplenism, renal insufficiency, antiplatelet antibodies, toxic effects of drugs (not dose-dependent), psychotropic drugs listed in the *Relevance* section above
Interfering factors	Platelet clumps or very large platelets make automated counts inaccurate; in these cases, manual inspection should be used.
	Thrombocytosis may be seen at high altitudes, in winter, or after strenuous exercise, trauma, or excitement.
	Thrombocytopenia may be observed before menstruation and during pregnancy.
Cross-references	**Complete Blood Count**
	Thrombocytopenia
	Thrombocytosis

American Association for Clinical Chemistry: Testing.com. Available at: https://www.testing.com. Accessed August 2021.

Fischbach FT, Fischbach MA: A Manual of Laboratory and Diagnostic Tests, 10th Edition. Philadelphia, PA, Wolters Kluwer Health/Lippincott Williams and Wilkins, 2018

Iyer KS, Dayal S: Modulators of platelet function in aging. Platelets 31(4):474–482, 2020

Polysomnography

Type of test	Neurophysiology
Background and explanation of test	Polysomnography is an overnight study in which multiple parameters are monitored while the patient sleeps, including electroencephalography, eye movements (measured by electro-oculogram), electrocardiography, electromyography, respiratory effort of chest and abdomen, oral/nasal airflow, and oxygen saturation. Digital data capture has simplified the detection of sleep-related events and the scoring of sleep stages and events.
	Although several disorders can be detected using polysomnography, the primary indication for this procedure is to confirm the clinical diagnosis of obstructive sleep apnea (OSA). For this purpose, apnea and hypopnea events are monitored. Apnea occurs when airflow stops for ≥10 seconds. Hypopnea occurs when airflow is reduced by ≥30% for ≥10 seconds with accompanying oxygen desaturation of ≥3%. The apnea-hypopnea index (AHI) is the sum of apneas and hypopneas per hour of sleep.
	To reduce cost and make testing more convenient, ambulatory (at-home) recording systems have been developed and are in use, but lab-based PSGs remain the gold standard. At-home testing can support but not exclude an OSA diagnosis.
Relevance to psychiatry and behavioral science	A PSG study can aid in diagnosing and characterizing several conditions that affect psychiatry patients, including nocturnal panic attacks, treatment-resistant depression in the context of sleep apnea, cognitive impairment with nocturnal desaturation, and various parasomnias. In cognitively healthy elderly patients, OSA has been shown to be associated with increased amyloid burden in follow-up.
Preparation of patient	The patient stays overnight in the sleep laboratory while undergoing monitoring. Video recording is also needed if the referring question relates to REM sleep behavior disorder or seizure. If the patient has OSA and the intention is to initiate continuous positive airway pressure (CPAP) treatment, CPAP can be used for part of the testing night to determine individual settings, although these "split-night" studies carry the risk of overestimating severity of sleep apnea in patients with mild disease.
Indications	• Evaluating sleep-disordered breathing • Confirming diagnosis of restless legs syndrome • Detecting periodic limb movements of sleep • Evaluating REM sleep behavior disorder • Confirming nocturnal seizures • Confirming nocturnal panic attacks (and excluding seizures) • Confirming other parasomnias, such as sleepwalking

Polysomnography *(continued)*

Indications *(continued)*	A PSG is also recommended for patients with a history of stroke, patients with a neuromuscular or pulmonary disorder with hypoventilation, and patients with congestive heart failure who take opioid medications.
Reference range	• Per laboratory report, normal values for sleep onset and offset times, hours of sleep, proportion of each sleep stage, and number of arousals during sleep • Absence of periodic leg movements • Oxygen saturation >90% • Absence of abnormal snoring • Absence of electrocardiographic rate and rhythm disturbances • AHI <5 apneas/hypopneas per hour in a patient with OSA symptoms (<10 per hour after age 60 years)
Critical value(s)	• Mild sleep apnea: AHI 5 to <15 • Moderate sleep apnea: AHI 15 to <30 • Severe sleep apnea: AHI ≥30
Abnormal test	• Apneas • Hypopneas • Desaturation • Disrupted sleep architecture • Abnormal leg movements • Abnormal behaviors
Interfering factors	Caffeine or other stimulants and sedative-hypnotic medications taken before testing can significantly interfere with test results.
Cross-references	**Obstructive Sleep Apnea** **Restless Legs Syndrome**

Andrade L, Paiva T: Ambulatory versus laboratory polysomnography in obstructive sleep apnea: comparative assessment of quality, clinical efficacy, treatment compliance, and quality of life. J Clin Sleep Med 14(8):1323–1331, 2018

Boulos MI, Jairam T, Kendzerska T, et al: Normal polysomnography parameters in healthy adults: a systematic review and meta-analysis. Lancet Respir Med 7(6):533–543, 2019

Kapur VK, Auckley DH, Chowdhuri S, et al: Clinical Practice Guideline for Diagnostic Testing for Adult Obstructive Sleep Apnea: an American Academy of Sleep Medicine clinical practice guideline. J Clin Sleep Med 13(3):479–504, 2017

Rouse JK, Shirley SR, Holley AB, et al: Split-night polysomnography overestimates apnea-hypopnea index in high-risk professions. Mil Med 184(5–6):e137–e140, 2019

Rundo JV, Downey R III: Polysomnography. Handb Clin Neurol 160:381–392, 2019

Sharma RA, Varga AW, Bubu OM, et al: Obstructive sleep apnea severity affects amyloid burden in cognitively normal elderly: a longitudinal study. Am J Respir Crit Care Med 197(7):933–943, 2018

Veasey SC, Rosen IM: Obstructive sleep apnea in adults. N Engl J Med 380(15):1442–1449, 2019

Positron emission tomography, brain

Type of test	Imaging, nuclear medicine
Background and explanation of test	In PET scanning, a gamma ray–emitting isotope (radionuclide) is coupled with a biologically active molecule or drug of interest, and the concentration of radionuclide activity is subsequently mapped to show the location of the coupled molecule/drug. If the coupled molecule is FDG, the scan yields information about tissue metabolic activity. Other isotopes are available for use with PET, including ^{15}O, ^{13}N, and ^{11}C, but ^{18}F coupled with glucose (FDG) is most often used in clinical scanning. ^{18}F has a long enough half-life that it is possible to produce the isotope at an off-site facility, which makes FDG more accessible to clinical imaging centers. In addition, it is less critical that the patient's mental state or activity be standardized with this isotope than with isotopes with very short half-lives, such as ^{15}O. PET scanning in clinical and research settings normally also includes anatomical imaging in the form of CT or MRI to co-register metabolic findings with anatomy.

Significant progress in the development of molecular probes over the past decade has enabled researchers to visualize brain pathology such as amyloid-β deposition, tau protein deposition, microglial activation and neuroinflammation, and synaptic density. For example, TSPO, a marker of neuroinflammation, has been found to be consistently elevated in unmedicated patients with major depression. Other insights have been gained from imaging dopaminergic, serotonergic, and other neuroreceptor functions in schizophrenia, depression, bipolar disorder, substance use disorders, eating disorders, OCD, ADHD, and autism spectrum disorder. Uniquely, PET can measure P-glycoprotein pump function in vivo, and this capability is expected to yield important insights about the blood-brain barrier in neuropsychiatric disease. |
| Relevance to psychiatry and behavioral science | Tracers for amyloid-β PET and tau PET have now been FDA approved.

Other applications of PET to neuropsychiatric diseases remain investigational. |
| Preparation of patient | Patients should follow a very-low-carbohydrate diet for 24 hours before scan and should not eat or drink anything but water for 6 hours before scan. Water should be encouraged, as much as tolerated. Routine medications should be taken. Diabetes medication should be taken no less than 4 hours before scan. |
| Indications | • Informing differential diagnosis of dementia subtypes

• Presurgical evaluation for epilepsy

• Detecting cancer

• Evaluating cardiac blood flow

• Research protocols |

Positron emission tomography, brain *(continued)*

Normal result	• Requires individual interpretation according to study protocol • In general, no abnormal accumulation of radiotracer and no unexpected gaps in visualization of tracer
Abnormal result	• Temporoparietal hypometabolism in Alzheimer's disease, often more marked in one hemisphere • Frontal or frontotemporal hypometabolism in frontal lobe dementia • Abnormal uptake reflecting deposition of amyloid and tau in neurodegenerative diseases • Increased uptake in vascular tumor • Abnormal uptake in seizure focus, dependent on time since seizure
Interfering factors	Hypoglycemia can affect glucose metabolism as imaged by FDG-PET. Movement of the patient of >1 cm can result in motion artifact.
Cross-references	**Dementia**

Cai Z, Li S, Matuskey D, et al: PET imaging of synaptic density: a new tool for investigation of neuropsychiatric diseases. Neurosci Lett 691:44–50, 2019

Coughlin JM, Horti AG, Pomper MG: Opportunities in precision psychiatry using PET neuroimaging in psychosis. Neurobiol Dis 131:104428, 2019

Gianni AD, De Donatis D, Valente S, et al: Eating disorders: do PET and SPECT have a role? A systematic review of the literature. Psychiatry Res Neuroimaging 300:111065, 2020

Hellwig S, Domschke K: Update on PET imaging biomarkers in the diagnosis of neuropsychiatric disorders. Curr Opin Neurol 32(4):539–547, 2019

Jain P, Chaney AM, Carlson ML, et al: Neuroinflammation PET imaging: current opinion and future directions. J Nucl Med 61(8):1107–1112, 2020

Leuzy A, Chiotis K, Lemoine L, et al: Tau PET imaging in neurodegenerative tauopathies: still a challenge. Mol Psychiatry 24(8):1112–1134, 2019

Meyer JH, Cervenka S, Kim, et al: Neuroinflammation in psychiatric disorders: PET imaging and promising new targets. Lancet Psychiatry 7(12):1064–1074, 2020

Mitelman SA: Transdiagnostic neuroimaging in psychiatry: a review. Psychiatry Res 277:23–38, 2019

Pagani M, Carletto S, Ostacoli L: PET and SPECT in psychiatry: the past and the future. Eur J Nucl Med Mol Imaging 46(10):1985–1987, 2019

Slough C, Masters SC, Hurley RA, Taber KH: Clinical positron emission tomography (PET) neuroimaging: advantages and limitations as a diagnostic tool. J Neuropsychiatry Clin Neurosci 28(2):A4–A71, 2016

Toyohara J: Importance of P-gp PET imaging in pharmacology. Curr Pharm Des 22(38):5830–5836, 2016

Potassium

Type of test	Blood
Background and explanation of test	Potassium is an electrolyte present in all body fluids but concentrated inside cells, where it functions to regulate water and acid-base balance, participates in nerve conduction, and stimulates contraction of muscle cells. Along with calcium and magnesium, potassium controls cardiac output (heart rate and force of contraction). Potassium is taken in from dietary sources and excreted primarily through the glomeruli of the kidneys. Mildly decreased potassium levels are common, particularly among patients treated with diuretic medications. Increased potassium levels result primarily from reduced renal function or cellular injury when intracellular potassium is released into the circulation.

Potassium can be assayed as an individual test but more often is checked as part of an electrolyte panel, renal panel, BMP, or CMP. |
Relevance to psychiatry and behavioral science	Severe hyperkalemia (high potassium) or hypokalemia (low potassium) can be life-threatening conditions requiring urgent intervention. Potassium may be increased with lithium treatment, with succinylcholine used for ECT, or in acute starvation (as in anorexia nervosa). Potassium may be decreased in chronic starvation, bulimia, psychogenic vomiting, anabolic steroid abuse, or alcohol use disorder. Patients with megaloblastic anemia treated with vitamin B_{12} or folate may become potassium depleted and thus require ongoing replacement.
Preparation of patient	Patients should avoid vigorous exercise before blood is drawn on the day of testing.
Indications	• *Symptoms of hypokalemia*: fatigue, constipation, muscle twitching, weakness, irregular heart rhythm • *Symptoms of hyperkalemia*: nausea, diarrhea, chest pain, muscle weakness, irregular heart rhythm • Admission laboratory workup • Routine component of health screening • Monitoring patients on diuretic medications • Monitoring kidney disease • Monitoring patients on dialysis or IV therapy
Reference range	3.5–5.1 mEq/L
Critical value(s)	<2 mEq/L associated with ventricular fibrillation

>7 mEq/L associated with muscular irritability (including myocardium, with peaked T waves) |

Potassium *(continued)*

Increased levels	• Renal failure, dehydration, renal obstruction, cellular injury (burns, trauma, surgery tissue ischemia, chemotherapy), intravascular hemolysis, metabolic acidosis, diabetic ketoacidosis, severe acute starvation (e.g., anorexia nervosa), status epilepticus, malignant hyperthermia, Addison's disease, rapid potassium infusion, acquired hyperkalemia (e.g., in SLE or sickle cell disease) • *Drugs:* NSAIDs, potassium-sparing diuretics, ACE inhibitors, and β-blockers
Decreased levels	• Chronic starvation, prolonged IV hydration without potassium replacement, prolonged vomiting or diarrhea, fluid loss from intestinal fistula, excessive loss of potassium in urine, loss from draining wounds, chronic heavy alcohol use, treatment of megaloblastic anemia with vitamin B_{12} or folate, cystic fibrosis • *Drugs:* corticosteroids, β-adrenergic agonists such as isoproterenol, β-adrenergic antagonists such as clonidine, antibiotics such as gentamicin and carbenicillin, and the antifungal agent amphotericin B
Interfering factors	Improper specimen handling is an important cause of spurious potassium elevation in outpatient settings in which blood must be transported to the laboratory. Regardless of setting, specimen hemolysis can be problematic. Use of a tourniquet and/or pumping the hand before drawing blood can elevate the potassium level by 20%. Patients with elevated WBC and platelet counts may also have spurious elevation of their potassium level. Some diurnal variation is seen in potassium levels, with values being 0.2–0.4 mEq/L higher in the afternoon and evening. Vigorous exercise can transiently increase potassium levels by 50%; this effect is enhanced by β-blockers.
Cross-references	**Anorexia Nervosa** **Bulimia Nervosa** **Hyperkalemia** **Hypokalemia**

American Association for Clinical Chemistry: Testing.com. Available at: https://www.testing.com. Accessed August 2021.

Dørup I: Magnesium and potassium deficiency: its diagnosis, occurrence and treatment in diuretic therapy and its consequences for growth, protein synthesis and growth factors. Acta Physiol Scand Suppl 618:1–55, 1994

Fischbach FT, Fischbach MA: A Manual of Laboratory and Diagnostic Tests, 10th Edition. Philadelphia, PA, Wolters Kluwer Health/Lippincott Williams and Wilkins, 2018

Saxena K: Clinical features and management of poisoning due to potassium chloride. Med Toxicol Adverse Drug Exp 4:429–443, 1989

Prealbumin

Type of test	Blood
Background and explanation of test	In the past, prealbumin was used as a general measure of nutritional status, but research has demonstrated that prealbumin levels reflect many other factors, including inflammation, infection, and trauma. For this reason, it is no longer recommended that prealbumin be used to detect malnutrition. The test may prove to have other uses, however; recent studies have shown the predictive value of prealbumin in diseases such as gastric cancer.
Relevance to psychiatry and behavioral science	Low prealbumin levels may be found in patients with AIDS, cancer, anorexia nervosa, and failure to thrive, but the utility of these findings is uncertain. Low prealbumin is a risk factor for development of delirium.
Preparation of patient	None needed
Indications	Specific indications to be determined.
Reference range	Adults: 18–45 mg/dL
Critical value(s)	None
Increased levels	High-dose steroids, adrenal gland hyperfunction, high-dose NSAIDs, Hodgkin's disease, shigellosis
Decreased levels	Protein-calorie undernutrition/malnutrition, inflammation, infection, trauma, hyperthyroidism, liver disease, cystic fibrosis, diabetes, protein-losing enteropathies, peritoneal dialysis, use of amiodarone or estrogens (including oral contraceptives)
Interfering factors	See discussion above.
Cross-references	None

American Association for Clinical Chemistry: Testing.com. Available at: https://www.testing.com. Accessed August 2021.

Hong Y, Seese L, Hickey G, et al: Preoperative prealbumin does not impact outcomes after left ventricular assist device implantation. J Card Surg 35(5):1029–1036, 2020

Zhang Z, Pereira SL, Luo M, Matheson EM: Evaluation of blood biomarkers associated with risk of malnutrition in older adults: a systematic review and meta-analysis. Nutrients 9(8):829, 2017

Zu H, Wang H, Li C, Xue Y: Preoperative prealbumin levels on admission as an independent predictive factor in patients with gastric cancer. Medicine (Baltimore) 99(11):e19196, 2020

Prolactin

Type of test	Blood
Background and explanation of test	Prolactin is an anterior pituitary hormone that functions primarily to promote lactation. Levels are normally high throughout pregnancy and just after childbirth and are then maintained at high levels by breastfeeding. The hormone is present in low concentrations in males and in nonpregnant females. Prolactin release from the pituitary is regulated at the level of the hypothalamus. Dopamine inhibits prolactin production, and when dopamine receptor antagonists are given, significant elevations can result. Other causes of elevation include pituitary tumors known as prolactinomas, epileptic seizures, and anorexia nervosa. Low prolactin levels can be found in conditions affecting the anterior pituitary, including craniopharyngiomas, tuberculosis, histoplasmosis, sarcoidosis, hemochromatosis, and a range of autoimmune conditions.
	In females, high prolactin levels are associated with low estrogen levels, amenorrhea, infertility, galactorrhea, painful sexual intercourse, reduced bone mineral density, and hirsutism. In males, high levels are associated with decreased libido, erectile dysfunction, infertility, and abnormal lack of body and facial hair. Headaches, visual impairment, and other hormonal deficiencies can be seen with pituitary tumors that compress surrounding tissues. Low prolactin levels normally do not require treatment.
Relevance to psychiatry and behavioral science	Serum prolactin levels can help to distinguish generalized tonic-clonic and complex partial seizures from psychogenic nonepileptic seizures. For this purpose, blood is drawn 10–20 minutes after the event, and a baseline level is checked the following day for comparison. A twofold or greater increase in prolactin associated with the event is characteristic of a true seizure. The gold standard for this differential diagnosis is video electroencephalography, but this technology is not universally available.
	First-generation antipsychotics, risperidone, and paliperidone are well known to cause serum prolactin elevations, with associated symptoms in patients. Aripiprazole and ziprasidone are thought to be relatively free of this effect. Other psychotropics that cause elevation include TCAs, the SSRIs citalopram and escitalopram, and other drugs listed below in the *Increased Levels* section.
Preparation of patient	Ideally, the blood sample is drawn 3–4 hours after morning awakening. For use in diagnosing epileptic seizures, the test sample is drawn 10–20 minutes after the suspected ictal event, and a baseline sample is drawn >6 hours after the event, often on the following day.
Indications	• Workup of suspected prolactin elevation based on clinical symptoms • Monitoring effects of antipsychotic and selected antidepressant drug therapy

Prolactin *(continued)*

Indications *(continued)*	• Distinguishing generalized tonic-clonic or complex partial seizures from psychogenic nonepileptic seizures • Determining cause of infertility and/or erectile dysfunction • Evaluating anterior pituitary function (with other hormones) • Follow-up of low testosterone level • Monitoring effectiveness of treatment for prolactinoma • Detecting recurrence of prolactinoma
Reference range	Nonpregnant adult females: <25 ng/mL Pregnant females: 80–400 ng/mL Adult males: <20 ng/mL
Critical value(s)	Level of >200 ng/mL in nonlactating females may indicate presence of a prolactinoma, although a normal level does not rule out prolactinoma. High levels may result from antipsychotic or other drug treatments.
Increased levels	• Prolactinoma • Pregnancy • Nursing • Hypothalamic disease • Hypothyroidism • Kidney disease • Other pituitary tumors and diseases • Polycystic ovary syndrome • Recent seizure • Cocaine withdrawal • *Drugs:* antipsychotics, other dopamine-blocking drugs (e.g., prochlorperazine, metoclopramide), TCAs, SSRIs, MAOIs, ramelteon, buspirone, alprazolam, morphine, estrogen, and herbal drugs (e.g., red clover, fenugreek, fennel)
Decreased levels	• Hypopituitarism • *Drugs:* dopamine, levodopa, ergot alkaloid derivatives
Interfering factors	Stress from illness, trauma, low blood sugar, strenuous exercise, or needle phobia can cause moderate increases in prolactin levels. Time of sample can affect results: levels rise during sleep and peak in early morning hours. Prolactin can form macromolecular complexes with IgG, leading to false-positive test results.
Cross-references	**Seizures**

Prolactin *(continued)*

American Association for Clinical Chemistry: Testing.com. Available at: https://www.testing.com. Accessed August 2021.

Park YM: Serum prolactin levels in patients with major depressive disorder receiving selective serotonin-reuptake inhibitor monotherapy for 3 months: a prospective study. Psychiatry Investig 14(3):368–371, 2017

Richa V, Rahul G, Sarika A: Macroprolactin: a frequent cause of misdiagnosed hyperprolactinemia in clinical practice. J Reprod Infertil 11(3):161–167, 2010

Torre DL, Falorni A: Pharmacological causes of hyperprolactinemia. Ther Clin Risk Manag 3(5):929–951, 2007

University of California San Francisco Health: Prolactin blood test. Medical Tests, August 19, 2018. Available at: https://www.ucsfhealth.org/medical-tests/prolactin-blood-test. Accessed August 2021.

Prostate-specific antigen (PSA)

Type of test	Blood
Background and explanation of test	PSA is a protein found in both normal prostate epithelial cells and prostate cancer cells that can be measured in the blood in both free and bound forms. The sum of the two forms—the total PSA—is variably increased in prostate carcinoma, hyperplasia, and inflammation and with leakage of prostatic fluid into the circulation. Use of PSA testing to detect clinically significant cancer has been a topic of controversy over several decades. The low sensitivity and specificity of the test has resulted in both missed diagnoses and overdiagnoses, the latter associated with morbidity from unnecessary biopsy and surgery. Attempts have been made to improve the test using PSA density and PSA change measures such as velocity and doubling time, but there is little agreement that these refinements have been successful.
	Where PSA testing has been discouraged, both advanced-stage diagnosis and mortality from prostate cancer have increased. Even so, consensus is lacking as to how to risk-stratify individual males for MRI study and biopsy. Detailed guidelines have recently been published by the European Association of Urology, noted in the reference list below.
	The American Cancer Society makes the following recommendations: males should be informed about the uncertainties, risks, and potential benefits of prostate cancer screening and then decide whether to be screened, in consultation with their health care provider. This discussion should take place at age 50 for males at average risk of prostate cancer who are expected to live another 10 years or longer. It should take place at age 45 for those at high risk, including Black males and those with a first-degree relative diagnosed at an early age (before age 65) with prostate cancer. It should take place at age 40 for males with more than one first-degree relative diagnosed at an early age. If testing is negative, retesting should take place every 2 years for those with a PSA level <2.5 ng/mL and yearly for those with a level ≥2.5 ng/mL.
Relevance to psychiatry and behavioral science	Psychiatrists who provide primary care for patients age ≥40 years need to be informed about the appropriate use of PSA testing and the interpretation of test results.
Preparation of patient	Blood sample should be collected prior to digital rectal exam and prior to prostate biopsy. Patients should avoid ejaculation and vigorous exercise in 48 hours before test.
Indications	• Screening for prostate cancer, as described above • Selecting patients for prostate biopsy or MRI • Workup for males with signs/symptoms suggestive of prostate cancer • Monitoring effectiveness of treatment for prostate cancer • Detecting recurrence of prostate cancer

Prostate-specific antigen (PSA) *(continued)*

Reference range	Age 40–49 years: 0.0–2.5 ng/mL
	Age 50–59 years: 0.0–3.5 ng/mL
	Age 60–69 years: 0.0–4.5 ng/mL
	Age 70–79 years: 0.0–6.5 ng/mL
	A single elevated PSA level should be confirmed with a second test several weeks later, before biopsy or other testing.
Critical value(s)	Total PSA levels >10 ng/mL indicate high risk of prostate cancer.
Increased levels	• Prostate cancer • Prostatic hypertrophy • Prostatic inflammation • Leakage of prostate fluid into circulation
Decreased levels	Not applicable
Interfering factors	PSA levels increase with age. In the absence of disease, Black males may have mildly to moderately increased PSA levels. Palpation of prostate on digital rectal exam increases PSA level. Both ejaculation and vigorous exercise involving the pelvis (e.g., cycling) may transiently increase PSA levels. High doses of chemotherapeutic drugs, such as cyclophosphamide and methotrexate, may increase or reduce PSA.
Cross-references	None

American Association for Clinical Chemistry: Testing.com. Available at: https://www.testing.com. Accessed September 2021.

Eyrich NW, Morgan TM, Tosoian JJ: Biomarkers for detection of clinically significant prostate cancer: contemporary clinical data and future directions. Transl Androl Urol 10(7):3091–3103, 2021

Fischbach FT, Fischbach MA: A Manual of Laboratory and Diagnostic Tests, 10th Edition. Philadelphia, PA, Wolters Kluwer Health/Lippincott Williams and Wilkins, 2018

Haverfield EV, Esplin ED, Aguilar SJ, et al: Physician-directed genetic screening to evaluate personal risk for medically actionable disorders: a large multi-center cohort study. BMC Med 19(1):199, 2021

Van Poppel H, Roobol MJ, Chapple CR, et al: Prostate-specific antigen testing as part of a risk-adapted early detection strategy for prostate cancer: European Association of Urology position and recommendations for 2021. Eur Urol 80(6):703–711, 2021

Protein, serum

Type of test	Blood
Background and explanation of test	Proteins have critical roles in the body as enzymes, hormones, and transporters and as constituents of cells, tissues, and organs. Two classes of protein are measured in blood: albumin and globulins. *Albumin*, which represents 60% of total protein, functions to maintain colloidal osmotic pressure within the vasculature and to transport drugs, hormones, and enzymes. It is produced in the liver, and its level can be dramatically reduced by liver disease, such as cirrhosis. The serum albumin level can also be reduced in kidney disease, when the nephron is no longer able to prevent loss of albumin in the urine. *Globulins* include antibodies, enzymes, and other essential proteins. Although measurement of total protein aids in the evaluation of nutritional status and can be helpful in screening for liver or kidney disease, it is more useful to know which component—albumin or globulins—is present in abnormal concentration.
Relevance to psychiatry and behavioral science	Total protein may be low in anorexia nervosa, failure to thrive in elderly patients, alcohol use disorder, and liver disease and postoperatively. Low protein values are frequently encountered among patients on medical/surgical units in the general hospital and represent a risk factor for the development of delirium. It is a commonly held misconception that a low protein level and correspondingly low protein binding of drugs result in increased drug action. In fact, reduced protein binding of drugs has little clinical effect, even among elderly patients. Unbound drug is available not only for distribution to the target organ but also for metabolism and excretion. What lowered protein binding does affect is the interpretation of the laboratory measurement of the total drug concentration; it is of potential concern that patients might develop symptoms of toxicity at apparently therapeutic drug levels when protein levels are low.
Preparation of patient	None needed
Indications	• Component of CMP • Evaluating nutritional status • Workup of signs/symptoms of liver or kidney disease • Evaluating edema
Reference range	6.0–8.0 g/dL
Critical value(s)	≤3 g/dL or ≥12 g/dL
Increased levels	• Dehydration • Viral infection (e.g., HIV, hepatitis B or C) • Multiple myeloma, other gammopathies • Waldenström's macroglobulinemia

Protein, serum _(continued)_

Increased levels _(continued)_	• Granulomatous diseases such as sarcoidosis • Collagen vascular diseases such as SLE and rheumatoid arthritis • Chronic inflammatory states • Chronic infections
Decreased levels	• Malnutrition • Malabsorption (celiac disease, inflammatory bowel disease) • Chronic or severe diarrhea • Postoperative state • Liver disease • Alcohol use disorder • Kidney disease • Burns, severe skin diseases • Protein-losing enteropathy or uropathy • Severe hemorrhage, with volume replacement • Heart failure • Hypothyroidism • Prolonged immobilization • Third trimester of pregnancy
Interfering factors	Spurious elevation in protein can be caused by specimen hemolysis, prolonged tourniquet application, or use of drugs such as anabolic steroids, androgens, corticosteroids, dextran, growth hormone, insulin, phenazopyridine, or progesterone. Spurious decrease in protein can be caused by sampling proximal to an IV catheter, massive infusion of crystalloid solution, or use of drugs such as ammonium ion, estrogen, or oral contraceptives.
Cross-references	**Albumin** **Anorexia Nervosa** **Cerebrospinal Fluid Protein** **Cirrhosis** **Comprehensive Metabolic Panel** **Urine Protein**

American Association for Clinical Chemistry: Testing.com. Available at: https://www.testing.com. Accessed September 2021.

Fuhrman MP, Charney P, Mueller CM: Hepatic proteins and nutrition assessment. J Am Diet Assoc 104:1258–1264, 2004

Jacobson SA, Pies RW, Katz IR: Clinical Manual of Geriatric Psychopharmacology. Washington, DC, American Psychiatric Publishing, 2007

Pyridoxine (vitamin B$_6$) level

Type of test	Blood
Background and explanation of test	Pyridoxine is a water-soluble vitamin and essential nutrient involved as a coenzyme in a large number of reactions regulating the metabolism of proteins, glucose, lipids, DNA, and neurotransmitters. It also has antioxidant and immune system functions. Research to date suggests that this vitamin has a role in processes as varied as cognitive decline in older adults, cancer risk, cardiovascular disease, late luteal phase dysphoric disorder, and morning sickness in pregnancy.
	Food sources of pyridoxine include fish, organ meats, beef, poultry, potatoes and other starchy vegetables, fortified cereals, and fruits other than citrus. Risk of deficiency is higher in pregnancy, in obese individuals, and in those with alcohol use disorder, malabsorption syndromes, impaired renal function, and autoimmune disorders such as rheumatoid arthritis and inflammatory bowel disease. In addition, certain antiepileptic drugs used in psychiatric practice increase the breakdown of pyridoxine, potentially causing deficiency; this is discussed in the following section.
	Adequacy of pyridoxine levels can be measured directly by testing for pyridoxal 5' phosphate, one of the vitamin's active forms. Values outside the reference range noted below are of potential concern because both deficiency and toxicity are seen. Deficiency is associated with dermatitis, cheilosis, glossitis, anemia, EEG abnormalities, depression, confusion, and poor immune system function. Toxicity, resulting from ≥1 g of oral pyridoxine daily for ≥12 months, can cause a severe, progressive sensory neuropathy with marked ataxia. Other toxic symptoms include photosensitivity, nausea, heartburn, and serious dermatological lesions.
Relevance to psychiatry and behavioral science	As noted above, pyridoxine levels outside the reference range are associated with depression, confusion, EEG abnormalities, and ataxia. Antiepileptic drugs known to increase the breakdown of pyridoxine include valproate, carbamazepine, and phenytoin.
Preparation of patient	8-hour or overnight fast is required.
Indications	Clinical suspicion of pyridoxine deficiency
Reference range	5–50 ng/mL
Critical value(s)	Deficiency: <5 ng/mL
	Toxicity: >50 ng/mL
Increased levels	Excessive supplementation
Decreased levels	• Pregnancy • Obesity • Alcohol use disorder • Autoimmune disorders • Cirrhosis

Pyridoxine (vitamin B₆) level *(continued)*

Decreased levels *(continued)*	• Hyperthyroidism
	• Malnutrition, eating disorders
	• Malabsorption
	• Chronic kidney disease
	• Congestive heart failure
	• *Drugs that antagonize pyridoxine or cause increased requirements*: TCAs, antiepileptic drugs, cycloserine, disulfiram, isoniazid, penicillamine, hydralazine, estrogens (including birth control pills), and theophylline
Interfering factors	Levels decrease with age, although age norms have not been published.
	Specimen handling affects results; the specimen must be received in the lab within 30 minutes of collection. Prolonged light exposure invalidates the results.
Cross-references	**Pyridoxine Deficiency**

ARUP Laboratories: Vitamin B₆ (pyridoxal 5-phosphate), in Lab Test Directory. Salt Lake City, UT, ARUP Laboratories, 2021. Available at: https://www.aruplab.com/Tests/Pub/0080111. Accessed September 2021.

Minovic I, Kieneker LM, Gansevoort RT, et al: Vitamin B₆, inflammation, and cardiovascular outcome in a population-based cohort: the Prevention of Renal and Vascular End-Stage Disease (PREVEND) study. Nutrients 12(9):2711, 2020

National Institutes of Health Office of Dietary Supplements: Vitamin B6: Fact Sheet for Health Professionals. Bethesda, MD, National Institutes of Health, 2021. Available at: https://ods.od.nih.gov/factsheets/VitaminB6-HealthProfessional. Accessed September 2021.

Odai T, Terauchi M, Suzuki R, et al: Depressive symptoms in middle-aged and elderly women are associated with a low intake of vitamin B6: a cross-sectional study. Nutrients 12(11):3437, 2020

Peterson CT, Rodionov DA, Osterman AL, Peterson SN: B vitamins and their role in immune regulation and cancer. Nutrients 12(11):3380, 2020

Romoli M, Perucca E, Sen A: Pyridoxine supplementation for levetiracetam-related neuropsychiatric adverse events: a systematic review. Epilepsy Behav 103(Pt A):106861, 2020

Schorgg P, Bärnighausen T, Rohrmann S, et al: Vitamin B₆ status among vegetarians: findings from a population-based survey. Nutrients 13(5):1627, 2021

Quantitative electroencephalogram (qEEG)

Type of test	Neurophysiology
Background and explanation of test	The qEEG represents a refinement and extension of conventional electroencephalography made possible by the introduction of digital data capture. The patient interface for a qEEG is the same as for an EEG, with the 10–20 electrode placement system used for both. qEEG can process raw EEG data to create new parameters, such as absolute and relative power in different frequency bands, spectral edge frequency, and signal coherence. Although qEEG has in the past been used largely in research settings, most new clinical EEG systems are now digital, with at least the theoretical potential to generate more sophisticated responses to referring questions. Digital systems retain the ability to generate analog displays of EEG data in real time, so that visual examination ("reading") can still take place as a check on qEEG findings. Digital systems can also generate spatial displays of data, often superimposed on an outline of the brain ("brain maps"). Depending on the referring question, qEEG may be analyzed and reported as numerical data, a series of brain maps, or a real-time tracing that includes activation procedures (hyperventilation and photic stimulation). Moreover, for conditions with persistent (nonperiodic) EEG correlates such as delirium, it would be possible to capture only a few seconds of qEEG for analysis, making this a preferred modality for patients who are unable to cooperate.
Relevance to psychiatry and behavioral science	See discussion in the **Electroencephalogram** entry. With qEEG, additional information can be obtained that allows three-dimensional dipole localization in seizure evaluation. In research settings, other data obtained include coherence of electrical signals among brain areas, providing a measure of functional connectivity that is particularly useful in the study of cognitive tasks and state changes.
Preparation of patient	Patients may need reassurance that qEEG only records electrical activity and does not deliver an electrical stimulus. The process of electrode application should be explained; application often includes use of collodion, an adhesive gel that requires vigorous cleansing for removal. Patients should avoid sedatives before testing. Sleep deprivation may be needed to ensure an adequate sleep sample is obtained (e.g., in the case of suspected seizures). Sleep deprivation protocol is to awaken the patient at 4:00 A.M. and then keep the patient awake without naps or stimulants until the time of testing.
Indications	• Detecting presence of epileptiform or ictal activity • Confirming diagnosis of delirium and monitoring course of delirium (serial studies) • Evaluating suspected functional neurological symptom presentations • Various research applications See **Electroencephalogram** entry for other indications.

Quantitative electroencephalogram (qEEG) *(continued)*

Reference range	• Alpha power (absolute and relative) highest over occipital areas; symmetric • No appreciable slow-wave (delta or theta) power in wakefulness • Other reference values per laboratory report
Critical value(s)	None
Abnormal test findings	• Increased delta and theta power in a generalized distribution may be consistent with delirium or medication effects. • Reduced alpha power in occipital areas may be consistent with dementia or medication effects. • Increased beta activity may be consistent with anxiety or sedative-hypnotic use or withdrawal. • Reduced coherence may indicate areas of neuronal loss or injury.
Interfering factors	Motion artifacts from eye movements may introduce delta power to frontotemporal areas. Muscle activity may introduce beta power. An EEG study that does not explicitly produce and document alerting stimuli for a patient with a depressed level of consciousness (e.g., suspected delirium) is considered incomplete. Many psychotropic drugs affect the EEG, usually introducing either slow-wave power (e.g., antipsychotics or mood stabilizers) or beta power (e.g., sedative-hypnotics or alcohol).
Cross-references	**Delirium** **Electroencephalogram**

Red blood cell (RBC) count

Type of test	Blood
Background and explanation of test	RBCs are the most numerous blood cells in the circulation. They are formed in bone marrow and have a life cycle of ~120 days. These cells function to carry hemoglobin bound to oxygen from the lungs to tissues and carbon dioxide from the tissues to the lungs.
Relevance to psychiatry and behavioral science	A low RBC count is associated with symptoms of fatigue, weakness, somnolence, anhedonia, and depression.
Preparation of patient	Fasting is not required. Patients should avoid dehydration and overhydration. Signs of severe anemia should be noted before blood is drawn. Note on requisition if the patient is receiving IV fluids.
Indications	• Routine component of CBC • Clinical suspicion of anemia or polycythemia
Reference range	Adult males: $4.5–5.5 \times 10^6/mm^3$ Adult females: $4.0–5.0 \times 10^6/mm^3$
Critical value(s)	None
Increased levels	*Primary erythrocytosis (increase in RBCs)* • Polycythemia vera (a myeloproliferative disorder) • Erythremic erythrocytosis (increased RBC production in bone marrow) *Secondary erythrocytosis* • Renal disease • Extrarenal tumors • High altitude • Pulmonary disease • Cardiovascular disease • Alveolar hypoventilation • Hemoglobinopathy • Tobacco use, carboxyhemoglobin *Relative erythrocytosis (decreased plasma volume)* • Dehydration (from vomiting, diarrhea) • Gaisböck syndrome
Decreased levels	• Anemia secondary to RBC destruction, blood loss, or dietary insufficiency of iron or vitamins essential to RBC production • Lymphoma, leukemia, or multiple myeloma • Hemorrhage • Chronic disease or infection • SLE, Addison's disease, rheumatic fever, and other diseases

Red blood cell (RBC) count *(continued)*

Interfering factors	Blood collection technique significantly affects the results. If the patient is recumbent during phlebotomy, the cell count is 5% lower. Results are elevated with prolonged venous stasis during phlebotomy. Lavender tube must be three-fourths full or the results will be invalid. A clotted sample will yield invalid results.
	Many psychotropic medications can cause spurious reductions in RBC count, including amitriptyline, amphetamine, barbiturates, bupropion, carbamazepine, chlordiazepoxide, chlorpromazine, clomipramine, clonazepam, desipramine, diphenhydramine, donepezil, fluphenazine, haloperidol, levodopa, MAOIs, meprobamate, mesoridazine, pemoline, phenobarbital, phenytoin, thioridazine, thiothixene, trazodone, and trifluoperazine.
Cross-references	**Anemia**
	Complete Blood Count
	Hematocrit
	Mean Corpuscular Volume

American Association for Clinical Chemistry: Testing.com. Available at: https://www.testing.com. Accessed September 2021.

Fischbach FT, Fischbach MA: A Manual of Laboratory and Diagnostic Tests, 10th Edition. Philadelphia, PA, Wolters Kluwer Health/Lippincott Williams and Wilkins, 2018

Renal function panel

Type of test	Blood
Background and explanation of test	The renal or kidney function panel consists of the following tests: albumin, BUN, calcium, total carbon dioxide, chloride, creatinine, glucose, phosphate, potassium, and sodium. A calculated anion gap value is often included.
	Risk factors for acute renal disease include a history of trauma, sepsis, hypotension, and reaction to contrast dye. Risk factors for chronic renal disease include hypertension, diabetes, atherosclerosis, familial kidney disease, polycystic kidneys, and use of nephrotoxic medications such as NSAIDs.
Relevance to psychiatry and behavioral science	Impaired renal function is associated with a range of neuropsychiatric symptoms, from fatigue and lethargy to delirium and coma. Cognitive impairment, sleep and appetite disturbances, and sexual dysfunction have also been reported.
	Because most psychotropic drugs are excreted at least partly by the kidneys, changes in renal function have definite pharmacokinetic effects. Lithium is eliminated only through the kidneys, such that the serum level is directly proportional to the GFR. Lithium and other drugs, such as gabapentin, can in turn affect kidney function. Lithium is associated with diabetes insipidus and, with long-term use, can cause tubulointerstitial disease. Use of lithium necessitates renal function monitoring, as described in the *Psychotropic Medications* chapter.
Preparation of patient	None needed
Indications	• Workup for a patient with risk factors for acute or chronic kidney disease • Monitoring a patient with diabetes for early renal dysfunction
Reference range	See entries for individual tests.
Critical value(s)	See entries for individual tests.
Increased levels	See entries for individual tests.
Decreased levels	See entries for individual tests.
Interfering factors	See entries for individual tests.
Cross-references	**Diabetes Insipidus** **Lithium** **Uremic Syndrome** See entries for component tests.

American Association for Clinical Chemistry: Testing.com. Available at: https://www.testing.com. Accessed September 2021.

ARUP Laboratories: Renal function panel, in Lab Test Directory. Salt Lake City, UT, ARUP Laboratories, 2021. Available at: https://ltd.aruplab.com/Tests/Pub/0020144. Accessed September 2021.

Reticulocyte count

Type of test	Blood
Background and explanation of test	Reticulocytes are immature RBCs formed in bone marrow that mature in the circulation, usually within 1–2 days. These cells provide one measure of the effectiveness of RBC production (erythropoiesis). The reticulocyte count is expressed as a percentage of the total RBC count.
	A better index of RBC production is the reticulocyte production index (RPI), which corrects for anemia and the premature shift of more immature reticulocytes from bone marrow to blood. The RPI is calculated using the following equation: $$RPI = \% \text{ reticulocytes} \times (\text{patient's hematocrit}/45) \times (1/\text{maturation time})$$ The maturation time varies with hematocrit; 45%=1 day, 35%=1.5 days, 25%=2.0 days, 15%=2.5 days. The RPI should increase with anemia; failure to increase suggests an inadequate bone marrow response.
Relevance to psychiatry and behavioral science	Reticulocyte count is decreased in alcohol use disorder and megaloblastic anemia (e.g., with vitamin B_{12} or folate deficiency).
Preparation of patient	None needed
Indications	• Diagnosing cause of anemia: bone marrow failure vs. bleeding or hemolysis • Monitoring effectiveness of treatment for anemia (pernicious anemia, folate deficiency, or iron deficiency) • Evaluating bone marrow recovery in aplastic anemia • Determining effects of radiation on bone marrow
Reference range	In the presence of anemia, an RPI >2 suggests effective bone marrow response.
Critical value(s)	None
Increased levels	• Posthemorrhage • Hemolytic anemia • After treatment of anemia
Decreased levels	• Iron deficiency anemia • Aplastic anemia • Pernicious anemia • Anemia of chronic disease • Radiation therapy • Bone marrow failure (e.g., from cancer) • Myelodysplastic syndromes • Alcohol use disorder

Reticulocyte count *(continued)*

Interfering factors	Improper specimen collection or handling may invalidate the results; this includes drawing blood after a recent transfusion or proximal to an IV catheter, or a hemolyzed sample.
	Drugs causing spurious elevations include antipyretics, chloroquine, levodopa, quinine, and sulfonamides.
	Drugs causing spurious reductions include several chemotherapeutic agents and sulfonamides.
Cross-references	**Anemia**
	Red Blood Cell Count

American Association for Clinical Chemistry: Testing.com. Available at: https://www.testing.com. Accessed September 2021.

Fischbach FT, Fischbach MA: A Manual of Laboratory and Diagnostic Tests, 10th Edition. Philadelphia, PA, Wolters Kluwer Health/Lippincott Williams and Wilkins, 2018

Serotonin transporter polymorphism

Type of test	Genetic
Background and explanation of test	The serotonin transporter terminates the actions of serotonin in the synaptic cleft by reuptake of this neurotransmitter into the presynaptic terminal where serotonin is recycled. The gene encoding the serotonin transporter is member 4 of solute carrier family 6, known by the shorthand *SLC6A4*. In humans, this gene is located on chromosome 17 (17q11). Among polymorphisms identified for this gene is a 44-base-pair insertion/deletion sequence in the promoter region known as 5-HTTLPR. Individuals with a deletion (the short or S allele) have a lower rate of serotonin transporter transcription than those with an insertion (the long or L allele). One clinical consequence of this difference is that individuals with the S allele, having lower transporter density on the presynaptic neuron, have fewer sites for drugs such as SSRIs to bind and would likely have a reduced response to treatment with these drugs.
	At this writing, *SLC6A4* 5-HTTLPR has been established as cost-effective in predicting efficacy and adverse effects with SSRI treatment, as noted below. Other polymorphisms in the serotonin transporter (e.g., rs25531 SNP) are under investigation to determine their clinical utility.
Relevance to psychiatry and behavioral science	The short or S allele confers an elevated risk of developing a major depressive episode after exposure to an adverse life event. This effect may be most pronounced early in the lifetime course of the illness. The S allele may also predict a poor outcome with antidepressant medication treatment, including delayed response, increased adverse effects, and/or induction of mania or rapid cycling in a patient with bipolar disease. It appears that these effects are seen mostly with purely serotonergic drugs such as SSRIs, so affected patients may be better treated with non-SSRI antidepressant drugs such as SNRIs or TCAs. The S allele is most common among Asians and Whites of European descent and least common among sub-Saharan Africans.
Preparation of patient	None needed
Indications	• Depression in a young patient of high-risk ethnicity • Depression in a patient with history of childhood abuse or neglect • Depression in a patient with serious recent life adversity • Question of bipolarity in a depressed patient awaiting treatment • Treatment-resistant depression
Positive test	Deletion identified (one or two S alleles)
Negative test	No deletion identified (two L alleles)
Interfering factors	None known
Cross-references	**Major Depressive Disorder**

Serotonin transporter polymorphism *(continued)*

Bradley P, Shiekh M, Mehra V, et al: Improved efficacy with targeted pharmacogenetic-guided treatment of patients with depression and anxiety: a randomized clinical trial demonstrating clinical utility. J Psychiatr Res 96:100–107, 2018

Le-Niculescu H, Roseberry K, Gill SS, et al: Precision medicine for mood disorders: objective assessment, risk prediction, pharmacogenomics, and repurposed drugs. Mol Psychiatry 26(7):2776–2804, 2021

Luddington NS, Mandadapu A, Husk M, et al: Clinical implications of genetic variation in the serotonin transporter promoter region: a review. Prim Care Companion J Clin Psychiatry 11(3):93–102, 2009

Oz MD, Baskak B, Uckun Z, et al: Association between serotonin 2A receptor (HTR2A), serotonin transporter (SLC6A4) and brain-derived neurotrophic factor (BDNF) gene polymorphisms and citalopram/sertraline induced sexual dysfunction in MDD patients. Pharmacogenomics J 20:443–450, 2020

Plenge P, Yang D, Salomon K, et al: The antidepressant drug vilazodone is an allosteric inhibitor of the serotonin transporter. Nat Commun 12(1):5063, 2021

Svensson JE, Svanborg C, Plavén-Sigray P, et al: Serotonin transporter availability increases in patients recovering from a depressive episode. Transl Psychiatry 11(1):264, 2021

Single-photon emission computed tomography

Type of test	Nuclear medicine
Background and explanation of test	SPECT brain scanning is a nuclear medicine procedure that evaluates cerebral blood flow, which is understood to reflect neuronal activity. A lipophilic radiopharmaceutical such as technetium-labeled hexamethylpropyleneamine oxime (99mTc-HMPAO) or ethylene cysteine diethylester (99mTc-ECD) is injected intravenously, and the labeled compound crosses the blood-brain barrier while continuing to emit gamma rays. An array of gamma-detecting cameras captures cerebral perfusion patterns in three dimensions. Molecular imaging is also made possible by injection of radiopharmaceuticals such as ioflupane ^{123}I, which binds to dopamine transporters and aids in the differential diagnosis of Parkinson's disease (PD).
	The SPECT procedure is like PET scanning, although the resulting contrast and spatial resolution have in the past been inferior to PET. Improvements in SPECT technology involving multiheaded gamma detectors have pushed the limits of resolution into the same range as PET. Moreover, SPECT is much less costly than PET, and the equipment is more readily available in clinical settings. SPECT is also less problematic for claustrophobic patients because the equipment is less confining. As with PET, SPECT is often performed in tandem with structural imaging such as CT or MRI.
Relevance to psychiatry and behavioral science	Indications for SPECT are like those for PET, although SPECT has been less studied and less validated than PET for psychiatric applications. Use of SPECT was constrained in the past because of its inability to investigate brain structures smaller than 1 cm. Despite this limitation, numerous studies have already demonstrated the utility of SPECT in distinguishing psychogenic nonepileptic seizures from epileptic seizures, in the differential diagnosis of dementia, in the evaluation of TBI, and in other neuropsychiatric conditions. It may be that the radiological tradition of reporting only hypoperfusion will have to be revisited for psychiatric applications, because several conditions have been found to involve increased regional blood flow.
Preparation of patient	Patients should eat before the procedure and take medications as usual but should avoid caffeine, nicotine, and alcohol. In addition, they should avoid drinking large amounts of liquid because of the need to remain still while the scan takes place. If sedation is needed, administer after tracer is injected.
Indications	• Distinguishing seizure from psychogenic nonepileptic seizure • Localizing epileptic foci before surgery • Diagnosing encephalitis • Detecting toxic encephalopathy (with global perfusion deficit) • Informing differential diagnosis of dementia subtypes

Single-photon emission computed tomography *(continued)*

Indications *(continued)*	• Detecting and evaluating cerebrovascular disease • Evaluating suspected TBI • Distinguishing PD from other movement disorders • Informing differential diagnosis of ADHD (controversial)
Normal result	Normal blood flow patterns
Abnormal result	• Globally reduced blood flow • Regionally or focally reduced blood flow • Focally increased blood flow
Interfering factors	Clinical value of SPECT scanning depends to a large extent on interpreter expertise. A commonly seen false-positive finding is crossed cerebellar diaschisis, in which reduced cerebellar blood flow is seen contralateral to supratentorial lesion, such as an infarct.
Cross-references	**Positron Emission Tomography, Brain**

Amen DG, Trujillo M, Newberg A, et al: Brain SPECT imaging in complex psychiatric cases: an evidence-based, underutilized tool. Open Neuroimag J 5:40–48, 2011

Fond G, Garosi A, Faugere M, et al: Peripheral inflammation is associated with brain SPECT perfusion changes in schizophrenia. Eur J Nucl Med Mol Imaging 49(3):905–912, 2022

Gallucci-Neto J, Brunoni AR, Ono CR, et al: Ictal SPECT in psychogenic nonepileptic and epileptic seizures. J Acad Consult Liaison Psychiatry 62(1):29–37, 2021

Henderson TA, Cohen P, van Lierop M, et al: A reckoning to keep doing what we are already doing with PET and SPECT functional neuroimaging. Am J Psychiatry 177(7):637–638, 2020

Miyagawa T, Przybelski SA, Maltais D, et al: The value of multimodal imaging with ^{123}I-FP-CIT SPECT in differential diagnosis of dementia with Lewy bodies and Alzheimer's disease dementia. Neurobiol Aging 99:11–18, 2021

Pagani M, Carletto S, Ostacoli L: PET and SPECT in psychiatry: the past and the future. Eur J Nucl Med Mol Imaging 46(10):1985–1987, 2019

Peitl V, Badžim VA, Šiško Markoš I, et al: Improvements of frontotemporal cerebral blood flow and cognitive functioning in patients with first episode of schizophrenia treated with long-acting aripiprazole. J Clin Psychopharmacol 41(6):638–643, 2021

Richieri R, Boyer L, Faget-Agius C, et al: Determinants of brain SPECT perfusion and connectivity in treatment-resistant depression. Psychiatry Res 231(2):134–140, 2015

Sodium

Type of test	Blood
Background and explanation of test	Sodium is the most abundant positively charged ion in the blood and has critical roles in neurotransmission, maintenance of osmotic pressure, and maintenance of acid-base balance. The sodium level reflects dietary intake less renal excretion, and a normal level is maintained through the actions of several hormones: aldosterone, which decreases renal sodium loss, natriuretic hormone, which increases renal sodium loss, and antidiuretic hormone (ADH), which increases resorption of water. As free body water increases or decreases, these hormones stimulate the kidney to compensate to restore sodium balance. In clinical practice, sodium levels are obtained to evaluate electrolytes, acid-base balance, water balance, water intoxication, and dehydration.
Relevance to psychiatry and behavioral science	Serum sodium abnormalities are found in several conditions seen in psychiatric practice, including polydipsia, lithium-induced diabetes insipidus, SIAD, beer potomania, and hypopituitarism. Drugs of abuse (e.g., amphetamines, Ecstasy, bath salts) can cause a life-threatening hyponatremia from increased ADH secretion, diaphoresis, and polydipsia. Psychotropic drugs associated with sodium derangements include antidepressants (e.g., SSRIs, TCAs), second-generation antipsychotics (e.g., aripiprazole, clozapine, olanzapine, risperidone, ziprasidone), carbamazepine, oxcarbazepine, lithium, phenothiazines, and opioids. Geriatric practitioners should be aware that age is a significant risk factor for hyponatremia, which is often associated with medications, SIAD, or endocrinopathy.
Preparation of patient	None needed
Indications	• Standard component of metabolic panels (BMP and CMP) and element of electrolyte panel • Admission workup and evaluation of delirium, seizure, and SIAD • Evaluating and monitoring electrolyte and acid-base disturbances, dehydration, and fluid overload • Evaluating and monitoring medication-induced effects
Reference range	≤90 years: 136–145 mEq/L >90 years: 132–146 mEq/L
Critical value(s)	<120 mEq/L or >160 mEq/L
Increased levels	• Dehydration with inadequate water intake • Excessive free water loss: excessive sweating, extensive thermal burns, diabetes insipidus, osmotic diuresis • Increased sodium intake in IV fluids (isotonic saline) • Decreased sodium loss: hyperaldosteronism (Cushing's syndrome, Conn's syndrome) • Tracheobronchitis

Sodium *(continued)*

Decreased levels	• Water intoxication, psychogenic polydipsia • SIAD • Treatment with thiazide diuretics and other drugs listed above • Third-space loss of sodium: ascites, peripheral edema, pleural effusion, loss through bowel lumen in ileus or obstruction • Increased free body water: excessive sodium-free oral, IV, or irrigant administration • Congestive heart failure • Increased sodium loss: Addison's disease, diarrhea, vomiting, sweating, burns, nasogastric suction, diuretic therapy, chronic renal insufficiency • Hyperlipidemia • Sodium-deficient diet • Hypothyroidism • Hyperglycemia: sodium decreases by 1.5–3.0 mEq/L for each 100 mg/dL increase in blood glucose
Interfering factors	Recent trauma, shock, or surgery can affect sodium values. A spurious reduction of sodium (pseudohyponatremia) can occur with certain assays in the presence of hyperproteinemia and hyperlipidemia due to decreased water content. Numerous non-psychotropic drugs affect sodium levels.
Cross-references	**Diabetes Insipidus** **Hypernatremia** **Hyponatremia** **Psychogenic Polydipsia** **Syndrome of Inappropriate Antidiuresis**

Adrogue HJ, Madias NE: Hyponatremia. N Engl J Med 342:1581–1589, 2000

Ali SN, Bazzano LA. Hyponatremia in association with second-generation antipsychotics: a systematic review of case reports. Ochsner J 18(3):230–235, 2018

Faria AC, Carmo H, Carvalho F, et al: Drinking to death: hyponatraemia induced by synthetic phenethylamines. Drug Alcohol Depend 212:108045, 2020

Filippatos TD, Makri A, Elisaf MS, Liamis G: Hyponatremia in the elderly: challenges and solutions. Clin Interv Aging 12:1957–1965, 2017

Lien YH, Shapiro JI: Hyponatremia: clinical diagnosis and management. Am J Med 120:653–658, 2007

Liu BA, Mittmann N, Knowles SR, et al: Hyponatremia and the syndrome of inappropriate secretion of antidiuretic hormone associated with the use of selective serotonin reuptake inhibitors: a review of spontaneous reports. CMAJ 155:519–527, 1996

Reynolds RM, Padfield PL, Seckl JR: Disorders of sodium balance. BMJ 332:702–705, 2006

Syphilis testing

Type of test	Blood, skin scraping from a visible lesion, CSF
Background and explanation of test	Antibody tests are used for the screening and diagnosis of syphilis. These are of two types: nontreponemal and treponemal. Nontreponemal tests do not detect antibodies to the bacteria that cause syphilis but instead detect other antibodies produced in the presence of syphilis infection. These tests are sensitive but not specific; false-positive results can occur with autoimmune disease, pregnancy, tuberculosis, and other conditions noted in the *Interfering Factors* section below. Nontreponemal tests include the RPR and VDRL tests. A positive result from either of these tests is confirmed with a more specific treponemal test.
	Treponemal tests detect antibodies directed to the *Treponema pallidum* organism. These tests include the FTA-ABS, the *T. pallidum* particle agglutination assay (TP-PA), the microhemagglutination assay for *T. pallidum* antibodies (MHA-TP), and various immunoassays. These tests are very specific for syphilis. Once treponemal antibodies form, however, they stay in the circulation indefinitely, so these tests cannot be used to distinguish a recent from a past infection. Nontreponemal antibodies, in contrast, disappear from the body with adequate treatment after ~3 years. FTA-ABS testing is useful 3–4 weeks after exposure. TP-PA testing is less often used but is more specific than FTA-ABS. If the treponemal test confirms infection, the disease should be staged and treated.
	Two methods of direct detection of *T. pallidum* include dark-field microscopy and molecular testing by PCR. Microscopy can be used in the early stages of syphilis with scrapings from a chancre. PCR can be used on scrapings, blood, or CSF.
	For suspected neurosyphilis, VDRL is performed on CSF. FTA-ABS, which is less specific than VDRL but highly sensitive, can be used to exclude neurosyphilis. PCR can be used to detect bacterial DNA in CSF or other samples.
Relevance to psychiatry and behavioral science	Among psychiatric patients, the risk of sexually transmitted infection (STI) is higher in those with alcohol or drug abuse or dependence, bipolar disorder, and certain personality disorders and in those who are HIV positive. With these risks in mind, appropriate vigilance regarding STI testing can be maintained. Neurosyphilis is associated with dementia, mood disorders, and behavioral changes.
Preparation of patient	None needed
Indications	• Chancre, skin rash, or other signs of syphilis as noted in the *Diseases and Conditions* chapter.
	• Screening a patient with another STI, such as gonorrhea
	• Screening a patient with newly diagnosed HIV infection
	• Screening for syphilis in pregnancy

Syphilis testing *(continued)*

Reference range	Negative or nonreactive
Positive test	Reactive RPR or VDRL and positive treponemal testing
Negative test	Nonreactive RPR or VDRL and negative treponemal testing
Interfering factors	False-positive RPR or VDRL results can be found in the presence of pneumonia, HIV disease, herpes simplex virus, malaria, primary antiphospholipid syndrome, IV drug use, SLE, Lyme disease, tuberculosis, rheumatoid arthritis, pregnancy, Hansen's disease, or other treponemal diseases. False-positive FTA-ABS results may occur in the presence of autoimmune disease, Hansen's disease, febrile illness, advanced age, Lyme disease, or other treponemal diseases.
Cross-references	**Syphilis**

American Association for Clinical Chemistry: Testing.com. Available at: https://www.testing.com. Accessed September 2021.

Clyne B, Jerrard DA: Syphilis testing. J Emerg Med 18:361–367, 2000

Young H: Guidelines for serological testing for syphilis. Sex Transm Infect 76:403–405, 2000

Temazepam level

Type of test	Blood
Background and explanation of test	Benzodiazepines are Schedule IV sedative-hypnotic drugs used to treat anxiety and insomnia. Temazepam is a drug with a slow onset of action and a half-life of up to 2 days. It is not extensively metabolized in the liver. In general, levels are checked when either overdose or noncompliance is suspected or to detect use without a prescription. In the latter case, a urine drug screen is more likely to be ordered than a blood level.
Relevance to psychiatry and behavioral science	Toxicity with chronic benzodiazepine ingestion may manifest as confusion, disorientation, memory impairment, ataxia, decreased reflexes, and dysarthria. With acute overdose, patients may exhibit somnolence, confusion, ataxia, decreased reflexes, vertigo, dysarthria, respiratory depression, and coma. Treatment of overdose is supportive. More serious consequences usually involve co-ingestion of alcohol or other sedatives, and in these cases, airway management is required. The choice to use flumazenil, an antagonist at the benzodiazepine receptor, is made on a case-by-case basis. Flumazenil does not affect the drug level. Activated charcoal is no longer recommended, and neither dialysis nor bowel irrigation has a role in treatment of overdose.
Preparation of patient	None needed
Indications	• Screening for drug use • Suspicion of overdose • Signs of toxicity in a treated patient • Suspected noncompliance with prescribed therapy
Reference range	0.4–0.9 µg/mL
Critical value(s)	Levels significantly above reference
Increased levels	• Overdose • Overuse
Decreased levels	Noncompliance
Interfering factors	None
Cross-references	**Benzodiazepines** **Urine Drug Screen**

Kang M, Galuska MA, Ghassemzadeh S: Benzodiazepine toxicity, in StatPearls. Treasure Island, FL, StatPearls Publishing, 2021. Available at: https://www.statpearls.com/ArticleLibrary/viewarticle/30312. Accessed September 2021.

Testosterone level

Type of test	Blood
Background and explanation of test	In response to stimulation by LH from the anterior pituitary, the testes secrete testosterone, a steroid hormone that in puberty stimulates the development of male sexual characteristics, including enlargement of the penis, growth of body hair, muscle development, and a deepening voice. In adult males, testosterone regulates sex drive and helps to maintain muscle mass. In females, testosterone is produced in small amounts by the ovaries and is converted to estradiol. In both sexes, testosterone is also secreted by the adrenal glands.
	Testosterone levels peak in the early morning hours (between 4:00 A.M. and 8:00 A.M.) and are lowest in the evening (between 4:00 P.M. and 8:00 P.M.). Most testosterone in the circulation is bound to protein; only about 1%–4% circulates as free testosterone.
	New guidelines for the diagnosis and management of testosterone deficiency were published by the American Urological Association in 2018 to guide replacement therapy for males with documented deficiency. This requires two separate morning tests showing a total testosterone level <300 ng/dL in conjunction with typical clinical signs/symptoms. If total testosterone is low, serum LH is measured. If LH is also low, serum prolactin is measured. These values determine the need for further testing or endocrinology referral.
Relevance to psychiatry and behavioral science	*Testosterone deficiency*
	In addition to classic symptoms of testosterone deficiency such as reduced sex drive, erectile dysfunction, and infertility, common symptoms of deficiency in males include fatigue, reduced energy, reduced endurance, diminished physical performance, reduced motivation, poor concentration, impaired memory, and irritability. Symptoms could be erroneously construed as a depressive episode.
	Obesity and the metabolic syndrome are associated with low total and free testosterone levels. The relationship is bidirectional. Waist circumference is a modifiable risk factor for low testosterone. Stress, which is implicated in both the metabolic syndrome and hypogonadism, is also associated with lowered testosterone levels.
	Alcoholism with cirrhosis is associated with low testosterone levels. Hypothalamic and pituitary disease can be associated with low testosterone levels and with tertiary or secondary hypogonadism, respectively.
	Psychotropic drugs associated with reduced testosterone levels include carbamazepine, conjugated estrogens, danazol, prednisone, dexamethasone, and medroxyprogesterone.

Testosterone level *(continued)*

Relevance to psychiatry and behavioral science *(continued)*	*Testosterone excess* Testosterone excess in males is associated with aggressive behavior, mood swings, irritability, impaired judgment, and euphoria. This is uncommon except in those taking steroids or testosterone to enhance athletic performance or to build muscle mass. Excess testosterone has numerous adverse physical effects, including heart muscle damage, liver disease, prostate enlargement, hypertension, edema, weight gain, headaches, high cholesterol, insomnia, and increased risk of blood clotting. Testosterone excess in females can be recognized clinically by the development of excess facial and body hair, male pattern baldness, acne, menstrual irregularities, deepening of the voice, and weight gain. Depression and anxiety are also seen. Psychotropic drugs associated with elevated testosterone levels include anabolic steroids, barbiturates, bromocriptine, danazol, estrogen/progestin, mifepristone, naloxone, phenytoin, and valproate.
Preparation of patient	None needed
Indications	*Males* • Erectile dysfunction • Reduced sex drive • Infertility • Hypogonadism • Cryptorchidism • Testicular tumor *Females* • Virilization, hirsutism • Reduced sex drive • Infertility • Workup for polycystic ovary syndrome *Transgender individuals* (female-to-male) • Monitoring testosterone levels to determine whether target male ranges have been achieved
Reference range	*Total testosterone* • Adult males: 270–1,070 ng/dL • Adult females: 15–70 ng/dL • Pregnant females: 3–4 times normal value • Postmenopausal females: 8–35 ng/dL *Free testosterone* • Adult males: 50–210 pg/mL • Adult females: 1.0–8.5 pg/mL

Testosterone level *(continued)*

Critical value(s)	Total testosterone <300 ng/dL in males on two separate morning tests supports the diagnosis of testosterone deficiency. Total testosterone >200 ng/dL in females suggests the presence of androgenic tumor, particularly in the presence of hirsutism.
Increased levels	*Increased total testosterone in males* • Hyperthyroidism • Adrenal tumors • Testicular tumors • Use of anabolic steroids • Androgen resistance syndromes • Congenital adrenal hyperplasia (infants and children) • Precocious puberty *Increased total testosterone in females* • Congenital adrenal hyperplasia • Ovarian tumor • Adrenal gland tumor • Idiopathic hirsutism • Hilar cell tumor • Trophoblastic disease of pregnancy • Testosterone exposure from testosterone topical products in a close contact *Increased free testosterone in females* • Polycystic ovary syndrome • Virilization
Decreased levels	*Decreased total testosterone in males* • Hypothalamic or pituitary disease • Genetic conditions such as Klinefelter's, Kallmann, Prader-Willi, and Down syndromes • Myotonic dystrophy with testicular failure • Chronic disease (e.g., diabetes, HIV, autoimmune disease) • Acquired testicular injury (mumps or physical injury, including chemotherapy or radiation) • Alcohol use disorder with cirrhosis • Chronic use of antidepressants or narcotics *Decreased free testosterone in males* • Hypogonadism • Normal age-related decline

Testosterone level *(continued)*

Interfering factors	Testosterone levels fluctuate in a diurnal pattern, so the time of sampling affects results. In addition, levels decrease with age and increase after exercise.
	Thyroid disease can increase or reduce the level of sex hormone–binding globulin and thereby influence the test results.
	Many laboratories use immunoassays that are not sufficiently sensitive to measure testosterone in patients with low values such as females and children, so samples from these patients should be sent to reference laboratories using mass spectroscopy techniques.
	Medications that affect results include all drugs that raise prolactin levels, anticonvulsants, estrogens, androgens, corticosteroids, digoxin, spironolactone, barbiturates, and other drugs listed above.
Cross-references	**Alcohol Use Disorder** **Cirrhosis** **Hypogonadism** **Klinefelter's Syndrome** **Metabolic Syndrome** **Prader-Willi Syndrome** **Thyrotoxicosis**

American Association for Clinical Chemistry: Testing.com. Available at: https://www.testing.com. Accessed September 2021

Hall SA, Esche GR, Araujo AB, et al: Correlates of low testosterone and symptomatic androgen deficiency in a population-based sample. J Clin Endocrinol Metab 93:3870–3877, 2008

Harvard Medical School: Testosterone: what it does and doesn't do. Harvard Health Publishing, August 29, 2019. Available at: https://www.health.harvard.edu/medications/testosterone--what-it-does-and-doesnt-do. Accessed September 2021.

Mayo Clinic Laboratories: Testosterone, Total and Free, Serum. Available at: https://www.mayocliniclabs.com/test-catalog/Overview/8508. Accessed September 2021.

Mulhall JP, Trost LW, Brannigan RE, et al: Evaluation and management of testosterone deficiency: AUA guideline. J Urol 200(2):423–432, 2018

Qaseem A, Horwitch CA, Vijan S, et al: Testosterone treatment in adult men with age-related low testosterone: a clinical guideline from the American College of Physicians. Ann Intern Med 172(2):126–133, 2020

Thiamine level

Type of test	Blood
Background and explanation of test	Thiamine (vitamin B_1) is a nutrient essential to carbohydrate metabolism for energy production and to protein and fat metabolism. Thiamine is also required for cognitive function, circulation, blood formation, normal growth, maintenance of muscle tone, and other processes. It acts as an antioxidant, protecting the body from the degenerative effects of aging, smoking, and alcohol consumption. Body stores of thiamine are limited, and deficiency can occur in as little as 10 days with inadequate dietary intake. Thiamine deficiency is commonly known as *beriberi*, with two types recognized: wet beriberi, which affects the heart and circulatory system, and dry beriberi, which affects the nervous system. Severe dry beriberi can be associated with Wernicke's encephalopathy, which can progress to Korsakoff's syndrome if untreated.
	Thiamine requirements are directly related to caloric intake, especially carbohydrates. Across the age spectrum, thiamine deficiency is underdiagnosed and thus undertreated. Populations at risk of deficiency are often seen by psychiatrists and behavioral health specialists, as noted below. When a patient with a potential deficiency presents to an emergency setting, thiamine must be replaced before glucose is administered to prevent precipitation of Wernicke's encephalopathy in a marginally deficient patient. A mnemonic for the correct order of therapy is *Thank God I gave thiamine before glucose!*
	It is the active form of thiamine—thiamine diphosphate (pyrophosphate)—that is measured in a sample of whole blood. It is not necessary to wait for the result before thiamine is administered, especially in the emergency setting. Overtreatment is preferred to undertreatment because thiamine has an excellent safety profile, whereas continuing deficiency can result in persistent neurocognitive impairment and is sometimes fatal.
Relevance to psychiatry and behavioral science	Individuals at risk of thiamine deficiency include those with alcohol use disorder (AUD), HIV/AIDS, rapid weight loss, anorexia nervosa, malnutrition due to other factors such as delusions of food poisoning, refeeding syndrome after starvation, hyperemesis gravidarum, or COVID-19 with protracted vomiting, as well as those who have undergone GI surgery, and elderly patients treated with diuretic drugs. Recent publications have highlighted the prevalence of thiamine deficiency in critically ill patients, particularly those with severe burns, septic shock, end-stage renal disease, and heart failure and those who have undergone major surgery.
	The classic triad of the Wernicke-Korsakoff syndrome—mental status changes, ocular signs, and ataxia—is not often seen, although it may be more prevalent among patients with anorexia than those with AUD.

Thiamine level *(continued)*

Relevance to psychiatry and behavioral science *(continued)*	Among ICU patients, deficiency can present with delirium only. Other neuropsychiatric signs include the sensorimotor dysfunction, vertigo, confusion, and coma. The presence of multiple signs and symptoms may suggest a late recognition of deficiency.
Preparation of patient	Patients should fast overnight and should abstain from alcohol for 24 hours before testing.
Indications	• Suspected thiamine deficiency in a patient at risk • Cardiac, neurological, or constitutional signs consistent with thiamine deficiency
Reference range	70–180 nmol/L
Critical value(s)	None
Increased levels	Toxicity is seen only with extremes of parenteral dosing.
Decreased levels	• AUD • Anorexia nervosa • Starvation, diets restricted to white rice or processed carbohydrates • Prolonged vomiting or diarrhea • Chronic illness, such as diabetes • Excessive consumption of raw fish or tea • Elderly patients • Long-term diuretic therapy • Cancer
Interfering factors	Barbiturates decrease thiamine levels.
Cross-references	**Thiamine Deficiency** **Wernicke's Encephalopathy and Wernicke-Korsakoff Syndrome**

ARUP Laboratories: Vitamin B_1 (thiamine), whole blood, in Lab Test Directory. Salt Lake City, UT, ARUP Laboratories, 2021. Available at: https://ltd.aruplab.com/Tests/Pub/0080388. Accessed September 2021.

Ghishan FK, Kiela PR: Vitamins and minerals in inflammatory bowel disease. Gastroenterol Clin North Am 46(4):797–808, 2017

Kho J, Mandal AKJ, Geraldes R, et al: COVID-19 encephalitis and Wernicke's encephalopathy. J Med Virol 93(9):5248–5251, 2021

Lange S, Medrzycka-Dabrowska W, Friganovic A, et al: Delirium in critical illness patients and the potential role of thiamine therapy in prevention and treatment: findings from a scoping review with implications for evidence-based practice. Int J Environ Res Public Health 18(16):8809, 2021

Lo Gullo A, Rifici C, Caliri S, et al: Refeeding syndrome in a woman with pancreatitis: a case report. J Int Med Res 49(2):300060520986675, 2021

Oudman E, Wijnia JW, Oey MJ, et al: Preventing Wernicke's encephalopathy in anorexia nervosa: a systematic review. Psychiatry Clin Neurosci 72(10):774–779, 2018

Polegato BF, Pereira AG, Azevedo PS, et al: Role of thiamine in health and disease. Nutr Clin Pract 34(4):558–564, 2019

Sinha S, Kataria A, Kolla BP, et al: Wernicke encephalopathy: clinical pearls. Mayo Clin Proc 94(6):1065–1072, 2019

Truong T, Hetzel F, Stiff KM, Husnain MG: Case of hypoactive delirium precipitated by thiamine deficiency. BMJ Case Rep 14(3):e239886, 2021

Thyroid function testing: free thyroxine

Type of test	Blood
Background and explanation of test	Thyroxine (T4) is a hormone produced in the thyroid gland and secreted in response to stimulation by TSH from the anterior pituitary. The small fraction of T4 that circulates in the unbound (free) form is metabolically active and has critical roles in determining the basal metabolic rate, release of calcium from bone, synthesis of proteins, and metabolism of lipids, carbohydrates, and vitamins. Through a feedback mechanism, the circulating T4 level influences the release of TSH and thyrotropin-releasing hormone (TRH) from the hypothalamus. The free T4 (FT4) level is measured in preference to total T4 because its measurement is not affected by blood protein levels. FT4 is usually ordered after an abnormal TSH test has been returned or when clinical suspicion of thyroid disease remains even when the TSH level is normal. TSH and FT4 together suggest the following diagnoses: • TSH high, FT4 low: hypothyroidism • TSH high, FT4 normal: subclinical hypothyroidism • TSH low, FT4 high: hyperthyroidism • TSH low, FT4 normal: subclinical hyperthyroidism • TSH low, FT4 low: nonthyroidal illness If TSH is high and FT4 is normal, thyroid antibodies are checked. If TSH is low and FT4 is high, thyroid antibodies are checked.
Relevance to psychiatry and behavioral science	Hyperthyroidism can cause delirium or psychiatric symptoms suggestive of primary mood disorders or psychosis. So-called apathetic hyperthyroidism is a syndrome affecting elderly patients that can be mistaken for other conditions. This is discussed further in the **Thyrotoxicosis** entry in the *Diseases and Conditions* chapter. Hypothyroidism is associated with fatigue, depressed mood, and memory impairment, symptoms not uncommonly attributed to primary depression. Normal FT4 with high or low TSH is consistent with subclinical thyroid disease, which can manifest as a fully developed or *formes frustes* picture of hyperthyroidism or hypothyroidism. Euthyroid sick syndrome, characterized by low FT4 and low TSH, commonly accompanies nonthyroidal illness in acutely ill patients, including those with COVID-19 infection. Of the psychotropic drugs noted in the *Interfering Factors* section below, lithium has the most significant effect on thyroid function and FT4 level.
Preparation of patient	Biotin supplements should be discontinued ≥2 days before testing.

Thyroid function testing: free thyroxine *(continued)*

Indications	<ul><li>Abnormal TSH result</li><li>Signs/symptoms of thyroid disease (even if TSH is normal)</li><li>Monitoring effects of treatment for thyroid illness</li></ul>
Reference range	Depends on the specific method used for assay; consult lab reference values.
Critical value(s)	<2 µg/dL or >20 µg/dL
Increased levels	<ul><li>Hyperthyroidism</li><li>Treated hypothyroidism</li></ul>
Decreased levels	<ul><li>Primary hypothyroidism</li><li>Secondary hypothyroidism (pituitary cause)</li><li>Tertiary hypothyroidism (hypothalamic cause)</li><li>Hypothyroidism treated with triiodothyronine (T3)</li><li>Late pregnancy</li></ul>
Interfering factors	FT4 levels fluctuate in pregnancy and in severe or chronic illness. Different reference ranges apply in pregnancy. Drugs that cause an increase in FT4 include amiodarone, aspirin, biotin, carbamazepine, furosemide, heparin, phenytoin, propranolol, X-ray contrast agents, and valproate. Drugs that cause a decrease in FT4 include lithium, carbamazepine, corticosteroids, estrogen, methadone, oral contraceptives, phenobarbital, and phenytoin.
Cross-references	**Hypothyroidism** **Thyroid Function Testing: Thyroid-Stimulating Hormone** **Thyrotoxicosis**

Benvenga S: L-T4 therapy in the presence of pharmacological interferents. Front Endocrinol (Lausanne) 11:607446, 2020

Bowen R, Benavides R, Colón-Franco JM, et al: Best practices in mitigating the risk of biotin interference with laboratory testing. Clin Biochem 74:1–11, 2019

Dworakowska D, Morley S, Mulholland N, Grossman AB: COVID-19-related thyroiditis: a novel disease entity? Clin Endocrinol (Oxf) 95(3):369–377, 2021

Roberts CG, Ladenson PW: Hypothyroidism. Lancet 363:793–803, 2004

Soh SB, Aw TC: Laboratory testing in thyroid conditions: pitfalls and clinical utility. Ann Lab Med 39(1):3–14, 2019

Spaulding SW, Lippes H: Hyperthyroidism: causes, clinical features, and diagnosis. Med Clin North Am 69:937–951, 1985

Ylli D, Wartofsky L, Burman KD: Evaluation and treatment of amiodarone-induced thyroid disorders. J Clin Endocrinol Metab 106(1):226–236, 2021

Thyroid function testing: thyroid-stimulating hormone (TSH)

Type of test	Blood
Background and explanation of test	TSH secreted by the anterior pituitary stimulates the thyroid gland to release stored triiodothyronine (T3) and thyroxine (T4), hormones responsible for the regulation of metabolism. TSH secretion is in turn regulated by thyrotropin-releasing hormone (TRH) from the hypothalamus and by feedback inhibition from T3 and T4. In the past, a combination of thyroid tests (thyroid panel) was used to screen for and diagnose thyroid disease, but the thyroid panel has now largely been replaced by the highly sensitive TSH assay for screening. If the TSH is normal in suspected thyroid disease, no further testing is indicated. If the TSH is not normal and the differential diagnosis includes subclinical thyroid disease or dysfunction of the hypothalamic-pituitary axis, however, free T4 should be measured along with TSH. TSH and free T4 (FT4) together suggest the following diagnoses: • TSH high, FT4 low: hypothyroidism • TSH high, FT4 normal: subclinical hypothyroidism • TSH low, FT4 high: hyperthyroidism • TSH low, FT4 normal: subclinical hyperthyroidism • TSH low, FT4 low: nonthyroidal illness
Relevance to psychiatry and behavioral science	Patients with hyperthyroidism can present with delirium or with psychiatric symptoms that suggest primary anxiety disorders, mood disorders, or psychosis. The geriatric syndrome of apathetic hyperthyroidism is described in the **Thyrotoxicosis** entry in the *Diseases and Conditions* chapter. Hypothyroidism is associated with fatigue, depressed mood, and memory impairment, symptoms that may improve with thyroid replacement. Even among patients with TSH values in the high-normal range, there is a higher frequency of depressive episodes, symptoms are more severe, and antidepressant treatment response can be suboptimal. Thyroid replacement with target TSH levels <2.5 mIU/L may be required to achieve remission, and this is true for patients with both bipolar and unipolar disease. Patients with treatment-resistant depression may benefit from thyroid supplementation titrated to a target TSH level as low as <2.0 mIU/L. Abnormal TSH with normal FT4 is consistent with subclinical thyroid disease, which can manifest as a fully developed or *formes frustes* picture of hyperthyroidism or hypothyroidism. Whether or how subclinical disease should be treated has been controversial. Recent reviews suggest that subclinical hypothyroidism in non-elderly patients should be treated when the TSH level is >4.0 mIU/L. For elderly patients, a higher TSH cutoff may be appropriate, although most healthy elderly persons have TSH levels <2.5 mIU/L.

Thyroid function testing: thyroid-stimulating hormone (TSH) *(continued)*

Relevance to psychiatry and behavioral science *(continued)*	In a recent study, more than half of hospitalized patients with COVID-19 were found to have a TSH level below the normal range. The level returned to normal with recovery from the viral illness.
Preparation of patient	Biotin supplements should be discontinued ≥2 days before testing.
Indications	• Diagnosing hypothyroidism or hyperthyroidism in a symptomatic patient • Screening for thyroid disease in patients at risk, such as females older than 50 years or patients treated with lithium • Evaluating the effects of thyroid nodule or goiter • Monitoring the efficacy of thyroid replacement therapy in a patient with hypothyroidism • Standard component of workup for patients with depression, memory impairment, or dementia
Reference range	0.5–5.0 mIU/L is understood to be the general reference range, but values differ slightly by lab, so the test report should be consulted. *Note:* With treatment for hypothyroid or hyperthyroid states, TSH may remain abnormal for up to 6 weeks after the euthyroid state has been attained.
Critical value(s)	<0.1 mIU/L indicates primary hyperthyroidism or exogenous thyrotoxicosis, with risk of atrial fibrillation (major risk factor for stroke).
Increased levels	• Primary hypothyroidism (≥100 times normal) • TSH-producing tumor (e.g., breast or lung) • Hashimoto's thyroiditis • Recovery phase of subacute thyroiditis or nonthyroidal illness • Insufficient thyroid replacement or thyroid hormone resistance in treated hypothyroid patients
Decreased levels	• Primary hyperthyroidism • Secondary hypothyroidism (pituitary disease) • Tertiary hypothyroidism (hypothalamic disease) • Subclinical hyperthyroidism (e.g., toxic multinodular goiter, treated Graves' disease) • Euthyroid sick syndrome • Overreplacement of thyroid hormone

Thyroid function testing: thyroid-stimulating hormone (TSH) *(continued)*

Interfering factors	TSH levels have normal diurnal variation that must be considered in the test interpretation.
	Numerous drugs—both psychotropic and non-psychotropic—have the potential to interfere with thyroid function assays; current and recently discontinued drugs should be listed on the lab requisition form.
	Two drugs that affect the thyroid itself are lithium and amiodarone, an antiarrhythmic drug.
	A recent meta-analysis found no impact of SSRI treatment on TSH levels. Iodinated contrast medium does not affect TSH level in patients with normal thyroid function. Carbamazepine and other enzyme inducers can increase metabolism of thyroid hormones and thereby cause an increase in TSH.
	TSH levels are known to increase with age, although this may indicate increasing thyroid dysfunction. Even though most elderly persons have TSH levels <2.5 mIU/L, some references suggest an upper limit of normal for TSH as high as 10 mIU/L for patients >80 years of age.
Cross-references	**Hypothyroidism**
	Thyroid Function Testing: Free Thyroxine
	Thyrotoxicosis

American Association for Clinical Chemistry: Testing.com. Available at: https://www.testing.com. Accessed September 2021.

Barbesino G: Thyroid function changes in the elderly and their relationship to cardiovascular health: a mini-review. Gerontology 65(1):1–8, 2019

Benvenga S: L-T4 therapy in the presence of pharmacological interferents. Front Endocrinol (Lausanne) 11:607446, 2020

Bowen R, Benavides R, Colón-Franco JM, et al: Best practices in mitigating the risk of biotin interference with laboratory testing. Clin Biochem 74:1–11, 2019

Caye A, Pilz LK, Maia AL, et al: The impact of selective serotonin reuptake inhibitors on the thyroid function among patients with major depressive disorder: a systematic review and meta-analysis. Eur Neuropsychopharmacol 33:139–145, 2020

Chen M, Zhou W, Xu W: Thyroid function analysis in 50 patients with COVID-19: a retrospective study. Thyroid 31(1):8–11, 2021

Chrysant SG: The current debate over treatment of subclinical hypothyroidism to prevent cardiovascular complications. Int J Clin Pract 74(7):e13499, 2020

Cohen BM, Sommer BR, Vuckovic A: Antidepressant-resistant depression in patients with comorbid subclinical hypothyroidism or high-normal TSH levels. Am J Psychiatry 175(7):598–604, 2018

Favresse J, Burlacu MC, Maiter D, Gruson D: Interferences with thyroid function immunoassays: clinical implications and detection algorithm. Endocr Rev 39(5):830–850, 2018

Soh SB, Aw TC: Laboratory testing in thyroid conditions: pitfalls and clinical utility. Ann Lab Med 39(1):3–14, 2019

Total iron-binding capacity (TIBC)

Type of test	Blood
Background and explanation of test	The TIBC is the maximum amount of iron that can be bound to transferrin, the protein in blood responsible for transporting iron to tissues. Iron is needed to produce hemoglobin and to transport oxygen, among other functions. In the TIBC test, iron is added to the patient's serum until the transferrin-binding sites are saturated, then the excess iron is removed, and the amount of bound iron remaining is measured. This value—TIBC—can be used with serum iron and transferrin levels in the evaluation of iron deficiency and iron overload states. However, transferrin saturation is actually a better measure of iron status, and this is calculated by dividing the serum iron by the TIBC and then multiplying by 100. The TIBC can be used to distinguish anemia (increased TIBC) from inflammatory conditions (normal TIBC).
Relevance to psychiatry and behavioral science	Patients with either hemochromatosis or iron deficiency anemia may present with fatigue, lethargy, and weakness, which could be mistaken for primary depression. In hemochromatosis, iron is deposited in the brain, increasing the risk of confusional states, cognitive dysfunction, mood disorders, dizziness, and tinnitus. There is some evidence that iron deposition may contribute to neurodegenerative diseases such as Alzheimer's disease. MRI studies have shown that iron levels in subcortical gray structures including the caudate, putamen, and globus pallidus are positively correlated with liver iron levels in elderly males.
Preparation of patient	Patients should fast for 12 hours before the test, with water permitted. Blood should be drawn in the morning, if possible.
Indications	• Anemia (microcytic, hypochromic) • Aiding in the diagnosis of iron deficiency anemia (see **Transferrin; Transferrin Saturation**) • Suspected hemochromatosis
Reference range	Adults: 250–450 µg/dL
Critical value(s)	None
Increased levels	• Iron deficiency anemia (microcytic) • Late pregnancy • Blood loss (acute and chronic) • Acute hepatitis • Use of oral contraceptives
Decreased levels	• Hemochromatosis • Non–iron deficiency anemia (chronic disease, infection) • Low protein levels (malnutrition, burns) • Cirrhosis • Renal disease

Total iron-binding capacity (TIBC) *(continued)*

Decreased levels *(continued)*	• Thalassemia • Hyperthyroidism • Use of ACTH, steroids, dextran, testosterone, asparaginase, or chloramphenicol
Interfering factors	TIBC and serum iron level may be normal in iron deficiency anemia if hemoglobin is >9 g/dL.
Cross-references	**Anemia** **Hemochromatosis** **Iron Level** **Transferrin; Transferrin Saturation**

American Association for Clinical Chemistry: Testing.com. Available at: https://www.testing.com. Accessed September 2021.

Auerbach M, Adamson JW: How we diagnose and treat iron deficiency anemia. Am J Hematol 91(1):31–38, 2016

Fischbach FT, Fischbach MA: A Manual of Laboratory and Diagnostic Tests, 10th Edition. Philadelphia, PA, Wolters Kluwer Health/Lippincott Williams and Wilkins, 2018

Killip S, Bennett JM, Chambers MD: Iron deficiency anemia. Am Fam Physician 75(5):671–678, 2007 [published correction appears in Am Fam Physician 78(8):914, 2008]

Pietrangelo A: Hereditary hemochromatosis: pathogenesis, diagnosis, and treatment. Gastroenterology 139:393–408, 2010

Zhu A, Kaneshiro M, Kaunitz JD: Evaluation and treatment of iron deficiency anemia: a gastroenterological perspective. Dig Dis Sci 55:548–559, 2010

Transferrin; transferrin saturation

Type of test	Blood
Background and explanation of test	Transferrin is a β-globulin and glycoprotein produced in the liver that transports dietary iron to storage depots and sites of hemoglobin synthesis. The transferrin test measures the level of blood transferrin, which depends on liver function and nutritional status. Transferrin saturation is calculated by dividing the serum iron level by the total iron-binding capacity (TIBC) and multiplying by 100. Normally, the saturation is between 20% and 50%. In iron deficiency, the iron level is low and the TIBC is increased, so the saturation can drop to a very low level. In hemochromatosis, the iron level is high and the TIBC is low or normal, so the saturation is high.
Relevance to psychiatry and behavioral science	Patients with either hemochromatosis or iron deficiency anemia may present with fatigue, lethargy, and weakness, which could be mistaken for primary depression. In hemochromatosis, iron is deposited in the brain, increasing the risk of confusional states, cognitive problems, mood disorders, dizziness, and tinnitus.
Preparation of patient	Patients should fast for 12 hours before testing, with water permitted.
Indications	• Aiding in the diagnosis of iron deficiency as the cause of anemia • Diagnosing hemochromatosis • Evaluating nutritional status • Evaluating liver function
Reference ranges	*Transferrin* • 200–400 mg/dL *Transferrin saturation* • Males: 10%–50% • Females: 15%–50%
Critical value(s)	None
Increased levels	*Transferrin* • Iron deficiency anemia • Pregnancy • Estrogen therapy *Transferrin saturation* • Hemochromatosis
Decreased levels	*Transferrin* • Anemia of chronic disease (microcytic) • Protein deficiency or loss • Chronic infection • Acute liver disease

Transferrin; transferrin saturation *(continued)*

Decreased levels *(continued)*	• Renal disease
	• Genetic disease
	• Hemochromatosis
	Transferrin saturation
	• Iron deficiency anemia
Interfering factors	Increased transferrin levels may be found with estrogen and oral contraceptive use.
	Decreased transferrin levels may be found with corticosteroid and testosterone use.
	Lipemic or hemolyzed specimens may invalidate testing.
Cross-references	**Anemia**
	Hemochromatosis
	Iron Level
	Total Iron-Binding Capacity

American Association for Clinical Chemistry: Testing.com. Available at: https://www.testing.com. Accessed September 2021.

ARUP Laboratories: Transferrin, serum, in Lab Test Directory. Salt Lake City, UT, ARUP Laboratories, 2021. Available at: https://ltd.aruplab.com/Tests/Pub/0050570. Accessed September 2021.

Auerbach M, Adamson JW: How we diagnose and treat iron deficiency anemia. Am J Hematol 91(1):31–38, 2016

Fischbach FT, Fischbach MA: A Manual of Laboratory and Diagnostic Tests, 10th Edition. Philadelphia, PA, Wolters Kluwer Health/Lippincott Williams and Wilkins, 2018

Killip S, Bennett JM, Chambers MD: Iron deficiency anemia. Am Fam Physician 75(5):671–678, 2007 [published correction appears in Am Fam Physician 78(8):914, 2008]

Pietrangelo A: Hereditary hemochromatosis: pathogenesis, diagnosis, and treatment. Gastroenterology 139:393–408, 2010

Zhu A, Kaneshiro M, Kaunitz JD: Evaluation and treatment of iron deficiency anemia: a gastroenterological perspective. Dig Dis Sci 55:548–559, 2010

Triglycerides

Type of test	Blood
Background and explanation of test	Most dietary fat intake is in the form of triglycerides (TGs), which are an important energy source for the body. At any given time, most TGs are stored in adipose tissue as glycerol, fatty acids, and monoglycerides. Lesser amounts are present in the circulation, and this is what the assay measures. After a meal, TG levels can increase dramatically as the body converts dietary energy into adipose tissue. Between meals, adipose tissue stores are reconverted to TGs to meet energy demands.
	High TG levels are associated with a heightened risk of heart disease and stroke. Certain medical and lifestyle factors are in turn associated with elevated TGs, including diabetes, kidney disease, sedentary lifestyle, smoking, excessive alcohol consumption, and being overweight.
	TGs and other lipids can be assayed with a fasting or non-fasting blood sample. A fasting sample is recommended for those with type 2 diabetes, excessive alcohol intake, or obesity. When TGs are measured, cholesterol is also measured because both represent risk factors for atherosclerotic disease, and the two can vary independently.
Relevance to psychiatry and behavioral science	TG levels may be elevated in alcohol use disorder, anorexia nervosa, and other conditions. In addition, psychotropic drugs such as mirtazapine, risperidone, and β-blockers are associated with TG elevations. Before such drugs are initiated, a fasting lipid profile should be obtained. High TG levels increase the patient's risk of pancreatitis and predict a more severe course of COVID-19 infection.
Preparation of patient	Routine non-fasting test requires no preparation.
	For fasting test, patients should abstain from food for 12 hours, with water permitted.
Indications	• Component of lipid panel, obtained every 4–6 years in healthy adults • Screening for patients with family history of lipid disorder • Assessing cardiovascular disease risk • Evaluating patients being considered for lipid-lowering treatments • Monitoring effects of lipid-lowering treatments • Assessing a patient with pancreatitis
Reference range	Normal: <150 mg/dL
	Mild elevation: 150–499 mg/dL
	Moderate elevation: 500–886 mg/dL
	Very high/Severe elevation: >886 mg/dL
	Note: These cutoffs apply to fasting samples.

Triglycerides *(continued)*

Critical value(s)	A level >500 mg/dL represents increased risk of pancreatitis.
	A level >5,000 mg/dL is associated with eruptive xanthoma, arcus cornealis, enlarged liver and spleen, and lipemia retinalis.
Increased levels	• Hyperlipoproteinemia
	• Alcohol use disorder
	• Liver disease, including fatty liver (non-alcoholic)
	• Kidney disease, nephrotic syndrome
	• Hypothyroidism
	• Type 2 diabetes
	• Pancreatitis
	• Glycogen storage disease
	• MI
	• Gout
	• Werner's syndrome
	• Down syndrome
	• Anorexia nervosa
Decreased levels	• Low-fat diet
	• Malnutrition
	• Malabsorption
	• Hyperthyroidism
	• Hyperparathyroidism
	• Severe stroke
Interfering factors	Food intake increases TG levels within hours of a meal. Alcohol use increases TG levels. Fasting TG levels may vary from day to day.
	Transient decrease occurs after strenuous exercise.
	Levels increase in pregnancy.
	Poorly controlled blood sugar in patients with diabetes can drive TG levels up.
	Levels increase with acute illnesses such as colds or influenza.
	Certain drugs increase TG levels, including β-blockers, corticosteroids, estrogens, furosemide, hydrochlorothiazide, interferon-α-2a, isotretinoin, mirtazapine, oral contraceptives, protease inhibitors, risperidone, and warfarin.
	Other drugs decrease triglyceride levels, including ACE inhibitors, hydroxychloroquine, indomethacin, insulin, levodopa, niacin, psyllium, and statins and other drugs used to treat high triglyceride levels.

Triglycerides (continued)

Cross-references	Cardiovascular Risk Assessment (Appendix C)
	Lipid Panel
	Metabolic Syndrome
	Pancreatitis, Acute

Arnett DK, Blumenthal RS, Albert MA, et al: 2019 ACC/AHA Guideline on the Primary Prevention of Cardiovascular Disease: a report of the American College of Cardiology/American Heart Association Task Force on Clinical Practice Guidelines. Circulation 140(11):e596–e646, 2019

Brunzell JD: Clinical practice: hypertriglyceridemia. N Engl J Med 357:1009–1017, 2007

Fischbach FT, Fischbach MA: A Manual of Laboratory and Diagnostic Tests, 10th Edition. Philadelphia, PA, Wolters Kluwer Health/Lippincott Williams and Wilkins, 2018

Lee Y, Siddiqui WJ: Cholesterol levels, in StatPearls. Treasure Island, FL, StatPearls Publishing, 2021. Available from: https://www.statpearls.com/ArticleLibrary/viewarticle/19466. Accessed September 2021.

Masana L, Correig E, Ibarretxe D, et al: Low HDL and high triglycerides predict COVID-19 severity. Sci Rep 11(1):7217, 2021

Nordestgaard BG: A test in context: lipid profile, fasting versus nonfasting. J Am Coll Cardiol 70(13):1637–1646, 2017

Troponins

Type of test	Blood
Background and explanation of test	Troponins are proteins found in the heart and skeletal muscle that regulate muscle contraction. Of three subtypes, only troponin I and troponin T have cardiac-specific forms (abbreviated as cTnI and cTnT); the form of troponin C is the same in both the heart and skeletal muscle. With cardiac muscle injury, cTnI and cTnT are released into the blood, where they can be measured. Since 2017, high-sensitivity tests for cTnI and cTnT have been available in the United States, and these assays are now the tests of choice to diagnose acute MI and other conditions. Most laboratories offer one test or the other, and although they are not interchangeable, they reflect the same information about myocardial injury. After an MI, the levels of these cardiac-specific troponins are elevated within hours of heart injury and remain elevated for 10–14 days. Serial measurements can help distinguish MI from other conditions such as myocarditis and cardiomyopathy.
Relevance to psychiatry and behavioral science	These high-sensitivity tests for cTnI and cTnT can detect very low serum troponin levels and small changes in levels within a short time. Recent research has found the tests useful in predicting adverse cardiovascular events in patients with arterial hypertension, pre-hypertension, and hypertensive crisis and in those with acute neurological injuries such as ischemic stroke. The term *stroke-heart syndrome* has been coined to emphasize the cardiac effects of stroke. Myocardial injury can also occur in other acute and severe neurological conditions involving the "brain-heart axis," including TBI, status epilepticus, intracerebral hemorrhage, and subarachnoid hemorrhage. The utility of these tests in psychiatric disease remains to be explored.
Indications	• Workup for chest pain • Suspected MI • New symptoms in patient with stable angina • Evaluating the cardiac complications of acute stroke and other acute neurological insults • Evaluating the severity of myocardial injury from other causes (e.g., COVID-19 infection) • Excluding myocardial injury in atypical chest pain syndromes
Preparation of patient	None needed
Reference range	Depends on the particular assay and technique; see laboratory reference values.
Critical value(s)	See laboratory reference values.
Increased levels	• MI • Unstable angina

Troponins *(continued)*

Increased levels *(continued)*	• Myocarditis • Cardiomyopathy • Congestive heart failure • Stroke-heart syndrome and other acute neurological conditions
Decreased levels	Not applicable
Interfering factors	Biotin may interfere with cTnT assay. Patients with chronic renal failure may have elevated high-sensitivity troponin levels (especially cTnT) in the absence of myocardial injury. Patients with chronic skeletal muscle injury (e.g., muscular dystrophy or chronic myositis) should be evaluated with cTnI for the same reason. Serial testing of these populations that show changing patterns may help distinguish abnormalities due to these chronic diseases from acute myocardial injury.
Cross-references	**Myocardial Infarction**

American Association for Clinical Chemistry: Lab Tests Online. Available at: https://www.testing.com. Accessed September 2021.

Azar RR, Sarkis A, Giannitsis E: A practical approach for the use of high-sensitivity cardiac troponin assays in the evaluation of patients with chest pain. Am J Cardiol 139:1–7, 2021

Bielecka-Dabrowa A, Cichocka-Radwan A, Lewek J, et al: Cardiac manifestations of COVID-19. Rev Cardiovasc Med 22(2):365–371, 2021

Chaulin A: Clinical and diagnostic value of highly sensitive cardiac troponins in arterial hypertension. Vasc Health Risk Manag 7:431–443, 2021

Frame IJ, Joshi PH, Mwangi C, et al: Susceptibility of cardiac troponin assays to biotin interference. Am J Clin Pathol 151(5):486–493, 2019

Mair J, Lindahl B, Müller C, et al: What to do when you question cardiac troponin values. Eur Heart J Acute Cardiovasc Care 7(6):577–586, 2018

Scheitz JF, Stengl H, Nolte CH, et al: Neurological update: use of cardiac troponin in patients with stroke. J Neurol 268(6):2284–2292, 2021

Tuberculosis (TB) testing

Type of test	Skin test (Mantoux, also known as purified protein derivative [PPD]) Blood test (IGRA) Sputum smear/culture Chest X-ray CSF Other body fluid or tissue samples, as indicated (e.g., biopsy tissue, urine, joint aspirate)
Background and explanation of test	Tests used to detect TB infection include the Mantoux test and the IGRA. The latter is a blood test that measures immune response to the presence of the TB bacillus. When the skin test or one of the IGRA tests is positive, a workup for TB disease is done, including a medical history, physical exam, chest X-ray, and sputum sampling for acid-fast bacilli (AFB). Other body fluids and tissues are sampled as indicated. For the Mantoux skin test, a small amount of PPD of TB antigens is injected under the skin of the forearm. If the person has been exposed to TB, antibodies will form an inflammatory skin reaction that is assessed by a trained professional 48–72 hours later. Skin tests are used in preference to blood tests for patients who have received the bacillus Calmette-Guérin (BCG) vaccine, and the IGRA is used for those who are unable to return for a reading of the skin test. When sputum is collected, a standard practice is to obtain three morning samples on consecutive days. Each sample is viewed immediately as a smear; if AFB are present on any smear, a mycobacterial infection is likely. The sample is cultured to identify the mycobacterium, and its sensitivity to various drugs is determined. Positive identification of a species may take days to weeks, and negative results of no mycobacterial growth may take up to 8 weeks. In patients treated for TB, AFB cultures can be used to monitor the effectiveness of treatment and to determine when the disease is no longer communicable.
Relevance to psychiatry and behavioral science	TB is a considerable public health risk for certain populations, including the homeless and those in nursing homes or correctional facilities. Elderly, very young, and immunocompromised patients are at particular risk. The index of suspicion for TB should be high in all psychiatric settings.
Preparation of patient	None needed
Indications	• Exposure to a person with active TB disease • HIV-positive or otherwise immunocompromised patient • Symptoms of active TB disease: persistent cough, sputum or phlegm (may be blood-tinged), unexplained weight loss, night sweats • Recent immigration from country where TB is endemic • Residence in long-term care facility

Tuberculosis (TB) testing *(continued)*

Indications *(continued)*	• Homelessness • Residence in correctional facility • IV drug use
Reference range	<10-mm area of induration on TB skin testing For IGRAs (blood tests), see report form. Sputum samples negative for AFB Chest X-ray negative for TB Other tissue/fluid samples negative for AFB
Critical value(s)	None
Positive test	*TB infection* indicated by positive skin test or blood test(s). *TB disease* indicated by positive chest X-ray or presence of AFB in sputum or other tissue.
Negative test	When AFB culture is negative in a patient suspected of having TB, either the patient does not have mycobacterial infection, the sampling did not successfully capture the bacilli, or the organism is present in some other body tissue. A negative culture several weeks after treatment indicates a positive response to treatment; in this case, the patient's infection is no longer communicable.
Interfering factors	IGRA tests require viable WBCs, so the blood sample must be refrigerated and sent to the lab on the same day. Several conditions decrease responsiveness to TB skin and blood tests: diabetes, silicosis, chronic renal failure, leukemia, and lymphoma. Treatment with immunosuppressive drugs also decreases responsiveness to TB skin test.
Cross-references	**Tuberculosis**

American Association for Clinical Chemistry: Testing.com. Available at: https://www.testing.com. Accessed September 2021.

ARUP Consult: Mycobacterium tuberculosis—tuberculosis, in ARUP Consult: The Physician's Guide to Laboratory Test Selection and Interpretation. Salt Lake City, UT, ARUP Laboratories, 2020. Available at: https://arupconsult.com/content/mycobacterium-tuberculosis. Accessed September 2021.

Carranza C, Pedraza-Sanchez S, de Oyarzabal-Mendez E, Torres M: Diagnosis for latent tuberculosis infection: new alternatives. Front Immunol 11:2006, 2020

Uric acid

Type of test	Blood
Background and explanation of test	Uric acid is produced by the degradation of injured and dying cells and the breakdown of dietary purines. Most is excreted by the kidneys and the remainder through the GI tract. Blood levels of uric acid can be elevated because of overproduction (e.g., with gout or leukemia) or underexcretion (e.g., with renal impairment). High uric acid levels are associated not only with gout but also with cardiovascular and cerebrovascular disease, hypertension, type 2 diabetes, chronic kidney disease, and the metabolic syndrome.
Relevance to psychiatry and behavioral science	Uric acid may be elevated in patients with alcohol use disorder. High levels are associated with heart attack, stroke, and vascular dementia. High levels likely have a role in the development of the metabolic syndrome, possibly because of proinflammatory and pro-oxidative effects.
Preparation of patient	Ideally, patients should fast for 8 hours and avoid strenuous exercise before testing.
Indications	• Suspected gout • Workup for recurrent kidney stones • Evaluating renal dysfunction • Monitoring effects of cytotoxic therapy (chemotherapy or radiation)
Reference range	Adult males: ≤7 mg/dL Adult females: ≤6 mg/dL Levels are based on the saturation point of uric acid used in gout management. Dose-dependent inflammatory action of uric acid occurs with levels >4 mg/dL.
Critical value(s)	>12 mg/dL
Increased levels	• Gout • Leukemia, lymphoma, multiple myeloma • Hemolytic anemia, sickle cell anemia • Polycythemia vera • Psoriasis • Cytotoxic therapy (e.g., chemotherapy, radiation) • Starvation, anorexia nervosa, severe dieting • Renal failure • Excessive alcohol consumption • Liver disease • Hyperlipidemia, obesity, metabolic syndrome • Metabolic acidosis, diabetic ketoacidosis

Uric acid (continued)

Increased levels (continued)	• Pernicious anemia
	• Kidney stones
	• Lead poisoning
	• Purine-rich diet (enriched with red meat, seafood)
	• *Drugs:* diuretics, β-blockers, low-dose aspirin
Decreased levels	• Fanconi syndrome
	• Wilson's disease
	• SIAD
	• Low-purine diet
	• Certain malignancies (e.g., Hodgkin's disease, broncho-genic carcinoma)
	• Xanthinuria
Interfering factors	High levels of stress and strenuous exercise cause increased uric acid levels.
Cross-references	**Alcohol Use Disorder**

American Association for Clinical Chemistry: Testing.com. Available at: https://www.testing.com. Accessed September 2021.

Borghi C, Agabiti-Rosei E, Johnson RJ, et al: Hyperuricaemia and gout in cardiovascular, metabolic and kidney disease. Eur J Intern Med 80:1–11, 2020

Cortese F, Scicchitano P, Cortese AM, et al: Uric acid in metabolic and cerebrovascular disorders: a review. Curr Vasc Pharmacol 18(6):610–618, 2020

Fischbach FT, Fischbach MA: A Manual of Laboratory and Diagnostic Tests, 10th Edition. Philadelphia, PA, Wolters Kluwer Health/Lippincott Williams and Wilkins, 2018

Kaul S, Gupta M, Bandyopadhyay D, et al: Gout pharmacotherapy in cardiovascular diseases: a review of utility and outcomes. Am J Cardiovasc Drugs 21(5):499–512, 2021

Lohr JW, Batuman V: Hyperuricemia. Medscape, July 1, 2022. Available at: https://emedicine.medscape.com/article/241767-overview. Accessed September 2021.

Maloberti A, Giannattasio C, Bombelli M, et al: Hyperuricemia and risk of cardiovascular outcomes: the experience of the URRAH (Uric Acid Right for Heart Health) Project. High Blood Press Cardiovasc Prev 27(2):121–128, 2020

Urinalysis

Type of test	Urine
Background and explanation of test	Urinalysis is a basic laboratory test most often used to evaluate urinary tract infection (UTI) or kidney dysfunction. Findings can also indicate glucose dysregulation, liver problems, and other conditions. A complete urinalysis reports the following characteristics of urine: color, appearance, specific gravity, pH, glucose, ketones, blood, protein, bilirubin, urobilinogen, nitrite, leukocyte esterase, and the results of a microscopic exam. The microscopic exam detects RBCs, WBCs, casts, crystals, and epithelial cells.
	Physical characteristics of the specimen are first noted, chemical tests are performed, and finally the specimen is examined microscopically. The first two steps can be done using a dipstick and automated methods, which makes this test quick and inexpensive. A urinalysis is often a standard component of the hospital admission workup or presurgical evaluation.
Relevance to psychiatry and behavioral science	Urinalysis is a routine component of the workup for mental status changes, particularly in elderly patients in nursing homes or hospital settings. UTIs can be associated with delirium, even in the absence of sepsis.
Preparation of patient	A first morning urine specimen may be requested because it is more concentrated and thus more likely to show abnormalities. If a random sample is used, it should be collected ≥4 hours after last voiding to ensure adequate contact time between bacteria and nitrates. Practice varies as to the amount collected; some labs request a 30–60 mL sample, whereas others request only 10 mL.
	If a midstream, clean-catch sample is requested, antibacterial wipes should be used to clean the area between the labia or around the meatus of the penis. A small amount of urine is voided to the toilet, then urine is captured in the container provided. Medications must be noted on the urinalysis request form to aid in crystal identification by the laboratory.
Indications	• Routine component of workup for hospital admission or preoperative surgical evaluation
	• Symptoms of UTI: irritation, burning, pain, change in frequency, or change in appearance of urine
	• Symptoms in elderly patients: fever, dysuria, incontinence, urgency, or change in frequency
	• Symptoms in catheterized patients: fever, rigors, vomiting, confusion, or costovertebral angle tenderness
	• Suspected pyelonephritis or kidney dysfunction
	• Screening for asymptomatic bacteriuria in pregnancy (at first antenatal visit)
Reference range	*Color*: pale yellow to amber
	Appearance: clear to slightly hazy

Urinalysis _(continued)_

Reference range _(continued)_	_Specific gravity_: 1.002–1.035;
	_pH_: 4.5–8.0
	Negative for glucose, ketones, blood, protein, bilirubin, urobilinogen, nitrite, and leukocyte esterase. Negative for casts or occasional hyaline. Negative or rare for RBCs. Negative for crystals. Negative or rare for WBCs. Few epithelial cells.
Critical value(s)	See entries for urinalysis components.
Increased levels	See entries for urinalysis components.
Decreased levels	See entries for urinalysis components.
Interfering factors	Improper specimen handling invalidates the results. Urine must be examined within 1 hour of collection or refrigerated immediately and examined within 24 hours. If the first morning specimen is not used, inadequate contact time can yield a false-negative nitrite test. Even with clean-catch specimens, feces, vaginal discharge, or menstrual blood can contaminate the specimen.
Cross-references	See entries for urinalysis components.
	Urinary Tract Infection

American Association for Clinical Chemistry: Testing.com. Available at: https://www.testing.com. Accessed October 2021.

Fischbach FT, Fischbach MA: A Manual of Laboratory and Diagnostic Tests, 10th Edition. Philadelphia, PA, Wolters Kluwer Health/Lippincott Williams and Wilkins, 2018

Simerville JA, Maxted WC, Pahira JJ: Urinalysis: a comprehensive review. Am Fam Physician 71:1153–1162, 2005

Urine appearance

Type of test	Component of routine urinalysis
Background and explanation of test	*Appearance* refers to the observed clarity of the specimen.
Relevance to psychiatry and behavioral science	See **Urinalysis**.
Preparation of patient	See **Urinalysis**.
Indications	See **Urinalysis**.
Reference range	Normally, fresh urine is clear to slightly hazy.
Abnormal test	• *Range*: hazy→slightly cloudy→cloudy→turbid→milky • Abnormal urine is often turbid or cloudy. These findings can indicate the presence of urinary tract infection.
Interfering factors	After a meal, normal urine can appear cloudy if allowed to stand, due to the presence of urates, carbonates, and phosphates. Vaginal discharge, semen, and fecal material all cause turbidity in urine. Skin cream, vaginal cream, talcum powder, and radiographic contrast dye may cause turbidity. Greasy turbidity can be seen with large amounts of fat in urine. Normal urine can develop haziness or turbidity after standing (even with refrigeration) due to precipitation of calcium oxalate or urate crystals.
Cross-references	**Urinalysis**

American Association for Clinical Chemistry: Testing.com. Available at: https://www.testing.com. Accessed October 2021.

Fischbach FT, Fischbach MA: A Manual of Laboratory and Diagnostic Tests, 10th Edition. Philadelphia, PA, Wolters Kluwer Health/Lippincott Williams and Wilkins, 2018

Simerville JA, Maxted WC, Pahira JJ: Urinalysis: a comprehensive review. Am Fam Physician 71:1153–1162, 2005

Urine bilirubin

Type of test	Component of routine urinalysis
Background and explanation of test	The presence of even trace amounts of bilirubin in the urine is not normal and should be investigated. Any disease process that results in increased conjugated bilirubin in the circulation can increase the level of bilirubin in urine.
	In the absence of disease, conjugated bilirubin is excreted through the GI tract. With hepatobiliary disease, it enters the circulation instead and is filtered and excreted by the kidneys. Urine bilirubin provides an early warning of hepatocellular disease or biliary obstruction (intrahepatic or extrahepatic). Bilirubin can appear in the urine before jaundice appears. In addition, the presence or absence of urinary bilirubin can help in determining the etiology of jaundice; urine bilirubin is absent in hemolytic disease.
Relevance to psychiatry and behavioral science	Urine bilirubin can be present in patients with hepatitis, cirrhosis, or (more rarely) hyperthyroidism. It may be useful in monitoring patients who are in treatment for drug/alcohol dependence. Several herbal remedies used by behavioral health patients can cause bilirubinuria, including kava kava, germander, and chaparral.
Preparation of patient	See **Urinalysis**.
Indications	• Component of routine urinalysis • Early diagnosis of hepatobiliary disease • Monitoring treatment for hepatitis
Reference range	Negative (<0.02 mg/dL)
Critical value(s)	None
Increased levels	• Hepatitis, cirrhosis, and other liver diseases • Obstructive biliary tract disease • Malignancy (liver or biliary tract) • Sepsis • Hyperthyroidism • Herbal medicines (kava kava, germander, chaparral)
Decreased levels	Not applicable
Interfering factors	Urine left standing causes false-negative results. Decreased sensitivity of the test is seen with the use of high doses of vitamin C or nitrates. Phenazopyridine (Pyridium)-like drugs or urochromes can turn urine amber or red and mask bilirubin reaction.
Cross-references	**Bilirubin** **Cirrhosis** **Hepatitis, Viral** **Urinalysis**

Urine bilirubin *(continued)*

American Association for Clinical Chemistry: Lab Tests Online. Available at: https://www.testing.com. Accessed October 2021.

Dasgupta A, Bernard DW: Herbal remedies: effects on clinical laboratory tests. Arch Pathol Lab Med 130(4):521–528, 2006

Fischbach FT, Fischbach MA: A Manual of Laboratory and Diagnostic Tests, 10th Edition. Philadelphia, PA, Wolters Kluwer Health/Lippincott Williams and Wilkins, 2018

Simerville JA, Maxted WC, Pahira JJ: Urinalysis: a comprehensive review. Am Fam Physician 71:1153–1162, 2005

Urine blood, hemoglobin, and myoglobin

Type of test	Component of routine urinalysis
Background and explanation of test	This part of the urinalysis detects RBCs, hemoglobin, and myoglobin. • *Hematuria* is present when intact RBCs are identified and indicates disease or trauma to the kidney or other part of the genitourinary system. • *Hemoglobinuria* is present when free hemoglobin is identified; this indicates either intravascular hemolysis that exceeds the capacity to metabolize or store excess free hemoglobin or lysis of RBCs in the urinary tract itself. • *Myoglobinuria* is present when the urine is positive for occult blood, but no RBCs are identified; this indicates injury to muscle tissue, with the excretion of muscle protein into the urine. Urine containing myoglobin can appear highly colored.
Relevance to psychiatry and behavioral science	Heavy smoking is associated with hematuria. NMS and ECT are known to cause myoglobinuria along with significantly elevated creatine kinase levels. Rhabdomyolysis with myoglobinuria is associated with succinylcholine, halogenated anesthetics, propofol, and corticosteroids.
Preparation of patient	See **Urinalysis**. Females should note whether they are menstruating at the time of sampling.
Indications	Component of routine urinalysis
Reference range	Negative (<10 erythrocytes/µL or <0.03 mg free hemoglobin/dL)
Critical value(s)	*Blood in urine is not a normal finding.* A positive test for blood should be confirmed on a second urine specimen. If the test is still positive, the cause should be investigated.
Increased levels	*Intact RBCs (hematuria)* Acute cystitis, lupus nephritis, kidney or genitourinary cancer, kidney or urinary tract stones, malignant hypertension, glomerulonephritis, pyelonephritis, trauma, polycystic kidney disease, leukemia, thrombocytopenia, strenuous exercise, benign recurrent (familial) hematuria, heavy smoking, drugs (nephrotoxins such as amphotericin, anticoagulants such as warfarin, hemolytic drugs such as aspirin) *Free hemoglobin (hemoglobinuria)* Extensive burns, bleeding after prostate surgery, transfusion of incompatible blood, malaria, certain poisons, hemolytic disorders (sickle cell anemia, thalassemia), kidney infarction, fava bean sensitivity, disseminated intravascular coagulation, strenuous exercise, paroxysmal hemoglobinuria, or hypotonic alkaline urine

Urine blood, hemoglobin, and myoglobin *(continued)*

Increased levels *(continued)*	*Myoglobinuria* NMS, ECT, trauma, intense physical activity, muscular dystrophy, malignant hyperthermia
Decreased levels	Not applicable
Interfering factors	Sensitivity of the test is reduced by high urine specific gravity or elevated urine protein. Menstrual blood or blood from urinary catheter trauma may contaminate the specimen. Bleach used to clean urine containers may cause false-positive results. Drugs causing false-positive results include bromides, copper, iodides, and oxidizing agents. High-dose vitamin C intake may cause false-negative results.
Cross-references	**Neuroleptic Malignant Syndrome** **Urinalysis** **Urinary Tract Infection** **Urine Red Blood Cells (RBCs) and RBC Casts**

American Association for Clinical Chemistry: Testing.com. Available at: https://www.testing.com. Accessed October 2021.

Angelini C, Marozzo R, Pegoraro V, Sacconi S: Diagnostic challenges in metabolic myopathies. Expert Rev Neurother 20(12):1287–1298, 2020

Barrons RW, Nguyen LT: Succinylcholine-induced rhabdomyolysis in adults: case report and review of the literature. J Pharm Pract 33(1):102–107, 2020

Cabral BMI, Edding SN, Portocarrero JP, Lerma EV: Rhabdomyolysis. Dis Mon 66(8):101015, 2020

Fischbach FT, Fischbach MA: A Manual of Laboratory and Diagnostic Tests, 10th Edition. Philadelphia, PA, Wolters Kluwer Health/Lippincott Williams and Wilkins, 2018

Laoutidis ZG, Kioulos KT: Antipsychotic-induced elevation of creatine kinase: a systematic review of the literature and recommendations for the clinical practice. Psychopharmacology (Berl) 231(22):4255–4270, 2014

Simerville JA, Maxted WC, Pahira JJ: Urinalysis: a comprehensive review. Am Fam Physician 71:1153–1162, 2005

Urine casts

Type of test	Component of routine urinalysis
Background and explanation of test	*Casts* are tube-shaped particles sometimes found in urine that are formed from coagulated proteins released in the distal convoluted tubule or collecting duct of the nephron. In the absence of pathology, only hyaline casts are seen. These are clear and few in number, although the number can increase with strenuous exercise. Other types of casts include cellular casts of WBCs or RBCs, granular casts, fatty casts, and waxy casts. Some types have specific pathological significance, as noted in the *Abnormal Test* section below. In general, low-flow, high-salt, and low-pH conditions in the nephron favor cast formation. To visualize casts, the urine sample is centrifuged, and a drop of the sediment is examined under low power. Phase-contrast microscopy is superior to bright field microscopy for this purpose.
Relevance to psychiatry and behavioral science	The synthetic cannabinoid commonly known as "spice" has been known to cause kidney injury in the form of acute tubular necrosis or acute interstitial nephritis, with granular casts formed. In COVID-19 infection, urinalysis findings have included myoglobin casts and cellular debris casts.
Preparation of patient	See **Urinalysis**.
Indications	Component of microscopic analysis of urine sediment included in complete urinalysis
Reference range	Broad, waxy casts: 0
	Fatty casts: 0
	Granular casts: 0–2
	Hyaline casts: 0–2
	RBC casts: 0
	WBC casts: 0
	Renal tubular epithelial casts: 0
Critical value(s)	None
Abnormal test	• Broad, waxy casts seen in urinary stasis, which occurs in renal failure.
	• Fatty casts indicate lipids in urine, usually in association with nephrotic syndrome.
	• Granular casts are a nonspecific sign of kidney disease.
	• Hyaline casts are caused by dehydration, exercise, or diuretic medication and are usually benign.
	• RBC casts indicate bleeding into the kidney tubule associated with glomerular disease, as found in SLE.
	• WBC casts indicate infection of the renal parenchyma, the most common cause being pyelonephritis.
	• Renal tubular epithelial casts indicate tubule injury associated with renal tubular necrosis, viral disease, or transplant rejection.

Urine casts *(continued)*

Interfering factors	Casts dissolve readily in alkaline or dilute urine. RBC casts may appear in urine after strenuous physical activity.
Cross-references	**Urinalysis**

American Association for Clinical Chemistry: Testing.com. Available at: https://www.testing.com. Accessed October 2021.

Fischbach FT, Fischbach MA: A Manual of Laboratory and Diagnostic Tests, 10th Edition. Philadelphia, PA, Wolters Kluwer Health/Lippincott Williams and Wilkins, 2018

Fogazzi GB, Delanghe J: Microscopic examination of urine sediment: phase contrast versus bright field. Clin Chim Acta 487:168–173, 2018

Simerville JA, Maxted WC, Pahira JJ: Urinalysis: a comprehensive review. Am Fam Physician 71:1153–1162, 2005

Zarifi C, Vyas S: Spice-y Kidney failure: a case report and systematic review of acute kidney injury attributable to the use of synthetic cannabis. Perm J 21:16–160, 2017

Urine color

Type of test	Component of routine urinalysis
Background and explanation of test	The color of normal urine comes from the pigment urochrome, a product of metabolism. The color can change with the use of certain drugs, ingestion of highly colored foods, and a limited number of diseases.
Relevance to psychiatry and behavioral science	Urine color may be a focus of concern for some somatizing patients. A limited group of psychotropic medications causes discoloration of the urine. Diseases causing urine discoloration include hepatitis, in which darkening of the urine is seen; acute intermittent porphyria, in which urine darkens on exposure to light; and Addison's disease. Other factors affecting urine color that may be of particular interest to psychiatrists and behavioral medicine clinicians are listed in the *Abnormal Findings* section below.
Preparation of patient	See **Urinalysis**.
Indications	See **Urinalysis**.
Reference range	Normally, urine is pale yellow to amber, depending on the patient's state of hydration. Straw-colored urine indicates low specific gravity. Amber urine indicates high specific gravity, usually with low urine output.
Critical findings	Red urine should be checked for hemoglobin; if present, the patient should be questioned about recent trauma, infection, or vigorous exercise. If occult blood is not present in red urine, the patient should be evaluated for porphyria. Other urine colors should be investigated using appropriate tests.
Abnormal findings	• *Colorless urine (suggests high urine output)*: large fluid intake, as with polydipsia; untreated diabetes with glycosuria; diabetes insipidus; excessive alcohol ingestion; diuretic therapy; or anxiety • *Dark yellow to amber urine*: bilirubin; urobilinogen; use of chlorpromazine, nitrofurantoin, or riboflavin; excessive ingestion of carrots or use of herbal remedies, such as cascara sagrada • *Orange urine*: concentrated urine as with dehydration; bile pigment; excessive ingestion of vitamin A or carrots; medications such as nitrofurantoin, used for urinary tract infection; use of phenothiazines, rifampin, heparin, or warfarin • *Green urine*: *Pseudomonas* infection; ingestion of chlorophyll, biliverdin, or certain vitamins or diuretics • *Red urine*: RBCs, hemoglobin, myoglobin, methemoglobin, oxyhemoglobin, porphyrins, malaria, or ingestion of beets, rhubarb, or senna (see also *Critical Findings* section above) • *Brown urine*: Addison's disease; presence of bile, myoglobin; use of levodopa, metronidazole, nitrofurantoin, or sulfonamides

Urine color *(continued)*

Abnormal findings *(continued)*	• *Black urine*: iron, melanin, methemoglobin, urobilinogen, or use of levodopa, chloroquine, metronidazole, senna, or herbal remedies such as cascara sagrada
	• *Blue urine*: use of amitriptyline, methylene blue, triamterene, or nitrofurantoin; *Pseudomonas* infection
	• *Milky urine*: cystinuria, presence of fat or abundant WBCs or phosphates
Interfering factors	Normal urine begins to darken on standing within 30 minutes.
Cross-references	**Urinalysis**

American Association for Clinical Chemistry: Testing.com. Available at: https://www.testing.com. Accessed October 2021.

Fischbach FT, Fischbach MA: A Manual of Laboratory and Diagnostic Tests, 10th Edition. Philadelphia, PA, Wolters Kluwer Health/Lippincott Williams and Wilkins, 2018

Simerville JA, Maxted WC, Pahira JJ: Urinalysis: a comprehensive review. Am Fam Physician 71:1153–1162, 2005

Urine crystals

Type of test	Component of routine urinalysis
Background and explanation of test	Crystals are a normal component of the urine that form when minerals are present in sufficient concentration, with urine protein often acting as a nidus for crystal formation. Different types of crystals are formed at different pH levels. Small numbers of magnesium ammonium phosphate crystals (struvite) are not harmful, but other types of crystals can be toxic and/or indicate the presence of systemic disease, as noted in the *Positive Test* section below. Dehydration as well as high-protein, high-salt diets can promote crystal formation. Aggregation of crystals can create kidney and lower urinary tract stones and may lead to hydronephrosis, pyelonephritis, or acute renal failure.
Relevance to psychiatry and behavioral science	Ethylene glycol poisoning is associated with calcium oxalate crystals. Commonly used medications (e.g., ampicillin and sulfonamides) and radiographic dyes can form crystals in the presence of dehydration.
Preparation of patient	Patients should not fast before testing but should continue their usual diet and hydration regimen. If crystals found on routine urinalysis are to be investigated further, a 24-hour urine sample should be requested.
Indications	Component of routine urinalysis as well as more detailed investigations with 24-hour urine sample
Reference range	The following crystals are considered normal or of no clinical significance: • *Acid urine*: amorphous urates, sodium urate • *Alkaline urine*: amorphous phosphates, calcium carbonate, and calcium phosphate Ammonium biurate crystals may be normal but require a second urine sample to confirm.
Critical value(s)	None
Positive test	• *Acid urine*: bilirubin crystals with elevated bilirubin levels; uric acid crystals with gout, increased purine metabolism, or Lesch-Nyhan syndrome • *Acid, neutral, or mildly alkaline urine*: calcium oxalate—may be normal, but large amounts in freshly voided specimen may suggest renal disease, liver disease, diabetes mellitus, ethylene glycol poisoning, or excessive doses of vitamin C • *Alkaline, neutral, or mildly acidic urine*: triple phosphate (struvite)—may be normal or may indicate urinary stasis with chronic cystitis, chronic pyelitis, or enlarged prostate
Negative test	None
Interfering factors	Urine must be examined immediately; urine left standing at room temperature yields invalid results.
Cross-references	**Urinalysis**

Urine crystals *(continued)*

American Association for Clinical Chemistry: Testing.com. Available at: https://www.testing.com. Accessed October 2021.

Cohen SM: Crystalluria and chronic kidney disease. Toxicol Pathol 46(8):949–955, 2018

Fischbach FT, Fischbach MA: A Manual of Laboratory and Diagnostic Tests, 10th Edition. Philadelphia, PA, Wolters Kluwer Health/Lippincott Williams and Wilkins, 2018

Rimer JD, Kolbach-Mandel AM, Ward MD, Wesson JA: The role of macromolecules in the formation of kidney stones. Urolithiasis 5(1):57–74, 2017

Simerville JA, Maxted WC, Pahira JJ: Urinalysis: a comprehensive review. Am Fam Physician 71:1153–1162, 2005

Williams JC Jr, Gambaro G, Rodgers A, et al: Urine and stone analysis for the investigation of the renal stone former: a consensus conference. Urolithiasis 49(1):1–16, 2021

Urine dipstick testing

Type of test	Urine
Background and explanation of test	Dipstick testing is a quick and inexpensive way to test urine for infection and other abnormalities without the need to involve the laboratory. Specific instructions for test kits must be followed to ensure the accuracy of the results, and interpretation is made in the context of clinical signs and symptoms.
Relevance to psychiatry and behavioral science	This test could be conducted in the outpatient office setting. It may be of particular use to physicians caring for geriatric patients.
Preparation of patient	Follow test kit instructions.
Indications	Suspected uncomplicated urinary tract infection (UTI)
Normal test	A dipstick test that is negative for leukocyte esterase (LE) and nitrite has a negative predictive value (i.e., absence of UTI) of ≥95%.
Abnormal test	• If either nitrite or LE *and* blood are positive, UTI is probable. • If nitrite, LE, blood, *and* protein are all negative, UTI is unlikely. Urethral syndrome may be present. • If nitrite is negative and *either* LE or blood is positive, UTI or urethral syndrome is probable. • If nitrite, LE, *and* blood are all negative *but* protein is positive, a diagnosis other than UTI should be suspected.
Interfering factors	If the test kit instructions are not followed, results may not be valid. Unless the first morning urine specimen is used, nitrite testing may yield false-negative results. If infecting bacteria do not reduce urinary nitrates, nitrite testing may yield false-negative results.
Cross-references	**Urinalysis** **Urinary Tract Infection** **Urine Blood, Hemoglobin, and Myoglobin** **Urine Leukocyte Esterase** **Urine Nitrite** **Urine Protein**

Devillé WL, Yzermans JC, van Duijn NP, et al: The urine dipstick test useful to rule out infections: a meta-analysis of the accuracy. BMC Urol 4:4, 2004

Fischbach FT, Fischbach MA: A Manual of Laboratory and Diagnostic Tests, 10th Edition. Philadelphia, PA, Wolters Kluwer Health/Lippincott Williams and Wilkins, 2018

Simerville JA, Maxted WC, Pahira JJ: Urinalysis: a comprehensive review. Am Fam Physician 71:1153–1162, 2005

Urine drug screen

Type of test	Urine
Background and explanation of test	Screening for drugs of abuse can be performed on blood, urine, hair, nails, and breath. Urine is most commonly used because it is easy to obtain and has a reasonable window of detection for clinical purposes. For initial screening, urine dipstick tests are often used. These are immunoassays that return positive results when specified thresholds are exceeded. These tests are prone to false-negative and false-positive results, so they must be followed up with more sensitive and specific tests that use gas chromatography/ mass spectrometry or high-performance liquid chromatography. These methods return quantitative results and identify the specific drugs detected.
	Although drug tests can be ordered individually, more often a standard panel of drugs is requested. For use in medical and mental health settings, that panel usually includes opioids, cocaine, amphetamines, barbiturates, benzodiazepines, phencyclidine (PCP), and cannabinoids (THC). Alcohol may or may not be included, depending on the laboratory protocol and panel requested. Standard panels often do not include "club drugs" such as MDMA (Ecstasy), gamma-hydroxybutyrate (GHB), flunitrazepam (Rohypnol), and ketamine or synthetic opioids such as fentanyl, methadone, and buprenorphine. Sensitivity to semisynthetic opioids such as oxycodone and hydrocodone may be low, such that specific drug testing may be needed. All of these issues should be discussed with the laboratory before the specimen is collected. For GHB, the half-life of the drug is so short that detection is always difficult.
	Complicating the interpretation of opioid screening results is the fact that some opioids are metabolized to other opioids, such that their presence may indicate metabolism rather than additional abuse. For example, if free morphine as a percentage of free codeine is <55%, the morphine may be a product of codeine metabolism. The detection of 6-acetylmorphine with morphine is definitive evidence of heroin use, but this intermediate metabolite is short-lived (<8 hours).
	Urine testing for buprenorphine can be requested, either to screen for illicit use or to confirm compliance with treatment. The major metabolite norbuprenorphine should be included. Urine methadone screening is subject to confounding by patients who are diverting the drug and then adding methadone itself to the urine sample. In this case, the metabolite EDDP (2-ethylidene-1,5-dimethyl-3,3-diphenylpyrrolidine) could be tested; its presence indicates that methadone has been taken and metabolized.

Urine drug screen *(continued)*

Background and explanation of test *(continued)*	Most urine assays for benzodiazepines are designed to detect only diazepam, nordiazepam, and oxazepam. Metabolites of alprazolam, lorazepam, and clonazepam are often not detected, but the parent drugs may be detectable if the cutoff for detection is lowered because only a small proportion of these drugs is excreted unchanged. A lower cutoff may also be required for very potent drugs, such as alprazolam, because only small doses are used.
	Interpretation of screening results for the stimulants amphetamine and methamphetamine is difficult because of poor specificity; positive results should be confirmed with quantitative testing. Methylphenidate detection requires a separate test. With cocaine, on the other hand, the detection of the metabolite benzoylecgonine is straightforward.
	Urine screening for marijuana use detects a metabolite of THC, with the window of detection dependent on the pattern of use, ranging from 3 days in a one-time user to 30 days in a heavy, chronic user. Positive results are unlikely to be found from passive inhalation. Testing for synthetic cannabinoids (e.g., Spice, K2) is not routine but can be specifically requested.
	Urine detection windows for various drugs are shown in a table prepared by ARUP Laboratories, which at this writing can be found at www.aruplab.com/files/resources/pain-management/DrugAnalytesPlasmaUrine.pdf.
Relevance to psychiatry and behavioral science	Urine drug screening is commonly used in the emergency setting and in general psychiatry and substance abuse treatment settings. Screening can detect illicit drug use or confirm compliance with treatment (e.g., with methadone). Screening can also flag possible diversion of prescribed medication. Use in occupational and forensic settings involves different protocols and detection cutoff levels and is not covered here. Unobserved urine sampling can result in false-negative results because of tampering (e.g., diluting urine). In these cases, a simultaneous urinalysis can assist in interpretation. A comprehensive history of recent substances used (including over-the-counter drugs) can help in the interpretation of false-positive results.
Preparation of patient	Patients should be informed of the reason for drug testing, and agreement should be made as to how the results will be used and who will see them. The consequences of interfering with drug testing (e.g., diluting urine) should be made clear.
Indications	• Patient in emergency setting with unexplained symptoms • Patient in emergency setting after an accident in which alcohol or substance use is suspected • Patient suspected of drug use • Pregnant patient at risk of drug use • Monitoring a known drug user

Urine drug screen *(continued)*

Reference range	Refer to lab documentation.
Critical value(s)	Not applicable
Positive test	Positive screening tests are confirmed by more sensitive and specific assays. Positive confirmation in the absence of confounding factors means the patient has ingested the drug.
Negative test	If the drug is not present or is present below the predetermined cutoff for positive test, the report is returned as "not detected."
	Note: A negative result does not necessarily mean the drug was never taken; it may have been eliminated by the time the test was taken or may have been present below the assay's detection limit. Dilution of urine and rapid drug metabolism both cause false-negative results. It is also possible that the drug taken was not included in the drug screening panel requested.
Interfering factors	*Amphetamines*: False-positive results may occur with aripiprazole, atomoxetine, bupropion, ephedrine, labetalol, MDMA (3,4-methylenedioxymethamphetamine), phentermine, pseudoephedrine, ranitidine, selegiline, trazodone, and Vicks inhalers.
	Benzodiazepines: False-positive results may occur with efavirenz and sertraline.
	Opioids: False-positive results may occur with dextromethorphan, diphenhydramine, rifampin, quinolone antibiotics, and poppy seeds.
	PCP: False-positive results may occur with dextromethorphan, doxylamine, ketamine, tramadol, and venlafaxine.
	THC: False-positive results may occur with dronabinol, efavirenz, and nabilone.
Cross-references	**Blood Alcohol Level**
	Drug Abuse

ARUP Laboratories: Drug Plasma Half-Life and Urine Detection Window. Salt Lake City, UT, ARUP Laboratories, 2021. Available at: https://www.aruplab.com/files/resources/pain-management/DrugAnalytesPlasmaUrine.pdf. Accessed June 2021

Dadiomov D: Laboratory testing for substance use disorders, in Absolute Addiction Psychiatry Review. Edited by Marienfeld C. Cham, Switzerland, Springer, 2020.

Moeller KE, Lee KC, Kissack JC: Urine drug screening: practical guide for clinicians. Mayo Clin Proc 83:66–76, 2008

Reisfield GM, Bertholf RL: "Practical guide" to urine drug screening clarified. Mayo Clin Proc 83:848–849, 2008

Urine epithelial cells and epithelial casts

Type of test	Component of routine urinalysis
Background and explanation of test	Three types of epithelial cells appear in urine: • Renal tubule epithelial cells, which may be seen with normal sloughing or may indicate renal disease. In acute tubular necrosis, epithelial cells containing large vacuoles known as *bubble cells* may be seen. When lipids cross the glomerulus, *oval fat bodies* may be seen. • Bladder or transitional epithelial cells • Squamous epithelial cells, mostly from the urethra and vagina Epithelial casts form from sloughed tubule cells that have degenerated. These casts are rare.
Relevance to psychiatry and behavioral science	Epithelial cells or casts are not a commonly encountered abnormality in psychiatric practice, although they may be found in heavy metal poisoning or aspirin overdose.
Preparation of patient	See **Urinalysis**.
Indications	Component of routine urinalysis
Reference range	Renal tubule epithelial cells: 0–3/hpf Renal tubule epithelial casts: 0 Squamous epithelial cells are common in normal urine.
Critical value(s)	None
Positive test	Renal tubule epithelial cells (>3/hpf): • Acute tubular necrosis • Acute glomerulonephritis • Pyelonephritis • Salicylate overdose • Impending allograft rejection • Viral infection (e.g., cytomegalovirus) • Heavy metal poisoning or other toxins Epithelial cell casts are also found with exposure to toxic agents or viruses.
Negative test	None
Interfering factors	None
Cross-references	**Urinalysis**

Fischbach FT, Fischbach MA: A Manual of Laboratory and Diagnostic Tests, 10th Edition. Philadelphia, PA, Wolters Kluwer Health/Lippincott Williams and Wilkins, 2018

Simerville JA, Maxted WC, Pahira JJ: Urinalysis: a comprehensive review. Am Fam Physician 71:1153–1162, 2005

Skoberne A, Konieczny A, Schiffer M: Glomerular epithelial cells in the urine: what has to be done to make them worthwhile? Am J Physiol Renal Physiol 296(2):F230–F241, 2009

Urine glucose

Type of test	Component of routine urinalysis
Background and explanation of test	Most glucose filtered by the glomerulus is reabsorbed in the proximal convoluted tubule. If blood glucose is high enough that the tubule's capacity is exceeded, glucose appears in the urine, a sign known as *glycosuria*. This occurs at a blood glucose level between 160 mg/dL and 180 mg/dL.
Relevance to psychiatry and behavioral science	Glycosuria occurs in several conditions of interest to psychiatrists and behavioral health clinicians. See *Increased Levels* section below.
Preparation of patient	See **Urinalysis**.
Indications	Component of routine urinalysis
Reference range	Random specimen: negative for glucose
Critical value(s)	Urine glucose >1,000 mg/dL (4+) indicates need to check blood glucose immediately and begin prompt treatment.
Increased levels	<ul><li>Diabetes mellitus</li><li>Endocrine disease (Cushing's syndrome, thyrotoxicosis)</li><li>Liver disease</li><li>Pancreatic disease</li><li>TBI</li><li>Stroke</li><li>Impaired tubular reabsorption (Fanconi syndrome, renal tubular disease)</li><li>Gestational diabetes</li></ul>
Decreased levels	Not applicable
Interfering factors	False-positive results (usually trace) may be seen with stress, MI, testing after heavy meal, or testing after IV glucose administration. Many drugs interfere with this assay.
Cross-references	**Urinalysis**

Fischbach FT, Fischbach MA: A Manual of Laboratory and Diagnostic Tests, 10th Edition. Philadelphia, PA, Wolters Kluwer Health/Lippincott Williams and Wilkins, 2018

Simerville JA, Maxted WC, Pahira JJ: Urinalysis: a comprehensive review. Am Fam Physician 71:1153–1162, 2005

Urine ketones

Type of test	Component of routine urinalysis
Background and explanation of test	Ketones are breakdown products of fats that are formed in the liver. Normally, ketones are completely metabolized, so they do not appear in the urine. When carbohydrate metabolism is altered such that fat is preferentially metabolized, excessive amounts of ketones are formed that do appear in the urine. Although ketonuria is most closely associated with diabetes mellitus, it can also occur in nondiabetic individuals who are fasting or on a ketogenic diet, after strenuous exercise, during acute illness, after certain types of anesthesia, with fever, with severe stress, or with pregnancy and lactation.
Relevance to psychiatry and behavioral science	Ketonuria in a patient with diabetes is an important sign that diabetes is not controlled and that medication and/or dietary intervention is needed. Prolonged vomiting or diarrhea in patients with purging behaviors can be associated with ketonuria. A false-positive result on urine ketone testing can occur with the use of valproate or phenothiazine drugs.
Preparation of patient	See **Urinalysis**.
Indications	• Component of routine urinalysis • Screening and monitoring of pregnant patient • Determining severity of acidosis • Various uses in patients with diabetes: monitoring elevated glucose in blood and/or urine, switching from insulin to oral hypoglycemic, monitoring patients taking oral hypoglycemic agents, distinguishing diabetic coma from insulin shock
Reference range	Negative or <0.2 mg/dL
Critical value(s)	>80 mg/dL signifies a large amount of urinary ketones.
Increased levels	• Diabetes—in diabetic patients, ketonuria indicates diabetes is not controlled and medication and/or dietary intervention is needed. • Starvation—in nondiabetic patients, ketonuria indicates fat metabolism in preference to carbohydrate metabolism. • Carbohydrate-restricted diet • Excessive amount of fat in diet • Renal glycosuria • Glycogen storage disease • Prolonged vomiting or diarrhea • Hyperthyroidism
Decreased levels	Not applicable

Urine ketones *(continued)*

Interfering factors	False-negative results can occur if urine is allowed to stand too long before analysis.
	False-positive results can occur with certain drugs: valproate, phenothiazines, levodopa, aspirin, insulin, metformin, acetylcysteine, captopril, niacin, isoniazid, phenazopyridine, penicillamine, and isopropyl alcohol, among others.
Cross-references	**Diabetes Mellitus**
	Urinalysis

American Association for Clinical Chemistry: Testing.com. Available at: https://www.testing.com. Accessed October 2021.

Fischbach FT, Fischbach MA: A Manual of Laboratory and Diagnostic Tests, 10th Edition. Philadelphia, PA, Wolters Kluwer Health/Lippincott Williams and Wilkins, 2018

Simerville JA, Maxted WC, Pahira JJ: Urinalysis: a comprehensive review. Am Fam Physician 71:1153–1162, 2005

Urine leukocyte esterase

Type of test	Component of routine urinalysis
Background and explanation of test	Urine dipstick testing detects the enzyme esterase that is released by leukocytes (WBCs). Positive results on dipstick analysis for leukocyte esterase (LE) should be followed up with a microscopic exam to look for WBCs and bacteria. Positive results on both nitrite and LE are highly suggestive of urinary tract infection (UTI) and should be followed up with a urine culture.
Relevance to psychiatry and behavioral science	Testing for LE is helpful in the detection of a UTI, which can be associated with delirium and other mental status changes, particularly in elderly patients.
Preparation of patient	See **Urinalysis**.
Indications	• Component of routine urinalysis • Clinical suspicion of UTI
Reference range	Negative for LE
Critical value(s)	None
Positive test	• Cystitis (bladder infection) • Acute pyelonephritis • Acute nephritis • Bladder tumor • SLE • Tuberculosis
Negative test	UTI is not likely present. Unless other evidence of a UTI is found, microscopic exam and culture are not indicated.
Interfering factors	False-positive results can occur with vaginal discharge, parasites, certain drugs (e.g., ampicillin, kanamycin), salicylate toxicity, or strenuous exercise. False-negative results can occur with large amounts of glucose or protein in the urine, high urine specific gravity, or certain drugs (e.g., tetracycline).
Cross-references	**Urinalysis** **Urinary Tract Infection** **Urine Dipstick Testing**

American Association for Clinical Chemistry: Testing.com. Available at: https://www.testing.com. Accessed October 2021.

Fischbach FT, Fischbach MA: A Manual of Laboratory and Diagnostic Tests, 10th Edition. Philadelphia, PA, Wolters Kluwer Health/Lippincott Williams and Wilkins, 2018

Simerville JA, Maxted WC, Pahira JJ: Urinalysis: a comprehensive review. Am Fam Physician 71:1153–1162, 2005

Urine microalbumin

Type of test	Urine (random "spot" specimen or 24-hour collection)
Background and explanation of test	A normally functioning kidney does not allow albumin or other proteins to pass into the urine, so the presence of albumin in a urine sample signals dysfunction of the glomerular filtration barrier. This albuminuria is now understood to reflect not only kidney disease but also risk of cardiovascular disease and vascular retinopathy. Microalbuminuria—now termed *moderately increased albuminuria*—is defined by an albumin excretion of 30–300 mg in a 24-hour urine collection. Macroalbuminuria or proteinuria—now termed *severely increased albuminuria*—is defined by an albumin excretion >300 mg in 24 hours. Individuals at risk of albuminuria include those with known kidney disease, diabetes, hypertension, obesity, or family history of chronic kidney disease. Those who are elderly or who belong to certain racial or ethnic groups also are at risk. The definitive test for urine albumin requires a 24-hour urine sample, but screening is usually done with a first-void morning urine specimen for which both albumin and creatinine are measured, and the albumin-to-creatinine ratio is determined. The urine dipstick has been considered an insensitive marker for albuminuria.
Relevance to psychiatry and behavioral science	Urine microalbumin has been underutilized for patients treated in behavioral health settings who are diabetic, hypertensive, or treated chronically with analgesic drugs.
Preparation of patient	Heavy exercise should be avoided before and during the 24-hour urine collection. Urine should not be collected during menstruation because blood contamination invalidates the results.
Indications	Detection of protein on urine dipstick testing Routine screening indicated for patients with the following conditions: • Diabetes (testing every 12 months) • Hypertension • Family history of kidney disease • Extensive analgesic use (including acetaminophen, aspirin, ibuprofen, and other NSAIDs)
Reference range	24-hour urine: <15 mg/24 hours Spot urine: <10 mg/L Albumin-to-creatinine ratio: • Males <10 mg/g • Females <15 mg/g
Critical value(s)	Moderately increased albuminuria: 30–300 mg/24 hours Severely increased albuminuria: >300 mg/24 hours

Urine microalbumin *(continued)*

Increased levels	• Diabetes
	• Hypertension
	• CNS infection
	• SLE
	• Kidney disease (glomerular or tubular)
	• Urinary tract infection
	• Congestive heart failure
	• Leukemia, lymphoma, multiple myeloma
	• Wilson's disease
	• Sickle cell disease
	• Acute infection, sepsis
	• Trauma
	• Hyperthyroidism
	• Vascular disease
	• Poisoning (turpentine, phosphorus, mercury, gold, lead, phenol, opiates, other drugs)
Decreased levels	Not applicable
Interfering factors	Strenuous exercise, fever, exposure to cold, dehydration, contrast dye within 3 days of testing, pregnancy
Cross-references	**Creatinine**
	Urine Protein

American Association for Clinical Chemistry: Testing.com. Available at: https://www.testing.com. Accessed October 2021.

Fischbach FT, Fischbach MA: A Manual of Laboratory and Diagnostic Tests, 10th Edition. Philadelphia, PA, Wolters Kluwer Health/Lippincott Williams and Wilkins, 2018

Lessey G, Stavropoulos K, Papademetriou V: Mild to moderate chronic kidney disease and cardiovascular events in patients with type 2 diabetes mellitus. Vasc Health Risk Manag 15:365–373, 2019

Márquez DF, Ruiz-Hurtado G, Segura J, Ruilope L: Microalbuminuria and cardiorenal risk: old and new evidence in different populations. F1000Res 8:F1000 Faculty Rev-1659, 2019

Weir MR: Microalbuminuria and cardiovascular disease. Clin J Am Soc Nephrol 2(3):581–590, 2007

Urine nitrite

Type of test	Component of routine urinalysis
Background and explanation of test	Nitrates normally present in urine can be converted to nitrites by certain gram-negative bacteria, causing a positive dipstick test that may indicate a urinary tract infection (UTI). A positive nitrite test is followed up by microscopic examination of the urine and, in some cases, by a urine culture. The latter is the gold standard for UTI diagnosis but is expensive and takes time to report. Because not all bacteria implicated in a UTI are capable of reducing nitrate, nitrite testing alone could produce a false-negative result. Nitrite results are therefore considered along with findings from the leukocyte esterase dipstick, microscopic examination for WBCs, and clinical signs and symptoms suggestive of a UTI.
Relevance to psychiatry and behavioral science	Testing for nitrite is helpful in the detection of a UTI, which can be associated with delirium and other mental status changes, particularly in elderly patients.
Preparation of patient	See **Urinalysis**. If a random sample is used, it should be collected ≥4 hours after the last voiding to ensure the adequate contact time between bacteria and nitrates.
Indications	• Component of routine urinalysis • Screening populations at risk of UTI: pregnant females, patients with diabetes, elderly patients, school-age children (particularly female), patients with recurrent UTI history • Monitoring treatment for UTI
Reference range	Negative on dipstick Microscopic exam: <10^3 bacteria/mL or ≤20 bacteria/hpf
Critical value(s)	None
Positive test	Significant bacteriuria present; perform urine culture.
Negative test	Does not necessarily signify absence of UTI, for the following reasons: • Infection is caused by bacteria that do not convert nitrate to nitrite (e.g., staphylococcus, streptococcus) • Urine is not present in bladder long enough for nitrate-to-nitrite conversion • Insufficient amounts of nitrate present in patient diet
Interfering factors	False-negative results can occur with high urine output, diabetes mellitus, SLE, sickle cell anemia, agammaglobulinemia, localized infection, use of certain drugs (antibiotics, anti-inflammatory drugs, high-dose vitamin C), or storage of dipsticks in a humid environment. False-positive results can occur with use of certain drugs (e.g., oral contraceptives or phenazopyridine). Improper specimen handling (e.g., delay in processing or failure to refrigerate) can invalidate the results.

Urine nitrite *(continued)*

Cross-references	**Urinalysis**
	Urinary Tract Infection

American Association for Clinical Chemistry: Testing.com. Available at: https://www.testing.com. Accessed October 2021.

Chu CM, Lowder JL: Diagnosis and treatment of urinary tract infections across age groups. Am J Obstet Gynecol 219(1):40–51, 2018

Fischbach FT, Fischbach MA: A Manual of Laboratory and Diagnostic Tests, 10th Edition. Philadelphia, PA, Wolters Kluwer Health/Lippincott Williams and Wilkins, 2018

Giesen LG, Cousins G, Dimitrov BD, et al: Predicting acute uncomplicated urinary tract infection in women: a systematic review of the diagnostic accuracy of symptoms and signs. BMC Fam Pract 11:78, 2010

Masajtis-Zagajewska A, Nowicki M: New markers of urinary tract infection. Clin Chim Acta 471:286–291, 2017

Urine pH

Type of test	Component of routine urinalysis
Background and explanation of test	Urine is typically slightly acidic, with a pH of ~6.0 and a normal range from 4.5 to 8. Diet and drugs both affect urine pH, as does any condition causing systemic acidosis or alkalosis. Urine pH can be manipulated in the management of kidney stones, which precipitate differently at particular pH values.
	Stones that precipitate in acidic urine include uric acid, calcium oxalate, cystine, and xanthine stones.
	Stones that precipitate in alkaline urine include calcium phosphate, calcium carbonate, and magnesium phosphate stones.
	Urine pH can also be adjusted to make medications such as streptomycin, neomycin, and kanamycin more effective in treating UTI because these drugs are more active in alkaline urine.
Relevance to psychiatry and behavioral science	See *Acidic Urine* and *Alkaline Urine* sections below.
Preparation of patient	See **Urinalysis**.
Indications	Component of routine urinalysis
Reference range	4.5–8.0 (average 6.0)
Critical value(s)	None
Acidic urine (pH <7.0)	• Fever • Metabolic acidosis • Diabetic ketosis • Diarrhea • Starvation • Uremia • Urinary tract infection (e.g., *Escherichia coli*) • Respiratory acidosis • Renal tuberculosis
Alkaline urine (pH >7.0)	• Urinary tract infection (e.g., *Proteus*, *Pseudomonas*) • Renal tubular acidosis • Chronic renal failure • Vomiting or gastric suctioning • Hyperventilation with respiratory alkalosis
Interfering factors	Urine allowed to stand before analysis becomes more alkaline. If urine pH is >9, another specimen is required.
	Urine becomes alkaline after eating and becomes acidic after overnight fasting.
	Urine becomes alkaline with diets high in citrus fruits, vegetables, and dairy products.

Urine pH *(continued)*

Interfering factors *(continued)*	Urine becomes acidic with diets high in meat products and cranberries.
	Specific medications can change urine pH:
	• Drugs that produce alkaline urine (high pH) include acetazolamide, potassium citrate, and sodium bicarbonate.
	• Drugs that produce acidic urine (low pH) include ammonium chloride, thiazide diuretics, and methenamine mandelate.
Cross-references	**Urinalysis**
	Urinary Tract Infection

American Association for Clinical Chemistry: Lab Tests Online. Available at: https://www.testing.com. Accessed October 2021.

Fischbach FT, Fischbach MA: A Manual of Laboratory and Diagnostic Tests, 10th Edition. Philadelphia, PA, Wolters Kluwer Health/Lippincott Williams and Wilkins, 2018

Simerville JA, Maxted WC, Pahira JJ: Urinalysis: a comprehensive review. Am Fam Physician 71:1153–1162, 2005

Urine protein

Type of test	Component of routine urinalysis
Background and explanation of test	The transient appearance of protein in the urine can occur with urinary tract infection, fever, stress, strenuous exercise, exposure to cold, or contamination with vaginal mucus. In addition, orthostatic proteinuria can be identified in patients younger than 30 years when urine that is sampled after the patient has been in the upright position shows significant protein, whereas urine sampled after the patient has been in the supine position does not. From the standpoint of the kidney, these findings are considered benign.

The persistence of anything more than trace proteinuria, on the other hand, can be a critical and early indicator of renal dysfunction. This type of proteinuria may be a consequence of primary renal disease or renal dysfunction secondary to conditions such as diabetes, vasculitis, amyloidosis, connective tissue disease, myeloma, congestive heart failure (CHF), or hypertension.

Qualitative urine protein testing is usually performed by dipstick, which primarily detects albumin. Follow-up could involve either a spot urine to determine the protein-to-creatinine ratio or a 24-hour urine collection. |
Relevance to psychiatry and behavioral science	Among many other conditions, persistent proteinuria may signal the presence of a disease such as vasculitis or CHF, which could present with psychiatric symptoms.
Preparation of patient	See **Urinalysis**.
Indications	Component of routine urinalysis
Reference range	Normal total protein excretion: • ≤10 mg/100 mL in a single specimen (a *negative* result) • ≤150 mg/24 hours (≤15 mg/dL) Some labs report semiquantitative test results for spot urine, interpreted as follows: • Trace: equivalent to 150 mg/24 hours • 1+: 200–500 mg/24 hours • 2+: 500–1,500 mg/24 hours • 3+: 2,000–5,000 mg/24 hours • 4+: 7,000 mg/24 hours
Critical value(s)	>150 mg/24 hours defines proteinuria (1+ to 4+). >2,000 mg/24 hours in adults usually indicates glomerular etiology. >3,500 mg/24 hours is consistent with nephrotic syndrome (with hypoalbuminemia, edema, and hyperlipidemia).

Urine protein *(continued)*

Increased levels	• Glomerular injury: glomerulonephritis, SLE, malignant hypertension, nephrotic syndrome, amyloidosis, and diabetes mellitus
	• Renal tubular dysfunction: pyelonephritis, Wilson's disease, and interstitial nephritis
	• Extrarenal causes: COVID-19 infection, CHF, increased serum proteins (multiple myeloma, lymphoma), sepsis, trauma, hyperthyroidism, cardiovascular disease, CNS lesions, renal transplant rejection, and poisoning by various substances (e.g., turpentine, opioids)
	• Proteinuria with increased WBCs: urinary tract infection
	• Proteinuria with increased WBCs and RBCs: inflammation of glomeruli (pyelonephritis)
Decreased levels	Not applicable
Interfering factors	Transient proteinuria is seen with the following conditions: strenuous exercise, seizures, emotional stress, cold exposure, fever, dehydration, certain food allergies, use of salicylates, premenstrual state, post-labor and delivery.
	False-positive urine protein is seen with alkaline urine, blood, vaginal discharge, and semen.
	False-negative urine protein is seen with very dilute urine.
	Because the dipstick primarily detects albumin, it would not detect abnormal proteins, such as Bence Jones proteins.
	Some renal diseases are not associated with proteinuria.
Cross-references	**Systemic Lupus Erythematosus**
	Thyrotoxicosis
	Urinalysis
	Urine Microalbumin
	Wilson's Disease

American Association for Clinical Chemistry: Testing.com. Available at: https://www.testing.com. Accessed October 2021.

George JA, Khoza S: SARS-CoV-2 infection and the kidneys: an evolving picture. Adv Exp Med Biol 1327:107–118, 2021

Haynes J, Haynes R: Proteinuria. BMJ 332(7536):284, 2006

Polkinghorne KR: Detection and measurement of urinary protein. Curr Opin Nephrol Hypertens 15(6):625–630, 2006

Urine red blood cells (RBCs) and RBC casts

Type of test	Component of routine urinalysis
Background and explanation of test	The presence of intact RBCs in the urine is termed *hematuria*, which is categorized as *gross* (visible to the naked eye) or *microscopic* (seen on microscopic urinalysis). The differential diagnosis for hematuria ranges from transient and benign etiologies to persistent and serious causes, such as urothelial carcinoma, as noted below. Urine dipstick testing is highly sensitive to hematuria but cannot distinguish intact RBCs from myoglobin or free hemoglobin, so a positive dipstick test must be followed by microscopic examination of the urine.
	Initial findings on urinalysis can help distinguish glomerular from non-glomerular causes of hematuria. A glomerular cause (arising from the kidney itself) is suggested by the presence of dysmorphic RBCs, significant proteinuria, and RBC casts and should prompt referral to a nephrologist.
	The risk of urothelial carcinoma increases with the number of RBCs found on high-power microscopy as well as older age, positive smoking history, and male sex.
Relevance to psychiatry and behavioral science	Behavioral health specialists are cautioned not to ignore urine blood. An initial separation of findings into glomerular versus non-glomerular origin can facilitate appropriate patient referral.
Preparation of patient	See **Urinalysis**.
Indications	Component of routine urinalysis
Reference range	RBCs: 0–3/hpf (40× magnification)
	RBC casts: 0/lpf (20× magnification)
Critical value(s)	Hematuria is defined as >3 RBCs/hpf.
	Presence of RBC casts indicates glomerular injury or, less commonly, severe tubular damage, among other conditions (e.g., congestive heart failure, malignant hypertension, lupus nephritis, acute bacterial endocarditis).
Abnormal test	Hematuria without other cells, casts, or protein suggests bleeding from the urinary tract. Common causes of isolated hematuria include stones, neoplasms, tuberculosis, trauma, and prostatitis. Blood clots with gross bleeding point to the urinary collecting system. WBCs present along with RBCs suggest the presence of infection.
Decreased levels	Not applicable
Interfering factors	A single urine specimen with hematuria can be found with menstruation, sexual intercourse, strenuous exercise, mild trauma, dehydration, allergy, or viral illness.
	Heavy smokers often have small numbers of RBCs in urine.
	Drugs associated with urine RBCs include aspirin, NSAIDs, heparin, amitriptyline, chlorpromazine, anticonvulsants, oral contraceptives, penicillin, and cyclophosphamide.

Urine red blood cells (RBCs) and RBC casts *(continued)*

Cross-references	Urinalysis
	Urinary Tract Infection
	Urine Blood, Hemoglobin, and Myoglobin

Barocas DA, Boorjian SA, Alvarez RD, et al: Microhematuria: AUA/SUFU guideline. J Urol 204:778, 2020

Becker GJ, Garigali G, Fogazzi GB: Advances in urine microscopy. Am J Kidney Dis 67(6):954–964, 2016

Fischbach FT, Fischbach MA: A Manual of Laboratory and Diagnostic Tests, 10th Edition. Philadelphia, PA, Wolters Kluwer Health/Lippincott Williams and Wilkins, 2018

Sharp VJ, Barnes KT, Erickson BA: Assessment of asymptomatic microscopic hematuria in adults. Am Fam Physician 88(11):747–754, 2013

Urine specific gravity

Type of test	Component of routine urinalysis
Background and explanation of test	Urine specific gravity (SG) is a measure of the density of urine, reflecting the kidney's ability to produce a concentrated or dilute urine in relation to plasma. It is proportional to urine osmolality. It can be performed by dipstick or in the laboratory.
Relevance to psychiatry and behavioral science	Urine SG can be a quick and readily available gauge of dehydration, overhydration (as with polydipsia), or urine osmolality.
Preparation of patient	See **Urinalysis**.
Indications	Component of routine urinalysis
Reference range	Normal kidney: 1.002–1.035

Normal hydration status: <1.007 |
Critical value(s)	SG >1.035 indicates contaminated specimen, high glucose concentration, or recent intake of radiopaque dyes or IV low-molecular-weight dextran.
Increased levels	SG >1.010 indicates relative dehydration.
Decreased levels	SG ≤1.022 after 12-hour fast (no food or water) indicates impaired renal concentrating ability, as in renal dysfunction or nephrogenic diabetes insipidus.
Interfering factors	Contaminated specimen
Cross-references	**Diabetes Insipidus**

Psychogenic Polydipsia

Urinalysis |

American Association for Clinical Chemistry: Testing.com. Available at: https://www.testing.com. Accessed October 2021.

Fischbach FT, Fischbach MA: A Manual of Laboratory and Diagnostic Tests, 10th Edition. Philadelphia, PA, Wolters Kluwer Health/Lippincott Williams and Wilkins, 2018

Simerville JA, Maxted WC, Pahira JJ: Urinalysis: a comprehensive review. Am Fam Physician 71:1153–1162, 2005

Urine white blood cells (WBCs) and WBC casts

Type of test	Component of routine urinalysis
Background and explanation of test	An increase in the number of WBCs in urine is termed *pyuria*. A significant increase suggests the presence of infection or inflammation, usually within the genitourinary system. Significant WBC elevation should be followed up with a urine culture.
Relevance to psychiatry and behavioral science	This test is helpful in the diagnosis of urinary tract infection (UTI), which can be associated with delirium and other mental status changes, particularly in elderly patients.
Preparation of patient	None needed
Indications	Component of routine urinalysis
Reference range	WBCs: 0–4/hpf. In females, slightly more WBCs can be normal. WBC casts: 0/lpf
Critical value(s)	>30 WBCs/hpf indicates the presence of acute bacterial infection in the genitourinary system. The presence of WBC casts requires further investigation to rule out pyelonephritis, which may otherwise be asymptomatic.
Increased levels	*Increased urine WBCs* • UTI or inflammation (e.g., of bladder, prostate, or urethra) • Renal disease (especially with WBC clumping) • Appendicitis • Pancreatitis • Strenuous exercise • SLE The presence of WBC casts may indicate disease of the kidney itself (most commonly pyelonephritis) or acute glomerulonephritis, interstitial nephritis, or lupus nephritis.
Decreased levels	Not applicable
Interfering factors	Vaginal secretions can cause false elevation in urine WBCs.
Cross-references	**Urinalysis** **Urinary Tract Infection**

American Association for Clinical Chemistry: Testing.com. Available at: https://www.testing.com. Accessed October 2021.

Fischbach FT, Fischbach MA: A Manual of Laboratory and Diagnostic Tests, 10th Edition. Philadelphia, PA, Wolters Kluwer Health/Lippincott Williams and Wilkins, 2018

Simerville JA, Maxted WC, Pahira JJ: Urinalysis: a comprehensive review. Am Fam Physician 71:1153–1162, 2005

Urobilinogen

Type of test	Component of routine urinalysis
Background and explanation of test	Bilirubin is converted to urobilinogen in the GI tract by bacterial enzymes. Some of this product is excreted in feces, and some travels in the portal circulation to the liver, where it is metabolized and excreted with bile. Traces of bilirubin that circumvent these processes are excreted in urine. Urobilinogen is increased in diseases associated with increased bilirubin levels and in diseases that prevent the liver from metabolizing bilirubin. Increased urobilinogen is one of the earliest signs of liver disease and of hemolytic disorders. • In the absence of disease, urine bilirubin is negative, and urobilinogen is normal. • In hemolytic disease, urine bilirubin is negative, and urobilinogen is increased. • In hepatic disease, urine bilirubin may be positive or negative, and urobilinogen is increased. • In biliary obstruction, urine bilirubin is positive, and urobilinogen is low or absent.
Relevance to psychiatry and behavioral science	Increased urobilinogen levels may be found in patients with hepatitis, cirrhosis, or pernicious anemia.
Preparation of patient	None needed
Indications	Component of routine urinalysis
Reference range	Random spot urine: 0.1–1 Ehrlich U/dL (<1 mg/dL)
Critical value(s)	None
Increased levels	• Increased rate of RBC destruction: hemolytic anemia, pernicious anemia, malaria • Hemorrhage into tissues: pulmonary infarction, excessive bruising • Hepatic injury: biliary disease, acute hepatitis, cirrhosis (viral or chemical) • Cholangitis
Decreased levels	• Partial or complete obstruction of bile ducts: gallstones, severe inflammation, or pancreatic cancer involving the head of the pancreas • Antibiotic therapy with suppression of gut flora and reduced conversion of bilirubin to urobilinogen
Interfering factors	Diurnal variation: peak urobilinogen excretion occurs from noon to 4:00 P.M. Urobilinogen decomposes quickly at room temperature when exposed to light. Highly colored urine affects reading of the test strip.
Cross-references	**Anemia** **Bilirubin**

Urobilinogen *(continued)*

Cross-references *(continued)*	**Cirrhosis**
	Hepatitis, Viral
	Urinalysis
	Urine Bilirubin

American Association for Clinical Chemistry: Testing.com. Available at: https://www.testing.com. Accessed October 2021.

Fischbach FT, Fischbach MA: A Manual of Laboratory and Diagnostic Tests, 10th Edition. Philadelphia, PA, Wolters Kluwer Health/Lippincott Williams and Wilkins, 2018

Simerville JA, Maxted WC, Pahira JJ: Urinalysis: a comprehensive review. Am Fam Physician 71:1153–1162, 2005

Valproate level

Type of test	Blood
Background and explanation of test	Valproate (sodium valproate, also known as valproic acid and divalproex sodium) is an antiepileptic drug indicated for generalized tonic-clonic, partial complex, and petit mal seizures. It is also used to treat bipolar disorder, mood instability in the context of dementia, TBI, myoclonus, and many other neuropsychiatric conditions. If there is any concern about altered protein binding in the valproate-treated patient, a free valproate rather than total valproate level should be checked.
Relevance to psychiatry and behavioral science	Reference ranges reported for valproate relate to seizure rather than behavioral indications. As a rule, levels correlate poorly with mood and behavioral control. The reason levels are checked in psychiatric practice is to monitor compliance (to exclude very low or zero levels) or toxicity (to exclude levels that are orders of magnitude above the upper limit of normal for seizure). Other labs are also monitored when valproate is used, as discussed in the **Valproate** entry in the *Psychotropic Medications* chapter.
Preparation of patient	To check level, patients taking valproate twice daily should be instructed to hold their morning dose until after blood is drawn. For patients taking divalproex extended-release formulation once daily in the morning, blood should be drawn before the morning dose. For those taking divalproex extended-release formulation once daily in the evening, blood should be drawn 18–21 hours after the last dose.
Indications	• Overdose • Signs/symptoms of valproate toxicity • Concern regarding noncompliance
Reference range	Total valproate: 50–125 µg/mL Free valproate: 6–22 µg/mL % Free valproate: 5%–18% (calculated)
Critical value(s)	Total valproate: >150 µg/mL Free valproate: >50 µg/mL
Increased levels	• Overdose • Hepatic insufficiency or failure
Decreased levels	Noncompliance
Interfering factors	Timing of blood draw influences results, as noted above. Coadministration of carbamazepine decreases valproate levels, and fluoxetine increases valproate levels, but these are actual level changes that do not represent test interference.

Valproate level *(continued)*

Cross-references	**Bipolar and Related Disorder Due to Another Medical Condition**
	Manic Episode
	Seizures
	Valproate

American Society of Health-System Pharmacists: AHFS Drug Information. Bethesda, MD, American Society of Health-System Pharmacists, 2016

Fleming J, Chetty M: Therapeutic monitoring of valproate in psychiatry: how far have we progressed? Clin Neuropharmacol 29(6):350–360, 2006

Reed RC, Dutta S: Does it really matter when a blood sample for valproic acid concentration is taken following once-daily administration of divalproex-ER? Ther Drug Monit 28(3):413–418, 2006

Vitamin B$_{12}$ level

Type of test	Blood
Background and explanation of test	Vitamin B$_{12}$ is required for protein synthesis, fat and carbohydrate metabolism, absorption and digestion of food, formation of RBCs, production of acetylcholine, maintenance of nerve cells, and fertility in females. Vitamin B$_{12}$ deficiency due to inadequate intake is rare in developed countries; deficiency usually is due to malabsorption—which is common in elderly patients—and can occur with conditions such as cystic fibrosis, pernicious anemia, reduced gastric acid production, excessive use of antacids, chronic use of histamine H$_2$ blockers, gastric bypass surgery, and other GI diseases such as tapeworm. Increased loss of B$_{12}$ may be seen in alcohol use disorder and in liver and kidney disease. Vitamin B$_{12}$ deficiency is associated with a megaloblastic anemia, in which fewer and larger RBCs are produced. The syndrome of subacute combined degeneration of the spinal cord due to B$_{12}$ deficiency is discussed in the **Vitamin B$_{12}$ Deficiency** entry in the *Diseases and Conditions* chapter.
Relevance to psychiatry and behavioral science	Vitamin B$_{12}$ deficiency is associated with a variety of symptoms of interest to psychiatrists and other behavioral health practitioners, including confusion, delirium, psychosis, somnolence, irritability, depression, mania, apathy, personality change, delusions, cognitive impairment (particularly involving memory), and the nonspecific symptoms of dizziness, weakness, and fatigue. Patients with vague neurological symptoms such as clumsiness, unsteadiness, tinnitus, speech impairment, or visual changes are sometimes misdiagnosed with functional neurological symptom disorders.
Preparation of patient	Patients should fast overnight before the test, and on the day of testing should hold heparin and avoid vitamin C, fluoride, and alcohol.
Indications	• Standard component of workup for dementia or memory impairment • Identifying cause of delirium • Evaluating mental status changes in an elderly patient • Identifying the cause of peripheral neuropathy • Presence of symptoms of subacute combined degeneration (weakness, sensory abnormalities) • Workup for macrocytic anemia (folate also measured) • Workup for macrocytosis (MCV >110 fL) • Evaluating nutritional status • Monitoring effectiveness of treatment for vitamin B$_{12}$ deficiency
Reference range	250–1,000 pg/mL

Vitamin B$_{12}$ level *(continued)*

Critical value(s)	For geriatric or adult patients with the neurological or psychiatric symptoms listed in *Relevance* section above, many clinicians prescribe vitamin B$_{12}$ supplementation when levels are <400 pg/mL. Among elderly patients, loss of muscle mass and strength are found with levels below this threshold.
Increased levels	• Supplementation • Leukemia • Liver dysfunction High B$_{12}$ levels are not associated with toxicity and are of uncertain significance.
Decreased levels	• Inadequate intake (e.g., strict vegetarian diet) • Poor absorption • Increased excretion
Interfering factors	Serum B$_{12}$ level may be increased by the use of chloral hydrate or omeprazole. Serum level may be decreased by the use of anticonvulsants, ascorbic acid, cholestyramine, chlorpromazine, colchicine, levodopa, metformin, neomycin, octreotide, oral contraceptives, ranitidine, or rifampin.
Cross-references	**Dementia** **Folate Deficiency** **Folate Level** **Vitamin B$_{12}$ Deficiency**

Andrès E, Loukili NH, Noel E, et al: Vitamin B$_{12}$ (cobalamin) deficiency in elderly patients. CMAJ 171(3):251–259, 2004

Ates Bulut E, Soysal P, Aydin AE, et al: Vitamin B$_{12}$ deficiency might be related to sarcopenia in older adults. Exp Gerontol 95:136–140, 2017

Fischbach FT, Fischbach MA: A Manual of Laboratory and Diagnostic Tests, 10th Edition. Philadelphia, PA, Wolters Kluwer Health/Lippincott Williams and Wilkins, 2018

Langan RC, Goodbred AJ: Vitamin B$_{12}$ deficiency: recognition and management. Am Fam Physician 96(6):384–389, 2017

Lerner V, Kanevsky M, Dwolatzky T, et al: Vitamin B$_{12}$ and folate serum levels in newly admitted psychiatric patients. Clin Nutr 25:60–67, 2006

Stabler SP: Clinical practice: vitamin B$_{12}$ deficiency. N Engl J Med 368(2):149–160, 2013

Zik C: Late-life vitamin B$_{12}$ deficiency. Clin Geriatr Med 35(3):319–325, 2019

Vitamin D level

Type of test	Blood
Background and explanation of test	Vitamin D is a fat-soluble vitamin ingested in foods and supplements and synthesized in the skin on exposure to sunlight. It becomes biologically active through hydroxylation in the liver and kidney. Vitamin D works with other hormones to regulate calcium balance through absorption from the GI tract and resorption from bone and to regulate phosphorus and magnesium absorption. Adequate levels of vitamin D are needed at all ages for bone growth and health. In older age, females are particularly prone to developing deficiency, especially those with dark skin, those who lack sunlight exposure, and those with malabsorption. The 25-hydroxy vitamin D level is recommended in preference to the 1,25-dihydroxy level in testing for deficiency.
Relevance to psychiatry and behavioral science	Low vitamin D levels have been associated with cognitive decline, Alzheimer's disease, and depression, although treatment studies have largely failed to demonstrate improvement with vitamin D replacement. Older adults are at particular risk of deficiency, which is especially common among females in nursing home settings. Other adverse effects of deficiency involve the musculoskeletal system and the heart. In addition, the risk of developing certain cancers and autoimmune diseases may be greater in deficient individuals.
Preparation of patient	None needed
Indications	• Detecting vitamin D deficiency in patients at risk • Confirming deficiency in patients with evidence of bone disease, bone or muscle weakness, or abnormal calcium, phosphorus, and/or PTH levels • Monitoring effectiveness of vitamin D replacement
Reference range	Adults: 30–80 ng/mL
Critical values	Toxicity is possible with 25-OH vitamin D levels >150 ng/mL. These high levels can be associated with tissue calcification (e.g., kidneys, vasculature), vomiting, constipation, anorexia, nausea, and severe electrolyte derangements.
Increased levels	Excessive supplementation
Decreased levels	• Inadequate vitamin D intake • Malabsorption of vitamin D • Inadequate sunlight exposure
Interfering factors	Drugs that decrease vitamin D levels include anticonvulsants (carbamazepine, phenytoin, primidone, phenobarbital), aluminum hydroxide, cholestyramine, glucocorticoids, isoniazid, rifampin, and mineral oil.
Cross-references	None

Vitamin D level *(continued)*

Anglin RE, Samaan Z, Walter SD, McDonald SD: Vitamin D deficiency and depression in adults: systematic review and meta-analysis. Br J Psychiatry 202:100–107, 2013

Annweiler C, Dursun E, Féron F, et al: Vitamin D and cognition in older adults: updated international recommendations. J Intern Med 277(1):45–57, 2015

ARUP Laboratories: Vitamin D, 25-hydroxy, in Lab Test Directory. Salt Lake City, UT, ARUP Laboratories, 2021. Available at: https://ltd.aruplab.com/Tests/Pub/0080379. Accessed October 2021.

Fischbach FT, Fischbach MA: A Manual of Laboratory and Diagnostic Tests, 10th Edition. Philadelphia, PA, Wolters Kluwer Health/Lippincott Williams and Wilkins, 2018

Goodwill AM, Szoeke C: A systematic review and meta-analysis of the effect of low vitamin D on cognition. J Am Geriatr Soc 65(10):2161–2168, 2017

Landel V, Annweiler C, Millet P, et al: Vitamin D, cognition and Alzheimer's disease: the therapeutic benefit is in the D-tails. J Alzheimers Dis 53(2):419–444, 2016

White blood cell (WBC) count

Type of test	Blood
Background and explanation of test	WBCs, or leukocytes, are cells of the immune system that reside in the lymphatic system, blood, and tissues. These cells have critical roles in fighting infection and ridding the body of foreign material. When these processes occur, more WBCs are produced by the bone marrow, and the WBC count increases, with the degree of elevation corresponding to the severity of the infection or intrusion. There are five types of WBCs—neutrophils, basophils, eosinophils, lymphocytes, and monocytes—present in stable proportions. Usually, when the WBC count is elevated, only one of the five types is increased in number. If all cell types are increased in number, it is more likely that hemoconcentration has occurred. The significance of elevation of each type of WBC is discussed in the individual WBC differential entries that follow. Conditions such as cancer and immune disorders and the use of medications such as clozapine can be associated with reduced WBC numbers because of decreased production or shortened survival of these cells. Whether WBC numbers are elevated or reduced, the pattern of abnormality—which type of WBC is affected—can suggest the underlying pathology. The WBC "differential" component of testing breaks down the numbers by each of the five cell types. A review of the blood smear also facilitates diagnosis because it can show abnormally formed or immature cells.
Relevance to psychiatry and behavioral science	Delirium is associated with conditions involving both elevated and decreased WBC levels. Lithium often causes an increase in WBC count. Clozapine and other psychotropic drugs can cause very low WBC counts, as discussed in the **White Blood Cell Count Differential: Neutrophils** entry. In general, patients with persistently low WBC numbers require special care, including protection from fresh fruits, vegetables, plants, and flowers; avoidance of intramuscular injections, rectal thermometers, and suppositories; and special care in using dental floss and razor blades.
Preparation of patient	Fasting is not required. Physiological stress should be avoided just before testing.
Indications	• Routine component of CBC • Ordered as individual test in certain clinical situations
Reference range	Black adults: $3.2–10.0 \times 10^3$ cells/mm^3; benign ethnic neutropenia shifts normal range in this population. All other adults: $4.5–10.5 \times 10^3$ cells/mm^3
Critical value(s)	Severe leukopenia $<2.0 \times 10^3$ cells/mm^3 Severe leukocytosis $>30.0 \times 10^3$ cells/mm^3

White blood cell (WBC) count *(continued)*

Increased levels	Leukocytosis (WBC count $>11.0 \times 10^3$ cells/mm^3) occurs in the following conditions: acute infection, leukemia, myeloproliferative disorders, tissue trauma, surgery, uremia, cancer (especially bronchogenic carcinoma), coma, eclampsia, thyrotoxicosis, ingestion of toxins, use of certain medications (lithium, corticosteroids, epinephrine, colony-stimulating factors, quinine), NMS, acute hemolysis, acute hemorrhage, post-splenectomy state, polycythemia vera, tissue necrosis, seizure, nausea and vomiting, physiological leukocytosis (e.g., from stress, exercise, pain, heat/cold), and sunlight exposure.
Decreased levels	Leukopenia (WBC count $<4.0 \times 10^3$ cells/mm^3) occurs in the following conditions: viral infections, bacterial infections, hypersplenism, primary bone marrow disorders (including leukemia, aplastic anemia, and pernicious anemia), and bone marrow depression by heavy metal intoxication, radiation, or drugs.
Interfering factors	A diurnal rhythm is seen, with early morning trough WBC levels and late-afternoon peaks. WBC values are also influenced by age, sex, exercise, medications, pregnancy, pain, temperature, altitude, and anesthesia. Any stress that increases the endogenous epinephrine level also increases the WBC level.
Cross-references	**Complete Blood Count** **White Blood Cell Count Differential: Basophil** **White Blood Cell Count Differential: Eosinophils** **White Blood Cell Count Differential: Lymphocytes** **White Blood Cell Count Differential: Monocytes** **White Blood Cell Count Differential: Neutrophils**

American Association for Clinical Chemistry: Lab Tests Online. Available at: https://www.testing.com. Accessed October 2021.

Fischbach FT, Fischbach MA: A Manual of Laboratory and Diagnostic Tests, 10th Edition. Philadelphia, PA, Wolters Kluwer Health/Lippincott Williams and Wilkins, 2018

Mank V, Brown K: Leukocytosis, in StatPearls. Treasure Island, FL, StatPearls Publishing, 2021. Available at: https://www.statpearls.com/ArticleLibrary/viewarticle/24216. Accessed October 2021.

Territo M: Overview of leukopenias, in Merck Manual Professional Version. Rahway, NJ, Merck & Co, 2021. Available at: https://www.merckmanuals.com/professional/hematology-and-oncology/leukopenias/overview-of-leukopenias. Accessed October 2021.

White blood cell (WBC) count differential: basophils

Type of test	Blood
Background and explanation of test	Basophils are circulating phagocytes with cytoplasmic granules containing histamine, heparin, and peroxidase. IgE binds with high affinity to the cell membrane of the basophil—and the mast cell, its tissue counterpart—and when a specific antigen interacts with that IgE, degranulation occurs, with release of inflammatory mediators.
	For this assay, each of the five types of WBCs is counted, and the value is expressed as a percentage of the total WBC count. Increases or decreases in the total WBC count and in each cell type have diagnostic importance. Although the percentage shows only the relative number of each cell type, the absolute number can be calculated by multiplying the percentage of that cell type by the total WBC count. The absolute value is used to determine whether the count of a particular cell type is increased.
	Each elevated WBC type is related to specific medical conditions. Basophils are associated with immediate hypersensitivity reactions, such as allergic asthma, and some delayed hypersensitivity reactions, such as contact allergies. They have a role in immune surveillance for bacteria, viruses, fungi, and parasites such as helminths that can infect the GI tract. In addition, basophils can help moderate the effects of venoms from certain snakes, scorpions, honeybees, and Gila monsters.
Relevance to psychiatry and behavioral science	Elevated basophil levels can be associated with collagen vascular diseases and hyperthyroidism. Injection of foreign protein, observed in cases of factitious disorder, may also cause basophil elevation. Low basophil levels may be seen with thyrotoxicosis.
	Certain psychotropic medications may cause spurious elevation of basophil levels, as noted in the *Interfering Factors* section below.
Preparation of patient	Fasting is not required. Any physiological stress should be avoided just before testing.
Indications	• WBC differential often included as routine component of CBC
	• WBC differential may be added when WBC count is abnormal, to help determine the source.
Reference range	15–50 cells/mm^3 0%–1% of total WBC count
Critical value(s)	None
Increased levels	*Basophilia* (>50 cells/mm^3) is associated with the following conditions: • Chicken pox • Tuberculosis

White blood cell (WBC) count differential: basophils *(continued)*

Increased levels *(continued)*	• Allergic reactions
	• Collagen vascular disease
	• Hyperthyroidism
	• Myelocytic leukemia
	• Acute basophilic leukemia
	• Myeloid metaplasia, myeloproliferative disorders
	• Hodgkin's disease
	• Injection of foreign protein
Decreased levels	Basopenia (<20 cells/mm^3) is associated with the following conditions:
	• Acute infection
	• Hyperthyroidism
	• Physiological stress (e.g., pregnancy, MI)
	• Prolonged steroid treatment
	• Chemotherapy
	• Radiation
	• Hereditary absence of basophils
Interfering factors	False elevation of basophil levels may be seen in patients treated with desipramine, paroxetine, triazolam, or venlafaxine.
Cross-references	**Complete Blood Count**
	White Blood Cell Count

Fischbach FT, Fischbach MA: A Manual of Laboratory and Diagnostic Tests, 10th Edition. Philadelphia, PA, Wolters Kluwer Health/Lippincott Williams and Wilkins, 2018

Kubo M: Mast cells and basophils in allergic inflammation. Curr Opin Immunol 54:74–79, 2018

McPherson RA, Pincus MR: Henry's Clinical Diagnosis and Management by Laboratory Methods, 24th Edition. Philadelphia, PA, Elsevier, 2022

Varricchi G, Raap U, Rivellese F, et al: Human mast cells and basophils: how are they similar how are they different? Immunol Rev 282(1):8–34, 2018

White blood cell (WBC) count differential: eosinophils

Type of test	Blood
Background and explanation of test	Eosinophils are phagocytes and inflammatory modulators produced in the bone marrow that move from blood to tissues, where they proliferate in response to immunological stimuli. Present in large numbers in tissues of the skin, lungs, and GI tract, these cells function to rid the body of parasites such as helminths, participate in allergic responses and asthma, and moderate inflammatory reactions from basophils and mast cells that have degranulated. For this assay, each of the five types of WBCs is counted, and the value is expressed as a percentage of the total WBC count. Increases or decreases in the total WBC count and in each cell type have diagnostic importance. Although the percentage shows only the relative number of each cell type, the absolute number can be calculated by multiplying the percentage of that cell type by the total WBC count. The absolute value is used to determine whether the count of a particular cell type is increased.
Relevance to psychiatry and behavioral science	Allergic reactions to psychotropic medications can cause eosinophilia. An epidemic of eosinophilia-myalgia syndrome (EMS) recognized in 1989 was linked to consumption of L-tryptophan from a single source that may have been adulterated during the manufacturing process. Patients experienced chronic myalgias, neuropathy, and skin induration in association with high eosinophil counts. Over a 6-month period, 1,500 people were affected and more than 30 people died. L-tryptophan sales were subsequently banned in the United States, and the epidemic subsided. In 2005, the ban was lifted. A new case of L-tryptophan-associated EMS was reported in 2011, raising the possibility that a small risk remains for L-tryptophan ingestion, possibly for individuals with unknown genetic risk.
Preparation of patient	Fasting is not required. Any physiological stress should be avoided just before testing.
Indications	• WBC differential often included as routine component of CBC • WBC differential may be added when WBC count is abnormal to help determine source.
Reference range	$0–0.35 \times 10^9$/L
Critical value(s)	Eosinophilia categorized by severity: • Mild: $0.35–<1.5 \times 10^9$/L • Moderate: $1.5–5 \times 10^9$/L • Severe: $>5 \times 10^9$/L Patients with mild eosinophilia lasting ≥6 months, those with moderate or severe eosinophilia, and those with increasing eosinophilia should be referred for specialist evaluation.

White blood cell (WBC) count differential: eosinophils *(continued)*

Increased levels	• Allergies, hay fever, asthma (most cases of eosinophilia)
	• Parasitic or fungal infections
	• Allergic drug reactions
	• Hematological malignancy
	• Atopic skin diseases (eczema, pemphigus)
	• Solid tumors
	• GI diseases (inflammatory bowel disease, celiac disease)
	• Lung diseases
	• Connective tissue diseases
	• Collagen vascular disease (SLE)
Decreased levels	Conditions associated with increased adrenal steroid levels:
	• Cushing's syndrome
	• Acute, severe bacterial infection
	• *Drugs:* corticosteroids, ACTH, epinephrine, thyroxine, or prostaglandins
Interfering factors	A diurnal rhythm seen, with the lowest eosinophil counts in the morning and the counts increasing from noon to midnight or later.
	Decreased counts are seen in physiological stress, including burns, postoperative states, ECT, and labor and delivery.
Cross-references	**Complete Blood Count**
	White Blood Cell Count

Allen JA, Peterson A, Sufit R, et al: Post-epidemic eosinophilia-myalgia syndrome associated with L-tryptophan. Arthritis Rheum 63(11):3633–3639, 2011

Fischbach FT, Fischbach MA: A Manual of Laboratory and Diagnostic Tests, 10th Edition. Philadelphia, PA, Wolters Kluwer Health/Lippincott Williams and Wilkins, 2018

McPherson RA, Pincus MR: Henry's Clinical Diagnosis and Management by Laboratory Methods, 24th Edition. Philadelphia, PA, Elsevier, 2022

Piera-Velazquez S, Wermuth PJ, Gomez-Reino JJ, et al: Chemical exposure-induced systemic fibrosing disorders: novel insights into systemic sclerosis etiology and pathogenesis. Semin Arthritis Rheum 50(6):1226–1237, 2020

White blood cell (WBC) count differential: lymphocytes

Type of test	Blood
Background and explanation of test	Small cells that migrate to sites of inflammation, lymphocytes have a central role in the immune response to infection, carcinogens, and foreign tissue as well as autoimmunity. The two main types of lymphocytes are B cells, responsible for the production of antibodies (humoral immunity), and T cells, which identify foreign material and process it for removal (cell-mediated immunity). All lymphocytes originate in the bone marrow, but T cells mature in the thymus gland. Most lymphocytes in the circulation are T cells, which have a life span of months to years, whereas B cells generally have a life span of days.
	B cells mediate the antigen-antibody response that is specific to the antigen. Cell-mediated immunity involving T cells includes defense against neoplasms and intracellular pathogens such as HIV and *Mycobacterium tuberculosis*, delayed hypersensitivity reactions, graft rejection, and graft-vs.-host reactions. Types of T cells include CD4+ helper cells, which assist B cells in making antibodies, and CD8+ cytotoxic cells, which are capable of destroying foreign material. In general, although the immune cells work in concert, extracellular pathogens are best handled by B cells, and intracellular pathogens are best handled by T cells.
	For this assay, each of the five types of WBCs is counted and the value is expressed as a percentage of the total WBC count. Increases or decreases in the total WBC count and in each cell type have diagnostic importance. Although the percentage shows only the relative number of each cell type, the absolute number can be calculated by multiplying the percentage of that cell type by the total WBC count. The absolute value is used to determine whether the count of a particular cell type is increased.
Relevance to psychiatry and behavioral science	In patients with HIV infection, CD4+ helper cell numbers in the circulation can be measured to determine immune status. The higher this CD4 count, the better the immune system function. Normal CD4 counts range from 500 to 1,500 cells/mm^3. When the count falls below 200 cells/mm^3, serious opportunistic infections may ensue. CD4 testing is no longer used to determine when antiretroviral therapy should begin, but it is used to monitor response to therapy.
Preparation of patient	Fasting is not required. Any physiological stress should be avoided just before testing.
Indications	• WBC differential often included as routine component of CBC • Specific subtype counts and assessment of functional activity of cells are performed in the evaluation of both lymphoproliferative states (e.g., leukemia, lymphoma) and immunodeficiency states (e.g., HIV infection, organ transplantation).

White blood cell (WBC) count differential: lymphocytes *(continued)*

Reference range	$1.0–4.8 \times 10^9$/L (20%–40% of total WBC count)
	Normal CD4-to-CD8 ratio >1
Critical value(s)	Lymphocyte count $<0.5 \times 10^9$/L: The patient should be protected from infection, especially viral.
	Lymphocyte count $>5.0 \times 10^9$/L unexplained by acute viral illness: The patient should be referred for specialist evaluation.
	High lymphocyte count in a patient also showing anemia or thrombocytopenia: The patient should be referred for specialist evaluation.
Increased levels	• Lymphatic leukemia or lymphoma
	• Infectious lymphocytosis
	• Infectious mononucleosis (with Downey cells and positive heterophile antibodies test)
	• Other viral diseases (respiratory tract infections, cytomegalovirus, measles, mumps, chickenpox, acute HIV infection, acute viral hepatitis, toxoplasmosis)
	• Certain bacterial diseases (tuberculosis, brucellosis, pertussis)
	• Crohn's disease, ulcerative colitis
	• Drug hypersensitivity or serum sickness
	• Hypoadrenalism, Addison's disease
	• Thyrotoxicosis
	• Neutropenia (relative lymphocytosis)
Decreased levels	• COVID-19 infection (decrease inversely proportional to disease severity)
	• AIDS, inherited immune disorders
	• Immunosuppression with drugs or radiation
	• Aplastic anemia
	• Hodgkin's disease, other malignancies
	• Severe debilitating illness
	• Advanced (miliary) tuberculosis, renal failure, SLE
	• ACTH-producing tumors
	• Lymphocyte loss through GI tract due to lymphatic obstruction
	• Congestive heart failure
Interfering factors	Lymphocyte values may increase after exercise, emotional stress, or menstruation.
	In general, Black patients may show a relative but not absolute increase in lymphocytes.

White blood cell (WBC) count differential: lymphocytes *(continued)*

Interfering factors *(continued)*	Psychotropic drugs associated with false lymphocyte elevations include gabapentin, haloperidol, levodopa, opioids, paroxetine, quazepam, triazolam, valproate, and venlafaxine.
	Psychotropic drugs associated with false lymphocyte reductions include alprazolam, aripiprazole, benzodiazepines, bupropion, folic acid, gabapentin, levetiracetam, lithium, mirtazapine, phenytoin, quazepam, thiamine, and triazolam.
Cross-references	**Complete Blood Count**
	HIV and AIDS
	Infectious Mononucleosis
	White Blood Cell Count

American Association for Clinical Chemistry: Testing.com. Available at: https://www.testing.com. Accessed October 2021

Akhavizadegan H, Hosamirudsari H, Alizadeh M, et al: Can laboratory tests at the time of admission guide us to the prognosis of patients with COVID-19? J Prev Med Hyg 62(2):E321–E325, 2021

Fischbach FT, Fischbach MA: A Manual of Laboratory and Diagnostic Tests, 10th Edition. Philadelphia, PA, Wolters Kluwer Health/Lippincott Williams and Wilkins, 2018

McPherson RA, Pincus MR: Henry's Clinical Diagnosis and Management by Laboratory Methods, 24th Edition. Philadelphia, PA, Elsevier, 2022

Palladino M: Complete blood count alterations in COVID-19 patients: a narrative review. Biochem Med (Zagreb) 31(3):030501, 2021

White blood cell (WBC) count differential: monocytes

Type of test	Blood
Background and explanation of test	Monocytes are WBCs uniquely poised for fast mobilization to sites of inflammation throughout the body. These cells have important biological functions involving humoral and cell-mediated immunity, surveillance of the internal environment, and orchestration of hematopoiesis. Pathogenic roles of monocytes have also been described, for example, in the formation of new blood vessels within atherosclerotic plaques and arterial walls.
	Historically, monocytes were thought to form in the bone marrow, circulate in the blood, and then move into tissues, where they were transformed into macrophages or dendritic cells. More recently, investigations have shown that most tissue macrophages have an embryonic origin and that conventional dendritic cells have a separate precursor in the bone marrow.
	For this assay, each of the five types of WBCs is counted and the value is expressed as a percentage of the total WBC count. Increases or decreases in the total WBC count and in each cell type have diagnostic importance. Although the percentage shows only the relative number of each cell type, the absolute number can be calculated by multiplying the percentage of that cell type by the total WBC count. The absolute value is used to determine whether the count of a particular cell type is increased.
Relevance to psychiatry and behavioral science	In recent years, a complex role for monocytes and other immune factors has been identified in a wide variety of psychiatric conditions, including TBI, PTSD, major depression, psychosis, Alzheimer's disease, HIV-associated neurocognitive impairment, and neuropathic pain, among others. Changes to the permeability of the blood-brain barrier may be implicated, but much more research is needed to demonstrate the clinical utility of these findings.
	Increased monocyte counts may be found in drug abusers with bacterial endocarditis or other infections and in patients with tuberculosis or syphilis. Several psychotropic drugs are associated with spurious changes to monocyte counts, as noted in the *Interfering Factors* section below.
Preparation of patient	Fasting is not required. Any physiological stress should be avoided just before testing.
Indications	• WBC differential may be included as routine component of CBC • WBC differential may be added when the WBC count is abnormal, to help determine source of abnormality.
Reference range	100–500 cells/mm^3 (3%–7% of total WBC count)
Critical value(s)	None

White blood cell (WBC) count differential: monocytes *(continued)*

Increased levels	• Bacterial infection
	• Tuberculosis
	• Subacute bacterial endocarditis
	• Syphilis
	Other established causes include leukemia, myeloproliferative disorders, carcinoma, lymphoma, recovery stage of neutropenia, lipid storage disease, surgical trauma, chronic ulcerative colitis, enteritis, sprue, collagen diseases, sarcoidosis, tetrachloroethane poisoning, and certain parasitic, mycotic, and rickettsial diseases.
Decreased levels	• HIV infection
	• Aplastic anemia
	• Overwhelming infection (with neutropenia)
	• Hairy cell leukemia
	• Steroid (prednisone) treatment
Interfering factors	Psychotropic drugs associated with falsely increased monocyte levels include alprazolam, chlorpromazine, haloperidol, paroxetine, and quazepam.
	Psychotropic drugs associated with falsely decreased monocyte levels include alprazolam and triazolam.
Cross-references	**Complete Blood Count**
	White Blood Cell Count

Fischbach FT, Fischbach MA: A Manual of Laboratory and Diagnostic Tests, 10th Edition. Philadelphia, PA, Wolters Kluwer Health/Lippincott Williams and Wilkins, 2018

Guilliams M, Mildner A, Yona S: Developmental and functional heterogeneity of monocytes. Immunity 49(4):595–613, 2018

Jaipersad AS, Lip GY, Silverman S, Shantsila E: The role of monocytes in angiogenesis and atherosclerosis. J Am Coll Cardiol 63(1):1–11, 2014

Malcangio M: Role of the immune system in neuropathic pain. Scand J Pain 20(1):33–37, 2019

Morris G, Fernandes BS, Puri BK, et al: Leaky brain in neurological and psychiatric disorders: drivers and consequences. Aust N Z J Psychiatry 52(10):924–948, 2018

Prinz M, Priller J: The role of peripheral immune cells in the CNS in steady state and disease. Nat Neurosci 20(2):136–144, 2017

White blood cell (WBC) count differential: neutrophils

Type of test	Blood
Background and explanation of test	Neutrophils—the most abundant WBC type in the circulation—are the body's primary defense against microbial invasion and important modulators of inflammation. These cells identify and destroy invading pathogens through phagocytosis, degranulation, cytokine expression, and the formation of neutrophil extracellular traps (NETs), which are fiber networks containing DNA, enzymes, and other toxic substances.
	Two populations of neutrophils of approximately equal size exist in the blood, one in rapid circulation and the other moving slowly along the inner walls of the vasculature (the "marginated pool"). These latter cells can be called up quickly in a process of demargination to assist at sites of infection or tissue injury.
	Mature neutrophils have an elongated, pinched nucleus said to be "segmented." Immature neutrophils have a band-shaped nucleus and are known as *bands* or *stabs*. When these latter forms are detected in a blood sample, a "left shift" toward more immature cells recruited from the bone marrow is noted. Recruitment of cells from the marginated pool, on the other hand, does not result in a left shift.
	The association of high neutrophil counts in peripheral blood—neutrophilia—with cancer and infection has been known for some time. Research has greatly increased understanding of the adverse effects of neutrophils in amplification of the inflammatory response and release of toxic molecules that can destroy surrounding tissue, contribute to microvascular thrombosis and cancer cell metastasis, and result in permanent injury to the lungs, heart, and kidneys. In severe cases of COVID-19, the formation of unregulated NETs is thought to give rise to the acute respiratory distress syndrome, thrombus formation, and other organ failures.
	Each of the five types of WBC is counted, and the value is expressed as a percentage of the total WBC count. Increases or decreases in the total WBC count and in each cell type have diagnostic importance. Although the percentage shows only the relative number of each cell type, the absolute number can be calculated by multiplying the percentage of that cell type by the total WBC count. The absolute value is used to determine whether the count of a particular cell type is increased.
Relevance to psychiatry and behavioral science	A decline in the number of neutrophils can occur with many psychotropic drugs, including the following:
	• *Antipsychotics*: amoxapine, chlorpromazine, clozapine, fluphenazine, haloperidol, perphenazine, prochlorperazine, risperidone, thiothixene, trifluoperazine
	• *Antidepressants*: desipramine, imipramine, mirtazapine
	• *Anticonvulsants*: carbamazepine, ethosuximide, phenytoin, valproate

White blood cell (WBC) count differential: neutrophils *(continued)*

Relevance to psychiatry and behavioral science *(continued)*	Severe neutropenia is defined by an ANC of <500 cells/mm^3. This condition is well established as an adverse effect of clozapine and occurs much more rarely with other psychotropic drugs. The risk of severe neutropenia is highest in the first 18 weeks of clozapine treatment, but the condition can occur at any time and is not dosage-dependent. Management of neutropenia is discussed in the **Clozapine** entry in the *Psychotropic Medications* chapter.
Preparation of patient	Fasting is not required. Any physiological stress should be avoided just before testing.
Indications	• WBC differential often included as routine component of CBC. • WBC differential may be added when WBC count is abnormal, to help determine source of abnormality. • Routine monitoring for patients treated with clozapine • Patient with fever, lymphadenopathy, or oral ulcerations
Reference range	3,000–7,000 cells/mm^3 (50% of total WBC count) 1,200–6,600 cells/mm^3 in adults with benign ethnic neutropenia. Individuals of African, Middle Eastern, and West Indian descent commonly have a lower baseline neutrophil count in the absence of disease. This is known as "benign ethnic neutropenia."
Critical value(s)	*Neutropenia*: • Mild: 1,000–1,500 cells/mm^3 • Moderate: 500–1,000 cells/mm^3 • Severe: <500 cells/mm^3 *Neutrophilia*: • >7,700 cells/mm^3
Increased levels	• *Infections*: acute bacterial infections, fungal and spirochetal infections, some parasitic and rickettsial infections • *Inflammation*: vasculitis, rheumatoid arthritis, pancreatitis, gout, acute asthma, hypersensitivity reactions, rheumatic fever • *Tissue necrosis*: MI, burns, tumors, lead or mercury poisoning, digitalis toxicity, venoms • Acute hemorrhage, hemolytic anemia, hemolytic transfusion reaction • Diabetic ketoacidosis, preeclampsia, uremia • Myeloproliferative diseases (e.g., leukemia) • Cancers such as carcinoma • Early viral infections, some parasitic infections

White blood cell (WBC) count differential: neutrophils (continued)

Increased levels (*continued*)	• Postoperative state • Smoking
Decreased levels	• *Decreased production*: genetic and stem cell disorders, acute overwhelming bacterial infections, viral infections, certain rickettsial and protozoal infections, drugs, chemicals, ionizing radiation, venoms, hematopoietic diseases (e.g., aplastic anemia, iron deficiency anemia) • *Decreased cell survival*: infections in patients with little marrow reserve (e.g., elderly), collagen vascular diseases (e.g., SLE), autoimmune disease, drug hypersensitivity, and splenic sequestration • *Pregnancy*: progressive decrease in segmented neutrophils until time of labor and delivery • Numerous drugs, including antimicrobial, analgesic, anti-inflammatory, cardiovascular, psychotropic, antihistamine, and antithyroid agents
Change in ratio	• *Degenerative shift to the left*: increase in the number of band forms without leukocytosis. This is found in certain overwhelming infections and has a poor prognosis. • *Regenerative shift to the left*: increase in the number of bands with leukocytosis. This is found in bacterial infections and has a good prognosis. • *Shift to the right*: decreased bands are seen, with increased segmented neutrophils. This is found in liver disease, megaloblastic anemia, hemolysis, use of drugs, cancer, and allergies. • *Hypersegmentation of neutrophils with no band forms*: This is found in pernicious anemia and other megaloblastic anemias and in chronic morphine addiction.
Interfering factors	Neutrophilia can be caused by physiological stress (excitement, intense emotion, heat/cold exposure, exercise, vomiting, menstruation, labor/delivery, or electric shock) or by administration of steroids, in which case the neutrophilia peaks in 4–6 hours and normalizes by 24 hours. Reduced neutrophilic response to infection or stress can be seen with old age or debility.
Cross-references	**Clozapine** **Complete Blood Count** **White Blood Cell Count**

Atallah-Yunes SA, Ready A, Newburger PE: Benign ethnic neutropenia. Blood Rev 37:100586, 2019

Borges L, Pithon-Curi TC, Curi R, Hatanaka E: COVID-19 and neutrophils: the relationship between hyperinflammation and neutrophil extracellular traps. Mediators Inflamm 2020:8829674, 2020

Castanheira FVS, Kubes P: Neutrophils and NETs in modulating acute and chronic inflammation. Blood 133(20):2178–2185, 2019

Fischbach FT, Fischbach MA: A Manual of Laboratory and Diagnostic Tests, 10th Edition. Philadelphia, PA, Wolters Kluwer Health/Lippincott Williams and Wilkins, 2018

White blood cell (WBC) count differential: neutrophils *(continued)*

Nader DN: Neutrophilia. Medscape, October 3, 2019. Available at: https://emedicine.medscape.com/article/208576-overview. Accessed October 2021.

Shaul ME, Fridlender ZG: Tumour-associated neutrophils in patients with cancer. Nat Rev Clin Oncol 16(10):601–620, 2019

Silvestre-Roig C, Braster Q, Ortega-Gomez A, Soehnlein O: Neutrophils as regulators of cardiovascular inflammation. Nat Rev Cardiol 17(6):327–340, 2020

Zuo Y, Yalavarthi S, Shi H, et al: Neutrophil extracellular traps in COVID-19. JCI Insight 5(11):e138999, 2020

CHAPTER 2
Diseases and Conditions

22q11.2 deletion syndrome

Clinical findings	The 22q11.2 deletion syndrome (which now subsumes DiGeorge and velocardiofacial syndrome) arises from a hemizygous microdeletion from the long arm of chromosome 22, in most cases affecting >100 genes. As could be expected, the effects of this deletion are numerous and varied, involving cardiac and palatal malformations; immune dysfunction; endocrine, genitourinary, and GI problems; and significant brain abnormalities associated with developmental delays, cognitive deficits, and neuropsychiatric illness. This is the most common microdeletion syndrome in humans, occurring in up to 1 in 2,000 live births. Prenatal and newborn screening for this condition began in the 1990s, and individuals born before that time may remain undiagnosed as adults.
	Children and adolescents with this syndrome exhibit various physical conditions and anomalies as well as developmental delays, learning disabilities, and variable degrees of intellectual disability. They are more likely than unaffected individuals to develop ADHD, autism spectrum disorder, anxiety disorders, mood disorders, and psychotic disorders/schizophrenia. Attention, executive function, working memory, visuospatial abilities, motor skills, and social skills are impaired. There is increased risk of behavioral disorders.
	Later in life, affected individuals are more likely to come to clinical attention because of neuropsychiatric problems. Mood episodes (both mania and depression), anxiety disorders, and psychosis are commonly seen. Because this deletion syndrome represents the strongest known molecular genetic risk factor for the development of psychosis, it is of particular interest to psychiatric researchers as a model for the study of schizophrenia.
	Some combination of the following abnormalities is seen, starting early in life:
	• Congenital heart disease
	• Malformation of the palate
	• Hypocalcemia
	• Immune deficiency
	• Learning difficulties
	• Facial dysmorphism in affected Whites (long face, malar flatness)
	• Dysphagia
	• Growth hormone deficiency
	• Autoimmune disease
	• Hearing loss and other sensory deficits
	• Numerous other structural abnormalities involving virtually all organ systems (e.g., thyroid, parathyroid, thymus)
	Personality and temperament are often characterized as follows:
	• Disinhibited and/or impulsive
	• Shy and/or socially withdrawn
	• Anxious
	• Socially awkward
	Cognitive and developmental problems include the following:
	• Intellectual disability (mild) in up to half of children
	• Substantially higher verbal than performance IQ scores

22q11.2 deletion syndrome *(continued)*

Clinical findings *(continued)*	• Developmental motor and language delays • Autism and autism spectrum disorders
Laboratory testing	At the initial visit for undiagnosed adults suspected of having 22q11.2 deletion syndrome: • Clinical genetic testing of the patient, offspring, and parents (siblings if the parents are unavailable). Consultation with a specialist in 22q11.2 deletion syndrome is advised for this purpose. Penetrance of deletion is complete, although the variability of clinical syndrome is marked. Anticipation is not known to occur. • Cognitive testing/capacity assessment • *Recommended laboratory tests*: CBC with differential, electrolytes, TSH, pH-corrected ionized calcium, magnesium, PTH, creatinine, LFTs, lipid profile, glucose, HbA1c Laboratory tests should be repeated at annual or biennial follow-up visits.

Antshel KM, Fremont W, Roizen NJ, et al: ADHD, major depressive disorder, and simple phobias are prevalent psychiatric conditions in youth with velocardiofacial syndrome. J Am Acad Child Adolesc Psychiatry 45:596–603, 2006

Davies RW, Fiksinski AM, Breetvelt EJ, et al: Using common genetic variation to examine phenotypic expression and risk prediction in 22q11.2 deletion syndrome. Nat Med 26(12):1912–1918, 2020

Fung WL, Butcher NJ, Costain G, et al: Practical guidelines for managing adults with 22q11.2 deletion syndrome. Genet Med 17(8):599–609, 2015

Gothelf D: Velocardiofacial syndrome. Child Adolesc Psychiatr Clin N Am 16(3):677–693, 2007

Green T, Gothelf D, Glaser B, et al: Psychiatric disorders and intellectual functioning throughout development in velocardiofacial (22q11.2 deletion) syndrome. J Am Acad Child Adolesc Psychiatry 48:1060–1068, 2009

Lajiness-O'Neill R, Beaulieu I, Asamoah A, et al: The neuropsychological phenotype of velocardiofacial syndrome (VCFS): relationship to psychopathology. Arch Clin Neuropsychol 21:175–184, 2006

McDonald-McGinn DM, Sullivan KE, Marino B, et al: 22q11.2 deletion syndrome. Nat Rev Dis Primers 1:15071, 2015

O'Rourke L, Murphy KC: Recent developments in understanding the relationship between 22q11.2 deletion syndrome and psychosis. Curr Opin Psychiatry 32(2):67–72, 2019

Tang KL, Antshel KM, Fremont WP, Kates WR: Behavioral and psychiatric phenotypes in 22q11.2 deletion syndrome. J Dev Behav Pediatr 36(8):639–650, 2015

Adrenal insufficiency (AI)

Clinical findings	AI is characterized by inadequate circulating cortisol levels, either from disease of the adrenal cortex itself (primary AI) or lack of stimulation by ACTH (central AI). Primary AI also involves inadequate aldosterone production. AI can present acutely or as a chronic illness. AI is most commonly caused by the use of exogenous glucocorticoid drugs that suppress the HPA axis. Other causes of AI include pituitary adenomas, autoimmune disease, TBI, and high-dose opioid treatment, among others. In the era of COVID-19, AI patients may be at particular risk because glucocorticoid levels can be insufficient for the severity of illness, so the systemic inflammatory response can be heightened. In these cases, a specific recommendation is made for the immediate doubling of cortisol replacement therapy.
	The acute presentation of AI—adrenal crisis—is characterized by an abrupt deterioration in health status, with hypotension, fever, rapidly progressive delirium, and stupor. With the administration of parenteral glucocorticoids, symptoms resolve over 1–2 hours. If the condition is not recognized and treated emergently, it can be fatal.
	Chronic adrenal insufficiency is more likely to be encountered in the psychiatric setting. Onset is insidious, and symptoms are nonspecific. *Clinical wisdom dictates that if you think of AI, you need to rule it out.* Prominent signs of chronic AI include the following: hypotension, orthostasis, weakness, weight loss, pain (myalgias, arthralgias), skin pigmentation (resembling tanning, especially in skin creases and around nipples), pigmentation of mucous membranes, vitiligo, loss of libido, amenorrhea, anorexia, nausea, vomiting, salt craving, and hair thinning.
	Most patients with AI have psychiatric symptoms, which include the following: depression, anxiety, mania, apathy, profound fatigue, confusion, poor concentration, executive dysfunction, delusions, hallucinations, agitation, aggression, disinhibition, social withdrawal, and sleep disturbances. EEG changes often seen to accompany mental status changes include diffuse slowing and bursts of sharp- and slow-wave discharges, which may persist after clinical symptoms have resolved.
Laboratory testing	The gold standard of testing for AI is the so-called short corticotropin test in which a dose of ACTH is administered parenterally, and serum cortisol is checked 30 and/or 60 minutes later. If the response to stimulation is subnormal, adrenal insufficiency is diagnosed, and a basal ACTH level is checked. If the ACTH level is high, primary adrenal insufficiency is diagnosed. If the ACTH level is low or low-normal, central adrenal insufficiency is diagnosed, and MRI of the brain is performed to evaluate the pituitary gland. Note that in acute secondary adrenal insufficiency due to pituitary stroke, results of the ACTH stimulation test may be normal. In the workup of the underlying cause of AI, autoantibodies against 21-hyroxylase are checked.
	Numerous other laboratory abnormalities are seen in AI, including low sodium, high potassium, high calcium, high bicarbonate, low bicarbonate with low pH (metabolic acidosis), elevated BUN, elevated creatinine, anemia, lymphocytosis, and eosinophilia.

Adrenal insufficiency (AI) *(continued)*

Almeida MQ, Mendonca BB: Adrenal insufficiency and glucocorticoid use during the COVID-19 pandemic. Clinics (Sao Paulo) 75:e2022, 2020

Anglin RE, Rosebush PI, Mazurek MF: The neuropsychiatric profile of Addison's disease: revisiting a forgotten phenomenon. J Neuropsychiatry Clin Neurosci 18(4):450–459, 2006

Bancos I, Hahner S, Tomlinson J, Arlt W: Diagnosis and management of adrenal insufficiency. Lancet Diabetes Endocrinol 3(3):216–226, 2015

Charmandari E, Nicolaides NC, Chrousos GP: Adrenal insufficiency. Lancet 383(9935):2152–2167, 2014

Donegan D: Opioid induced adrenal insufficiency: what is new? Curr Opin Endocrinol Diabetes Obes 26(3):133–138, 2019

Pazderska A, Pearce SH: Adrenal insufficiency: recognition and management. Clin Med (Lond) 17(3):258–262, 2017

Rushworth RL, Torpy DJ, Falhammar H: Adrenal crisis. N Engl J Med 381(9):852–861, 2019

Alcohol use disorder (AUD)

Clinical findings	The patient and/or informant reports a pattern of excessive drinking:
	• For males, 4+ drinks daily or 15 drinks weekly
	• For females and older males: 3+ drinks daily or 8 drinks weekly
	• For pregnant individuals: any drinking
	• Binge drinking: 5+ drinks for males and 4+ drinks for females within 2 hours
	A patient may admit to wanting to stop drinking but being unable to do so. They are secretive about drinking and engage in risky behaviors, such as drunk driving. The patient and/or informant reports problems in relationships, at school, or at work because of the patient's drinking, and the patient may have become dangerous or violent while drunk. They may be in denial about the seriousness of the problem. The patient may have a history of alcohol withdrawal when drinking was stopped, with symptoms ranging from mild shaking and anxiety to delirium tremens, with fever, unstable vital signs, and confusion.
	On examination, patients may be in a disheveled and agitated state with unstable vital signs or may have a normal appearance. Alcohol on the breath may be covered up by mouthwash or aftershave. In a long-time heavy drinker, examination may reveal tremor, slurring of speech, hyperactive deep tendon reflexes, incoordination, gait instability, muscle wasting, peripheral neuropathy, or cognitive impairment affecting memory and executive functions. With the onset of liver disease, fetor hepaticus, asterixis, gynecomastia, hepatosplenomegaly, ascites, testicular atrophy, and skin changes become prominent. The latter include jaundice, spider telangiectasia, palmar erythema, caput medusa, ecchymoses, nail changes such as clubbing, hyperpigmentation, porphyria cutanea tarda, exacerbation of rosacea (with rhinophyma), psoriasis, seborrhea, skin infections, and excoriation due to pruritus.
Laboratory testing	Laboratory abnormalities supporting a diagnosis of AUD suspected on clinical grounds include the following:
	• *Elevated GGT (>47 U/L in males or >25 U/L in females) consistent with 4+ drinks daily for 4 weeks or more.* It takes 2–3 weeks of abstinence to normalize the GGT level. Elevation of GGT has high sensitivity for liver disease but low specificity in the evaluation of etiology. Specificity improves through patient selection; although GGT assay would have little use in screening for alcoholic liver disease, it would be highly useful in confirming recent drinking in a chronic drinker who is in treatment and is supposedly abstinent. In males, GGT is used alone for this indication. In females, it is best used in tandem with CDT. Specificity also improves when elevated GGT is found in combination with an AST-to-ALT ratio >2, which is consistent with alcoholic liver disease.
	• *Elevated CDT ≥2.6%.* Test is positive in people drinking 50–80 g of ethanol daily for a minimum of several weeks. In general, the specificity of the test is high (97%), but the sensitivity is variable (65%–95%). Sensitivity can be improved without loss of specificity when GGT is measured in conjunction with CDT because the combined test is positive in people drinking ≥40 g of ethanol daily. With 2–4 weeks of abstinence, CDT value normalizes.
	• Ratio of AST to ALT >2:1
	• Elevated MCV (>101 fL, although age- and sex-dependent)

Alcohol use disorder (AUD) *(continued)*

Laboratory testing *(continued)*	• Elevated uric acid level (≥7 mg/dL, although this is age- and sex-dependent).
	• Elevated total homocysteine level (>15 μmol/L).
	• Elevated phosphatidylethanol (PEth). This refers to a group of phospholipids formed in the presence of ethanol and incorporated into membranes of RBCs. PEth has a half-life of 4–10 days and a window of detection of 2–4 weeks (longer in chronic, heavy drinkers). Serial PEth testing is useful in monitoring abstinence in known drinkers over time. Although a reference range is not yet established, a level >20 ng/mL is considered evidence of moderate to heavy drinking. False elevations can be seen in patients with advanced liver disease.
	Recent drinking can be confirmed using breath analysis, saliva ethanol, urine ethanol, or blood alcohol level (BAL). Urine ethylglucuronide could also be measured; this metabolite of ethanol remains positive in urine for 2–3 days, longer than ethanol itself. GGT and/or CDT can often be useful, as noted above.
	In patients with known alcohol dependence or abuse, the BAL can be useful in diagnosing intoxication or withdrawal (the latter when BAL is zero in the presence of relevant signs and symptoms). Other common blood lab abnormalities in patients with AUD include hypomagnesemia, hypophosphatemia, hypoglycemia, anemia, thrombocytopenia, and hypoprothrombinemia.
	In patients with alcohol-related dementia, CT or MRI may show generalized atrophy (both cortical and central atrophy, the latter evidenced by ventricular enlargement). Atrophy may decrease to some extent with abstinence. In patients with cerebellar signs, CT or MRI may show atrophy of cerebellar cortex, most often in the anterior and superior segments of the vermis. Radiologists should be alerted to clinical findings suggestive of cerebellar involvement.
	Clinical diagnosis of alcohol-related polyneuropathy can be confirmed by EMG, with single-fiber study complementing conventional needle EMG. In acute alcoholic myopathy, AST and creatine kinase can be elevated in the presence of painful muscle weakness. Chronic alcohol-related myopathy, which is progressive with continued drinking, can be diagnosed by EMG or NCT. Patients with recurrent seizures or who are "found down" may develop rhabdomyolysis with myoglobinuria and acute renal failure.

American Psychiatric Association: Diagnostic and Statistical Manual of Mental Disorders, 5th Edition, Text Revision. Washington, DC, American Psychiatric Association, 2022

Andresen-Streichert H, Müller A, Glahn A, et al: Alcohol biomarkers in clinical and forensic contexts. Dtsch Arztebl Int 115(18):309–315, 2018

Brust JC: A 74-year-old man with memory loss and neuropathy who enjoys alcoholic beverages. JAMA 299:1046–1054, 2008

Chrostek L, Cylwik B, Szmitkowski M, et al: The diagnostic accuracy of carbohydrate-deficient transferrin, sialic acid and commonly used markers of alcohol abuse during abstinence. Clin Chim Acta 364:167–171, 2006

Helander A, Böttcher M, Dahmen N, Beck O: Elimination characteristics of the alcohol biomarker phosphatidylethanol (PEth) in blood during alcohol detoxification. Alcohol Alcohol 54(3):251–257, 2019

Neumann J, Beck O, Helander A, Böttcher M: Performance of PEth compared with other alcohol biomarkers in subjects presenting for occupational and pre-employment medical examination. Alcohol Alcohol 55(4):401–408, 2020

Alcohol use disorder (AUD) *(continued)*

Nguyen VL, Haber PS, Seth D: Applications and challenges for the use of phosphatidylethanol testing in liver disease patients (mini review). Alcohol Clin Exp Res 42(2):238–243, 2018

Rinck D, Frieling H, Freitag A, et al: Combinations of carbohydrate-deficient transferrin, mean corpuscular erythrocyte volume, gamma-glutamyltransferase, homocysteine and folate increase the significance of biological markers in alcohol dependent patients. Drug Alcohol Depend 89:60–65, 2007

Sillanaukee P: Laboratory markers of alcohol abuse. Alcohol Alcohol 31:613–616, 1996

Ulwelling W, Smith K: The PEth blood test in the security environment: what it is; why it is important; and interpretative guidelines. J Forensic Sci 63(6):1634–1640, 2018

Aluminum toxicity

Clinical findings	Because aluminum is found everywhere in the environment, exposure occurs naturally through ingestion of food, drinking water, or certain over-the-counter drugs such as antacids; use of aluminum-containing cookware; food packaging; cosmetics such as antiperspirants, sun creams, and toothpaste; and some vaccines. Under normal circumstances, these sources pose little health risk because only a small fraction of aluminum is absorbed through the GI tract and skin. Thus, although the tolerable weekly intake set by the European Food Safety Authority of 1 mg of aluminum per kilogram of body weight can easily be exceeded by food intake alone, this fact is of little clinical significance; internal exposure measured by aluminum levels in the urine or blood provides a better measure of toxicity.
	Potentially toxic exposure to aluminum occurs in occupations such as aluminum welding and processing. Historically, this level of exposure was also found among renal dialysis patients treated with aluminum-containing dialysis fluids, but this exposure has been mitigated since the year 2000 by a change in dialysate constituents and is now rare. Environmental exposure from industrial emissions, hazardous waste sites, and contaminated well water still occurs. Worth noting is the fact that reverse osmosis water filters remove almost 100% of aluminum from drinking water. In addition, exposure from vaccine adjuvants is minimal; aluminum levels in blood and urine from vaccinated patients are the same as those from unvaccinated patients. COVID-19 vaccines approved in the United States do not contain aluminum.
	Neurotoxic effects of significant aluminum exposure were identified in a cohort of dialysis patients studied before 2000. At the molecular level, aluminum induces oxidative stress, modifies calcium signaling pathways in the hippocampus, and reduces synthesis of acetylcholine. Clinical symptoms include disorientation, memory impairment, apraxia, speech impairment, seizures, and dementia. Neuropathological study shows neuronal loss and vascular changes, all of which are minimal. Amyloid plaques and neurofibrillary tangles are not evident. In those who survive, neurotoxic effects are at least partially reversed with elimination of exposure.
	With industrial exposure associated with toxic urine and blood levels, neuropsychological changes in concentration, learning, and memory have been found. In addition, industrial exposure to aluminum can give rise to *metal fume fever*, a flu-like illness with headache, fever/chills, myalgias, cough, chest tightness, and a metallic taste in the mouth. Onset of this syndrome can be delayed for several hours, and symptoms can last for 1–2 days. Chronic exposure to fine aluminum dust can cause pulmonary fibrosis.
	Elevated aluminum concentrations have been found in the brain tissue of patients with Alzheimer's disease (AD), autism spectrum disorder, and epilepsy. This does not necessarily imply causation; aluminum has a high affinity for proteins, which it is able to cross-link. Numerous studies have failed to establish a connection between aluminum levels and AD, and other potential disease links to aluminum have been less well studied. One case of adult-onset epilepsy was reported from a 1988 water poisoning event in the Cornish town of Camelford, but in that fatal case, both exposure and aluminum levels in the brain tissue were extremely high.

Aluminum toxicity (continued)

Clinical findings (continued)	A critical reading of the literature would suggest there is currently no convincing evidence that aluminum accumulation causes AD. The specific encephalopathy caused by aluminum toxicity is distinct from AD.
	Concern has also arisen in relation to aluminum exposure and breast cancer. Although aluminum levels tend to be higher in cancerous tissue, the metal does not appear to trigger tumor formation but instead is stored to a greater degree in cancerous tissue. More research is needed to resolve remaining questions regarding metal exposure and breast cancer.
Laboratory testing	Aluminum is found in the blood (serum) and urine of all individuals. The upper limit of normal (ULN) for the general population is <5 µg/L in serum and <15 µg/L in urine. Some sources use <7 µg/L as the ULN for urine. For routine screening and testing of dialysis patients using phosphate binders, serum is the specimen of choice. For chronic exposure and monitoring, urine is the specimen of choice. Elevated levels should be confirmed on a second specimen because the sample is very susceptible to environmental contamination during collection. In addition, medications and nutritional supplements may interfere with the test and should be discontinued if possible before sampling. With occupational exposure, early changes found on neuropsychological testing corresponded to serum aluminum levels of ≥13 µg/L and urine levels of ≥120 µg/L. For aluminum workers, testing before employment and annually thereafter is recommended.

ARUP Laboratories: Aluminum, serum, in Laboratory Test Directory. Salt Lake City, UT, ARUP Laboratories, 2021. Available at: https://ltd.aruplab.com/Tests/Pub/0099266. Accessed December 2021.

Goullé JP, Grangeot-Keros L: Aluminum and vaccines: Current state of knowledge. Med Mal Infect 50(1):16–21, 2020

Klotz K, Weistenhöfer W, Neff F, et al: The health effects of aluminum exposure. Dtsch Arztebl Int 114(39):653–659, 2017

Principi N, Esposito S: Aluminum in vaccines: does it create a safety problem? Vaccine 36(39):5825–5831, 2018

Schifman RB, Luevano DR: Aluminum toxicity: evaluation of 16-year trend among 14,919 patients and 45,480 results. Arch Pathol Lab Med 142(6):742–746, 2018

Alzheimer's disease (AD)

Clinical findings	AD is a neurodegenerative disorder with an insidious onset and gradual progression from a preclinical stage, in which only neuropathological abnormalities are identified, to late-stage dementia, in which the person has lost the ability to function independently. Long before cognitive symptoms are noticed, the affected individual may exhibit apathy, changes in mood, heightened anxiety, or sleep problems. Although the earliest cognitive changes are commonly seen in day-to-day memory functions (with distant memories preserved while recent memories are lost), non-amnestic presentations with first symptoms in language, visuospatial function, or executive functions are also recognized.
	Criteria for the diagnosis of dementia formulated by the National Institute on Aging–Alzheimer's Association (NIA-AA) include the following:
	• The presence of cognitive or neuropsychiatric symptoms that interfere with function, represent a decline, and are not explained by delirium or major psychiatric disorder.
	• Cognitive impairment detected through history and testing (bedside mental status exam or neuropsychological testing).
	• Impairment involving two or more of the following domains:
	• Ability to acquire and remember new information
	• Reasoning, handling of complex tasks, judgment
	• Visuospatial abilities
	• Language functions (speaking, reading, writing)
	• Personality, behavior, comportment
	Criteria for probable AD formulated by the NIA-AA include the following:
	• Meets the above criteria for dementia, with insidious onset and gradual progression.
	• Prominent cognitive deficits in one of the following domains along with at least one other cognitive domain: memory, language, visuospatial function, or executive function.
	• No evidence of substantial cerebrovascular disease, core features of dementia with Lewy bodies, prominent features of behavioral variant FTD, prominent features of non-AD primary progressive aphasia, or another disease or medication that substantially affects cognition.
Laboratory testing	Standard laboratory testing for patients undergoing workup for dementia includes the following blood tests: TSH, vitamin B_{12}, homocysteine, CBC with differential, CMP, ESR, and CRP. Abnormal findings in any of these tests could reveal conditions that might contribute to cognitive changes. In addition, brain MRI without gadolinium is performed to evaluate atrophy, infarcts, white matter changes, microhemorrhages, and conditions such as hydrocephalus or mass lesions. If MRI is not available, noncontrast head CT is recommended. Atrophy in AD involves the hippocampal areas and temporoparietal cortices.
	Depending on patient demographics or other findings from history or physical exam, further testing may be indicated, such as the following: antinuclear antibody testing, HbA1c, lipid profile, folate, ammonia, lead, Lyme antibodies, RPR, HIV, serum protein electrophoresis, MMA, PT, and PTT. Chest X-ray or sleep study may be needed.

Alzheimer's disease (AD) *(continued)*

Laboratory testing *(continued)*	If the evaluation is inconclusive as to the cause of dementia or the presentation is atypical, early onset, or rapidly progressive, more comprehensive testing may be needed. This would include blood tests for TPOAb, antithyroglobulin antibodies, and apoliprotein E testing. CSF would be tested for AD biomarkers (low amyloid-β_{42}, elevated tau, elevated phospho-tau, and amyloid-tau index <1). Some labs might now test for soluble triggering receptor expressed on myeloid cells 2 (TREM2) in CSF, which is a proxy of microglial activity and associated with the rate of AD progression. FDG-PET or SPECT imaging showing bilateral temporoparietal hypometabolism would be helpful in supporting an AD diagnosis and distinguishing AD from frontotemporal degeneration. Amyloid and tau PET imaging showing excessive and widespread binding would also increase diagnostic certainty. Familial autosomal dominant AD is a rare, early onset (before age 65 years) condition caused by mutations in the amyloid precursor protein, presenilin 1, or presenilin 2 genes. In cases in which these mutations have been inherited, AD is certain to develop. Much more common is sporadic, late-onset AD, for which scores of susceptibility genes have been recognized. The most important genetic risk for late-onset disease is the ε4 allele of *APOE*, which is strongly associated with accelerated amyloid-β deposition in the brain and a higher risk of developing AD.

Altuna-Azkargorta M, Mendioroz-Iriarte M: Blood biomarkers in Alzheimer's disease. Neurologia (Engl Ed) 36(9):704–710, 2021

American Psychiatric Association: Diagnostic and Statistical Manual of Mental Disorders, 5th Edition, Text Revision. Washington, DC, American Psychiatric Association, 2022

Atri A: The Alzheimer's disease clinical spectrum: diagnosis and management. Med Clin North Am 103(2):263–293, 2019

de Leon MJ, DeSanti S, Zinkowski R, et al: MRI and CSF studies in the early diagnosis of Alzheimer's disease. J Intern Med 256:205–223, 2004

Edwin TH, Henjum K, Nilsson LNG, et al: A high cerebrospinal fluid soluble TREM2 level is associated with slow clinical progression of Alzheimer's disease. Alzheimers Dement (Amst) 12(1):e12128, 2020

McKhann GM, Knopman DS, Chertkow H, et al: The diagnosis of dementia due to Alzheimer's disease: recommendations from the National Institute on Aging-Alzheimer's Association workgroups on diagnostic guidelines for Alzheimer's disease. Alzheimers Dement 7(3):263–269, 2011

Waldemar G, Dubois B, Emre M, et al: Recommendations for the diagnosis and management of Alzheimer's disease and other disorders associated with dementia: EFNS guideline. Eur J Neurol 14:e1–e26, 2007

Anemia

Clinical findings	Anemia refers to a deficiency of RBCs in the body, reflected by a low hemoglobin level. It can arise acutely (e.g., with hemorrhage) or develop slowly (e.g., with chronic kidney disease). Three mechanisms account for most cases: inadequate RBC production, blood loss, and RBC destruction (hemolysis).
	Iron deficiency is the most common cause of anemia. Chronic iron deficiency anemia can be associated with symptoms such as burning paresthesias of the tongue, smooth tongue, sores at the angles of the mouth, spoon-shaped nails, and cognitive dysfunction. Of interest to behavioral health professionals, these findings may occur in patients with pica (i.e., ingestion of dirt, clay, or other substances). Other causes of anemia include vitamin B_{12} deficiency, folate deficiency, anemia associated with inflammation, aplastic anemia, bone marrow disease such as leukemia, hemolytic anemia, and sickle cell anemia. Psychotropic medications such as quetiapine have been associated with hemolytic anemia.
	The classic symptoms of anemia are fatigue, weakness, and pallor. A robust association with depression has been noted. Sleep disorders are often reported, including restless legs syndrome and periodic limb movements of sleep. A slowly developing anemia that is still mild may be asymptomatic, but as anemia becomes more severe, symptoms such as headache, dizziness, palpitations, chest pain, shortness of breath, and exercise intolerance may be seen. With acute blood loss, volume depletion and hypoperfusion become evident. With acute intravascular hemolysis, signs and symptoms also include jaundice, back pain, and free hemoglobin in the plasma and urine. In these cases, renal failure may ensue. Particular attention should be paid to pregnant patients during their first 30 weeks of pregnancy, when anemia is associated with an increased risk of neurodevelopmental disorders in the offspring. In elderly patients, anemia increases the risk of cardiovascular disease, cognitive impairment, falls with fracture, and reduced quality of life.
	A useful physical sign can be elicited by asking patients to hyperextend their hand; if the palmar creases are lighter than the surrounding skin, the hemoglobin level usually is <8 g/dL.
Laboratory testing	Reference hemoglobin ranges are as follows: • Adult females: 12.1–15.1 g/dL • Adult males: 13.8–17.2 g/dL Panic hemoglobin values include the following: • <5.0 g/dL associated with heart failure and death • >20 g/dL associated with capillary clogging *Diagnostic algorithm for anemia*: 1. Check CBC with platelets and differential (including RBC indices and morphology on manual differential), and check reticulocytes (number and percentage). 2. If anemia is present on CBC (hemoglobin <13 g/dL in males or <12 g/dL in females), check reticulocyte index (also called reticulocyte production index).

Anemia *(continued)*

Laboratory testing *(continued)*	3. If reticulocyte index is normal, classify anemia by RBC indices (MCV, mean corpuscular hemoglobin concentration [MCHC]):
	• *Microcytic, hypochromic*: iron deficiency anemia, sideroblastic anemia, or thalassemia
	• *Normocytic, normochromic*: inflammation, autoimmune disease, chronic kidney disease, endocrine disease, critical illness, or bone marrow disease
	• *Macrocytic*: vitamin B_{12} deficiency, folate deficiency, alcohol use disorder, drug effects, hypothyroidism, myelodysplasia
	4. If reticulocyte index is ≥2.5, look at peripheral smear for fragmented cells.
	• *If not present*: acute blood loss (hemorrhage)
	• *If present*: intravascular hemolysis, autoimmune destruction, sickle cell disease, or other hemolytic anemias
	5. To distinguish among causes of normocytic, normochromic anemia, check serum iron, total iron-binding capacity (TIBC), and ferritin levels.
	6. To distinguish among causes of microcytic, hypochromic anemia, look at peripheral smear.
	• If smear is abnormal, consider thalassemia, sideroblastic anemia, or bone marrow disease
	• If smear is normal, check serum iron, TIBC, and ferritin levels.
	• Low/normal TIBC and iron, normal/high ferritin = inflammation or chronic disease.
	• High TIBC, low iron, low ferritin = iron deficiency. Serum ferritin <15 ng/mL confirms diagnosis of iron deficiency, and >100 ng/mL excludes diagnosis.
	To monitor recovery with iron supplementation in iron deficiency anemia, the patient's hemoglobin is checked after 3 weeks to confirm response and after 9 weeks to confirm recovery when the source of iron deficiency has been identified and corrected. With iron supplementation, the hemoglobin level should rise by ~2 g/dL every 3 weeks. To ensure iron stores have been replenished, iron supplementation should continue for 3–6 months from the time hemoglobin normalizes.

Gafter-Gvili A, Schechter A, Rozen-Zvi B: Iron deficiency anemia in chronic kidney disease. Acta Haematol 142(1):44–50, 2019

Hidese S, Saito K, Asano S, Kunugi H: Association between iron-deficiency anemia and depression: a web-based Japanese investigation. Psychiatry Clin Neurosci 72(7):513–521, 2018

Leung W, Singh I, McWilliams S, et al: Iron deficiency and sleep: a scoping review. Sleep Med Rev 51:101274, 2020

Phillips J, Henderson AC: Hemolytic anemia: evaluation and differential diagnosis. Am Fam Physician 98(6):354–361, 2018

Stauder R, Valent P, Theurl I: Anemia at older age: etiologies, clinical implications, and management. Blood 131(5):505–514, 2018

Vulser H, Wiernik E, Hoertel N, et al: Association between depression and anemia in otherwise healthy adults. Acta Psychiatr Scand 134(2):150–160, 2016

Wiegersma AM, Dalman C, Lee BK, et al: Association of prenatal maternal anemia with neurodevelopmental disorders. JAMA Psychiatry 76(12):1294–1304, 2019

Anorexia nervosa (AN)

Clinical findings	AN is characterized by a self-imposed restriction of food intake with significantly low body weight, fear of gaining weight, and body image distortion. High morbidity and mortality rates in this condition arise from malnutrition and its various medical complications, as well as coexisting psychiatric disorders, including suicide. The disorder predominantly affects women, with a mean age at onset of 18 years, but is typically resistant to treatment so that recovery occurs only gradually, over years to decades. Genetic and psychosocial factors underlie the condition, which may be sustained by changes in neural architecture.

Two types of AN are recognized: the restricting type and the binge eating/purging type, with the latter including either binge-eating or purging behaviors such as self-induced vomiting or misuse of laxatives, diuretics, or enemas. Crossover between types is common in the course of the illness, so type is determined by current symptoms rather than symptom history. The binge-eating/purging type is distinguished from bulimia nervosa by the maintenance of normal weight in the latter condition.

Physical findings among adults presenting with AN include low body weight (BMI ≤17.5), bradycardia, orthostatic hypotension, dehydration, muscle wasting, and lanugo. Dental erosion, hand calluses, and salivary gland hypertrophy may be seen in those with purging behaviors. Psychiatric comorbidities include major depression, anxiety disorders, OCD, trauma-related disorders, and substance misuse. The suicide rate is among individuals with AN is 18 times that of control subjects.

Medical complications of AN affect all organ systems. Cardiac signs include serious bradycardia during sleep, prolonged QT, heart muscle wasting with dysrhythmias and sudden death, changes in left ventricular function, pericardial and valvular pathology, and dysregulation of peripheral vascular contractility. Injury to hepatocytes can lead to acute liver failure associated with encephalopathy and coagulation problems. Other potential complications include a decline in the GFR, bone marrow atrophy, difficulty standing because of loss of muscle mass, osteoporosis, and cerebral atrophy. The latter finding usually improves with weight restoration. |
| Laboratory testing | For all patients with AN, consider the following:

• Urinalysis: On presentation, check urine sample before the patient is weighed to determine specific gravity (reflecting hydration status), pH, presence of ketones, and evidence of kidney injury.

• CBC with differential: low cell counts due to bone marrow atrophy, with relative lymphocytosis. Rarely, platelet count is also low.

• Chemistries: high bicarbonate, normal calcium, and low values for sodium, potassium, chloride, phosphorus, magnesium, glucose, and albumin. High BUN and creatinine reflect prerenal azotemia.

For malnourished and severely symptomatic patients:

• ECG: bradycardia, prolongation of QT interval, nonspecific ST-segment changes, U waves, and, in severe cases, dysrhythmias, including ventricular fibrillation and asystole. In presence of severe sinus bradycardia or junctional rhythm, marked prolongation of corrected QT interval, or syncope, admission to telemetry unit is recommended. |

Anorexia nervosa (AN) *(continued)*

Laboratory testing *(continued)*	• LFTs: elevated AST, ALT, lactate dehydrogenase, ALP • Thiamine: low, although testing may not capture deficiency For patients underweight >6 months: • DEXA scan for osteoporosis/osteopenia • Estradiol level in females, testosterone level in males Nonroutine assessments: • Serum amylase level: elevation indicates persistent or recurrent vomiting • Thyroid function tests: high TSH, low thyroxine consistent with hypothyroidism • Lipids: increased low-density lipoprotein cholesterol and total cholesterol arising from loss of body fat (increased lipolysis) • LH and FSH levels for persistent amenorrhea at normal weight • Brain MRI or CT to detect brain atrophy • Fecal occult blood testing

American Psychiatric Association: Diagnostic and Statistical Manual of Mental Disorders, 5th Edition, Text Revision. Washington, DC, American Psychiatric Association, 2022

Dobrescu SR, Dinkler L, Gillberg C, et al: Anorexia nervosa: 30-year outcome. Br J Psychiatr 216(2):97–104, 2020

Eddy KT, Tabri N, Thomas JJ, et al: Recovery from anorexia nervosa and bulimia nervosa at 22-year follow-up. J Clin Psychiatry 78(2):184–189, 2017

Gibson D, Workman C, Mehler PS: Medical complications of anorexia nervosa and bulimia nervosa. Psychiatr Clin North Am 42(2):263–274, 2019

Harrington BC, Jimerson M, Haxton C, Jimerson DC: Initial evaluation, diagnosis, and treatment of anorexia nervosa and bulimia nervosa. Am Fam Physician 91(1):46–52, 2015

Mitchell JE, Peterson C: Anorexia nervosa. N Engl J Med 382(14):1343–1351, 2020

Rosen E, Bakshi N, Watters A, et al: Hepatic complications of anorexia nervosa. Dig Dis Sci 62(11):2977–2981, 2017

Sachs KV, Harnke B, Mehler PS, Krantz MJ: Cardiovascular complications of anorexia nervosa: a systematic review. Int J Eat Disord 49(3):238–248, 2016

Treasure J, Zipfel S, Micali N, et al: Anorexia nervosa. Nat Rev Dis Primers 1:15074, 2015

Volpe U, Tortorella A, Manchia M, et al: Eating disorders: what age at onset? Psychiatry Res 238:225–227, 2016

Weinbrenner T, Züger M, Jacoby GE, et al: Lipoprotein metabolism in patients with anorexia nervosa: a case-control study investigating the mechanisms leading to hypercholesterolaemia. Br J Nutr 91(6):959–969, 2004

Westmoreland P, Krantz MJ, Mehler PS: Medical complications of anorexia nervosa and bulimia. Am J Med 129(1):30–37, 2016

Zipfel S, Giel KE, Bulik CM, et al: Anorexia nervosa: aetiology, assessment, and treatment. Lancet Psychiatry 2(12):1099–1111, 2015

Antiphospholipid syndrome (APS)

Clinical findings	APS is a systemic autoimmune disease characterized by thrombotic or obstetrical events that occur in patients with persistent antiphospholipid (aPL) antibodies. The syndrome is often found in association with other autoimmune diseases such as SLE but also can be seen in the absence of other autoimmune symptoms. The diagnosis of APS is made when both clinical manifestations and laboratory abnormalities (positive aPL tests) are present.
	Neurological presentations of APS are well recognized. These include stroke/TIA, cognitive dysfunction, subcortical white matter changes, dementia, delirium, seizures, headaches, chorea, transverse myelitis, Guillain-Barré syndrome, a "multiple sclerosis-like" syndrome, and motor neuropathy. Stroke occurring in a young adult should raise suspicion for APS. TIA can manifest as amaurosis fugax, vertigo, transient global amnesia, transient paresthesias, or weakness. Subcortical white matter lesions may be seen on MRI in the absence of symptoms. Headaches are often recurrent and refractory to usual treatment but may respond well to anticoagulation. In general, psychiatric presentations are not well recognized, but psychosis, mania, treatment-resistant bipolar disorder, and depression have been reported. APS-associated psychosis is characterized by acute onset, female sex, older age at onset, and comorbid medical conditions.
	Obstetrical presentations of APS include fetal loss after the tenth week of gestation, recurrent early miscarriages, intrauterine growth restriction, and preeclampsia. Other clinical presentations of APS include deep venous thrombosis, pulmonary embolism, thrombocytopenia, hemolytic anemia, MI, cardiac valve vegetations/thickening, nephropathy, superficial thrombophlebitis, livedo reticularis/racemosa, and livedoid vasculopathy with cutaneous ulceration.
Laboratory testing	aPL antibodies include lupus anticoagulant, anticardiolipin, and anti-β-2 glycoprotein 1. Of the three tests, lupus anticoagulant has the strongest correlation with clinical events, but all three tests are performed to facilitate risk stratification. Persistence of antibodies is determined by testing on two or more occasions ≥12 weeks apart. If a patient with autoimmune symptoms does not test positive, the test is repeated because antibodies can develop at any time. In addition, false-positive results can be seen with current infections, prior syphilis infection, or the use of anticoagulants.
	Laboratory criteria indicating a positive aPL antibody test include any one or a combination of the following: • Lupus anticoagulant present in plasma on two or more occasions ≥12 weeks apart • Anticardiolipin antibody of IgG and/or IgM isotype in serum or plasma, present in medium to high titer (>40 GPL or MPL, or >99th percentile) on two or more occasions ≥12 weeks apart • Anti-β-2 glycoprotein 1 antibody of IgG and/or IgM isotype in serum or plasma (in titer >99th percentile) on two or more occasions ≥12 weeks apart

Antiphospholipid syndrome (APS) *(continued)*

Laboratory testing *(continued)*	In addition to APS, the differential diagnosis for a positive test includes SLE and other autoimmune disorders, HIV, certain cancers, and advanced age. Infections and drugs such as phenothiazines and procainamide may cause a transient positive test. aPL antibodies have been identified in patients with COVID-19 infection, but it is not known whether they are involved in thrombotic events. At present, aPL antibodies have no role in COVID-19 diagnosis or management. Available data suggest that mRNA vaccines for COVID-19 appear to be well tolerated in patients with aPL antibodies or APS.
	Thrombocytopenia is also present in 20% of APS cases, usually mild (>100,000 platelets/μL).
	INR is monitored in patients treated for APS with anticoagulants, although there is some controversy as to target INR level.

Aneja J, Kuppili PP, Paul K, et al: Antiphospholipid syndrome presenting as treatment resistant bipolar disorder and thrombocytopenia in a young male. J Neuroimmunol 343:577238, 2020

Avari JN, Young RC: A patient with bipolar disorder and antiphospholipid syndrome. J Geriatr Psychiatry Neurol 25(1):26–28, 2012

Devreese K, Hoylaerts MF: Challenges in the diagnosis of the antiphospholipid syndrome. Clin Chem 56:930–940, 2010

Erkan D, Lockshin MD: Non-criteria manifestations of antiphospholipid syndrome. Lupus 19:424–427, 2010

Garcia D, Erkan D: Diagnosis and management of the antiphospholipid syndrome. N Engl J Med 378(21):2010–2021, 2018

Gris JC, Nobile B, Bouvier S: Neuropsychiatric presentations of antiphospholipid antibodies. Thromb Res 135(suppl 1):S56–S59, 2015

Hallab A, Naveed S, Altibi A, et al: Association of psychosis with antiphospholipid antibody syndrome: a systematic review of clinical studies. Gen Hosp Psychiatry 50:137–147, 2018

Muscal E, Brey RL: Antiphospholipid syndrome and the brain in pediatric and adult patients. Lupus 19:406–411, 2010

Petri M: Antiphospholipid syndrome. Transl Res 225:70–81, 2020

Sammaritano LR: Antiphospholipid syndrome. Best Pract Res Clin Rheumatol 34(1):101463, 2020

Sayar Z, Moll R, Isenberg D, Cohen H: Thrombotic antiphospholipid syndrome: a practical guide to diagnosis and management. Thromb Res 198:213–221, 2021

Yelnik CM, Kozora E, Appenzeller S: Cognitive disorders and antiphospholipid antibodies. Autoimmun Rev 15(12):1193–1198, 2016

Yelnik CM, Kozora E, Appenzeller S: Non-stroke central neurologic manifestations in antiphospholipid syndrome. Curr Rheumatol Rep 18(2):11, 2016

Anxiety disorder due to another medical condition; substance/medication-induced anxiety disorder

Clinical findings	Secondary anxiety may be chronic and unremitting or episodic. Causes of chronic anxiety include chronic obstructive pulmonary disease, hyperthyroidism, hypocalcemia, congestive heart failure, TBI, dementia, and stroke (especially in the left frontal area). Drugs associated with chronic anxiety include stimulants, yohimbine, and antidepressants in certain patients (especially if the dose is excessive). Withdrawal from clonidine, anticholinergic drugs, alcohol, sedative-hypnotics, or nicotine is also associated with this condition.
	Causes of episodic anxiety include Parkinson's disease (during "off" periods), angina (especially in females), asthma, paroxysmal atrial tachycardia, pheochromocytoma, hypoglycemia, substance abuse or withdrawal, simple partial seizures, pulmonary emboli, and mastocytosis. Drugs associated with episodic anxiety include sympathomimetics, caffeine, cocaine, amphetamines, marijuana, and hallucinogens. Also associated is withdrawal from alcohol, which may occur at a particular time every day after the previous night's drinking.
Laboratory testing	Basic laboratory workup for anxiety includes only a metabolic panel (BMP or CMP) to check calcium and glucose levels, and TSH. Depending on patient characteristics and history, other elements of the evaluation might include one or more of the following: • ECG, Holter monitoring, cardiac stress testing, and/or echocardiogram • Chest X-ray, pulmonary function tests, and/or arterial blood gases • GGT with or without CDT for suspicion of covert drinking • Plasma free metanephrines • Urine porphyrin precursors (aminolevulinic acid [ALA] and porphobilinogen [PBG]) • Pulmonary CT scan • EEG

American Psychiatric Association: Diagnostic and Statistical Manual of Mental Disorders, 5th Edition, Text Revision. Washington, DC, American Psychiatric Association, 2022

Attention-deficit/hyperactivity disorder in adults

Clinical findings	In adults, a formal DSM-5-TR diagnosis of ADHD requires the presence of five symptoms across the domains of attention and hyperactivity, with several symptoms present before age 12 years. Although most adults fail to meet the full diagnostic criteria, up to 70% have persistent symptoms or functional impairment. Only 25% of adults currently diagnosed with ADHD received the diagnosis in childhood. Although the disorder is more common in young males than in young females, in adults the ratio is closer to 1:1.
	With aging, the motor unrest seen in children and adolescents declines, whereas problems with sustained attention, executive function, and impulsivity persist. Prominent symptoms in adult patients include emotional dysregulation, sleep/wake disturbances, and impulsivity, with the latter underlying an increased incidence of motor vehicle accidents, violent crimes, and risky sexual activity. The lifetime risk of suicide is increased four- to fivefold. Comorbid mood, anxiety, and/or substance abuse disorders are the rule and may obscure the ADHD diagnosis.
	Evaluation of adults with suspected ADHD relies mainly on the patient interview, using a checklist such as the *Adult ADHD Self-Report Scale* and its accompanying instructions, which constitute a semistructured interview. Ancillary reports from family and others familiar with the patient are helpful but not always available. Increasingly, ADHD is identified during neuropsychological testing in memory disorder clinics when disproportionate impairment is found in attentional and executive functions, and further history reveals several symptoms of childhood onset.
Laboratory testing	Laboratory testing in the diagnosis of ADHD is limited to ruling out underlying diseases that could account for symptoms, including drug use, TBI, epilepsy, hydrocephalus, brain aneurysm or arteriovenous malformation, stroke, HIV, thyroid disease, lead poisoning, visual or hearing loss, or pediatric autoimmune neuropsychiatric disorders associated with streptococcal infections (PANDAS).
	ADHD has a significant genetic component, with a heritability of 0.8, but only a few genes have been associated with this condition, and at present there are no accepted genetic biomarkers. Gene-environment interactions may have inflated these heritability estimates. Half of adults with ADHD exhibit executive function impairment on neuropsychological testing, including deficits in sustained attention and set shifting, working memory, planning ability, and inhibitory control. Other abnormalities are seen in the regulation of arousal, reaction time variability, and temporal processing. Structural brain abnormalities seen in ADHD include reduced global brain volume and reduced volume in the prefrontal, cerebellar, and subcortical regions. Volume loss is positively correlated with severity of ADHD symptoms. Correspondingly, functional imaging has demonstrated reduced activation in the prefrontal cortex, anterior cingulate gyrus, and associated parietal, striatal, and cerebellar areas. PET studies have shown dysfunction in both the dopaminergic and noradrenergic pathways. Although these findings are useful in understanding the pathophysiology of ADHD, as of this writing they are not used in formal diagnosis.

Attention-deficit/hyperactivity disorder in adults *(continued)*

American Psychiatric Association: Diagnostic and Statistical Manual of Mental Disorders, 5th Edition, Text Revision. Washington, DC, American Psychiatric Association, 2022

Anbarasan D, Kitchin M, Adler LA: Screening for adult ADHD. Curr Psychiatry Rep 22(12):72, 2020

Banaschewski T, Becker K, Döpfner M, et al: Attention-deficit/hyperactivity disorder. Dtsch Arztebl Int 114(9):149–159, 2017

Colvin MK, Stern TA: Diagnosis, evaluation, and treatment of attention-deficit/hyperactivity disorder. J Clin Psychiatry 76(9):e1148, 2015

Jain R, Jain S, Montano CB: Addressing diagnosis and treatment gaps in adults with attention-deficit/hyperactivity disorder. Prim Care Companion CNS Disord 19(5):17nr02153, 2017

Magnin E, Maurs C: Attention-deficit/hyperactivity disorder during adulthood. Rev Neurol (Paris) 173(7–8):506–515, 2017

Matthews M, Nigg JT, Fair DA: Attention deficit hyperactivity disorder. Curr Top Behav Neurosci 16:235–266, 2014

Posner J, Polanczyk GV, Sonuga-Barke E: Attention-deficit hyperactivity disorder. Lancet 395(10222):450–462, 2020

Thapar A, Cooper M: Attention deficit hyperactivity disorder. Lancet 387(10024):1240–1250, 2016

Volkow ND, Swanson JM: Clinical practice: adult attention deficit-hyperactivity disorder. N Engl J Med 369(20):1935–1944, 2013

Young JL, Goodman DW: Adult Attention-deficit/hyperactivity disorder diagnosis, management, and treatment in the DSM-5 era. Prim Care Companion CNS Disord 18(6):10.4088/PCC.16r02000, 2016

Autism spectrum disorder (ASD)

Clinical findings	ASD is a neurodevelopmental disorder affecting ~1 in 68 children. The disorder is characterized by persistent deficits in social communication and interaction and by restricted, repetitive patterns of behavior, interests, or activities. It is highly heterogeneous in presentation and course. In a community sample, one-third of adults diagnosed with ASD as children who had normal or higher intelligence no longer reported ASD symptoms. Adults with ASD coupled with intellectual disability, on the other hand, required daily support.
	Specific ASD symptoms in adults include social anxiety; difficulty with social interactions; problems making friends and maintaining friendships; difficulty discerning the emotions of others, including facial expressions and body language; problems regulating emotions; hypersensitivity to touch, sounds, or smells; monotonic speech; difficulty with changes to routines; inflexible thinking; and a limited range of interests. Some individuals demonstrate exceptional abilities in a particular field of expertise.
	Currently, diagnosis of ASD is clinical, based on childhood and adult symptoms reported by the patient (and an informant, if possible). Instruments such as the Autism Diagnostic Observation Schedule, Second Edition (ADOS-2), and the Social Responsiveness Scale, Second Edition (SRS-2), facilitate the process. If symptoms were not present in childhood, another diagnosis is considered. In addition, other conditions that could give rise to symptoms should be excluded. Emerging evidence suggests that eye-tracking data can be used to distinguish adults with so-called high-functioning autism from healthy control subjects.
	Risk factors for the development of ASD are numerous and may include conception by in vitro fertilization, advanced paternal or maternal age, prenatal exposure to air pollution and other teratogens, gestational diabetes, smoking, alcohol consumption, infections (especially rubella), preeclampsia, and maternal nutritional deficiencies (folic acid, iron, fatty acids, vitamins), among others. Furthermore, mounting evidence suggests that individuals with ASD have a reduced ability to eliminate toxic metals such as aluminum and mercury and that the accumulation of these elements contributes to ASD symptoms.
	The most common comorbidities in ASD include anxiety, depression, sleep disorders, learning disability, developmental coordination disorder, intellectual disability, OCD, ADHD, epilepsy, GI disorders, immune system disorders, and FXS. ASD traits are also highly prevalent among eating disorder patients.
Laboratory testing	Laboratory testing cannot be used to diagnose ASD, but genetic testing can in some cases identify its cause. ASD is known to be a multifactorial genetic disease that does not conform to classical Mendelian inheritance. Most affected individuals have multiple interacting genes underlying the phenotype. The most frequently ordered test for individuals presenting with clinical features of ASD is the chromosomal microarray (CMA), which checks for extra or missing parts on chromosomes to account for the development of ASD. CMA can identify a genetic cause in 5%–14% of cases. Affected individuals should also be tested for FXS, and affected females should be tested for Rett syndrome. If these tests do not identify a cause for ASD, whole exome sequencing or whole genome sequencing may be recommended.

Autism spectrum disorder (ASD) *(continued)*

Adamou M, Jones SL, Wetherhill S: Predicting diagnostic outcome in adult autism spectrum disorder using the Autism Diagnostic Observation Schedule, Second Edition. BMC Psychiatry 21(1):24, 2021

American Psychiatric Association: Diagnostic and Statistical Manual of Mental Disorders, 5th Edition, Text Revision. Washington, DC, American Psychiatric Association, 2022

Baj J, Flieger W, Flieger M, et al: Autism spectrum disorder: trace elements imbalances and the pathogenesis and severity of autistic symptoms. Neurosci Biobehav Rev 129:117–132, 2021

Bentz M, Westwood H, Jepsen JRM, et al: The autism diagnostic observation schedule: patterns in individuals with anorexia nervosa. Eur Eat Disord Rev 28(5):571–579, 2020

Fernandez BA, Scherer SW: Syndromic autism spectrum disorders: moving from a clinically defined to a molecularly defined approach. Dialogues Clin Neurosci 19(4):353–371, 2017

Kreiman BL, Boles RG: State of the art of genetic testing for patients with autism: a practical guide for clinicians. Semin Pediatr Neurol 34:100804, 2020

Lintas C, Persico AM: Autistic phenotypes and genetic testing: state-of-the-art for the clinical geneticist. J Med Genet 46:1–8, 2009

Lord C, Elsabbagh M, Baird G, Veenstra-Vanderweele J: Autism spectrum disorder. Lancet 392(10146):508–520, 2018

Styles M, Alsharshani D, Samara M, et al: Risk factors, diagnosis, prognosis and treatment of autism. Front Biosci (Landmark Ed) 25:1682–1717, 2020

Tammimies K, Marshall CR, Walker S, et al: Molecular diagnostic yield of chromosomal microarray analysis and whole-exome sequencing in children with autism spectrum disorder. JAMA 314(9):895–903, 2015

Bipolar and related disorder due to another medical condition

Clinical findings	This condition—also known as secondary mania (SM)—is characterized by a prominent and persistent period of abnormally elevated, expansive, or irritable mood and abnormally increased activity or energy. There is evidence from the history, physical examination, or laboratory findings that the disturbance is the direct pathophysiological consequence of another medical condition. Usually, the onset of mania is acute to subacute, in tandem with the presentation of the medical condition. SM is more likely in patients with atypical features, such as first episode after age 40 years, single episode, treatment resistance, unusual symptoms (e.g., visual or olfactory hallucinations, clouded consciousness, disorientation, marked memory impairment), focal neurological signs, or soft neurological signs (e.g., astereognosis or dysdiadochokinesia). Known causes of SM include the following: • Cushing's disease • Hypothyroidism or hyperthyroidism • Vitamin B_{12} deficiency • Hemodialysis • Multiple sclerosis • SLE • Stroke • TBI • Postpartum state • Infection: influenza, encephalitis, neurosyphilis, HIV/AIDS • Brain tumor • Primary CNS lymphoma • Epilepsy • Neurodegenerative diseases: prion disease, FTD, Huntington's disease • Post-neurosurgery state • Calcification of the basal ganglia: idiopathic (Fahr's disease) or secondary to hypoparathyroidism or other conditions Brain lesions most often involve hypoactivity or disconnection of right hemisphere structures or excitatory lesions such as epileptic foci in left hemisphere structures.
Laboratory testing	The cause of SM may be apparent, based on the history or physical examination. If not, the following laboratory investigations should be considered: • CMP • CBC with differential and platelets • TSH • Vitamin B_{12} level • Brain MRI or head CT • EEG • 24-hour urine free cortisol level with follow-up testing • Urine toxicology • HIV testing

Bipolar and related disorder due to another medical condition *(continued)*

Laboratory testing *(continued)*	• Syphilis serology (RPR or VDRL) • Antinuclear antibody with follow-up testing

American Psychiatric Association: Diagnostic and Statistical Manual of Mental Disorders, 5th Edition, Text Revision. Washington, DC, American Psychiatric Association, 2022

Bergink V, Rasgon N, Wisner KL: Postpartum psychosis: madness, mania, and melancholia in motherhood. Am J Psychiatry 173(12):1179–1188, 2016

Satzer D, Bond DJ: Mania secondary to focal brain lesions: implications for understanding the functional neuroanatomy of bipolar disorder. Bipolar Disord 18(3):205–220, 2016

Torales J, González I, Barrios I, et al: Manic episodes due to medical illnesses: a literature review. J Nerv Ment Dis 206(9):733–738, 2018

Wang C, Fipps DC: Primary CNS lymphoma and secondary causes of mania: a case report and literature review. J Neuropsychiatry Clin Neurosci 34(1):84–88, 2022

Brain abscess

Clinical findings	Brain abscess is a focal bacterial, fungal, or parasitic infection that begins as an area of cerebritis and evolves into an encapsulated area of pus. The condition develops from the spread of pathogens from adjacent tissues or hematogenous dissemination. Patients at risk include those with a history of trauma, dental abscess, otitis media, IV drug abuse, endocarditis, immunodeficiency, or bronchiectasis. Abscess is more common in males and in children, adolescents, and young adults.
	Classic signs of brain abscess include fever, headache, and focal neurological deficits, but seizures and altered mental status are also commonly seen, the latter presaging a poor outcome. Onset is usually subacute. Specific focal signs depend on the location of the lesion(s), with frontotemporal or frontoparietal areas most often affected. Multiple lesions may be seen with a hematogenous origin.
	If the abscess is left untreated, intracranial pressure may eventually increase so that meningeal signs develop. Projectile vomiting can occur. Rupture of the abscess into the ventricular space carries a high risk of obstructive hydrocephalus and is fatal in up to 85% of cases.
Laboratory testing	Sonneville et al. (2017) proposed an algorithm for the workup of suspected brain abscess, as follows:
	1. Presence of clinical signs/symptoms noted above.
	2. While awaiting brain imaging, consider predisposing conditions (e.g., endocarditis, dental infection).
	3. Brain MRI if readily available. If not, urgent CT with contrast.
	4. If CT does not detect abscess, perform MRI.
	5. Obtain blood cultures before initiating antibacterial treatment.
	6. Consider HIV testing, especially if lesions are bilateral (indicating possible toxoplasmosis).
	7. Stereotactic aspiration of all abscesses ≥2.5 cm. If no abscess ≥2.5 cm, at least one ≥1 cm.
	8. Microbiology: routine, with or without molecular testing, and with specific tests for tuberculosis, fungus, etc., as indicated.
	Other laboratory abnormalities in affected patients include leukocytosis and elevated ESR. Lumbar puncture is contraindicated. EEG may show focal slowing. Follow-up EEG after treatment is recommended because many patients develop seizures in the following year.

Brook I: Microbiology and treatment of brain abscess. J Clin Neurosci 38:8–12, 2017

Brouwer MC, van de Beek D: Epidemiology, diagnosis, and treatment of brain abscesses. Curr Opin Infect Dis 30(1):129–134, 2017

Cantiera M, Tattevin P, Sonneville R: Brain abscess in immunocompetent adult patients. Rev Neurol (Paris) 175(7–8):469–474, 2019

Chow F: Brain and spinal epidural abscess. Continuum (Minneap Minn) 24(5):1327–1348, 2018

Sonneville R, Ruimy R, Benzonana N, et al: An update on bacterial brain abscess in immunocompetent patients. Clin Microbiol Infect 23(9):614–620, 2017

Brain tumor

Clinical findings	The most commonly diagnosed brain tumors are gliomas, meningiomas, and metastases from distant cancers such as melanoma and lung, breast, or kidney cancer. These tumors range from benign, slow-growing meningiomas to malignant, aggressive glioblastomas. Tumor-related symptoms depend on the location, size, and growth rate of the tumor as well as the extent of surrounding inflammation and edema. Common neuropsychiatric symptoms include headache, fatigue, cognitive changes, personality and behavioral changes, and focal signs such as hemiparesis. Frequent complications include epilepsy, stroke, venous thromboembolism, endocrine dysfunction, infection, and radiation necrosis secondary to treatment. Increasingly, genomic data are used along with histopathological findings to inform the classification and treatment of brain tumors.
Laboratory testing	For patients with suspected brain tumors, MRI with contrast is used in preference to CT unless there is some contraindication to MRI. The neuroradiologist should be asked for specific information about the size, constitution, surrounding tissue, and vascularity of the tumor, as well as the likely tumor type based on these characteristics and its location. In selected cases (e.g., suspected lymphoma), if neuroimaging study did not show any evidence of increased intracranial pressure, lumbar puncture may be performed to visualize cancer cells or tumor markers.
	Biopsy of tumor tissue is usually accomplished via craniotomy at the time the tumor is removed. Alternatively, stereotactic biopsy may be used to confirm the diagnosis and identify the specific tumor type. This involves insertion of a needle through a small hole rather than craniotomy and is used for tumors thought to be radiation-sensitive or for masses that are inaccessible to surgery.
	EEG may show focal slowing or epileptiform activity around the site of the tumor. Ictal (seizure) activity may be captured. At present, PET scanning is not routinely used for brain tumor diagnosis but occasionally may be used for tumor grading or for more precise tissue targeting for surgery. In treated cases, PET can also help distinguish delayed radiation encephalopathy from recurrent tumor.
	Other lab tests may be indicated in the diagnostic workup if metastatic disease is suspected (e.g., if multiple tumor foci are identified) and the primary remains unknown. These include CT of the chest, abdomen, and pelvis; CT of the neck if thyroid cancer is suspected; mammogram; ultrasound of the testes; and stool testing for occult blood. Certain brain tumors are associated with SIAD; see **Syndrome of Inappropriate Antidiuresis** entry for details of lab workup.

Louis DN, Perry A, Wesseling P, et al: The 2021 WHO Classification of Tumors of the Central Nervous System: a summary. Neuro Oncol 23(8):1231–1251, 2021

McFaline-Figueroa JR, Lee EQ: Brain tumors. Am J Med 131(8):874–882, 2018

Ostrom QT, Wright CH, Barnholtz-Sloan JS: Brain metastases: epidemiology. Handb Clin Neurol 149:27–42, 2018

Perez A, Huse JT: The evolving classification of diffuse gliomas: World Health Organization updates for 2021. Curr Neurol Neurosci Rep 21(12):67, 2021

Schiff D, Alyahya M: Neurological and medical complications in brain tumor patients. Curr Neurol Neurosci Rep 20(8):33, 2020 [published correction appears in Curr Neurol Neurosci Rep 20(9):40, 2020]

Vargo MM: Brain tumors and metastases. Phys Med Rehabil Clin N Am 28(1):115–141, 2017

Bulimia nervosa (BN)

Clinical findings	BN is characterized by cycles of recurrent binge eating and recurrent compensatory behaviors, such as self-induced vomiting, food restriction, and compulsive exercise. Affected individuals are not underweight but have a variety of health problems related to irregular eating and purging. The disorder commonly begins in adolescence or young adulthood and has a crude mortality rate of 2% per decade. Both the incidence of BN and the severity of existing cases worsened during the COVID-19 pandemic. Members of the LGBTQ+ community may be disproportionately affected by this condition.
	Psychological symptoms of BN include a preoccupation with body shape and weight, negative body image, feeling of loss of control over eating, and excessive guilt, self-hate, and self-criticism. Executive function impairment is identified on neuropsychological testing. Patients are often seen as perfectionists, with their self-worth determined by their current weight. Impulsivity and lack of emotional control become highly problematic when the patient becomes self-injurious. Psychiatric comorbidities include major depression, anxiety disorders, substance abuse, and borderline personality disorder, and the risk of suicide is significant.
	Physical signs include weight fluctuation, dehydration, electrolyte derangements, cardiac dysrhythmias, and amenorrhea or menstrual irregularity. Osteopenia can develop with episodes of weight loss and sex steroid suppression. With recurrent vomiting, scarring of the dorsum of the hand, erosion of dental enamel, dental caries, throat and mouth ulcers, parotid gland enlargement, Mallory-Weiss tears, and/or esophageal rupture can be seen. Cardiac and skeletal myopathies can occur secondary to abuse of syrup of ipecac. Laxative dependence and rectal prolapse from recurrent diarrhea may develop.
Laboratory testing	Electrolyte abnormalities in BN may include the following: • Low magnesium • Low potassium • Low sodium • Low chloride • Elevated phosphate • Metabolic alkalosis and elevated salivary amylase with vomiting • Metabolic acidosis with laxative or diuretic use Cardiomyopathy may be present on echocardiogram in cases of chronic ipecac ingestion to induce vomiting.

American Psychiatric Association: Diagnostic and Statistical Manual of Mental Disorders, 5th Edition, Text Revision. Washington, DC, American Psychiatric Association, 2022

Gibson D, Workman C, Mehler PS: Medical complications of anorexia nervosa and bulimia nervosa. Psychiatr Clin North Am 42(2):263–274, 2019

Hay P: Current approach to eating disorders: a clinical update. Intern Med J 50(1):24–29, 2020

Hirst RB, Beard CL, Colby KA, et al: Anorexia nervosa and bulimia nervosa: a meta-analysis of executive functioning. Neurosci Biobehav Rev 83:678–690, 2017

Strumia R: Dermatologic signs in patients with eating disorders. Am J Clin Dermatol 6:165–173, 2005

Treasure J, Claudino AM, Zucker N: Eating disorders. Lancet 375:583–593, 2010

Wade TD: Recent research on bulimia nervosa. Psychiatr Clin North Am 42(1):21–32, 2019

Catatonia

Clinical findings	The DSM-5 classification of catatonia includes the following two categories:
	1. Catatonia associated with another mental disorder (neurodevelopmental, psychotic, bipolar, depressive, or other disorder)
	2. Catatonic disorder due to another medical condition
	In addition, an unspecified catatonia and two other schizophrenia spectrum categories are listed.
	The clinical presentation of catatonia is dominated by at least three of the following symptoms:
	• Stupor—no psychomotor activity and/or not actively relating to the environment
	• Catalepsy—a limb remains in whatever position it is placed
	• Waxy flexibility—resistance of a limb to movement by examiner
	• Mutism—no or little verbal response (item is excluded if patient is aphasic)
	• Negativism—no response or opposition to instructions or verbal stimuli
	• Posturing—spontaneous, active maintenance of a posture against gravity
	• Mannerism—odd caricature of a normal action
	• Stereotypy—frequent, repetitive, non-goal-directed movement
	• Agitation that is not influenced by external stimuli
	• Grimacing
	• Echolalia—mimicking another's speech
	• Echopraxia—mimicking another's movements
	An instrument such as the Bush-Francis Catatonia Rating Scale can be helpful in screening for catatonia and determining its severity. A careful history may implicate medications or drugs in the disorder.
	A wide range of medical conditions have been found to underlie catatonic disorder, including neurological conditions such as encephalitis, non-convulsive status epilepticus, Parkinson's disease, cerebrovascular disease, head trauma, and brain neoplasm; metabolic conditions, such as thyroid disease, renal failure, hepatic encephalopathy, ketoacidosis, and electrolyte derangements; intoxication with substances such as Ecstasy, amphetamines, and phencyclidine; and withdrawal from benzodiazepines, alcohol, or other sedative-hypnotics. Of note, COVID-19 infection has been associated with catatonic disorder with underlying anti-NMDAR encephalitis.
Laboratory testing	Recommended tests to exclude medical or substance-related causes of catatonia include the following:
	• CBC with differential and platelets
	• CMP
	• Creatine kinase
	• Thyroid function tests
	• Urinalysis
	• Urine toxicology screen
	• Brain imaging: MRI or CT

Catatonia *(continued)*

Laboratory testing *(continued)*	• EEG (to exclude non-convulsive status epilepticus)
	• CSF studies (if no evidence of increased intracranial pressure)
	In addition, a fibrin D-dimer level is recommended to determine the risk of venous thromboembolism. A greatly elevated D-dimer level may be found in immobile patients.

American Psychiatric Association: Diagnostic and Statistical Manual of Mental Disorders, 5th Edition, Text Revision. Washington, DC, American Psychiatric Association, 2022

Brar K, Kaushik SS, Lippmann S: Catatonia update. Prim Care Companion CNS Disord 19(5):16br02023, 2017

Bush G, Fink M, Petrides G, et al: Catatonia, I: rating scale and standardized examination. Acta Psychiatr Scand 93(2):129–136, 1996

Francis A: Catatonia: diagnosis, classification and treatment. Curr Psychiatry Rep 12:180–185, 2010

Rajan S, Kaas B, Moukheiber E: Movement disorders emergencies. Semin Neurol 39(1):125–136, 2019

Vasilevska V, Guest PC, Bernstein HG, et al: Molecular mimicry of NMDA receptors may contribute to neuropsychiatric symptoms in severe COVID-19 cases. J Neuroinflammation 18(1):245, 2021

Central pontine myelinolysis (CPM)

Clinical findings	CPM is a potentially fatal neurological condition most often caused by overly rapid correction of hyponatremia, with shifts of small molecules and fluid in the brain that result in the destruction of myelin. Although the pons is particularly susceptible to injury, other areas of the brain can be affected, resulting in extrapontine myelinolysis (EPM). The two conditions are now subsumed under the term osmotic demyelination syndrome (ODS).
	Patients with chronic hyponatremia (>48 hours) are at higher risk of ODS. Other populations at risk include those with alcohol use disorder, malnutrition, history of liver transplant, eating disorders, serious burns, or HIV/AIDS; elderly patients; and those undergoing renal dialysis. Of interest to psychiatrists, severe hyponatremia can develop when the club drug Ecstasy is consumed along with excessive free water intake, placing patients at risk of ODS with sodium correction.
	Symptoms of ODS begin 2–3 days after hyponatremia is corrected, with additional symptoms arising over the following 1–2 weeks, the pattern partly dependent on the location of demyelination:
	• General symptoms of ODS include encephalopathy, seizure, catatonia, mutism, apathy, lethargy, primitive reflexes, cognitive dysfunction, and psychiatric symptoms such as depression, mania, disinhibition, and emotional lability.
	• EPM is characterized by movement disorders including the akinetic-rigid syndromes, tremor, dystonia, chorea, choreoathetosis, myoclonus, opsoclonus, gait disorders, and ataxia.
	• CPM is characterized by cranial nerve abnormalities (dysarthria, dysphagia, pupillary and ocular motility disorders), delirium, apathy, cognitive dysfunction, loss of reflexes, and the locked-in syndrome (in which the patient is awake and aware but is unable to move, show facial expression, speak, or communicate except by eye movements).
	With timely and effective intervention, morbidity and mortality of ODS have improved, but one-third to one-half of patients will still require some at-home care, be fully dependent, or die from the condition. It is also possible for affected patients to develop late-appearing symptoms such as behavioral problems, intellectual impairment, or movement disorders such as parkinsonism. Predictors of poor outcome include prior liver transplant as well as severe hyponatremia (<114 mEq/L), hypokalemia, and severe lack of awareness on presentation.
Laboratory testing	Workup for the cause of hyponatremia (serum sodium <135 mEq/L) is discussed in the **Hyponatremia** entry.
	When ODS is suspected, brain MRI should be obtained as early as possible. Head CT could be used if brain MRI is not available, although CT is significantly less sensitive. MRI with diffusion-weighted imaging is most likely to show early changes. T2-weighted images show hyperintense (bright) areas where demyelination has occurred.
	Other laboratory tests include the following:
	• Serum sodium performed serially during correction
	• Serum potassium

Central pontine myelinolysis (CPM) *(continued)*

Laboratory testing *(continued)*	• LFTs • Nutritional evaluation (serum vitamin B_{12}, MMA, folic acid, and phosphate)

Filippatos TD, Makri A, Elisaf MS, Liamis G: Hyponatremia in the elderly: challenges and solutions. Clin Interv Aging 12:1957–1965, 2017

Hoorn EJ, Zietse R: Diagnosis and treatment of hyponatremia: compilation of the guidelines. J Am Soc Nephrol 28(5):1340–1349, 2017

Lambeck J, Hieber M, Drebing A, Niesen WD: Central pontine myelinosis and osmotic demyelination syndrome. Dtsch Arztebl Int 116(35–36):600–606, 2019

Vladimirov T, Dreikorn M, Stahl K: Central pontine myelinolysis in a patient with bulimia: case report and literature review. Clin Neurol Neurosurg 192:105722, 2020

Chronic fatigue syndrome (CFS)

Clinical findings	CFS, also known as myalgic encephalomyelitis/chronic fatigue syndrome (ME/CFS), is characterized by disabling fatigue lasting 6 months or longer, nonrestorative sleep, post-exertional malaise, and either cognitive dysfunction or orthostatic intolerance. Fatigue results in a substantial reduction or impairment in the ability to engage in premorbid levels of occupational, educational, social, or personal activities. Fatigue may be profound and is not alleviated with rest. Currently, the condition is considered a complex, multisystem neuroimmune disease.
	Other symptoms associated with CFS but not required for the diagnosis include sore throat, tender lymph nodes, myalgia, arthralgia, headache, paresthesias, hypersensitivity to sensory stimuli, and other symptoms of dysautonomia (nausea, palpitations, cold hands and feet, irritable bladder, and irritable bowel).
	Certain medical conditions exclude the diagnosis of CFS, including untreated sleep apnea, cancer, hypothyroidism, major psychiatric disorder (schizophrenia spectrum disorder, bipolar disorder, eating disorder, or substance abuse), and severe obesity. Other conditions that do not exclude the diagnosis include fibromyalgia, somatic symptom disorders, treated hypothyroidism, and slightly elevated antinuclear antibodies. About one-third of individuals diagnosed with CFS also meet criteria for fibromyalgia.
	Despite substantial research effort, the cause of CFS is still unknown. Evidence of increased intracranial pressure, reduced cerebral blood flow, and endothelial cell dysfunction has been found, but a generally accepted unifying hypothesis has not been advanced. Moreover, although Epstein-Barr virus (EBV) and other pathogens have been implicated in CFS, it appears that the condition is not caused by a single infectious agent. Instead, it is thought that severe infections with pathogens such as EBV, Ross River virus, or *Coxiella burnetti* may contribute to later development of CFS in a subset of cases. The same may be true for the post-acute sequelae syndrome of COVID-19 infection ("long-haul" COVID-19).
Laboratory testing	The basic workup for CFS includes the following tests: <ul><li>CBC with differential</li><li>ESR</li><li>CMP (with LFTs)</li><li>Serum globulin</li><li>Phosphorus</li><li>TSH (ultra-sensitive)</li><li>Urinalysis</li></ul> In selected cases, the following tests may be indicated: <ul><li>Estradiol or testosterone level</li><li>Echocardiogram (to determine ejection fraction)</li><li>Polysomnography</li><li>Maintenance of wakefulness test (to exclude narcolepsy)</li><li>Arterial blood gases</li><li>Lyme disease testing</li><li>Rheumatoid factor, antinuclear antibody</li></ul>

Chronic fatigue syndrome (CFS) *(continued)*

Carod-Artal FJ: Post-COVID-19 syndrome: epidemiology, diagnostic criteria and pathogenic mechanisms involved. Rev Neurol 72(11):384–396, 2021

Lim EJ, Son CG: Review of case definitions for myalgic encephalomyelitis/chronic fatigue syndrome (ME/CFS). J Transl Med 18(1):289, 2020

Natelson BH: Myalgic Encephalomyelitis/Chronic fatigue syndrome and fibromyalgia: definitions, similarities, and differences. Clin Ther 41(4):612–618, 2019

Sandler CX, Lloyd AR: Chronic fatigue syndrome: progress and possibilities. Med J Aust 212(9):428–433, 2020

Tleyjeh IM, Saddik B, Ramakrishnan RK, et al: Long term predictors of breathlessness, exercise intolerance, chronic fatigue and well-being in hospitalized patients with COVID-19: a cohort study with 4 months median follow-up. J Infect Public Health 15(1):21–28, 2022

Wirth KJ, Scheibenbogen C, Paul F: An attempt to explain the neurological symptoms of myalgic encephalomyelitis/chronic fatigue syndrome. J Transl Med 19(1):471, 2021

Chronic traumatic encephalopathy (CTE)

Clinical findings	CTE is a neurodegenerative disease affecting those who have experienced repetitive head trauma such as military personnel; football, hockey and soccer players; boxers; and survivors of domestic abuse. The cumulative head trauma burden must be substantial, even though individual impacts may not have been associated with signs of concussion. CTE is characterized by cognitive, neuropsychiatric, and motor impairments that are progressive, ultimately leading to functional dependence and dementia. Symptoms typically begin after a clear period of stable functioning after head injury exposure ends. A definitive diagnosis of CTE requires confirmation by neuropathological examination showing a particular pattern of hyperphosphorylated tau deposition in neurofibrillary tangles. Core clinical features include the following: • Cognitive deficits are common in CTE, mostly affecting episodic memory, executive function, and attention. • Language, visuospatial function, and other domains may also be involved. • Neurobehavioral dysregulation is also common and may be severe, including explosiveness, impulsivity, rage, violent outbursts, severe irritability, or emotional lability. • Condition progressively worsens over a period of at least 1 year in the absence of continued exposure to head injury. Other signs and symptoms that are not included in the core criteria but can support the diagnosis are as follows: • *Psychiatric*: anxiety, pervasive worries, excessive fears, agitation, obsessive-compulsive behavior, depression, apathy, anhedonia, hopelessness, suicidal ideation and behavior, suspicion, delusional jealousy, and paranoid ideation. • *Motor*: gait and balance problems, dysarthria, parkinsonism (bradykinesia, rigidity, resting tremor, and parkinsonian gait).
Laboratory testing	A spectrum of pathology is seen, reflecting the progression of hyperphosphorylated tau deposition across time, with accompanying axonal disruption and loss. What begins as focal perivascular tangle formation in the frontal neocortex progresses to severe tauopathy involving widespread brain regions (including the medial temporal lobe), enabling the staging of pathology from I to IV. Clinical-pathological correlation has shown that early disease (pathological stage I) is associated with headache and problems with attention and concentration. In pathological stage II, additional symptoms of depression, explosivity, and short-term memory loss are seen. In stage III, executive dysfunction and cognitive impairment are noted. In stage IV, dementia with word-finding difficulty and aggression are seen. In severe CTE, other pathological changes are seen, including accumulation of amyloid-β, α-synuclein, and TDP-43 (transactive response DNA binding protein 43 kDa). Common comorbid pathological diagnoses include motor neuron disease, Alzheimer's disease, frontotemporal lobar degeneration, and Lewy body disease.

Chronic traumatic encephalopathy (CTE) *(continued)*

Laboratory testing *(continued)*	Neuroimaging shows white matter hyperintensities on FLAIR sequences corresponding to neuropathological changes of white matter rarefaction, arteriolosclerosis, and phosphorylated tau accumulation.
	Increased CSF phosphorylated tau-231 may prove to be a sensitive biomarker of CTE.

Bieniek KF, Cairns NJ, Crary JF, et al: The second NINDS/NIBIB consensus meeting to define neuropathological criteria for the diagnosis of chronic traumatic encephalopathy. J Neuropathol Exp Neurol 80(3):210–219, 2021

Katz DI, Bernick C, Dodick DW, et al: National Institute of Neurological Disorders and Stroke consensus diagnostic criteria for traumatic encephalopathy syndrome. Neurology 96(18):848–863, 2021

Mariani M, Alosco ML, Mez J, Stern RA: Clinical presentation of chronic traumatic encephalopathy. Semin Neurol 40(4):370–383, 2020

McKee AC, Stern RA, Nowinski CJ, et al: The spectrum of disease in chronic traumatic encephalopathy. Brain 136(Pt 1):43–64, 2013 [published correction appears in Brain 136(Pt 10):e255, 2013]

Mez J, Daneshvar DH, Kiernan PT, et al: Clinicopathological evaluation of chronic traumatic encephalopathy in players of American football. JAMA 318(4):360–370, 2017

Mez J, Stern RA, McKee AC: Chronic traumatic encephalopathy. Semin Neurol 40(4):351–352, 2020

Mufson EJ, Kelley C, Perez SE: Chronic traumatic encephalopathy and the nucleus basalis of Meynert. Handb Clin Neurol 182:9–29, 2021

Stein TD, Crary JF: Chronic traumatic encephalopathy and neuropathological comorbidities. Semin Neurol 40(4):384–393, 2020

Turk KW, Geada A, Alvarez VE, et al: A comparison between tau and amyloid-beta cerebrospinal fluid biomarkers in chronic traumatic encephalopathy and Alzheimer disease. Alzheimers Res Ther 14(1):28, 2022

Uretsky M, Bouix S, Killiany RJ, et al: Association between antemortem FLAIR white matter hyperintensities and neuropathology in brain donors exposed to repetitive head impacts. Neurology 98(1):e27–e39, 2022

Cirrhosis

Clinical findings	Cirrhosis refers to a pathological state of the liver in which normal tissue is replaced by fibrous tissue and regenerative nodules after a prolonged period of inflammation. Initially, the condition is asymptomatic and in its earliest stages may be reversible. Symptoms emerge when compensatory processes fail. The most common causes of cirrhosis are viral hepatitis, alcoholic liver disease, and non-alcoholic fatty liver disease/steatohepatitis. Other causes include storage diseases such as Wilson's disease, immune-mediated conditions such as primary biliary cholangitis, and cardiovascular disease such as congestive heart failure.
	Symptoms seen as compensatory processes begin to fail include drowsiness, fatigue, cognitive changes, confusion, weakness, sleep problems, loss of appetite, weight loss, and abdominal discomfort. With decompensation, jaundice, portal hypertension (with ascites and peripheral edema), hepatic encephalopathy, and bleeding are seen.
	On physical exam, most of the signs of cirrhosis are noted outside the abdomen. These include fetor hepaticus, parotid gland enlargement, spider angiomas, icterus, gynecomastia, asterixis, palmar erythema, Dupuytren contracture, splenomegaly, abdominal venous patterns indicating portal hypertension, ecchymoses, petechiae, edema, testicular atrophy, and skin excoriation due to pruritus.
Laboratory testing	Initial testing includes the following: • CBC with platelets • CMP • Ferritin • Transferrin saturation • GGT • Total bilirubin • PT/INR • Abdominal ultrasound Testing to determine the etiology of cirrhosis includes the following: • Chronic hepatitis B: hepatitis B surface antigen, and hepatitis B core antibody; if either is positive, hepatitis B virus DNA • Chronic hepatitis C: anti-hepatitis C antibody; if positive, hepatitis C virus RNA • Non-alcoholic fatty liver disease: lipid panel, HbA1c • Autoimmune hepatitis: antinuclear antibodies, smooth muscle antibodies Although liver biopsy has been the gold standard for confirming and staging fibrosis, less invasive strategies are now routinely used, including the estimation of fibrosis based on basic blood tests (e.g., the Fibrosis-4 Index for Liver Fibrosis and the Non-Alcoholic Fatty Liver Disease Fibrosis Score, both accessible at www.mdcalc.com). In addition, more specific blood tests that incorporate direct measures of fibrosis include hyaluronic acid and the *N*-terminal propeptide of type III collagen.

Cirrhosis *(continued)*

Laboratory testing *(continued)*	A widely used, noninvasive testing method known as transient elastography is replacing biopsy for patients with either minimal or advanced disease. Transient elastography measures liver stiffness through the abdominal wall using pulse-echo ultrasound acquisition. The procedure takes 5–10 minutes, and results are available at the point of care. Liver biopsy may still be needed for patients with intermediate stages of disease.
	Both laboratory and clinical data are used to provide information about prognosis using the Child-Pugh Score for Cirrhosis Mortality and for transplant planning using the MELD Score (Model for End-stage Liver Disease), both accessible at www.mdcalc.com.
	Patients with diagnosed cirrhosis should undergo ultrasound screening every 6 months for hepatocellular carcinoma.

Ginès P, Krag A, Abraldes JG, et al: Liver cirrhosis. Lancet 398(10308):1359–1376, 2021

Loomba R, Adams LA: Advances in non-invasive assessment of hepatic fibrosis. Gut 69(7):1343–1352, 2020

Smith A, Baumgartner K, Bositis C: Cirrhosis: diagnosis and management. Am Fam Physician 100(12):759–770, 2019

Stanford Medicine: Stanford Medicine 25: Liver disease, head to foot. Stanford, CA, Stanford Medicine, 2022. Available at: https://stanfordmedicine25.stanford.edu/the25/liverdisease.html. Accessed January 2022.

COVID-19

Clinical findings	Coronavirus disease 2019 (COVID-19) caused by the severe acute respiratory syndrome coronavirus-2 (SARS-CoV-2) is associated with a wide range of clinical presentations, from asymptomatic disease to septic shock and multiorgan failure. Exposure occurs mainly via short-range airborne transmission and, to a lesser extent, from aerosolized particles that persist in poorly ventilated indoor settings (long-range airborne transmission). Contact exposure from touching contaminated surfaces may also occur. An infected person is contagious for 2 days before and—in severe cases—up to 20 days after symptoms first appear. Mask-wearing, physical distancing, and hand hygiene reduce transmission rates.
	Symptoms of infection occur from 2 to 14 days after exposure and primarily involve the respiratory system. Both direct infection and inflammatory responses are implicated. Common symptoms include fever, cough, shortness of breath, chest tightness, sputum production, hemoptysis, fatigue, anosmia, hypogeusia, sore throat, diarrhea, nausea, vomiting, anorexia, abdominal pain, and myalgias. Symptoms requiring urgent intervention include breathing difficulty, persistent chest pain or pressure, new-onset confusion, inability to awaken or stay awake, and discoloration of the skin, lips, or nail beds suggestive of hypoxia. Increasingly, reports have emerged of cardiac, renal, hepatic, endocrine, hematological, and nervous system involvement, resulting in an extremely wide range of clinical and laboratory abnormalities. In severe cases, permanent injury to the lungs, heart, kidneys, and nervous system are seen.
	Nervous system involvement—"neuro-COVID"—includes the central, peripheral, and autonomic nervous systems. Signs and symptoms include the following: • Headache • Impaired consciousness • Delirium • Generalized myoclonus • Stroke—ischemic and hemorrhagic • Venous sinus thrombosis • Meningitis and encephalitis • Seizures—secondary to electrolyte derangements, hypoxia, organ failure, or stroke • Neurogenic respiratory failure • Dysautonomia—with orthostasis, hypotension, and vasovagal syncope • New-onset myasthenia gravis • Optic neuritis • Cranial polyneuropathy • Sensorineural hearing loss • Guillain-Barré syndrome • Transverse myelitis

COVID-19 *(continued)*

Clinical findings *(continued)*	So-called *long-haul COVID* may develop weeks to months after initial infection, the result of either persistent low-grade inflammation or neurodegeneration. Prominent symptoms include fatigue, myalgia, headache, chest pain, tachycardia, cough, shortness of breath, poor concentration, tremor, muscle twitching, insomnia, and depression. At 6 months, significant disability is seen in >50% of those affected, while impaired cognition is seen in almost 70%. Long-lasting symptoms include persistent anosmia/dysgeusia, memory problems, anxiety, and depression.
Laboratory testing	Testing for current COVID-19 infection involves antigen testing, performed either with a rapid test or a laboratory-based test. A swab is taken from the nose or posterior pharynx to provide the sample. For the rapid test, which can be done at home (or at a pharmacy or health care facility), it is only necessary to follow the package instructions. Results are available within ~15 minutes. For the laboratory test, the reverse transcription–PCR method is used, which is the gold standard of testing. The results take 1 or more days to return.
	Antibody tests are used to determine whether someone was previously exposed to or infected with COVID-19. Because it takes at least 12 days for the body to generate sufficient antibody levels to be detected, these tests are not useful to the person who is concerned about current infection.
	Chest imaging such as chest X-ray, CT scan, and lung ultrasound can be used to support the diagnosis of COVID-19. The classic finding on chest CT is that of ground-glass opacities, along with consolidation of tissue and "crazy paving," referring to ground-glass opacities with superimposed intralobular septal thickening. Findings are distributed to the periphery of both lungs. Chest CT can also reveal lymphadenopathy, nodules, cystic changes, and pleural effusions. These findings are not specific to COVID-19 but can also occur with other types of infection. These findings may be detectable before COVID-19 symptoms are apparent.
	As could be expected with such widespread organ involvement, laboratory abnormalities in COVID-19 are frequent and sometimes severe. Abnormalities include elevated PT, lactate dehydrogenase, D-dimer, ALT, CRP, and creatine kinase. Early in the course of the infection, a large reduction in CD4 and CD8 lymphocytes can be seen. ICU patients may have high levels of inflammatory mediators, indicators of coagulation activation and cellular immune deficiency, and evidence of myocardial, hepatic, and renal injury. A poor prognosis is heralded by elevations in serum ferritin, D-dimer, neutrophil count, BUN, and creatinine.

Aghagoli G, Gallo Marin B, et al: Neurological involvement in COVID-19 and potential mechanisms: a review. Neurocrit Care 34(3):1062–1071, 2021

Alsharif W, Qurashi A: Effectiveness of COVID-19 diagnosis and management tools: a review. Radiography (Lond) 27(2):682–687, 2021

Andalib S, Biller J, Di Napoli M, et al: Peripheral nervous system manifestations associated with COVID-19. Curr Neurol Neurosci Rep 21(3):9, 2021

Baig AM: Deleterious outcomes in long-hauler COVID-19: the effects of SARS-CoV-2 on the CNS in chronic COVID syndrome. ACS Chem Neurosci 11(24):4017–4020, 2020

Chaumont H, Meppiel E, Roze E, et al: Long-term outcomes after NeuroCOVID: a 6-month follow-up study on 60 patients. Rev Neurol (Paris) 178(1–2):137–143, 2022

COVID-19 *(continued)*

Divani AA, Andalib S, Biller J, et al: Central nervous system manifestations associated with COVID-19. Curr Neurol Neurosci Rep 20(12):60, 2020 [published correction appears in Curr Neurol Neurosci Rep 20(12):66, 2020]

Schroeder ME, Manderski MT, Amro C, et al: Large gathering attendance is associated with increased odds of contracting COVID-19: a survey based study. J Prev 43(2):157–166, 2022

West R, Kobokovich A, Connell N, Gronvall GK: COVID-19 antibody tests: a valuable public health tool with limited relevance to individuals. Trends Microbiol 29(3):214–223, 2021

Whittaker A, Anson M, Harky A: Neurological manifestations of COVID-19: a systematic review and current update. Acta Neurol Scand 142(1):14–22, 2020

Creutzfeldt-Jakob disease (CJD)

Clinical findings	CJD is a rapidly progressive and fatal neurodegenerative disease caused by an alteration in a naturally occurring prion protein (PrP^c) to an abnormal form termed *scrapie prion protein* (PrP^{Sc}). As with other prion diseases, most cases of CJD are sporadic, but genetic and acquired forms also exist. Sporadic CJD (sCJD) is classified into six subcategories based on the genotype of the prion protein at codon 129 and the molecular signature of PrP^{Sc} on Western blot analysis. Established risk factors for sCJD include only increasing age and methionine homozygosity at prion protein codon 129.
	The category of acquired CJD includes the variant CJD associated with ingestion of red meat infected with bovine spongiform encephalopathy (BSE; "mad cow disease") and iatrogenic forms. The incidence of variant CJD has declined dramatically with measures to eradicate BSE in animals. Iatrogenic CJD has been associated with corneal transplantation, contaminated EEG depth electrodes, contaminated growth hormone preparations, and surgical procedures including dura mater grafts. With increased awareness and infection control measures, iatrogenic cases have also declined, but cases could still emerge because the latency for some infections is as high as 25 years or longer.
	An immune-mediated encephalitis with severe neurological symptoms closely mimicking sCJD has been reported in COVID-19 infection. This syndrome was fully reversed with immunotherapy.
	The diagnosis of sCJD is made based on clinical and laboratory findings specified in the CDC guidelines available at www.cdc.gov/prions/cjd/diagnostic-criteria.html.
	Clinical findings include the following:
	• Rapidly progressive dementia
	• Myoclonus
	• Visual or cerebellar signs
	• Motor signs: pyramidal or extrapyramidal
	• Akinetic mutism
	Cognitive dysfunction primarily involves memory loss but also aphasia and frontal/executive dysfunction. Myoclonus is spontaneous or stimulus-responsive ("startle"). Visual signs may include blurring, decreased acuity, hemianopia, or cortical blindness. Cerebellar signs include limb ataxia and wide-based, unsteady, and irregular gait. Motor signs include weakness, reflex abnormalities, changes in muscle tone, and abnormal movements. Akinetic mutism is defined by the loss of movement and speech. Typically, the disease progresses from cognitive dysfunction to cerebellar signs to myoclonus and akinetic mutism to death, in rapid sequence.
Laboratory testing	Two developments in laboratory testing have significantly improved early diagnostic capability: real-time quaking-induced conversion (RT-QuIC) and MRI diffusion-weighted imaging. In RT-QuIC, a sample such as CSF is subjected to vigorous shaking that breaks up prion protein aggregates for further incubation and the amplification of misfolded proteins. Now in its second generation, this test is highly sensitive and specific for sCJD, and a positive RT-QuIC in combination with characteristic clinical findings is sufficient for a diagnosis of probable sCJD. The RT-QuIC test should be performed as soon as prion disease is suspected.

Creutzfeldt-Jakob disease (CJD) *(continued)*

Laboratory testing *(continued)*	Other tissues that can be used for testing with RT-QuIC include olfactory mucosa and skin samples. An analogous technique, protein misfolding cyclic amplification (PMCA), has high diagnostic accuracy for variant CJD using CSF, blood, or urine samples.
	MRI diffusion-weighted imaging has greatly increased the value of MRI in the early diagnosis of sCJD, when hyperintensities are seen in the cortex and basal ganglia, with sparing of the perirolandic and hippocampal areas. Depending on the molecular subtype of sCJD, other patterns may be seen. Usually, these hyperintense lesions do not exhibit swelling and do not enhance with contrast. The hyperintensities can be seen to diminish with disease progression, possibly reflecting neuronal loss. Of note, MRI FLAIR imaging could alternatively be used to meet the CDC's diagnostic criteria for positive imaging result.
	Other laboratory tests of use in the diagnosis of sCJD include electroencephalography and CSF analysis. Although the classic EEG finding is that of periodic sharp wave complexes, waking EEGs evolve with disease progression from non-specific patterns of generalized slowing and frontal intermittent rhythmic delta activity, to paroxysmal patterns resembling triphasic waves, to this pattern of periodic sharp waves. Stimulus-induced rhythmic, periodic, or ictal discharges (SIRPIDs) may be seen in the transition from sleep to wake states.
	CSF with a positive 14-3-3 assay may be helpful in diagnosing patients with a disease duration of <2 years who have a high pretest probability of sCJD. False-positive results can be seen in acute stroke, encephalitis, and other dementias.

Atarashi R, Sano K, Satoh K, Nishida N: Real-time quaking-induced conversion: a highly sensitive assay for prion detection. Prion 5(3):150–153, 2011

Beretta S, Stabile A, Balducci C, et al: COVID-19-associated immune-mediated encephalitis mimicking acute-onset Creutzfeldt-Jakob disease. Ann Clin Transl Neurol 8(12):2314–2318, 2021

Centers for Disease Control and Prevention: Prion Diseases: CDC's Diagnostic Criteria for Creutzfeldt-Jakob Disease (CJD). Atlanta, GA, Centers for Disease Control and Prevention, 2018. Available at: https://www.cdc.gov/prions/cjd/diagnostic-criteria.html. Accessed January 2022.

Figgie MP Jr, Appleby BS: Clinical use of improved diagnostic testing for detection of prion disease. Viruses 13(5):789, 2021

Gelisse P, Crespel A, Luigi Gigli G, Kaplan PW: Stimulus-induced rhythmic or periodic intermittent discharges (SIRPIDs) in patients with triphasic waves and Creutzfeldt-Jakob disease. Clin Neurophysiol 132(8):1757–1769, 2021

Nakhleh R, Tessema ST, Mahgoub A: Creutzfeldt-Jakob disease as a cause of dementia. BMJ Case Rep 14(5):e240020, 2021

Park HY, Kim M, Suh CH, et al: Diagnostic value of diffusion-weighted brain magnetic resonance imaging in patients with sporadic Creutzfeldt-Jakob disease: a systematic review and meta-analysis. Eur Radiol 31(12):9073–9085, 2021

Tokumaru AM, Saito Y, Murayma S: Diffusion-weighted imaging is key to diagnosing specific diseases. Magn Reson Imaging Clin N Am 29(2):163–183, 2021

Cushing's syndrome (CS)

Clinical findings	CS is characterized by signs and symptoms resulting from excess circulating cortisol levels, most commonly due to the use of glucocorticoid drugs (exogenous CS) or the presence of an ACTH-secreting pituitary tumor. The latter is known as Cushing's disease (CD). Other endogenous causes of CS include adrenal tumors and tumors of the lung, pancreas, ovary, thyroid, or thymus gland. Two forms of endogenous CS are recognized: ACTH-dependent, in which the overproduction of ACTH drives cortisol production (as in CD and these other tumors with ectopic ACTH release), and ACTH-independent, in which the adrenal glands produce cortisol autonomously. Recognition and early treatment of CS and CD are critical because these conditions are associated with increased mortality and morbidity, the latter including hypertension, the metabolic syndrome, osteoporosis with fracture, opportunistic infections, and several important neuropsychiatric disorders.
	Presenting signs of CS include the following: • Central obesity • Fat deposition in the face and upper back • Thin skin with wide purple striae • Hirsutism • Acne • Proximal muscle weakness • Hypertension • Glucose intolerance, diabetes • Psychiatric: irritability, emotional lability, fatigue, depression, anxiety, mania, psychosis, cognitive deficits, and sleep disturbances
	With mild hypercortisolism, physical signs of CS might not be present, but hypertension, diabetes, and osteoporosis coexisting in a non-elderly patient might raise the index of suspicion.
	Of the psychiatric disorders associated with CS, depression and anxiety are the most common, whereas mania and psychosis are rare. Mania is most often associated with the use of exogenous steroids. When depression occurs, cortisol levels tend to be higher and CS symptoms more severe. When psychotic symptoms develop, they tend to be treatment resistant. Patients with depression or psychosis may present a risk of suicide at any time in the course of illness. In general, psychiatric symptoms improve or resolve with treatment of CS that effectively lowers peripheral cortisol levels, but improvement in cognitive deficits appears to be more variable. This likely depends on the duration and the severity of elevated cortisol levels before treatment, among other factors. Multiple cognitive domains have been found to be affected, including attention, memory, executive function, verbal fluency, processing speed, and social cognition.
	In the era of COVID-19, special considerations apply to patients presenting with suspected hypercortisolism. This population is considered at particular risk for contracting COVID-19 and represents a high-risk group if infection occurs. Accordingly, diagnostic algorithms have been streamlined so that cases requiring urgent intervention are flagged.

Cushing's syndrome (CS) *(continued)*

Laboratory testing	Laboratory confirmation of endogenous CS involves the following steps: 1. Confirm elevated peripheral cortisol levels. 2. Distinguish ACTH-dependent from ACTH-independent cases. 3. Distinguish pituitary from ectopic sources of ACTH in ACTH-dependent cases. To confirm elevated peripheral cortisol levels, 24-hour urine free cortisol is measured. The reference range will depend on the methods used in testing, so local laboratory references should be consulted. If cortisol is elevated, a low-dose dexamethasone suppression test (DST) is performed to document the lack of feedback inhibition of cortisol on the HPA axis. Oral dexamethasone 1 mg is given between 11:00 P.M. and midnight, and plasma cortisol is checked at 8:00 A.M. the next day. If the result is normal or equivocal, a high-dose DST may be performed over 2 nights using 4 mg of dexamethasone and checking plasma cortisol at 8:00 A.M. the second morning. Late-night salivary cortisol level is measured to document the loss of normal diurnal variation in cortisol. When the diagnosis of CS has been confirmed, an ACTH level is obtained to determine whether excessive ACTH secretion is the cause. A normal or high ACTH level suggests ACTH-dependent CS because high cortisol levels would usually suppress ACTH. A low ACTH level suggests ACTH-independent CS arising from an adrenal source. If the diagnosis of ACTH-dependent CS is confirmed, then a high-resolution pituitary MRI with gadolinium is performed to identify pituitary lesions such as adenomas. These lesions are usually microadenomas (<10 mm) and may be difficult to visualize. If the study is equivocal, it may be necessary to take blood samples from the inferior petrosal sinuses draining blood from the pituitary to check ACTH levels for comparison with peripheral blood. Alternatively, a corticotropin-releasing hormone (CRH) stimulation test could be performed. Pituitary adenomas causing CD will respond to CRH stimulation, whereas ectopic ACTH-secreting tumors will not. Neuroimaging studies of CS and CD have shown significant volume reductions in the hippocampus, anterior cingulate cortex, and medial frontal gyrus. Although hippocampal volume appears to be at least partly restored with successful treatment, these reduced cortical volumes may be persistent. In addition, widespread white matter changes are observed, with some evidence of underlying demyelination.

Barbot M, Zilio M, Scaroni C: Cushing's syndrome: overview of clinical presentation, diagnostic tools and complications. Best Pract Res Clin Endocrinol Metab 34(2):101380, 2020

Bauduin SEEC, van der Wee NJA, van der Werff SJA: Structural brain abnormalities in Cushing's syndrome. Curr Opin Endocrinol Diabetes Obes 25(4):285–289, 2018

Berlinska A, Swiatkowska-Stodulska R, Sworczak K: Old problem, new concerns: hypercortisolemia in the time of COVID-19. Front Endocrinol (Lausanne) 12:711612, 2021

Fujii Y, Mizoguchi Y, Masuoka J, et al: Cushing's syndrome and psychosis: a case report and literature review. Prim Care Companion CNS Disord 20(5):18br02279, 2018

Lonser RR, Nieman L, Oldfield EH: Cushing's disease: pathobiology, diagnosis, and management. J Neurosurg 126(2):404–417, 2017

Cushing's syndrome (CS) *(continued)*

Nieman LK: Diagnosis of Cushing's syndrome in the modern era. Endocrinol Metab Clin North Am 47(2):259–273, 2018

Pivonello R, De Martino MC, De Leo M, et al: Cushing's disease. Endocrine 56(1):10–18, 2017

Ragnarsson O: Cushing's syndrome—disease monitoring: recurrence, surveillance with biomarkers or imaging studies. Best Pract Res Clin Endocrinol Metab 34(2):101382, 2020

Santos A, Webb SM, Resmini E: Psychological complications of Cushing's syndrome. Curr Opin Endocrinol Diabetes Obes 28(3):325–329, 2021

Wagner-Bartak NA, Baiomy A, Habra MA, et al: Cushing syndrome: diagnostic workup and imaging features, with clinical and pathologic correlation. AJR Am J Roentgenol 209(1):19–32, 2017

Delirium

Clinical findings	According to DSM-5, delirium is characterized by a disturbance in attention and awareness that develops acutely, represents a change from baseline function, and tends to fluctuate over the course of the day. At least one other cognitive disturbance must be present in orientation, memory, language, visuospatial ability, or perception, and there must be evidence of an underlying condition or conditions to explain the disturbance. Symptoms often become more florid in the evening or nighttime hours, and sleep disruption is common and can be so severe that daytime and nighttime activity patterns are reversed. Changes in perception can take the form of florid visual hallucinations. Although not part of the formal criteria, delusions are often present and, coupled with disorientation, can drive disruptive behaviors such as attempted elopement. In the case of etiologies such as alcohol withdrawal, autonomic signs are seen.
	DSM-5 categorizes delirium etiologies as substance intoxication, substance withdrawal, medication-induced, due to another medical condition, or due to multiple etiologies. Underlying diseases commonly include infection (particularly sepsis, pneumonia, or urinary tract infection), metabolic derangement, electrolyte disturbance, dehydration, cardiac dysrhythmia, heart failure, stroke, MI, TBI, alcohol/sedative withdrawal, status epilepticus, and medication toxicity (e.g., with opioids or anticholinergics). Delirium also commonly occurs following major surgery, particularly heart surgery.
	Delirium is seen in COVID-19 infection, particularly in severe cases with pulmonary involvement but also in seemingly mild cases without respiratory symptoms. Both direct brain effects from viral entry and indirect effects from inflammatory mechanisms have been implicated. Delirium that emerges during hospitalization for COVID-19 may herald CNS invasion and a worsening prognosis.
	Validated clinical instruments that are useful in diagnosing and monitoring delirium include the following: • 4AT Rapid Clinical Test for Delirium (www.the4at.com/4at-download) • Confusion Assessment Method (americandeliriumsociety.org/wp-content/uploads/2021/08/CAM-Long_Training-Manual.pdf) • Intensive Care Delirium Screening Checklist (www.lhsc.on.ca/media/8367/download)
Laboratory testing	Laboratory testing is performed to determine the cause or causes of delirium. Basic tests include the following: • CMP • CBC with differential and platelets • Urinalysis (especially in females) In elderly patients and in non-elderly patients with cardiopulmonary symptoms, an ECG and chest X-ray are also performed.

Delirium *(continued)*

Laboratory testing *(continued)*	An EEG may be helpful if the diagnosis of the syndrome of delirium itself is in doubt, particularly if there is a pre-delirium baseline EEG study available for comparison. EEGs are very sensitive to delirium if the test is conducted with proper alerting procedures and is interpreted by an experienced electroencephalographer. The EEG may also reveal the presence of non-convulsive status epilepticus, with persistent symptoms of disturbed attention and awareness. If the basic workup is unrevealing of a substantial cause of delirium, the following laboratory studies should be considered: • ESR or CRP • Serum ammonia level • HIV testing • Antinuclear antibody test • Vitamin B_{12} and folate levels • RPR • Urine toxicology • Blood alcohol level • Medication levels • Brain MRI or head CT • EEG • CSF analysis • Blood cultures • Urine porphyrins • Arterial blood gases

American Psychiatric Association: Diagnostic and Statistical Manual of Mental Disorders, 5th Edition, Text Revision. Washington, DC, American Psychiatric Association, 2022

Hawkins M, Sockalingam S, Bonato S, et al: A rapid review of the pathoetiology, presentation, and management of delirium in adults with COVID-19. J Psychosom Res 141:110350, 2020

Hshieh TT, Inouye SK, Oh ES: Delirium in the elderly. Clin Geriatr Med 36(2):183–199, 2020

Jacobson S, Jerrier H: EEG in delirium. Semin Clin Neuropsychiatry 5:86–92, 2000

Klimiec-Moskal E, Slowik A, Dziedzic T: Delirium and subsyndromal delirium are associated with the long-term risk of death after ischaemic stroke. Aging Clin Exp Res 34(6):1459–1462, 2022

Kotfis K, Williams Roberson S, Wilson J, et al: COVID-19: what do we need to know about ICU delirium during the SARS-CoV-2 pandemic? Anaesthesiol Intensive Ther 52(2):132–138, 2020

Marcantonio ER: Delirium in hospitalized older adults. N Engl J Med 377(15):1456–1466, 2017

Mattison MLP: Delirium. Ann Intern Med 173(7):ITC49–ITC64, 2020

Thom RP, Levy-Carrick NC, Bui M, Silbersweig D: Delirium. Am J Psychiatry 176(10):785–793, 2019

White L, Jackson T: Delirium and COVID-19: a narrative review of emerging evidence. Anaesthesia 77(Suppl 1):49–58, 2022

Dementia

Clinical findings	Dementia—DSM-5-TR major neurocognitive disorder—is a syndrome defined by a decline in cognition that is sufficient to interfere with independent daily functioning and is caused by a range of neurological, neuropsychiatric, and medical conditions. The primary dementias most likely to be encountered clinically include Alzheimer's disease (AD), vascular dementia (VaD), dementia with Lewy bodies (DLB), frontotemporal dementia (FTD), and Creutzfeldt-Jakob disease (CJD). Importantly, the differential diagnosis of dementia also involves myriad secondary syndromes in which potentially reversible cognitive dysfunction develops because of toxic exposure or vitamin deficiencies, for example, and these must be excluded in the workup. The syndromic diagnosis of "dementia" is insufficient for adequate patient care; efforts must be made to identify the underlying diseases or conditions.
	The history of the present illness obtained from the patient and a reliable informant arguably contains most of the information needed for diagnosis. An insidious onset of episodic memory problems with gradual progression suggests the possibility of AD. A subacute onset and stepwise progression of deficits suggests cerebrovascular disease. Early dream enactment behaviors, prominent visual hallucinations, and/or parkinsonism suggests Lewy body disease. Prominent disinhibition often mistaken for a primary psychiatric disorder suggests the possibility of behavioral variant frontotemporal dementia (bvFTD). A very rapidly progressive course characterizes CJD.
	Other critical elements of the history relate to contributing medical conditions such as hypertension, hyperlipidemia, diabetes, history of TBI, Parkinson's disease (PD), and stroke. Alcohol and drug use should be quantified. Use of medications affecting cognition such as hypnotic and anticholinergic drugs should be specifically queried. Any family history of dementia, particularly early onset dementia in a first-degree relative, should be noted. This could suggest the presence of a genetic form of dementia requiring a separate line of testing.
	The mental status examination is a rich source of information about the patient's present state, starting with their appearance and general behavior, which can be disheveled and disinhibited in patients with bvFTD. Impairments in speech, motor activity, affect, thinking, and perception all provide evidence in support of disease affecting different brain regions. Certain patients, including those with AD, may demonstrate a remarkable lack of insight, possibly suggesting frontal system involvement.
	The gold standard of cognitive testing involves a neuropsychological battery directed toward suspected causes of dementia as well as common alternatives. Because this level of testing is not universally available, a clinical screen can be used as an initial proxy measure. At present, the most commonly used cognitive screening tool is the Montreal Cognitive Assessment (MoCA; www.parkinsons.va.gov/resources/MOCA-Test-English.pdf), which takes about 10 minutes and yields a range of scores from 1 to 30, with a score <24 generally considered the cutoff for needed follow-up. It should be noted that if a screen such as the MoCA is used, seemingly trivial individual deficits such as in cube copying or naming may represent whole domains of impairment that would be found on more detailed testing.

Dementia *(continued)*

Clinical findings *(continued)*	The physical exam may reveal abnormalities such as focal neurological deficits, parkinsonism, evidence of cerebrovascular disease, or evidence of alcohol or drug use that may be contributing to the patient's cognitive problems.
Laboratory testing	The following tests should be performed for all patients presenting with cognitive issues: • CBC with differential • CMP (includes glucose, electrolytes, LFTs, and kidney function tests) • TSH • Vitamin B_{12} and folate levels • Structural brain imaging: MRI or CT to identify cortical and hippocampal atrophy, masses, strokes, white matter disease, NPH, and other lesions Depending on the patient's history and exam findings, the following tests may be considered: • Urine toxicology screen • HIV testing • FTA-ABS—not RPR or VDRL, both of which are often negative in patients with dementia due to neurosyphilis • Chest X-ray • EEG to identify non-convulsive status epilepticus, periodic complexes of CJD • CSF for oligoclonal bands, CSF culture for infection, results of high-volume CSF removal in NPH • CSF amyloid-β and tau levels in suspected AD • CSF for real-time quaking-induced conversion (RT-QuIC) analysis and MRI diffusion-weighted imaging in suspected CJD • PET scan in suspected AD • PET or SPECT scan in vascular dementia or FTD • PET or SPECT scan in suspected DLB or PD dementia • Iodine MIBG cardiac scintigraphy showing low uptake of MIBG in suspected DLB or PD dementia Other tests that may be useful in selected cases: • Parathyroid function • Adrenal function • Heavy metal screening • ESR or CRP • Angiogram • Genetic testing for young patients with first-degree relatives with early onset dementia (and others) Note that brain biopsy is indicated only rarely. Specialized tests for AD are discussed in the **Alzheimer's Disease** entry.

Dementia *(continued)*

American Psychiatric Association: Diagnostic and Statistical Manual of Mental Disorders, 5th Edition, Text Revision. Washington, DC, American Psychiatric Association, 2022

Arvanitakis Z, Shah RC, Bennett DA: Diagnosis and management of dementia: review. JAMA 322(16):1589–1599, 2019

Gale SA, Acar D, Daffner KR: Dementia. Am J Med 131(10):1161–1169, 2018

Gorelick PB, Scuteri A, Black SE, et al: Vascular contributions to cognitive impairment and dementia: a statement for healthcare professionals from the American Heart Association/American Stroke Association. Stroke 42(9):2672–2713, 2011

Mak E, Su L, Williams GB, O'Brien JT: Neuroimaging correlates of cognitive impairment and dementia in Parkinson's disease. Parkinsonism Relat Disord 21(8):862–870, 2015

McKeith IG, Boeve BF, Dickson DW, et al: Diagnosis and management of dementia with Lewy bodies: fourth consensus report of the DLB Consortium. Neurology 89(1):88–100, 2017

Ricci M, Cimini A, Chiaravalloti A, et al: Positron emission tomography (PET) and neuroimaging in the personalized approach to neurodegenerative causes of dementia. Int J Mol Sci 21(20):7481, 2020

Younes K, Miller BL: Frontotemporal dementia: neuropathology, genetics, neuroimaging, and treatments. Psychiatr Clin North Am 43(2):331–344, 2020

Yousaf T, Dervenoulas G, Valkimadi PE, Politis M: Neuroimaging in Lewy body dementia. J Neurol 266(1):1–26, 2019

Dementia with Lewy bodies (DLB)

Clinical findings	DLB—one of the most common of the neurodegenerative dementias—is caused by the aggregation of misfolded α-synuclein protein inside neurons of the central and peripheral nervous systems. The essential feature of DLB is dementia, defined as progressive cognitive decline that interferes with function. Deficits may be particularly prominent on tests of attention, executive function, and visuospatial ability. Memory impairment may not be prominent in early stages but is usually evident with progression.
	Core features of DLB include fluctuating cognition (attention and alertness), recurrent visual hallucinations that are well formed and detailed, REM sleep behavior disorder (RBD; which may precede cognitive decline) and spontaneous parkinsonism. Fluctuation of symptoms, recurrent visual hallucinations, and RBD typically occur early and may be persistent.
	Supportive clinical features include severe neuroleptic sensitivity, postural instability, repeated falls, syncope or other episodes of unresponsiveness, severe autonomic dysfunction (with constipation, orthostatic hypotension, and urinary incontinence), hypersomnia, hyposmia, hallucinations in other modalities, systematized delusions, apathy, anxiety, and depression.
	In distinguishing DLB from Parkinson's disease dementia (PDD), a "1-year rule" applies: If parkinsonism develops more than 1 year before cognitive changes, PDD is diagnosed. If parkinsonism develops concurrently with cognitive changes (or within 1 year), DLB is diagnosed.
	Prodromes to DLB have been identified in which signs and symptoms indicate that DLB will eventually develop. Although less well studied, three such prodromal DLB syndromes have been proposed: • Mild cognitive impairment with Lewy bodies (MCI-LB) • Delirium-onset prodrome • Psychiatric-onset prodrome
	Because the first symptoms may be seen ≥15 years before dementia ensues, these prodromes are very likely to come to the attention of psychiatrists and other behavioral health specialists.
	In MCI-LB, objective evidence of cognitive impairment is seen in one or more domains, most likely in attention-executive and/or visual processing. Impairment on tasks of attention, processing speed, and verbal fluency typically constitute the attention-executive deficits, and impairment on tasks of visual discrimination, assembly, and figure drawing typically constitute the visual perceptual and spatial deficits. If memory is affected, deficits in at least one other domain are seen. Functional status is preserved or minimally affected. Fluctuating cognition is seen, with varying levels of attention and alertness. Recurrent visual hallucinations may be observed, and RBD may be present. Features of spontaneous parkinsonism are seen, including rigidity, bradykinesia, and/or resting tremor.
	The delirium-onset prodrome of DLB should be suspected when delirium is recurrent or prolonged, in cases where no cause of delirium is identified, and in patients with progressive cognitive impairment after delirium resolves. Care should be taken to identify this subpopulation because antipsychotic and anticholinergic drugs can be harmful for these patients. Biomarkers noted below may be useful in this context.

Dementia with Lewy bodies (DLB) *(continued)*

Clinical findings *(continued)*	The psychiatric-onset prodrome of DLB most often takes the form of late-onset major depression or psychosis. Psychosis may be florid, with vivid visual hallucinations and hallucinations in other modalities and systematized delusions such as Capgras syndrome or phantom boarder syndrome. Other presentations reported include apathy and anxiety. Mild cognitive dysfunction can be present but is not predominant and may fluctuate over time. Complicating surveillance for symptoms of Lewy body pathology in this context is the fact that psychomotor retardation resembles the bradykinesia of parkinsonism. Moreover, parkinsonism can be induced by antipsychotic medications, and RBD can be induced by antidepressant medications. Biomarkers noted below may be useful in the differential diagnosis.
Laboratory testing	Biomarkers indicative of DLB include the following: • Reduced dopamine transporter uptake in basal ganglia on SPECT or PET imaging • Abnormally low uptake on ^{123}iodine-MIBG myocardial scintigraphy • PSG confirming REM sleep without atonia Biomarkers that support the diagnosis of DLB include the following: • Relative preservation of medial temporal lobe structures on CT or MRI • Generalized low uptake on SPECT or PET scan with reduced occipital activity • FDG-PET showing preserved metabolism of the posterior cingulate cortex (the "cingulate island sign") • Prominent posterior slow-wave activity on EEG with periodic fluctuations in the pre-alpha/theta range

American Psychiatric Association: Diagnostic and Statistical Manual of Mental Disorders, 5th Edition, Text Revision. Washington, DC, American Psychiatric Association, 2022

Fukatsu T, Kanemoto K: Phantom boarder symptom in elderly Japanese. Psychogeriatrics 22(1):108–112, 2022

Leys F, Wenning GK, Fanciulli A: The role of cardiovascular autonomic failure in the differential diagnosis of alpha-synucleinopathies. Neurol Sci 43(1):187–198, 2022

McKeith IG: Consensus guidelines for the clinical and pathologic diagnosis of dementia with Lewy bodies (DLB): report of the Consortium on DLB International Workshop. J Alzheimers Dis 9:417–423, 2006

McKeith IG, Boeve BF, Dickson DW, et al: Diagnosis and management of dementia with Lewy bodies: fourth consensus report of the DLB Consortium. Neurology 89(1):88–100, 2017

Taylor JP, McKeith IG, Burn DJ, et al: New evidence on the management of Lewy body dementia. Lancet Neurol 19(2):157–169, 2020

Depressive disorder due to another medical condition

Clinical findings	This diagnosis differs from that of primary depressive disorder in that it is based on a more limited set of criteria and is characterized by additional signs and symptoms attributable to the medical disorder. The depression itself involves only a prominent and persistent period of depressed mood or markedly diminished interest in usual activities. The presence of a medical condition that could be linked to the depression by some physiological mechanism must be established, and this requires comprehensive evaluation of the patient's medical history, family history, current substance abuse and medications, physical and mental status exams, and laboratory testing. A temporal relationship between the depressive disorder and the medical condition is helpful, as is the presence of atypical features of depression.
	Medical conditions known to be associated with depressive disorder include the following:
	• Endocrine diseases—Addison's disease, Cushing's syndrome, hyperparathyroidism, hypothyroidism
	• Vitamin deficiencies—Vitamin B_{12}, folate
	• Neurological diseases—stroke; TBI; epilepsy; multiple sclerosis; or Alzheimer's, Parkinson's, Huntington's, or Wilson's disease
	• Infections—CJD, HIV, hepatitis C, neurosyphilis, Lyme disease, West Nile virus
	• Malignancies—pancreatic cancer, paraneoplastic syndromes
Laboratory testing	Laboratory testing for all patients includes the following:
	• CMP
	• CBC with differential and platelets
	• Vitamin B_{12} and folate levels
	• TSH
	Further testing depends on the results of the clinical evaluation and the initial lab results. This may include any of the following (as well as other disease-specific tests):
	• Urinalysis
	• Urine toxicology screen
	• RPR
	• HIV testing
	• Blood alcohol level
	• Therapeutic medication levels (for TCAs or mood stabilizers)
	• Urine pregnancy testing, if indicated
	• ECG
	• Brain MRI or head CT

American Psychiatric Association: Diagnostic and Statistical Manual of Mental Disorders, 5th Edition, Text Revision. Washington, DC, American Psychiatric Association, 2022

Carroll VK, Rado JT: Is a medical illness causing your patient's depression? Endocrine, neurologic, infectious, or malignant processes could cause mood symptoms. Curr Psychiatry 8(8):43, 2009

Deng J, Zhou F, Hou W, et al: The prevalence of depression, anxiety, and sleep disturbances in COVID-19 patients: a meta-analysis. Ann NY Acad Sci 1486(1):90–111, 2021

Marsh L: Depression and Parkinson's disease: current knowledge. Curr Neurol Neurosci Rep 13(12):409, 2013

Robinson RG, Jorge RE. Post-stroke depression: a review. Am J Psychiatry 173(3):221–231, 2016

Seoud T, Syed A, Carleton N, et al: Depression before and after a diagnosis of pancreatic cancer: results from a national, population-based study. Pancreas 49(8):1117–1122, 2020

Diabetes insipidus (DI)

Clinical findings	DI is a disease characterized by the passage of large volumes of dilute urine, more than 3 L in 24 hours. The condition is classified into one of several forms:
	• *Central or neurogenic DI* results from a deficiency of antidiuretic hormone (ADH), which is produced in the hypothalamus and stored in the pituitary gland. It arises from injury to the hypothalamus or the pituitary gland. Causes include head injury, stroke, tumor, surgery, infection, inflammation, aneurysm, and diseases such as Langerhans cell histiocytosis.
	• *Nephrogenic DI* results from resistance of the kidneys to the actions of ADH. It arises when the distal renal tubules are unable to reabsorb filtered water. Causes include urinary tract blockage, chronic kidney disease, hypercalcemia, hypokalemia, and lithium treatment.
	• *Primary polydipsia* results from excessive water intake despite normal ADH secretion and action. This condition is identified in patients with major psychiatric disorders and in health enthusiasts. Excessive drinking can also arise from injury to the hypothalamus or pituitary gland resulting in a low thirst threshold (dipsogenic DI).
	• *Gestational DI* results from overexpression of an enzyme from the placenta that metabolizes ADH, causing a deficiency. It is usually mild and resolves with labor and delivery but can recur with a subsequent pregnancy.
	Signs and symptoms of DI include polyuria (>3 L/day), nocturia, severe thirst, colorless urine, dehydration, weakness, and myalgias. Fatigue, dizziness, confusion, nausea, and, rarely, loss of consciousness can occur with dehydration. Physical examination may be normal or may reveal evidence of dehydration, bladder enlargement, or hydronephrosis (with flank pain or tenderness, pain radiating to the genitals, and/or bladder enlargement).
Laboratory testing	DI is defined as the passage of large volumes (>3 L/24 hours) of dilute urine (<300 mOsm/kg). Laboratory testing includes the following elements:
	• 24-hour urine collection for urine volume determination
	• Urine specific gravity
	• Simultaneous measurements of plasma and urinary osmolality
	• Serum electrolytes and glucose
	• Plasma ADH level
	• Challenge tests, such as infusion of hypertonic saline stimulating copeptin (a proxy for ADH), that can distinguish central DI from primary polydipsia; water deprivation tests to ensure dehydration and maximal stimulation of ADH are less often used in current practice.
	• MRI of pituitary gland and/or hypothalamus and assay of pituitary hormones other than ADH
	• Genetic testing if there is evidence of familial DI

Goo YJ, Song SH, Kwon OI, et al: Venous thromboembolism and severe hypernatremia in a patient with lithium-induced nephrogenic diabetes insipidus and acute kidney injury. Ann Palliat Med 11(8):2756–2760, 2021

Refardt J, Winzeler B, Christ-Crain M: Copeptin and its role in the diagnosis of diabetes insipidus and the syndrome of inappropriate antidiuresis. Clin Endocrinol (Oxf) 91(1):22–32, 2019

Diabetes insipidus (DI) *(continued)*

Refardt J, Winzeler B, Christ-Crain M: Diabetes insipidus: an update. Endocrinol Metab Clin North Am 49(3):517–531, 2020

Schernthaner-Reiter MH, Stratakis CA, Luger A: Genetics of diabetes insipidus. Endocrinol Metab Clin North Am 46(2):305–334, 2017

Yuen KCJ, Sharf V, Smith E, et al: Sodium and water perturbations in patients who had an acute stroke: clinical relevance and management strategies for the neurologist. Stroke Vasc Neurol 7(3):258–266, 2022

Diabetes mellitus (DM)

Clinical findings	DM refers to several metabolic disorders characterized by persistent hyperglycemia arising from impaired insulin secretion, insulin resistance, or both. DM is classified as type 1 (absolute insulin deficiency), type 2 (insulin resistance/decreased insulin response with relative insulin deficiency), gestational, and other (which includes a variety of conditions such as pancreatitis and drug-induced diabetes). Historically, type 1 DM was thought to occur only in children and type 2 only in adults, but it is now recognized that either type can occur at any age; thus, terms such as *adult-onset diabetes* and *non-insulin-dependent diabetes* have fallen out of use. The term *latent autoimmune diabetes of adulthood* (LADA) is in current use and refers to an adult-onset form of type 1 DM.
	Obesity is the primary risk factor for type 2 DM. Patients with type 2 DM who are not overweight may show a redistribution of body fat to the abdominal area. Other risk factors include increasing age, sedentary lifestyle, hypertension, dyslipidemia, positive family history of type 2 DM, and ethnicity (higher risk for those of Black, American Indian, Hispanic/Latino, or Asian race/ethnicity). The presence of depression or sleep disturbance presents additional risk. A quick screening measure for risk factors is available from the CDC at www.cdc.gov/prediabetes/takethetest.
	Undiagnosed and untreated DM is a major public health problem. Whereas type 1 DM usually presents with recognizable signs of hyperglycemia (polyuria, polydipsia, polyphagia, ketoacidosis), type 2 DM can remain silent for years because hyperglycemia develops only gradually as insulin secretion becomes insufficient to overcome insulin resistance. When hyperglycemia has developed, however, patients with either form of DM can develop the same complications: neuropathy, retinopathy, vasculopathy, sexual dysfunction, kidney disease, and cognitive impairment from cerebral small vessel disease.
	Links between DM and psychiatric disease or psychological factors are many and complex. Mounting evidence suggests a shared pathogenesis of depression and type 2 DM involving overactivation of innate immunity with a cytokine-mediated inflammatory response, and possibly HPA axis dysregulation. The presence of DM doubles the risk of depression, and depression is associated with treatment nonadherence, poor glycemic control, and diabetic complications. Anxiety disorders are also associated with poor glycemic control. Eating disorders present a unique risk of complications of DM when insulin is withheld by patients as a means to lose weight. Minor and major neurocognitive disorders may result from a variety of DM-related brain insults, including vascular disease, oxidative stress, neuroinflammation, apoptosis, reduction of neurotrophic factors, and mitochondrial dysfunction, among others.
Laboratory testing	American Diabetes Association (ADA) guidelines suggest screening for DM in adults age ≥45 years and in individuals with multiple risk factors regardless of age. The same tests are used for screening and diagnosis.
	Testing for diabetes/prediabetes in asymptomatic adults should be considered for those who are overweight or obese (BMI ≥25 kg/m², or ≥23 kg/m² in those of Asian ethnicity) who have one or more of the following risk factors: <ul><li>First-degree relative with DM</li><li>High-risk race/ethnicity (Black, American Indian, Hispanic/Latino, or Asian)</li></ul>

Diabetes mellitus (DM) *(continued)*

Laboratory testing *(continued)*	• History of cardiovascular disease
	• Hypertension (≥140/90 or on treatment)
	• High-density lipoprotein cholesterol <35 mg/dL and/or triglyceride level >250 mg/dL
	• Female with polycystic ovary syndrome
	• Sedentary lifestyle
	• Other conditions associated with insulin resistance (e.g., acanthosis nigricans)
	For asymptomatic patients with a normal test result, testing should be repeated every 3 years. This interval can be shortened in those with obesity or other risks. Patients with prediabetes should be tested annually. Females with a history of gestational DM should have lifelong testing at least every 3 years. Patients with HIV should be tested before antiretroviral treatment, 1–3 months after starting treatment, and every 6–12 months thereafter.
	Test results used in the ADA diagnostic criteria for type 2 DM include any the following:
	• Fasting plasma glucose (FPG) ≥126 mg/dL
	• 2-hour plasma glucose level ≥200 mg/dL during a 75-g oral glucose tolerance test (OGTT)
	• Random plasma glucose level ≥200 mg/dL in a patient with symptoms of hyperglycemia or hyperglycemic crisis
	• HbA1c level ≥6.5%
	Regardless of the test used, diagnosis requires two abnormal results, either from same blood sample or a different sample. An FPG test requires fasting for 8 hours. The 2-hour OGTT is a standard test for gestational diabetes at 24–28 weeks of pregnancy.
	The HbA1c test is used to assess glycemic control, with the result reflecting average glucose values over preceding 3 months. The test is not as sensitive as FPG or OGTT in detecting DM. The HbA1c test should be performed at initial assessment and every 3 months thereafter until the glycemic target has been attained. At that point, testing should be done at least every 6 months in those with good control and every 3 months otherwise.
	The diagnosis of type 1 DM differs from that of type 2 in the early stages of type 1 disease (involving autoantibodies), but the two algorithms converge when abnormal glucose levels are seen. The persistence of two or more autoantibodies predicts the onset of clinical diabetes. FPG rather than HbA1c testing is used to diagnose acute onset of type 1 DM.
	Further testing for complications of DM includes the following:
	• Screening for diabetic kidney disease: urine albumin and GFR at least annually in patients with type 1 DM for ≥5 years or type 2 DM and hypertension
	• Eye exam (dilated retinal exam) every 1–2 years to evaluate retinopathy
	• Screening for hypogonadism with a morning serum testosterone measurement in males with symptoms such as reduced libido or erectile dysfunction

Diabetes mellitus (DM) *(continued)*

| Laboratory testing *(continued)* | • Attention to liver function, with further testing (e.g., with elastography) as indicated |
| | • Regular screening for psychiatric disorders such as depression and anxiety |

American Diabetes Association: Classification and diagnosis of diabetes: standards of medical care in diabetes—2021. Diabetes Care 44(Suppl 1):S15–S33, 2021

ARUP Consult: Diabetes mellitus, in ARUP Consult: The Physician's Guide to Laboratory Test Selection and Interpretation. Salt Lake City, UT, ARUP Laboratories, 2022. Available at: https://arupconsult.com/content/diabetes-mellitus. Accessed April 2022.

Garrett C, Doherty A: Diabetes and mental health. Clin Med (Lond) 14(6):669–672, 2014

Hamed SA: Brain injury with diabetes mellitus: evidence, mechanisms and treatment implications. Expert Rev Clin Pharmacol 10(4):409–428, 2017

Holingue C, Wennberg A, Berger S, et al: Disturbed sleep and diabetes: a potential nexus of dementia risk. Metabolism 84:85–93, 2018

Moulton CD, Pickup JC, Ismail K: The link between depression and diabetes: the search for shared mechanisms. Lancet Diabetes Endocrinol 3(6):461–471, 2015

Park M, Reynolds CF III: Depression among older adults with diabetes mellitus. Clin Geriatr Med 31(1):117–137, 2015

Petersmann A, Müller-Wieland D, Müller UA, et al: Definition, classification and diagnosis of diabetes mellitus. Exp Clin Endocrinol Diabetes 127(Suppl 1):S1–S7, 2019

Tang Q, Li S, Yang Z, et al: A narrative review of multimodal imaging of white matter lesions in type-2 diabetes mellitus. Ann Palliat Med 10(12):12867–12876, 2021

Down syndrome (DS)

Clinical findings	DS is a common genetic disorder caused by abnormal cell division resulting in an extra copy of chromosome 21 (trisomy 21). Mosaicism and partial trisomy 21 also occur. DS is associated with varying degrees of intellectual disability, characteristic physical findings, and a range of cardiovascular, neuropsychiatric, endocrine, autoimmune, and musculoskeletal disorders. The most important risk factor for DS is advanced maternal age. The life expectancy of affected individuals is ~60 years.
	Many of the physical features of DS are recognizable at birth, such as upslanted palpebral fissures, flat nasal bridge, nuchal folds, single palmar flexion crease, clinodactyly of the fifth finger, and muscular hypotonia. The phenotype also includes short stature and, in some cases, atlantoaxial instability.
	Medical conditions affecting individuals with DS more often than the general population include the following:
	• Congenital heart disease—particularly ventricular septal defect and atrioventricular septal defect
	• Pulmonary hypertension—attributable in part to congenital heart disease and upper airway obstruction
	• Obstructive sleep apnea
	• Endocrine disorders—obesity, hypogonadism (with or without infertility), accelerated bone loss with aging
	• Hematological/oncological disorders—myeloid leukemia, acute lymphoblastic leukemia, and transient abnormal myelopoiesis (in newborns)
	• Autoimmune disease—thyroid dysfunction, celiac disease, juvenile arthritis, type 1 diabetes mellitus, Addison's disease, hemolytic anemia, dermatomyositis, alopecia, vitiligo
	• Immune dysregulation—involving both innate and adaptive immunity; infection is common, particularly respiratory (increased risk for COVID-19 infection)
	• Hearing and vision problems
	• Neurological—dysphagia, seizures, Alzheimer's disease (AD) (early onset), moyamoya disease, cerebellar hypoplasia (causing hypotonia, motor incoordination)
	• Psychiatric—autism, anxiety disorders, depression, OCD, ADHD, eating disorders, catatonia, psychosis, Down syndrome disintegrative disorder (DSDD)
	Trisomy at chromosome 21 results in the overproduction and early brain deposition of amyloid-β protein. Patients with DS show histopathological features of AD starting around age 40 years. Many remain asymptomatic, however, with noticeable cognitive decline starting decades later. Dementia may be more likely to develop in patients with seizures.
	DSDD is a developmental regression characterized by a loss of previously acquired adaptive, cognitive, and social functions. Onset is subacute, with symptoms including mutism, catatonia, dementia, depression, and autistic features. The disorder may enter a chronic phase in which the individual does not return to baseline functioning.
	The cause of DSDD is not known; autoimmune mechanisms, neuroinflammation, psychiatric disease, and psychological stress have been implicated.

Down syndrome (DS) *(continued)*

Laboratory testing	Cell-free DNA screening has replaced other screening tests for prenatal diagnosis of DS. In this test, a sample of the mother's blood is drawn after 10 weeks of pregnancy, and fetal DNA is measured to determine whether DNA from chromosome 21 is overrepresented. Results normally take 1–2 weeks to return. A positive test can be followed up with more invasive procedures of chorionic villus sampling or amniocentesis, which provide definitive diagnosis.
	If DS is suspected in an undiagnosed child, fluorescence in situ hybridization (FISH) of chromosome 21 can be performed to diagnose trisomy. This can be followed up by a karyotype to determine the specific genetic cause (translocation or nondisjunction), which is needed for genetic counseling.
	The numerous medical conditions associated with DS require diagnostic workup based on clinical signs and symptoms, such that practitioners must not only maintain a high index of suspicion but also have a thorough understanding of comorbidities. For example, if symptoms of celiac disease are present, testing of levels of IgA antibodies to tissue transglutaminase 2 is recommended. EEG is recommended if there is any suspicion of seizure. Hearing and vision should be tested regularly, and TSH blood testing performed annually.

Antonarakis SE, Skotko BG, Rafii MS, et al: Down syndrome. Nat Rev Dis Primers 6(1):9, 2020

Arumugam A, Raja K, Venugopalan M, et al: Down syndrome: a narrative review with a focus on anatomical features. Clin Anat 29(5):568–577, 2016

Ballard C, Mobley W, Hardy J, et al: Dementia in Down's syndrome. Lancet Neurol 15(6):622–636, 2016

Bull MJ: Down syndrome. N Engl J Med 382(24):2344–2352, 2020

Dard R, Janel N, Vialard F: COVID-19 and Down's syndrome: are we heading for a disaster? Eur J Hum Genet 28(11):1477–1478, 2020

Rosso M, Fremion E, Santoro SL, et al: Down syndrome disintegrative disorder: a clinical regression syndrome of increasing importance. Pediatrics 145(6):e20192939, 2020

Santoro JD, Pagarkar D, Chu DT, et al: Neurologic complications of Down syndrome: a systematic review. J Neurol 268(12):4495–4509, 2021

Whooten R, Schmitt J, Schwartz A: Endocrine manifestations of Down syndrome. Curr Opin Endocrinol Diabetes Obes 25(1):61–66, 2018

DRESS syndrome

Clinical findings	The DRESS syndrome—drug reaction with eosinophilia and systemic symptoms—is a severe drug rash associated with fever, lymphadenopathy, internal organ involvement, and hematological abnormalities. Internal organs affected include the liver, kidneys, lungs, heart, and pancreas. Encephalitis and meningitis may be seen. The syndrome has a 10% or greater mortality rate, even with early recognition and treatment. DRESS has been underrecognized in psychiatry, even though many of the implicated drugs are psychotropics. The pathogenesis of DRESS is not known but may involve an interaction of genetics, viral reactivation (herpesvirus, Epstein-Barr virus, cytomegalovirus), and medication.
	Psychotropic drugs commonly implicated in DRESS include carbamazepine, lamotrigine, phenytoin, valproate, and phenobarbital. Less commonly, bupropion, mirtazapine, amitriptyline, oxcarbazepine, gabapentin, benzodiazepines, clomipramine, quetiapine, clozapine, olanzapine, aripiprazole, and certain antiretroviral drugs have been reported. Retrospective reviews have demonstrated that DRESS is grossly underreported with psychotropics.
	The DRESS rash typically appears 2–8 weeks after the drug is initiated, with earlier presentations seen with drug rechallenge. Classically described as morbilliform, the rash is now known to have various presentations, including urticarial, targetoid (erythema multiforme–like), pustular, and others. The rash spreads rapidly to involve more than 50% of the skin. In about one-third of cases, gross facial edema accompanies the rash. Lymphadenopathy typically involves more than one node, with enlargement often ≥1 cm.
	The internal organ most affected in DRESS is the liver, with presenting features of hepatitis, jaundice, or asymptomatic transaminitis. The pattern of injury can be hepatocellular, cholestatic, or mixed. Kidney involvement takes the form of acute interstitial nephritis with proteinuria, hematuria, and sterile pyuria. Pulmonary manifestations include pneumonia, effusions, nodules, and acute respiratory distress. Myocarditis associated with DRESS may develop in association with the rash or as a late manifestation, up to 4 months after first symptoms. Myocarditis may be asymptomatic, requiring a high index of suspicion in patients with other elements of the syndrome. Pancreatic involvement can be acute or late-appearing and may involve endocrine more than exocrine functions. Hematological signs include eosinophilia, leukocytosis, lymphocytopenia, and atypical lymphocytes.
	Several autoimmune conditions are late-appearing sequelae of DRESS. The most common is autoimmune thyroiditis, which may manifest at any time from several weeks to 3 years after initial symptoms. Other syndromes include SLE, diabetes mellitus type 1, and autoimmune hemolytic anemia.
	The scoring system developed by the European Registry of Severe Cutaneous Adverse Reactions (RegiSCAR) has been used for the formal diagnosis of DRESS. It should be noted that *formes frustes* of DRESS can be seen. The RegiSCAR with scoring is reproduced in the paper by Cho et al. (2017) in the reference list below.

DRESS syndrome *(continued)*

Clinical findings *(continued)*	Key criteria are as follows: • Acute skin rash • Fever ≥38.5°C • Lymphadenopathy (≥1 cm) in at least two sites • Internal organ involvement (one or more organs) • Hematological abnormalities (lymphocytes, eosinophils, platelets)
Laboratory testing	For laboratory confirmation of the diagnosis of DRESS, the following tests are recommended: • CBC with differential and platelets (including search for atypical lymphocytes) • CRP • LFTs • Creatinine, glucose, calcium • Urinalysis for protein, cells • Creatine kinase, troponin • ECG Other tests are recommended by different specialists, mainly to evaluate internal organ involvement. These include thyroid function tests, echocardiogram, lipase, PTH, serum ferritin, triglycerides, blood cultures, chest X-ray, head CT or brain MRI, and CSF analysis. In addition, PCR testing for herpesvirus 6, herpesvirus 7, cytomegalovirus, and Epstein-Barr virus may be suggested.

Bommersbach TJ, Lapid MI, Leung JG, et al: Management of psychotropic drug–induced DRESS syndrome: a systematic review. Mayo Clin Proc 91(6):787–801, 2016

Cardones AR: Drug reaction with eosinophilia and systemic symptoms (DRESS) syndrome. Clin Dermatol 38(6):702–711, 2020

Cho YT, Yang CW, Chu CY: Drug reaction with eosinophilia and systemic symptoms (DRESS): an interplay among drugs, viruses, and immune system. Int J Mol Sci 18(6):1243, 2017

de Filippis R, Soldevila-Matías P, De Fazio P, et al: Clozapine-related drug reaction with eosinophilia and systemic symptoms (DRESS) syndrome: a systematic review. Expert Rev Clin Pharmacol 13(8):875–883, 2020

de Filippis R, Soldevila-Matías P, Guinart D, et al: Unravelling cases of clozapine-related drug reaction with eosinophilia and systemic symptoms (DRESS) in patients reported otherwise: a systematic review. J Psychopharmacol 35(9):1062–1073, 2021

Isaacs M, Cardones AR, Rahnama-Moghadam S: DRESS syndrome: clinical myths and pearls. Cutis 102(5):322–326, 2018

Jevtic D, Dumic I, Nordin T, et al: Less known gastrointestinal manifestations of drug reaction with eosinophilia and systemic symptoms (DRESS) syndrome: a systematic review of the literature. J Clin Med 10(18):4287, 2021

Taleb S, Zgueb Y, Ouali U, et al: Drug reaction with eosinophilia and systemic symptoms syndrome related to aripiprazole therapy. J Clin Psychopharmacol 39(6):691–693, 2019

Drug abuse

Clinical findings	Testing rates for drugs of abuse declined precipitously during the COVID-19 pandemic, and although some testing programs are now back on track, available evidence suggests that positivity rates for heroin, non-prescribed fentanyl, and combinations of these drugs with stimulants and sedative-hypnotics have all increased significantly. Not surprisingly, the extreme stressors of the pandemic have been linked to the rise in abuse and to disruption of treatment for those with preexisting substance-related diagnoses.
	Cannabis use is also on the rise worldwide, and in the United States this trend is fueled by state-level legalization. Neither harms predicted by opponents of legalization nor benefits predicted by advocates have materialized in any substantial way, except that tax revenues have exceeded expectations.
	This section provides a list of clinical findings linked to classes of commonly abused drugs. More information on laboratory testing can be found in the **Urine Drug Screen** entry in the *Laboratory Tests* chapter.
	Amphetamines
	With mild to moderate intoxication, symptoms include talkativeness, grandiosity, vigilance, suspiciousness, mydriasis, elevated blood pressure (both systolic and diastolic), tachycardia or reflex bradycardia, and hyperreflexia. With severe intoxication, symptoms include agitation, bizarre behavior, auditory and tactile hallucinations, delusions, bruxism, choreoathetosis, dystonia, fever, diaphoresis, nausea, vomiting, diarrhea, abdominal cramping, delirium, and assaultive behavior.
	Among high-dose users, psychosis may develop that takes days to weeks to resolve despite abstinence, and even low-dose use can cause recurrence of psychotic symptoms because of sensitization. On the other hand, tolerance to euphoric effects is common, causing dosage escalation in chronic users.
	Withdrawal symptoms include dysphoria, fatigue, irritability, agitation, insomnia or hypersomnia, and suicidal ideation. Medical complications of amphetamine abuse include seizures, hypertensive encephalopathy, cardiac dysrhythmias, MI, cardiomyopathy, hemorrhagic and ischemic stroke, and rhabdomyolysis. Methamphetamine abusers may develop a subcortical dementia that persists even with long abstinence.
	Cannabis (marijuana and derivatives)
	With intoxication, the following signs and symptoms may be observed: silly affect, depersonalization, derealization, sensory distortions, memory impairment, carbohydrate craving, injected sclerae, mild ataxia, tachycardia, elevated supine blood pressure, and orthostatic hypotension. Panic symptoms commonly occur. Psychosis is much less common; when present, symptoms include persecutory delusions and auditory and visual hallucinations. Psychotic symptoms may take several days to resolve with abstinence.
	Cocaine
	With usual doses, signs and symptoms include hyperactivity, talkativeness, vigilance, grandiosity, anorexia, insomnia, increased libido, tachycardia, mydriasis, and hypertension.

Drug abuse *(continued)*

| Clinical findings *(continued)* | With higher doses (usually from smoking or IV administration), signs and symptoms include agitation, hallucinations (visual and tactile), impotence, nausea, vomiting, choreoathetosis, and delirium with high risk of aggressive and assaultive behaviors. With abstinence, symptoms of fatigue, depression, irritability, and anxiety are seen. With prolonged use, psychosis can occur during intoxication, with persecutory delusions and auditory hallucinations. Comorbid alcohol or opioid abuse is common. Medical complications are the same as with amphetamines, except for the additional complication of necrosis of the nasal septum among users who ingest cocaine intranasally.

Hallucinogens

With intoxication, psychosis with delusions, visual illusions, and hallucinations occurs in the context of a clear sensorium. The patient reports synesthetic experiences, depersonalization, and derealization. With 3,4-methylenedioxymethamphetamine (MDMA, Ecstasy), the patient exhibits signs of emotionality and increased empathic experience. With any hallucinogen, anxiety, panic, and dysphoric delusions can occur. Signs include mild elevation of temperature, tachycardia, hypertension, mydriasis, fine tremor, incoordination, and hyperreflexia. With MDMA, bruxism is also seen.

Inhalants

Inhalant abuse usually begins in childhood or adolescence, more often in males. Products inhaled include glue, paint thinner, gasoline, cleaning products (some containing methanol), aerosol propellants (e.g., contained in canned whipped cream), fingernail polish or polish remover, and typewriter correction fluid. A rag saturated with the product is held over the mouth and nose or placed in a bag for inhalation. Common signs of inhalant abuse include scleral injection, rhinorrhea, chemical odor on the breath, paint or stains on clothing, and sores around the mouth. Signs of intoxication include drunken appearance, drowsiness, dizziness, ataxia, dysarthria, diplopia, nystagmus, confusion, visual hallucinations, and delusions. With continued use, agitation, irritability, and impulsivity may be seen. In severe intoxication, coma can occur. Medical complications such as ventricular arrhythmias, bronchospasm, and seizures can occur. With long-term use, dementia may develop with amnesia, frontal lobe dysfunction, and cerebellar signs. Atrophy and white matter changes consistent with demyelination may be seen on brain MRI.

Opioids

With intoxication, signs and symptoms include drowsiness, inattention, elation, dysarthria, miosis, absent bowel sounds, constipation, urinary retention, and pruritus. With overdose, most patients are lethargic or comatose. Miosis may be noted, giving way to mydriasis if respiratory depression worsens and cerebral anoxia develops. Seizures may occur, and death by respiratory arrest is a common outcome. Individuals who survive an episode of anoxia may have postanoxic leukoencephalopathy with residual cognitive impairment. With regular use, tolerance develops to all symptoms of intoxication except miosis and constipation. |
|---|---|

Drug abuse *(continued)*

Clinical findings *(continued)*	Withdrawal symptoms include yawning, lacrimation, diaphoresis, rhinorrhea, dysphoria, irritability, insomnia, nausea, vomiting, diarrhea, abdominal cramping, piloerection ("gooseflesh"), intense muscle and bone pain, myoclonus, mydriasis, tachycardia, and hypertension. Medical complications are numerous with long-standing abuse.
	Sedative-hypnotics
	Symptoms of mild to moderate intoxication include euphoria, emotional lability, impaired judgment, impulsivity, slowed reaction time, drowsiness, lethargy, dysarthria, nystagmus, incoordination, ataxia, and blackouts. With more severe intoxication, particularly with alcohol co-ingestion, stupor, coma, respiratory depression, and death may occur.
	Withdrawal symptoms include anxiety, irritability, tachycardia, hypertension, tremor, diaphoresis, subjective weakness, nausea and vomiting, insomnia, and seizures. With prolonged high-dose use, withdrawal delirium may be seen, with fever, visual and tactile hallucinations, delusions, catatonia, and severe agitation. Other complications of sedative abuse include falls with fracture and motor vehicle accidents.
Laboratory testing	See **Urine Drug Screen** in the *Laboratory Tests* chapter for detailed information about testing.
	Screening for drug use first involves an immunoassay, which is inexpensive and available at the point of care but provides only qualitative information and is subject to false-positive and false-negative results. A positive result is considered provisional until confirmed in the laboratory by methods such as gas or liquid chromatography–tandem mass spectrometry.
	The most common means of tampering with urine drug specimens in the workplace and forensic settings is dilution of the sample. Validity checks performed in the laboratory—including measurement of urine creatinine and specific gravity—can determine whether dilution has occurred. Urine pH and other assays can be used to determine whether the specimen has been adulterated. False-positives on urine drug testing in a commercial laboratory do not result from eating poppy seeds (for opiates) or passive smoke inhalation (for cannabis).
	When opioids are prescribed long-term for pain syndromes, misuse can be flagged by aberrant behaviors such as lost prescriptions, repeated requests for early refills, or unauthorized dose escalations. Although prescription drug monitoring programs help considerably with misuse issues, frequent drug testing may be needed based on risk level. Testing is recommended every 1–3 months for patients at high risk because of a known substance abuse problem, mental health condition, aberrant behaviors, or use of high opioid dosage (>120 morphine mg equivalent). For patients without such risk factors, testing may be scheduled every 6–12 months.

American Psychiatric Association: Diagnostic and Statistical Manual of Mental Disorders, 5th Edition, Text Revision. Washington, DC, American Psychiatric Association, 2022

Dadiomov D: Laboratory testing for substance use disorders, in Absolute Addiction Psychiatry Review. Edited by Marienfeld C. Cham, Switzerland, Springer, 2020

Lin SY, Lee HH, Lee JF, Chen BH: Urine specimen validity test for drug abuse testing in workplace and court settings. J Food Drug Anal 26(1):380–384, 2018

Moeller KE, Kissack JC, Atayee RS, Lee KC: Clinical interpretation of urine drug tests: what clinicians need to know about urine drug screens. Mayo Clin Proc 92(5):774–796, 2017

Drug abuse *(continued)*

Niles JK, Gudin J, Radcliff J, Kaufman HW: The opioid epidemic within the COVID-19 pandemic: drug testing in 2020. Popul Health Manag 24(S1):S43–S51, 2021

Sazegar P: Cannabis essentials: tools for clinical practice. Am Fam Physician 104(6):598–608, 2021

Vogel EA, Chieng A, Robinson A, et al: Associations between substance use problems and stress during COVID-19. J Stud Alcohol Drugs 82(6):776–781, 2021

Drug-induced liver injury (DILI)

Clinical findings	Prescribed and over-the-counter drugs, herbal drugs, and dietary supplements are all known to have adverse effects on the liver, with asymptomatic elevation of liver enzymes being the most common manifestation and liver failure resulting in either transplant or death being the most serious. DILI is the most frequent cause of acute liver failure in the United States and other developed countries.
	Liver effects can be intrinsic to the drug, as with acetaminophen; these effects are dose-related and predictable and usually occur early, within 1–5 days. Idiosyncratic reactions, on the other hand, occur unpredictably with a wide range of drugs at therapeutic as well as toxic drug levels. Usual onset of idiosyncratic reactions is in 5–90 days (sooner with prior drug exposure). DILI comprises both intrinsic and idiosyncratic forms. The patterns of liver involvement in DILI can be hepatocellular, cholestatic, or mixed.
	The class of drugs most often implicated in DILI is the antibiotics, although herbal drugs and dietary supplements are increasingly recognized as causative. Of psychotropic drugs, all classes of antidepressants, many antipsychotics, several mood stabilizers/anticonvulsants, and other drugs are implicated. Among the antidepressants, fatal hepatotoxicity has been reported with nefazodone, trazodone, duloxetine, bupropion, and sertraline. SSRI antidepressants have the least potential toxicity. Among the antipsychotics, clozapine and olanzapine are associated with the most severe hepatotoxicity. The National Library of Medicine maintains an online database known as LiverTox (available at www.ncbi.nlm.nih.gov/books/NBK547852) that provides information on liver injury with reference to specific drugs.
	Known risk factors for DILI include older age, female sex, and race, with Asians at greater risk than Blacks, who are at greater risk than Whites. It is still controversial as to whether preexisting liver disease is a risk factor, but regular alcohol use and chronic hepatitis are noted as factors in some studies. In the United States, DILI presents with jaundice in 70% of cases. Most patients recover with drug discontinuation, but 17% develop chronic DILI and 10% require transplant and/or die from the disease.
	DILI should be suspected in any patient with a new elevation of liver enzymes. All drugs consumed in the prior 3 months should be reviewed, including herbals, over-the-counter drugs, and time-limited drugs that have run their course. The temporal association of symptoms with the use of the suspected drug(s) should be confirmed. Additional information can be inferred from the improvement seen with drug discontinuation. A positive response to corticosteroids and recurrence when steroids are withdrawn help to diagnose autoimmune hepatitis rather than DILI. Liver enzymes usually fall within days to weeks, with <10% of patients developing chronic disease.
Laboratory testing	• The most useful tests in the diagnosis and monitoring of DILI are ALT, AST, ALP, and total bilirubin.
	• At the initial visit, classify liver injury by calculating the R value (ALT divided by ALP). If the R value is ≥5, the pattern is hepatocellular. If the R value is ≤2, the pattern is cholestatic. If the R value is <5 and >2, the pattern is mixed.

Drug-induced liver injury (DILI) *(continued)*

Laboratory testing *(continued)*	<ul><li>A hepatocellular pattern can also be identified by an isolated elevation of ALT ≥5 times the upper limit of normal (ULN).</li><li>A cholestatic pattern can also be identified by an isolated elevation of ALP ≥2 times the ULN.</li><li>If AST or ALT is >3 times the ULN, ALP is normal on initial testing, and patient is jaundiced, the mortality rate is 10%.</li><li>In hepatocellular DILI, a serum bilirubin ≥3 times the ULN in the absence of biliary obstruction or Gilbert's syndrome carries a 5%–50% mortality rate.</li><li>Further testing for patients with the hepatocellular pattern includes hepatitis C virus RNA and IgM anti–hepatitis E virus in addition to hepatitis A virus and hepatitis B virus and autoimmune serology.</li><li>Further testing for patients with the cholestatic or mixed pattern includes ultrasound and cholangiography.</li><li>Tests used to distinguish DILI from autoimmune hepatitis include antibodies (e.g., antinuclear antibody testing) for autoimmune hepatitis and HLA genotyping for DILI.</li><li>Although liver imaging in DILI typically is normal, abdominal ultrasound is recommended to exclude biliary obstruction and any focal liver abnormalities.</li><li>Elastography may be used to exclude other causes of liver disease such as fatty liver disease.</li><li>Liver biopsy may be needed in exceptional cases.</li></ul>

Chalasani NP, Maddur H, Russo MW, et al: ACG clinical guideline: diagnosis and management of idiosyncratic drug-induced liver injury. Am J Gastroenterol 116(5):878–898, 2021

Dias CL, Fonseca L, Gadelha A, Noto C: Clozapine-induced hepatotoxicity: a life threatening situation. Schizophr Res 235:3–4, 2021

Druschky K, Toto S, Bleich S, et al: Severe drug-induced liver injury in patients under treatment with antipsychotic drugs: data from the AMSP study. World J Biol Psychiatry 22(5):373–386, 2021

European Association for the Study of the Liver: EASL clinical practice guidelines: drug-induced liver injury. J Hepatol 70(6):1222–1261, 2019

Katarey D, Verma S: Drug-induced liver injury. Clin Med (Lond) 16(Suppl 6):s104–s109, 2016

Kumachev A, Wu PE: Drug-induced liver injury. CMAJ 193(9):E310, 2021

Lee BT, Odin JA, Grewal P: An approach to drug-induced liver injury from the geriatric perspective. Curr Gastroenterol Rep 23(4):6, 2021

McGill MR, Jaeschke H: Biomarkers of drug-induced liver injury. Adv Pharmacol 85:221–239, 2019

National Library of Medicine: National Center for Biotechnology Information: LiverTox. Available at: https://www.ncbi.nlm.nih.gov/books/NBK547852. Accessed April 2022.

Nikogosyan G, Orias D, Goebert D, et al: Acute aripiprazole-associated liver injury. J Clin Psychopharmacol 41(3):344–346, 2021

Park SH, Ishino R: Liver injury associated with antidepressants. Curr Drug Saf 8(3):207–223, 2013

Voican CS, Corruble E, Naveau S, Perlemuter G: Antidepressant-induced liver injury: a review for clinicians. Am J Psychiatry 171(4):404–415, 2014

Dysphagia

Clinical findings	Swallowing is a complex motor function involving nuclei of the brainstem, cranial nerves, striated muscles of the tongue, and smooth muscles of the pharynx and esophagus. The three phases of swallowing—oral, pharyngeal, and esophageal—must be coordinated for efficient swallowing to occur. The workup of dysphagia is performed to distinguish oropharyngeal from esophageal origins.
	Oropharyngeal dysphagia is characterized by difficulty initiating swallowing, with coughing and choking and risk of aspiration. This type of dysphagia is most often associated with neurogenic causes including stroke, dementia, and Parkinson's disease. Esophageal dysphagia is characterized by the subjective report that food feels "stuck" in the chest, pain with swallowing (odynophagia), regurgitation of food, wheezing, hoarseness, drooling, coughing, and choking. This type of dysphagia is most often associated with gastroesophageal reflux disease and functional esophageal disorders. Chronic opioid use can also cause this type of dysphagia. Dysphagia for solid food indicates mechanical obstruction at the level of the esophagus or the base of the tongue. Dysphagia for liquids indicates neurogenic dysphagia, but this type can progress to include dysphagia for solid food.
	Bedside evaluation for dysphagia includes a cranial nerve exam and auscultation of the lungs. An informal first-pass water test can be performed in which 50 mL of water is swallowed in 5-mL aliquots. With this test, oropharyngeal symptoms may become immediately apparent. An evaluation by a speech-language pathologist could then provide sufficient information to determine which of several instrumented tests might be indicated.
Laboratory testing	Commonly used instrumented tests for dysphagia include the modified barium swallow (MBS) and fiberoptic endoscopic evaluation of swallowing (FEES). High-resolution manometry is used to evaluate the function of pharyngeal muscles and the upper esophageal sphincter in patients with suspected oropharyngeal dysphagia. Upper GI endoscopy is the first test used for patients with suspected esophageal dysphagia. Manometry can also be used to evaluate the competence of the lower esophageal sphincter in these patients.

Babaei A, Szabo A, Shad S, Massey BT: Chronic daily opioid exposure is associated with dysphagia, esophageal outflow obstruction, and disordered peristalsis. Neurogastroenterol Motil 31(7):e13601, 2019

Jones CA, Colletti CM, Ding MC: Post-stroke dysphagia: recent insights and unanswered questions. Curr Neurol Neurosci Rep 20(12):61, 2020

Rommel N, Hamdy S: Oropharyngeal dysphagia: manifestations and diagnosis. Nat Rev Gastroenterol Hepatol 13(1):49–59, 2016

Suttrup I, Warnecke T: Dysphagia in Parkinson's disease. Dysphagia 31(1):24–32, 2016

Wilkinson JM, Codipilly DC, Wilfahrt RP: Dysphagia: evaluation and collaborative management. Am Fam Physician 103(2):97–106, 2021

Encephalitis, viral

Clinical findings	Encephalitis refers to brain inflammation caused by infection or autoimmunity with consequent neurological dysfunction. The clinical diagnosis requires the presence of altered mental status (decreased level of consciousness, lethargy, or personality change) for ≥24 hours without an identified alternative cause, in conjunction with two or more of the following criteria:
	• Fever ≥100.4°F within the 72 hours before or after presentation
	• Seizures (generalized or partial) not explained by a preexisting seizure disorder
	• New focal neurological signs (e.g., aphasia, ataxia, cranial nerve palsies)
	• CSF WBC count ≥5/mm^3
	• Neuroimaging evidence of an abnormality of brain parenchyma (new or acute)
	• EEG abnormalities consistent with encephalitis and not attributable to another cause
	Meningitis commonly accompanies encephalitis, with additional symptoms including nuchal rigidity, vomiting, and photophobia. Psychotic symptoms (e.g., hallucinations and agitation) can be seen with the mental status alterations of encephalitis, which is consistent with a delirium syndrome. Dysregulation of the HPA axis can lead to diabetes insipidus, SIAD, and other problems.
	In half of encephalitis cases, no cause is identified. Of the identified causes, viruses are the most commonly implicated. In the United States, most cases of viral encephalitis are caused by herpes simplex virus (HSV) type 1 or 2, varicella zoster virus, enteroviruses, or arboviruses transmitted from infected animals to humans by tick or mosquito bites. Rabies is a very rare cause of encephalitis in humans.
	Because HSV is the most common cause of sporadic fatal encephalitis in the Western world, the first step in the differential diagnosis is to distinguish HSV from other viral causes. This is done by laboratory testing, as discussed below. Clinical features favoring HSV include older age, acute presentation, fever, and GI symptoms. HSV encephalitis occurs across the age spectrum and lacks a seasonal or geographical pattern.
	Enterovirus-related encephalitis occurs sporadically or in outbreaks that typically occur during the summer months. Presenting symptoms include diarrhea, vomiting, and viral exanthems such as herpangina and hand-foot-and-mouth disease.
	Arthropod-borne viruses—arboviruses—causing encephalitis in humans in North America include the mosquito-borne eastern equine, western equine, Venezuelan equine, Chikungunya, Jamestown, California, St. Louis, La Crosse, and West Nile viruses, as well as the tick-borne Powassan. Arbovirus encephalitis occurs seasonally, with the incidence dependent on geographical region. Zika virus was once a concern for pregnant females because of associated birth defects such as microcephaly in offspring, but Zika has not been transmitted by mosquitoes in the continental United States since 2018.

Encephalitis, viral *(continued)*

Laboratory testing	In 2013, the International Encephalitis Consortium published guidelines for the laboratory workup of encephalitis in adults. Recommendations for routine studies are as follows: 1. CSF: • Collect ≥20 mL if possible and freeze ≥5–10 mL if possible • Check opening pressure, WBC count with differential, RBC count, protein, and glucose • Gram stain and bacterial culture • HSV 1/2 PCR (consider HSV CSF IgG and IgM also, if available) • Varicella zoster virus (VZV) PCR (consider VZV IgG and IgM also if available) • Enterovirus PCR • Cryptococcal antigen and/or India ink staining • Oligoclonal bands and IgG index • VDRL for syphilis 2. Serum: • Blood cultures • HIV serology (consider RNA) • Treponemal testing (RPR, specific treponemal test) • Hold acute serum and collect convalescent serum 10–14 days later for paired antibody testing 3. Imaging: • Brain imaging (MRI preferred to CT) • Chest imaging (X-ray and/or CT) 4. Neurophysiology: • EEG Other tissues/fluids (e.g., stool culture, biopsy of skin lesions) are tested if there is extra-CNS involvement. Conditional studies are recommended based on host factors, geographical factors, season and exposure, and the presence of specific signs and symptoms. See Venkatesan et al. (2013) reference cited below for complete guidelines.

Kennedy PGE, Quan PL, Lipkin WI: Viral encephalitis of unknown cause: current perspective and recent advances. Viruses 9(6):138, 2017

Tyler KL: Acute viral encephalitis. N Engl J Med 379(6):557–566, 2018

Venkatesan A, Tunkel AR, Bloch KC, et al: Case definitions, diagnostic algorithms, and priorities in encephalitis: consensus statement of the International Encephalitis Consortium. Clin Infect Dis 57(8):1114–1128, 2013

Wright WF, Pinto CN, Palisoc K, Baghli S: Viral (aseptic) meningitis: a review. J Neurol Sci 398:176–183, 2019

Ethylene glycol poisoning

Clinical findings	Ethylene glycol is an odorless, sweet-tasting substance that is found in certain detergents, paints, de-icing products, brake fluid, and anti-freeze. It can be accidentally ingested by children, intentionally taken in overdose, or abused as a substance in place of ethanol. The lethal dose varies according to the dilution of ethylene glycol ingested, whether alcohol is also ingested, whether vomiting occurs, and the adequacy of renal excretion. Ingestion of as little as 4 fl oz of ethylene glycol has been found to be fatal for an average-sized adult. Even so, if the patient presents to the emergency room without delay and is rapidly diagnosed and treated, a good outcome is possible even with a large ingestion.
	Three stages of ethylene glycol toxicity are recognized:
	Stage 1: Predominately CNS manifestations (30 minutes–12 hours after ingestion)
	In this stage, the patient may report epigastric pain and nausea, and soon appears to be inebriated. Symptoms such as lethargy, weakness, incoordination, slurred speech, dizziness, headache, euphoria, or unusual behavior may be observed. These effects are caused by unmetabolized ethylene glycol in the circulation. Over time, CNS symptoms can worsen to include seizures (status epilepticus), myoclonus, stupor, coma, cranial nerve deficits, quadriplegia, and brain death.
	Stage 2: Cardiopulmonary manifestations (12–24 hours after ingestion)
	As ethylene glycol is metabolized to its toxic metabolites, cardiopulmonary failure can develop. Rapid deep breathing is often seen, a compensation for the developing metabolic acidosis. CNS depression may be extreme, such that airway protection by intubation is required. Pulmonary edema and respiratory failure may occur. Heart rate and blood pressure abnormalities as well as congestive heart failure can develop. These effects are caused by direct effects of toxic metabolites or by deposition of oxalate crystals in the cardiovascular and pulmonary systems. This is the stage at which death occurs in fatal cases.
	Stage 3: Renal manifestations (24–72 hours after ingestion)
	Patients who survive the first two stages often develop acute renal failure, which can be oliguric, anuric, or non-oliguric. Microscopic or gross hematuria can be seen, and hemodialysis may be indicated. These effects are caused by obstructive nephropathy or acute tubular necrosis (ATN) due to calcium oxalate, ATN due to other causes, direct toxicity of ethylene glycol metabolites, focal hemorrhagic cortical necrosis, and interstitial nephritis.
	A fourth stage of delayed-onset neuropathy develops in some patients, with cranial nerve deficits that are most marked in the facial and auditory nerves, gait problems, dysmetria, ankle clonus, extensor plantar reflexes, and an ascending motor/sensory neuropathy.
Laboratory testing	An ethylene glycol level >20 mg/dL confirms toxicity, but the turn-around time for test is usually 1–4 days.
	Classic laboratory abnormalities in ethylene glycol poisoning include metabolic acidosis, increased anion gap, and increased osmolar gap, but specific findings depend on time of blood draw.

Ethylene glycol poisoning *(continued)*

Laboratory testing *(continued)*	Ethylene glycol itself has low molecular weight and little intrinsic toxicity such that large molar concentrations can develop in the circulation in the hours immediately after ingestion. Initially, plasma osmolality increases in proportion to its concentration. At this stage, an increased osmolar gap with a normal anion gap and the absence of metabolic acidosis would be found. Subsequently, the osmolar gap returns to normal as metabolic acidosis progresses and the anion gap increases, indicating the presence of toxic metabolites.
	Other laboratory findings that may assist in the diagnosis of toxicity include falsely elevated lactate levels and calcium oxalate monohydrate crystals in urine. In addition, hypocalcemia and thrombocytopenia can be seen. If antifreeze ingestion is suspected, urine could be subjected to ultraviolet illumination to see if it fluoresces; this is due to the presence of sodium fluorescein being added to antifreeze formulations, presumably to help identify automotive fluid leaks.
	Brain imaging abnormalities in ethylene glycol poisoning involve the basal ganglia, thalamus, brainstem, and white matter. In stage 1, diffuse cerebral edema is seen, and subsequently on CT scan hypodensities are noted in the basal ganglia, thalamus, and brainstem. MRI is more sensitive to these changes, showing hyperintensities on T2-weighted images in these same areas as well as the amygdala and hippocampus. Restricted diffusion in deep white matter is consistent with cytotoxic edema.

ARUP Laboratories: Ethylene glycol, in Laboratory Test Directory. Salt Lake City, UT, ARUP Laboratories, 2021. Available at: https://www.aruplab.com/Tests/Pub/0090110. Accessed June 2021.

Esumi R, Suzuki K, Ishikura K, Imai H: Challenges in diagnosing comatose patients with ethylene glycol poisoning. Am J Med 134(2):e127–e128, 2021

Malhotra A, Mongelluzzo G, Wu X, et al: Ethylene glycol toxicity: MRI brain findings. Clin Neuroradiol 27(1):109–113, 2017

Poirier-Blanchette L, Simard C, Schwartz BC: Spurious point-of-care lactate elevation in ethylene glycol intoxication: rediscovering a clinical pearl. BMJ Case Rep 14(2):e239936, 2021

Sheta HM, Al-Najami I, Christensen HD, Madsen JS: Rapid diagnosis of ethylene glycol poisoning by urine microscopy. Am J Case Rep 19:689–693, 2018

Fatty liver disease

Clinical findings	Two types of fatty liver disease are recognized: alcoholic fatty liver disease and non-alcoholic fatty liver disease (NAFLD; also known as metabolic-associated fatty liver disease). Alcoholic fatty liver disease develops in heavy alcohol users because the metabolism of alcohol generates intermediates such as acetaldehyde that are injurious to liver cells. Without intervention, alcoholic fatty liver disease is likely to progress to hepatitis and cirrhosis.
	NAFLD refers to the accumulation of fat in liver cells among patients with risk factors for the metabolic syndrome and insulin resistance, including obesity, type 2 diabetes, hypertension, and hyperlipidemia. This type of fatty liver disease can also progress to steatohepatitis (non-alcoholic steatohepatitis, or NASH), with inflammation and liver cell injury leading to fibrosis, cirrhosis, and cancer. NAFLD has become a major public health problem in the United States, with almost 25% of adults affected.
	Most cases of fatty liver disease are clinically silent until later stages. Early symptoms are nonspecific and include only fatigue and right upper quadrant discomfort. Alcoholic fatty liver disease might be suspected based on history or physical exam findings such as labile hypertension. NAFLD might be suspected because features of the metabolic syndrome are present. Detection of fatty liver often involves the finding of elevated liver enzymes on routine blood testing, and diagnosis of fatty liver requires further laboratory studies as discussed below.
Laboratory testing	Tests used to diagnose fatty liver disease include LFTs, abdominal imaging, and elastography. In NAFLD, mild elevation in AST and ALT is seen in conjunction with GGT up to 3 times the upper limit of normal. In alcoholic liver disease, AST elevation is greater than ALT elevation in a ratio of more than 2:1. Abdominal imaging—ultrasound, CT, and MRI—yields information about liver anatomy, including fatty content and nodularity.
	Elastography is a noninvasive testing method that measures liver stiffness through the abdominal wall using ultrasound (vibration-controlled transient elastography, or VCTE) or MRI (magnetic resonance elastography, or MRE). These techniques are useful for patients with either minimal or advanced fibrotic disease.
	Estimation of degree of fibrosis can be obtained noninvasively using published formulas based on results of blood tests. The Fibrosis-4 Index for Liver Fibrosis uses AST, ALT, platelet count, and age, whereas the Non-Alcoholic Fatty Liver Disease Fibrosis Score uses AST, ALT, platelet count, albumin, abnormal fasting glucose, BMI, and age. Both instruments are accessible at www.mdcalc.com. Another formula for predicting moderate fibrosis and cirrhosis is the Enhanced Liver Fibrosis Score, obtained from measured values of tissue inhibitor of metalloproteinase-1 (TIMP-1), amino-terminal propeptide of type III procollagen (PIIINP), and hyaluronic acid (HA). These formulas can be used in combination to determine the presence of advanced fibrosis, which is associated with hepatic decompensation including ascites, variceal bleeding, and encephalopathy, as well as hepatocellular carcinoma.

Fatty liver disease *(continued)*

Fuster D, Samet JH: Alcohol use in patients with chronic liver disease. N Engl J Med 379(13):1251–1261, 2018

Juo YY, Livingston EH: Testing for nonalcoholic fatty liver disease. JAMA 322(18):1836, 2019

Neuschwander-Tetri BA: Non-alcoholic fatty liver disease. BMC Med 15(1):45, 2017

Sanyal AJ, Van Natta ML, Clark J, et al: Prospective study of outcomes in adults with nonalcoholic fatty liver disease. N Engl J Med 385(17):1559–1569, 2021

Sheka AC, Adeyi O, Thompson J, et al: Nonalcoholic steatohepatitis: a review. JAMA 323(12):1175–1183, 2020 [published correction appears in JAMA 323(16):1619, 2020]

Younossi ZM, Felix S, Jeffers T, et al: Performance of the Enhanced Liver Fibrosis Test to estimate advanced fibrosis among patients with nonalcoholic fatty liver disease. JAMA Netw Open 4(9):e2123923, 2021

Folate deficiency

Clinical findings	Folate (vitamin B_9) is an essential nutrient that plays a critical role in the synthesis of DNA, RNA, proteins, and RBCs. Deficiency of folate affects cell division and can result in the accumulation of toxic metabolites such as homocysteine. Foods that contain folate include leafy green vegetables, fresh fruit, beans, whole grains, seafood, and eggs. Folic acid is a synthetic form of folate used in supplements and fortified foods.
	Folate deficiency has well-established associations with malnutrition, alcohol use disorder, malabsorption syndromes, pregnancy, hemodialysis treatment, and the use of anticonvulsant drugs. Less well-known and less common is the association of deficiency with antibodies to the folate receptor-1 found on the basolateral endothelial surface of the choroid plexus, which is responsible for transporting folate across the blood-brain barrier into the CSF. When these antibodies bind to the receptor, it is unable to transport folate such that cerebral folate deficiency develops. This deficiency can be present even while peripheral folate levels are normal. This antibody-mediated cerebral folate deficiency is well known in infants and young children but also can occur in adults.
	Signs and symptoms of peripheral folate deficiency include the following: megaloblastic anemia, dementia, peripheral neuropathy (particularly reduced vibration sense in lower extremities), weakness, ataxia, positive Romberg testing, and paraplegia with abnormal deep tendon reflexes and extensor plantar responses. Nausea, vomiting, diarrhea, headache, and shortness of breath may also be seen. Signs and symptoms of cerebral folate deficiency in adults include cerebral calcifications, white matter lesions on MRI, pyramidal symptoms (spasticity, weakness, hyperreflexia), movement disorders (e.g., myoclonus), cerebellar dysfunction, and cognitive impairment.
	Folate deficiency has been identified in half of stroke survivors and at high rates among patients with schizophrenia. Low folate levels present a risk factor for dementia, particularly in the presence of elevated homocysteine levels. Cerebral folate deficiency has been identified in patients with treatment-refractory depression in whom serum folate levels were normal. Notes on unpublished cases indicate that cerebral folate deficiency can present in adolescents as catatonic schizophrenia and in adults as myoclonus and dementia. Cerebral folate deficiency should be included in the differential diagnosis for patients with cognitive impairment, neurological signs, brain calcifications, and white matter lesions seen on MRI.
Laboratory testing	Reference values for adults: • Serum folate: 3–13 ng/mL • RBC folate: 140–628 ng/mL • CSF 5-MTHF (5-methyltetrahydrofolate): 40–120 nmol/L Macrocytic anemia is seen, with hypersegmented neutrophils and macro-ovalocytes. Either serum or RBC folate can be assayed; serum folate testing is more widely available, whereas RBC folate testing more closely reflects tissue levels. Plasma homocysteine, which is even more sensitive, is increased in folate deficiency but is nonspecific.

Folate deficiency *(continued)*

Laboratory testing *(continued)*	Before folate therapy is initiated, vitamin B_{12} deficiency should be excluded with a normal B_{12} level and a normal MMA level. These deficiencies may occur in tandem, and replacement of folate alone may result in clinical worsening.
	To monitor the effectiveness of folate replacement, a CBC should be performed after 2 weeks to document increase in hemoglobin and decrease in MCV; another CBC should be performed after 8 weeks to document resolution of anemia.
	Long-term folate replacement is not necessary unless the cause persists (e.g., malnutrition); long-term monitoring is usually not needed.
	Workup for cerebral folate deficiency includes measurement of 5-MTHF and assay of serum for binding and blocking folate receptor antibodies.

Baroni L, Bonetto C, Rizzo G, et al: Association between cognitive impairment and vitamin B12, folate, and homocysteine status in elderly adults: a retrospective study. J Alzheimers Dis 70(2):443–453, 2019

Cao B, Wang DF, Xu MY, et al: Lower folate levels in schizophrenia: a meta-analysis. Psychiatry Res 245:1–7, 2016

Masingue M, Benoist JF, Roze E, et al: Cerebral folate deficiency in adults: a heterogeneous potentially treatable condition. J Neurol Sci 396:112–118, 2019

McPherson RA, Pincus MR: Henry's Clinical Diagnosis and Management by Laboratory Methods, 24th Edition Philadelphia, PA, Elsevier, 2022

Pan LA, Martin P, Zimmer T, et al: Neurometabolic disorders: potentially treatable abnormalities in patients with treatment-refractory depression and suicidal behavior. Am J Psychiatry 174(1):42–50, 2017

Pascoe MC, Linden T: Folate and MMA predict cognitive impairment in elderly stroke survivors: a cross sectional study. Psychiatry Res 243:49–52, 2016

Pope S, Artuch R, Heales S, Rahman S: Cerebral folate deficiency: analytical tests and differential diagnosis. J Inherit Metab Dis 42(4):655–672, 2019

Ramaekers V, Sequeira JM, Quadros EV: Clinical recognition and aspects of the cerebral folate deficiency syndromes. Clin Chem Lab Med 51(3):497–511, 2013

Reynolds EH: The neurology of folic acid deficiency. Handb Clin Neurol 120:927–943, 2014

Sanvisens A, Zuluaga P, Pineda M, et al: Folate deficiency in patients seeking treatment of alcohol use disorder. Drug Alcohol Depend 180:417–422, 2017

Sobczynska-Malefora A, Harrington DJ: Laboratory assessment of folate (vitamin B_9) status. J Clin Pathol 71(11):949–956, 2018

Williams Barnhardt E, Jacque M, Sharma TR: Brief reversible psychosis and altered mental status in a patient with folate deficiency: a case report. Prim Care Companion CNS Disord 18(1):10.4088/PCC.15l01839, 2016

Fragile X syndrome (FXS)

Clinical findings	FXS—the most common heritable form of intellectual disability—results from the expansion of a segment of DNA known as a CGG (cytosine-guanine-guanine) trinucleotide repeat in the non-coding region of the fragile X mental retardation 1 gene (*FMR1*). This excess DNA gives rise to excess *FMR1*-mRNA, which is toxic to cells and disrupts basic cellular functions. The clinical consequences of the expansion depend on the number of repeats in *FMR1*: 55–200 repeats represent a premutation, whereas >200–1,000 repeats represent a full mutation.
	The full mutation results in FXS, a neurodevelopmental disorder characterized by intellectual disability and autism spectrum disorder (ASD). Girls are usually less severely affected than boys. In addition to autistic behaviors and subaverage intellectual function, signs and symptoms include physical characteristics such as large head circumference, long narrow face, prominent jaw and forehead, protruding ears, finger joint laxity, flat feet, and macro-orchidism in boys after puberty. Anxiety, social avoidance, hyperactivity, ADHD, and seizures are seen. Specific behaviors include hand flapping, hand biting, and temper tantrums, as well as (after puberty) impulsivity, distractibility, and perseverative speech. Affected adults have increased rates of hypertension, obesity, parkinsonism, GI disorders, and mood disorders. MRI in adults shows reduced volume of the cerebellar vermis and enlargement of the caudate nucleus and lateral ventricles.
	Fragile X premutation–associated conditions (FXPAC) include the following:
	• Fragile X tremor/ataxia syndrome (FXTAS) is a progressive disease with onset usually after age 50 years that is characterized by kinetic tremor and/or cerebellar ataxia, with additional symptoms including parkinsonism, autonomic dysfunction, proximal leg muscle weakness, peripheral neuropathy, and cognitive impairment involving memory and executive functions. MRI abnormalities that may be identified well before clinical symptoms include reduced volume in the cerebellum and brainstem and white matter changes.
	• Fragile X–associated neuropsychiatric disorders (FXAND) are associated with developmental problems such as ASD, ADHD, depression, OCD, and anxiety disorders. These conditions are seen in both adults and children. Adults are also observed to have chronic fatigue, fibromyalgia, autoimmune dysfunction, migraine syndromes, and central pain syndromes. It has been proposed that the term FXAND be replaced by two terms: fragile X-associated neuropsychiatric conditions (FXANC) and fragile X various associated conditions (FXVAC) to reflect the non-neuropsychiatric nature of some of these symptoms.
	• Fragile X–associated primary ovarian insufficiency (FXPOI) in its most severe form is characterized by irregular or absent menstrual periods and elevated FSH levels before age 40 years, low estrogen levels, early menopause, and early osteoporosis.

Fragile X syndrome (FXS) *(continued)*

Laboratory testing	PCR is used to identify expansions of CGG trinucleotide repeat in *FMR1*: • >200–1,000 repeats—full mutation • 55–200 repeats—premutation • 59–200 repeats—premutation with risk of FXTAS Methylation-specific PCR is then performed for CGG repeats >100 to distinguish premutation from full mutation alleles.

ARUP Laboratories: Fragile X syndrome, in Laboratory Test Directory. Salt Lake City, UT, ARUP Laboratories, Test Directory, 2022. Available at: https://arupconsult.com/ati/fragile-x-syndrome. Accessed January 2022.

Grigsby J, Brega AG, Bennett RE, et al: Clinically significant psychiatric symptoms among male carriers of the fragile X premutation, with and without FXTAS, and the mediating influence of executive functioning. Clin Neuropsychol 30(6):944–959, 2016

Hagerman RJ, Hagerman P. Fragile X-associated tremor/ataxia syndrome: features, mechanisms and management. Nat Rev Neurol 12(7):403–412, 2016

Hagerman RJ, Jackson C, Amiri K, et al: Girls with fragile X syndrome: physical and neurocognitive status and outcome. Pediatrics 89(3):395–400, 1992

Hall DA, Berry-Kravis E: Fragile X syndrome and fragile X-associated tremor ataxia syndrome. Handb Clin Neurol 147:377–391, 2018

Johnson K, Herring J, Richstein J: Fragile X premutation associated conditions (FXPAC). Front Pediatr 8:266, 2020

Salcedo-Arellano MJ, Dufour B, McLennan Y, et al: Fragile X syndrome and associated disorders: clinical aspects and pathology. Neurobiol Dis 136:104740, 2020

Santos E, Emeka-Nwonovo C, Wang JY, et al: Developmental aspects of FXAND in a man with the *FMR1* premutation. Mol Genet Genomic Med 8(2):e1050, 2020

Frontotemporal dementia (FTD)

Clinical findings	FTD refers to a group of neurodegenerative disorders with progressive deficits in behavior, executive function, and language arising from pathology in the frontal lobes, anterior temporal lobes, or both. FTD is a leading cause of early onset dementia and the third-most-common form of dementia overall. Up to 50% of cases are familial, involving mutations in chromosome 9 open reading frame 72 (*C9orf72*), microtubule-associated protein tau (*MAPT*), or progranulin (*GRN*). *C9orf72* mutation is the most common, and this and the *GRN* mutation have been associated with presentations that look like primary psychiatric disorders. Several disorders related to FTD—FTD-motor neuron disease, progressive supranuclear palsy, and corticobasal syndrome—are not discussed further in this section.
	FTD is classified into three subtypes:
	• Behavioral variant FTD (bvFTD)
	• Nonfluent variant primary progressive aphasia (nfvPPA)
	• Semantic variant primary progressive aphasia (svPPA)
	svPPA is characterized by impaired object naming and impaired single-word comprehension, along with impaired object knowledge (especially for low-frequency or low-familiarity items), surface dyslexia or dysgraphia (difficulty reading or spelling words with atypical sound-letter associations such as "colonel" or "island"), and sparing of repetition, grammaticality, and motor aspects of speech. A reverse temporal gradient of recall may be observed, with poor recall of distant autobiographical memories and spared recent memory. nfvPPA is characterized by either agrammatism or speech apraxia (effortful, halting speech with inconsistent sound errors and distortions) or both, along with impaired comprehension of syntactically complex sentences and sparing of single-word comprehension and/or object knowledge. bvFTD is characterized by early behavioral and executive deficits. As FTD progresses and brain pathology spreads, these three variants converge such that global cognitive impairment is seen. Motor deficits are seen, including motor neuron disease in a subset of patients. Although the rate of progression varies among patients, death is expected 7–8 years after onset of symptoms, usually due to intercurrent infection such as pneumonia.
	bvFTD is characterized by progressive deterioration of behavior and/or cognition as noted by history or observation. Symptoms of possible bvFTD include the following:
	• Early behavioral disinhibition
	• Early apathy or inertia
	• Early loss of sympathy or empathy
	• Early perseverative, stereotyped, or compulsive/ritualistic behavior
	• Hyperorality and dietary changes
	• Neuropsychological profile of executive/generation deficits with relative sparing of memory and visuospatial functions
	Probable bvFTD can be diagnosed when three or more symptoms of possible bvFTD are present, functional decline is noted, and neuroimaging results are consistent with bvFTD.

Frontotemporal dementia (FTD) *(continued)*

Clinical findings *(continued)*	Definite bvFTD can be diagnosed with additional histopathological evidence of frontotemporal lobar degeneration on biopsy or postmortem exam or in the presence of a known pathogenic mutation.
	Among those meeting criteria for possible bvFTD are a subset of patients who show little progression of behavioral and cognitive impairment. This syndrome—termed *bvFTD phenocopy*—is difficult to distinguish clinically from bvFTD at presentation, except that MRI and PET findings appear normal. Affected individuals are more likely to be young males lacking motor features and family history of FTD. These patients tend to have a better prognosis than typical bvFTD patients, as if their pathology were on a spectrum midway between bvFTD and normal.
	Patients with *C9orf72* mutations present clinically with bvFTD, amyotrophic lateral sclerosis (ALS), or a combination of the two, or with prodromal psychiatric syndromes. *C9orf72* mutations give rise to repeat expansions, with carrier status reported to be associated with bipolar disorder, OCD, and schizophrenia in the years preceding FTD diagnosis. In more than half of carriers, delusions and hallucinations (primarily auditory) are observed and are often severe. Patients with *GRN* mutations may exhibit visual hallucinations and delusions, and there appears to be an association of these mutations with late-onset bipolar I disorder that evolves into bvFTD.
	Motor symptoms are most often seen in patients with bvFTD, including early parkinsonism and motor neuron disease, the latter ranging from mild symptoms to the fully developed syndrome of dysarthria, dysphagia, pseudobulbar affect, and upper and lower motor neuron signs.
Laboratory testing	*Genetic testing*
	Up to 50% of bvFTD cases are familial, most involving mutations in *C9orf72*, *MAPT*, or *GRN*. The *C9orf72* mutation is the most common, and this and the *GRN* mutation have been associated with presentations that resemble primary psychiatric disorders. The *GRN* and *MAPT* mutations are seen almost without exception in individuals who have a strong family history, whereas the *C9orf72* mutation is also seen in sporadic disease. *C9orf72* mutations give rise to repeat expansions, with >200 repeats considered pathogenic and ≤30 repeats considered normal.
	Recommendations for testing are as follows:
	• Genetic testing (all FTD mutations) in patients with probable bvFTD and at least one first-degree relative with bvFTD, late-onset primary psychiatric disorder, ALS, or other early onset neurodegenerative disease
	• *C9orf72* screening in all patients with possible or probable bvFTD, regardless of family history
	• *C9orf72* screening in patients with late-onset primary psychiatric disease and at least one first-degree relative with FTD or ALS
	• Strongly consider *C9orf72* screening in all patients with suspected bvFTD that does not meet the full diagnostic criteria if there are prominent psychiatric symptoms or the patient has a family history of late-onset primary psychiatric disease.
	• *GRN* screening for patients with primary progressive aphasia, both familial and sporadic

Frontotemporal dementia (FTD) *(continued)*

Laboratory testing *(continued)*	*Neuroimaging*
	Structural imaging
	• Structural neuroimaging is a requisite component of the workup for FTD, with MRI preferred to CT.
	• In bvFTD, disproportionate atrophy is seen in the frontal (especially right frontal) and anterior temporal areas, with the severity dependent on the disease stage.
	• In nfvPPA, degeneration is typically seen in the left inferior frontal gyrus, insula, and premotor areas.
	• In svPPA, bilateral anterior temporal atrophy is seen, left more than right.
	Functional imaging
	• Functional neuroimaging findings parallel those of structural imaging, with hypoperfusion (SPECT) or hypometabolism (PET) in specific areas dependent on subtype of FTD.
	• FDG-PET imaging can help distinguish FTD from Alzheimer's disease (AD).
	• In bvFTD, FDG-PET shows glucose hypometabolism in orbitofrontal, dorsomedial, and dorsolateral prefrontal areas, anterior temporal pole, and basal ganglia. These may be detectable before clinical criteria are met.
	CSF analysis
	• Analysis of CSF for amyloid-β_{42}, tau, and phosphorylated-tau is recommended to exclude AD.
	• CSF neurofilament light chain assay can help to distinguish bvFTD from primary psychiatric disorders. Neurofilaments are constituents of the axonal skeleton, and their presence in CSF is a marker for neurodegeneration.

American Psychiatric Association: Diagnostic and Statistical Manual of Mental Disorders, 5th Edition, Text Revision. Washington, DC, American Psychiatric Association, 2022

Bang J, Spina S, Miller BL: Frontotemporal dementia. Lancet 386(10004):1672–1682, 2015

Cipriani G, Danti S, Nuti A, et al: Is that schizophrenia or frontotemporal dementia? Supporting clinicians in making the right diagnosis. Acta Neurol Belg 120(4):799–804, 2020

Mendez MF, Parand L, Akhlaghipour G: Bipolar disorder among patients diagnosed with frontotemporal dementia. J Neuropsychiatry Clin Neurosci 32(4):376–384, 2020

Nobili F, Arbizu J, Bouwman F, et al: European Association of Nuclear Medicine and European Academy of Neurology recommendations for the use of brain 18F-fluorodeoxyglucose positron emission tomography in neurodegenerative cognitive impairment and dementia: Delphi consensus. Eur J Neurol 25(10):1201–1217, 2018

Olney NT, Spina S, Miller BL: Frontotemporal dementia. Neurol Clin 35(2):339–374, 2017

Olszewska DA, Lonergan R, Fallon EM, Lynch T: Genetics of frontotemporal dementia. Curr Neurol Neurosci Rep 16(12):107, 2016

Onyike CU, Huey ED: Frontotemporal dementia and psychiatry. Int Rev Psychiatry 25(2):127–129, 2013

Paquin V, Therriault J, Pascoal TA, et al: Frontal variant of Alzheimer disease differentiated from frontotemporal dementia using in vivo amyloid and tau imaging. Cogn Behav Neurol 33(4):288–293, 2020

Power C, Lawlor BA: The behavioral variant frontotemporal dementia phenocopy syndrome: a review. J Geriatr Psychiatry Neurol 34(3):196–208, 2021

Pressman PS, Matlock D, Ducharme S: Distinguishing behavioral variant frontotemporal dementia from primary psychiatric disorders: a review of recently published consensus recommendations from the Neuropsychiatric International Consortium for Frontotemporal Dementia. J Neuropsychiatry Clin Neurosci 33(2):152–156, 2021

Frontotemporal dementia (FTD) *(continued)*

Saracino D, Ferrieux S, Noguès-Lassiaille M, et al: Primary progressive aphasia associated with GRN mutations: new insights into the nonamyloid logopenic variant. Neurology 97(1):e88–e102, 2021

Seeley WW: Behavioral variant frontotemporal dementia. Continuum (Minneap Minn) 25(1):76–100, 2019

Swift IJ, Sogorb-Esteve A, Heller C, et al: Fluid biomarkers in frontotemporal dementia: past, present and future. J Neurol Neurosurg Psychiatry 92(2):204–215, 2021

van der Ende EL, Jackson JL, White A, et al: Unravelling the clinical spectrum and the role of repeat length in C9orf72 repeat expansions. J Neurol Neurosurg Psychiatry 92:502–509, 2021

Generalized anxiety disorder (GAD)

Clinical findings	GAD is characterized in DSM-5 by excessive anxiety and worry about numerous events or activities that occur more days than not for at least 6 months. The individual finds the symptoms difficult to control. The anxiety and worry are associated with three or more of the following symptoms:
	• Restlessness or feeling "keyed up" or "on edge"
	• Easy fatigue
	• Difficulty concentrating or "mind going blank"
	• Irritability
	• Muscle tension
	• Sleep disturbance
	These symptoms cause significant distress or impairment in social, occupational, or other areas of function. The disturbance is not attributable to the physiological effects of a substance or another medical condition and is not better explained by another psychiatric disorder.
	The alternative diagnosis of anxiety associated with another medical condition should be given if the patient's history, laboratory findings, or physical examination reveals a specific medical condition judged to be causative. The alternative diagnosis of substance/medication-induced anxiety disorder should be given if a drug of abuse or exposure to a toxin is judged to be causative. These conditions are more closely associated with panic disorder and anxiety, but several common abnormalities should be excluded as contributing factors to GAD. Although the identification of biomarkers of GAD is an active area of investigation, findings have not yet been adequately validated for clinical use.
Laboratory testing	The basic laboratory workup for GAD includes only TSH and a metabolic panel (BMP or CMP) to check calcium and glucose levels. Further testing may be indicated to exclude medical conditions causing or contributing to anxiety. Depending on patient characteristics and history, further evaluation might include one or more of the following:
	• ECG, Holter monitoring, cardiac stress testing, and/or echocardiogram
	• Chest X-ray, pulmonary function tests, and/or arterial blood gases
	• GGT with or without CDT for suspicion of covert drinking
	• Plasma free metanephrines
	• Urine porphyrin precursors
	• Pulmonary CT scan
	• EEG

American Psychiatric Association: Diagnostic and Statistical Manual of Mental Disorders, 5th Edition, Text Revision. Washington, DC, American Psychiatric Association, 2022

Hilbert K, Lueken U, Muehlhan M, Beesdo-Baum K: Separating generalized anxiety disorder from major depression using clinical, hormonal, and structural MRI data: a multimodal machine learning study. Brain Behav 7(3):e00633, 2017

Maron E, Nutt D: Biological markers of generalized anxiety disorder. Dialogues Clin Neurosci 19(2):147–158, 2017

Tomasi J, Lisoway AJ, Zai CC, et al: Towards precision medicine in generalized anxiety disorder: review of genetics and pharmaco(epi)genetics. J Psychiatr Res 119:33–47, 2019

Hashimoto's encephalopathy

Clinical findings	Hashimoto's encephalopathy is an autoimmune disorder characterized by an acute to subacute onset of confusion with altered consciousness seen in association with antithyroid antibodies and a positive response to steroid treatment. The relationship of the syndrome to thyroid function itself is poorly understood, and there is no agreement as to whether response to steroids is universal, even though some have advocated renaming it as *steroid-responsive encephalopathy associated with autoimmune thyroiditis* (SREAT). In fact, the same syndrome is also associated with Graves' disease, and antithyroid antibodies are also found in multiple sclerosis, neuromyelitis optica, and other causes of autoimmune encephalitis.
	Two general presenting patterns are recognized:
	• Acute—multiple recurrent episodes of focal neurological signs that develop acutely to subacutely in association with variable cognitive impairment and alteration of consciousness. This presentation is sometimes called "stroke-like."
	• Diffuse—a progressive condition characterized by slowly worsening cognitive impairment with confusion, hallucinations, somnolence, and dementia. Some patients in this category present in coma.
	Other neuropsychiatric symptoms that can be seen in either group include the following:
	• Psychosis—visual hallucinations and delusions (usually paranoid) in up to one-third of patients. Psychiatric symptoms are the only symptoms in up to a quarter of patients
	• Seizures—focal or generalized tonic-clonic seizures in up to two-thirds of patients, often the presenting symptom and including status epilepticus in some patients
	• Pyramidal tract signs—diffuse hyperreflexia, spasticity, and other signs in most patients
	• Other motor signs—tremor and myoclonus, which can be focal or multifocal
	Hashimoto's encephalopathy is more common in females and in at least one case series has been linked to the HLA b8 DRw3 haplotype. The long-term course of illness may be self-limited, relapsing-remitting, or progressive. Limited data from pathological examination have shown lymphocytic infiltration surrounding small arterioles and venules in the brain.
Laboratory testing	Although most patients have either normal thyroid function or mild hypothyroidism, laboratory values reported in the literature reflect a range of function from overt hypothyroidism to overt hyperthyroidism. Elevated thyroid antibodies in serum include anti-TPOAb and/or antithyroglobulin antibody. Level of antibody elevation does not correlate well with symptom severity, and antibody levels decline with treatment in some cases but not in others. In addition, antibodies are present in ≤20% of the healthy population, so they are not specific to Hashimoto's encephalopathy.
	CSF analysis is abnormal in most cases, showing elevation of protein and a lymphocytic pleocytosis. CSF glucose is normal, and other findings are inconsistent.

Hashimoto's encephalopathy *(continued)*

Laboratory testing *(continued)*	EEG shows nonspecific slowing of background activity in most patients that resolves with steroid treatment, although EEG improvement may lag behind clinical improvement. Epileptiform or ictal activity may be captured. Brain MRI is usually normal or shows incidental or nonspecific findings. FDG-PET can be used to determine degree of brain inflammation in patients who present with limbic encephalitis, showing hypermetabolism in affected areas.
	The following tests are recommended for workup of suspected Hashimoto's encephalopathy:
	• Thyroid function tests—TSH and free T4
	• Laboratory testing for the usual causes of delirium, acute psychosis, new-onset cognitive impairment, or seizures, depending on presentation
	• CSF analysis for protein and cell counts, in addition to infection workup
	• EEG to exclude epileptiform or ictal activity
	• MRI with gadolinium contrast to exclude brain abscess or other pathology that could explain symptoms

Churilov LP, Sobolevskaia PA, Stroev YI: Thyroid gland and brain: enigma of Hashimoto's encephalopathy. Best Pract Res Clin Endocrinol Metab 33(6):101364, 2019

Crotty GF, Doherty C, Solomon IH, et al: Learning from history: Lord Brain and Hashimoto's encephalopathy. Pract Neurol 19(4):316–320, 2019

Laurent C, Capron J, Quillerou B, et al: Steroid-responsive encephalopathy associated with autoimmune thyroiditis (SREAT): characteristics, treatment and outcome in 251 cases from the literature. Autoimmun Rev 15(12):1129–1133, 2016

Mattozzi S, Sabater L, Escudero D, et al: Hashimoto encephalopathy in the 21st century. Neurology 94(2):e217–e224, 2020

Nagano M, Kobayashi K, Yamada-Otani M, et al: Hashimoto's encephalopathy presenting with smoldering limbic encephalitis. Intern Med 58(8):1167–1172, 2019

Tsai CH, Yu KT, Chan HY, Chan CH: Hashimoto's encephalopathy presenting as catatonia in a bipolar patient. Asian J Psychiatr 66:102895, 2021

Zhou JY, Xu B, Lopes J, et al: Hashimoto encephalopathy: literature review. Acta Neurol Scand 135(3):285–290, 2017

Headache

Clinical findings	Headaches can be classified as primary or secondary. Primary headaches include migraines, tension-type, cluster, and other headaches, such as from cold stimuli. In some patients, these headaches are associated with specific activities such as exercise, sex, or coughing. In addition, primary headaches can be aggravated by poor sleep, stress, bad posture, dehydration, nitrate-containing foods, and alcohol (particularly red wine). Secondary headaches are symptomatic of diseases or conditions activating pain-sensitive pathways of the head, such as head or neck trauma, infection, intracranial mass, vascular disease including brain hemorrhage or carotid artery dissection, severe hypertension, sinusitis, and dental problems. These conditions range from benign to serious and require a careful clinical evaluation, particularly in older, pregnant, or immunocompromised patients.
	Red flags for dangerous headaches requiring urgent workup include the following:
	• First or worst-ever headache
	• Worsening headache pattern
	• Headache triggered by cough, exertion, or sex
	• Headache with change in personality or mental status
	• Seizures
	• Meningeal signs
	• Temporal tenderness
	• Focal neurological signs
	• Papilledema
	• Sudden-onset "thunderclap" headache
	• Systemic illness, fever, rash with headache
	• New headache in a patient with cancer, HIV disease, Lyme disease
	Migraine headaches can be distinguished from other headache types by their severity, location, duration, and the presence of nausea, photophobia, phonophobia (sensitivity to sounds), and pulsating pain. The mnemonic POUND can be used to recall some features at the bedside, including Pulsatile, One-day duration (4–72 hours), Unilateral, Nausea/vomiting, and Disabling intensity. Migraines are often exacerbated by exertion. Some patients experience an aura, usually preceding the headache, with visual, sensory, or speech symptoms that are short-lived and reversible.
	Tension-type headaches are the most common headache type, characterized by mild to moderate aching pain, often with a feeling of tightness around the head and tenderness of scalp, neck, and shoulder muscles. Pain is not exacerbated by exertion.
	Cluster headaches are usually unilateral, with pain occurring behind the eye and in the temporal area, jaw, teeth, and neck, accompanied by ipsilateral autonomic signs such as lacrimation, nasal congestion, eyelid edema, or forehead sweating. Headaches occur several times a day, each lasting 15 minutes to 3 hours, with the series of headaches lasting 6–12 weeks. Cluster headaches are associated with depression, sleep apnea, restless legs syndrome, and asthma. These headaches are often so severe that affected patients commonly have suicidal ideation, and their risk of attempted suicide is elevated.

Headache *(continued)*

Clinical findings *(continued)*	In addition to their association with depression, headaches are also seen with anxiety, panic disorder, and chronic traumatic encephalopathy. A recently recognized syndrome that presents with severe headache—reversible cerebral vasoconstriction—is associated with the use of serotonergic drugs. This syndrome involves local constriction of cerebral arteries and can cause ischemic brain injury.
Laboratory testing	The most important laboratory test to consider in the workup of headache is neuroimaging, either head CT or brain MRI. In general, patients presenting with acute headache undergo CT, whereas those with chronic headache undergo MRI. In the absence of the red flags noted above, however, patients with a recognizable headache pattern and a history of headaches do not require imaging.
	Patients presenting with acute-onset severe headache should undergo urgent CT without contrast. If a lumbar puncture is anticipated in a patient with suspected subarachnoid hemorrhage or meningitis, CT should in all cases be performed before lumbar puncture, regardless of neurological exam findings. Immunocompromised patients with severe headache should undergo MRI with and without contrast.
	Other tests used in headache workup include ESR and CRP if temporal arteritis or other inflammatory process is suspected. Angiography (CT or magnetic resonance) may be needed to examine blood vessels.

Arca KN, Halker Singh RB: Dehydration and headache. Curr Pain Headache Rep 25(8):56, 2021

Arca KN, Halker Singh RB: The hypertensive headache: a review. Curr Pain Headache Rep 23(5):30, 2019

de Vries Lentsch S, Louter MA, van Oosterhout W, et al: Depressive symptoms during the different phases of a migraine attack: a prospective diary study. J Affect Disord 297:502–507, 2022

Giri S, Tronvik EA, Hagen K: The bidirectional temporal relationship between headache and affective disorders: longitudinal data from the HUNT studies. J Headache Pain 23(1):14, 2022

Hainer BL, Matheson EM: Approach to acute headache in adults. Am Fam Physician 87(10):682–687, 2013

Kopel D, Peeler C, Zhu S: Headache emergencies. Neurol Clin 39(2):355–372, 2021

Manning T, Bartow C, Dunlap M, et al: Reversible cerebral vasoconstriction syndrome associated with fluoxetine. J Acad Consult Liaison Psychiatry 62(6):634–644, 2021

Palmieri A, Valentinis L, Zanchin G: Update on headache and brain tumors. Cephalalgia 41(4):431–437, 2021

Hemochromatosis

Clinical findings	Hemochromatosis is a condition of iron overload affecting the liver, heart, endocrine pancreas, bones, joints, skin, and pituitary gland. It can be hereditary or acquired, the latter due to chronic liver disease or recurrent blood transfusions, among other causes. The hereditary form is found primarily among Whites of northern European descent and is often identified only after years of iron deposition (after age 40 in males and age 60 in females). The most common form of hereditary disease is now known to be caused by a deficiency of hepcidin, a protein produced by hepatocytes that is responsible for the regulation of iron absorption, recycling, and release into the circulation. This discovery has prompted the development of new treatments in the form of hepcidin inducers, with the promise of effective treatment without repeated phlebotomy.
	Complications of iron overload include steatohepatitis, liver fibrosis, cirrhosis, hepatocellular carcinoma, type 2 diabetes, supraventricular arrhythmias, congestive heart failure, dilated cardiomyopathy, pulmonary hypertension, hypogonadism, impotence, hypothyroidism, arthritis, osteoporosis, and premature death from liver or heart failure. The brain is mostly spared by actions of the blood-brain barrier. End-organ damage can be limited by early recognition and treatment, so the index of suspicion should be high in patients presenting with multiple symptoms involving different organ systems.
	Clinical signs of hemochromatosis seen on physical exam include the following: • Arthritis • Melanoderma (bronzing of the skin) • Nail changes (white nails, flat nails, spoon nails) • Hepatomegaly • Cardiac arrhythmia • Congestive heart failure
Laboratory testing	*Blood tests* • Fasting transferrin saturation >45% • Ferritin >300 ng/mL for males; >200 ng/mL for females • Liver enzymes variably elevated • Blood glucose may be elevated *Radiology* • MRI to evaluate iron excess in liver, spleen, and pancreas (liver biopsy no longer required) • X-ray to evaluate chondrocalcinosis of the wrists or knees or subchondral arthropathy *Electrophysiology* • ECG to detect arrhythmias and other abnormalities *Genetic testing* • Genotyping: C282Y and H63D • Genetic testing for other types of hereditary hemochromatosis is costly and not often useful except in specialist clinics. • First-degree relatives of patients with hereditary hemochromatosis should be offered genetic testing after age 18.

Hemochromatosis *(continued)*

Brissot P, Pietrangelo A, Adams PC: Haemochromatosis. Nat Rev Dis Primers 4:18016, 2018

Golfeyz S, Lewis S, Weisberg IS: Hemochromatosis: pathophysiology, evaluation, and management of hepatic iron overload with a focus on MRI. Expert Rev Gastroenterol Hepatol 12(8):767–778, 2018

Hamada Y, Hirano E, Sugimoto K, et al: A farewell to phlebotomy-use of placenta-derived drugs Laennec and Porcine for improving hereditary hemochromatosis without phlebotomy: a case report. J Med Case Rep 16(1):26, 2022

Hum RM, Ho P: Hereditary haemochromatosis presenting to rheumatology clinic as inflammatory arthritis. BMJ Case Rep 15(1):e246236, 2022

Kane SF, Roberts C, Paulus R: Hereditary hemochromatosis: rapid evidence review. Am Fam Physician 104(3):263–270, 2021

Udani K, Chris-Olaiya A, Ohadugha C, et al: Cardiovascular manifestations in hospitalized patients with hemochromatosis in the United States. Int J Cardiol 342:117–124, 2021

Hepatic encephalopathy (HE)

Clinical findings	HE is a syndrome of neuropsychiatric impairment associated with advanced liver disease. Onset can be acute, chronic, or acute-on-chronic. Acute HE arising from acute liver failure is a fulminant condition associated with cerebral edema and coma. Chronic HE, which develops in the context of cirrhosis or portosystemic shunt, can be persistent or recurrent, with episodes precipitated by intercurrent illness such as GI bleeding or infection. Severe chronic HE in cirrhosis is also a serious condition, carrying a <50% survival rate at 1 year.
	Signs and symptoms of HE depend on the stage or grade of illness as described in the West Haven criteria:
	• Grade 0: No abnormalities detected
	• Grade 1: Trivial lack of awareness, lethargy, apathy, slowing, irritability, anxiety or euphoria, shortened attention span, acalculia
	• Grade 2: Disorientation to time, inappropriate behaviors, obvious personality changes, cognitive deficits, slurred speech, asterixis
	• Grade 3: Somnolence to stupor, marked confusion, amnesia, incomprehensible speech, bizarre behavior, inability to perform mental tasks
	• Grade 4: Coma with or without response to painful stimuli
	The term "minimal HE" has been used to describe patients who have subtle cognitive impairment that is only detectable by neuropsychological testing. Because these patients have problems with complex and sustained attention and slowed reaction times, they may be unfit to drive or to hold certain kinds of employment. Another distinction is drawn between "covert" and "overt" HE, with Grades 0 and 1 considered covert and Grades 2–4 overt.
Laboratory testing	Diagnosis of HE is made based on clinical findings. Although ammonia level may be elevated, degree of elevation does not correlate well with severity of encephalopathy except in acute HE. Ammonia level is also subject to test interference.
	EEG shows generalized slowing, slowing of posterior dominant frequency, triphasic waves, and, in some cases, epileptiform activity.
	Even in patients with known underlying liver disease, the following possible precipitants should be investigated in acute HE:
	• Hyponatremia
	• Hypokalemia
	• Alkalosis
	• Dehydration
	• Hypoglycemia
	• Renal insufficiency
	• Infection (e.g., spontaneous bacterial peritonitis)
	• Blood in the GI tract
	• Use of alcohol or drugs such as benzodiazepines or opioids

Dharel N, Bajaj JS: Definition and nomenclature of hepatic encephalopathy. J Clin Exp Hepatol 5(Suppl 1):S37–S41, 2015

Karanfilian BV, Park T, Senatore F, Rustgi VK: Minimal hepatic encephalopathy. Clin Liver Dis 24(2):209–218, 2020

Kullmann F, Hollerbach S, Lock G, et al: Brain electrical activity mapping of EEG for the diagnosis of (sub)clinical hepatic encephalopathy in chronic liver disease. Eur J Gastroenterol Hepatol 13:513–522, 2001

Hepatic encephalopathy (HE)

Rose CF, Amodio P, Bajaj JS, et al: Hepatic encephalopathy: novel insights into classification, pathophysiology and therapy. J Hepatol 73(6):1526–1547, 2020

Rudler M, Weiss N, Bouzbib C, Thabut D: Diagnosis and management of hepatic encephalopathy. Clin Liver Dis 25(2):393–417, 2021

Weissenborn K: Hepatic encephalopathy: definition, clinical grading and diagnostic principles. Drugs 79(Suppl 1):5–9, 2019

Wijdicks EF: Hepatic encephalopathy. N Engl J Med 375(17):1660–1670, 2016

Hepatitis, viral

Clinical findings	Viral hepatitis is an inflammation of the liver most commonly caused by one of five hepatitis viruses designated A, B, C, D, and E. Symptoms usually begin acutely and range in severity from a minor flu-like illness to fulminant hepatic failure, depending on the particular virus and the host response. Symptoms include loss of appetite, malaise, fatigue, fever, nausea, vomiting, right upper quadrant pain, dark urine, light-colored stool, joint pain, and jaundice. Patients who smoke may report a distaste for cigarettes. In most cases, patients recover in 1–2 months even without treatment, although some patients with hepatitis B or C develop chronic liver disease with risk of cirrhosis, liver failure, and/or hepatocellular carcinoma. Viral hepatitis has high seroprevalence among patients in psychiatric care.
	• Hepatitis A virus (HAV)—the most common cause of acute viral hepatitis—is transmitted by the fecal-oral route, when even microscopic amounts of fecal material are ingested in food or drink or picked up from objects touched by an infected person. Foodborne outbreaks occur with fresh or frozen food contaminated during harvesting, processing, handling, or cooking. Symptoms are usually mild, although fulminant hepatic failure has been reported. Complete recovery is seen in nearly all patients at 6 months. An effective vaccine is widely available.
	• Hepatitis B virus (HBV)—the second most common cause of acute viral hepatitis—is transmitted when blood, semen, or other body fluids from an infected person enter the body of a person not infected. Examples include sexual contact or sharing needles or syringes, toothbrushes, razors, or any other object contaminated with even microscopic amounts of blood. HBV has high seroprevalence among methadone clinic patients. Although many people do not know they are infected, HBV can cause very severe symptoms including fulminant liver failure, particularly with hepatitis D co-infection. In addition, HBV infection can become chronic, and up to 25% of this population develops cirrhosis, liver failure, or hepatocellular carcinoma. An effective vaccine is widely available and is recommended for many groups, as listed in published guidelines.
	• Hepatitis C virus (HCV) is transmitted when blood from an infected person enters the body of a person who is not infected. Examples include sharing needles or syringes or a history of blood transfusion or organ transplant before 1992 (when HCV was eliminated from the blood supply). Exposure from sexual contact is rare. HCV infection is often associated with neuropsychiatric syndromes such as cognitive impairment, stroke, and peripheral neuropathy. Although HCV infection can cause a mild illness, more than half of patients develop a chronic infection. HCV is a leading indication for liver transplant and a leading cause of hepatocellular carcinoma. There is no vaccine available.
	• Hepatitis D virus (HDV)—found only among patients with hepatitis B infection—is transmitted through contact with infected blood. A high index of suspicion for HDV infection is needed in patients with risk factors for HBV because HBV/HDV co-infection carries a higher risk of rapidly progressive disease with cirrhosis, liver failure, and hepatocellular carcinoma.

Hepatitis, viral *(continued)*

Clinical findings *(continued)*	• Hepatitis E virus (HEV)—a common and likely underdiagnosed cause of acute viral hepatitis—is transmitted by the fecal-oral route. This virus has several genotypes, some of which also infect animals. Most infections are mild and self-limited, but the genotypes also infecting animals are reported to cause chronic hepatitis in immunocompromised patients. The minority of patients who progress to acute liver failure are usually malnourished or pregnant or have preexisting chronic liver disease. HEV infection can precipitate acute-on-chronic liver failure. In addition, HEV can involve the CNS and kidneys. CNS infection has been associated with Guillain-Barré syndrome, meningoencephalitis, and brachial plexus neuritis.
Laboratory testing	When a patient with no prior history of hepatitis presents with signs and symptoms suggestive of acute infectious hepatitis, a screening panel should be ordered. In the United States, screening is carried out for HAV, HBV, and HCV infection simultaneously, except in the case of known exposure to a specific type. The panel includes the following tests: • HAV antibody, IgM • HBV core antibody, IgM • HBV surface antigen with reflex to confirmation • HCV antibody If the patient presents with signs and symptoms suggestive of acute hepatitis and has a known history of HBV infection, they are tested for co-infection with HDV. If the patient presents with signs and symptoms like those of HAV but is seronegative for HAV, testing for HEV by HEV IgM antibody may be indicated. Other tests are performed to detect liver injury, including liver enzymes and blood clotting measures. The CDC recommends screening for HBV for the following populations: • People born in countries with 2% or higher HBV prevalence • People born in the United States not vaccinated as infants whose parents were born in regions with high rates of HBV infection (hepatitis B surface antigen [HBsAg] prevalence of ≥8%) • Men who have sex with men • People who inject drugs • People with HIV • Household and sexual contacts of people with HBV • People requiring immunosuppressive therapy • People with end-stage renal disease (including hemodialysis patients) • Blood and tissue donors • People with elevated ALT levels (≥19 IU/L for females and ≥30 IU/L for males) • Pregnant females (HBsAg only) • Infants born to HBV-infected mothers (HBsAg and antibody to HBsAg only)

Hepatitis, viral *(continued)*

Laboratory testing *(continued)*	The CDC recommends universal screening for HCV for the following populations: • Screening at least once in a lifetime for all adults age ≥18 years, except in settings where the prevalence of HCV infection (HCV RNA positivity) is <0.1% • Screening for all pregnant females during each pregnancy, except in settings where the prevalence of HCV infection (HCV RNA positivity) is <0.1% The CDC recommends one-time HCV testing regardless of age or setting prevalence among people with recognized conditions or exposures: • People with HIV • People who have ever injected drugs and shared needles, syringes, or other drug preparation equipment, including those who injected once or a few times many years ago • People with selected medical conditions, including people who have ever received maintenance hemodialysis and people with persistently abnormal ALT levels • Prior recipients of transfusions or organ transplants, including people who received clotting factor concentrates produced before 1987, people who received a transfusion of blood or blood components before July 1992, people who received an organ transplant before July 1992, and people who were notified that they received blood from a donor who later tested positive for HCV infection • Health care, emergency medical, and public safety personnel after needle sticks, sharps, or mucosal exposures to HCV-positive blood • Children born to mothers with HCV infection The CDC recommends routine periodic testing for people with ongoing risk factors, while risk factors persist: • People who currently inject drugs and share needles, syringes, or other drug preparation equipment • People with selected medical conditions, including people who have ever received maintenance hemodialysis Any person who requests HCV testing should receive it, regardless of disclosure of risk, because many persons may be reluctant to disclose stigmatizing risks.

Abutaleb A, Kottilil S: Hepatitis A: epidemiology, natural history, unusual clinical manifestations, and prevention. Gastroenterol Clin North Am 49(2):191–199, 2020

Almeida PH, Matielo CEL, Curvelo LA, et al: Update on the management and treatment of viral hepatitis. World J Gastroenterol 27(23):3249–3261, 2021

American Association for Clinical Chemistry: Lab Tests Online. Available at: https://www.testing.com. Accessed July 2021.

Bart G, Piccolo P, Zhang L, et al: Markers for hepatitis A, B and C in methadone maintained patients: an unexpectedly high co-infection with silent hepatitis B. Addiction 103:681–686, 2008

Castaneda D, Gonzalez AJ, Alomari M, et al: From hepatitis A to E: a critical review of viral hepatitis. World J Gastroenterol 27(16):1691–1715, 2021

Choi JW, Son HJ, Lee SS, et al: Acute hepatitis E virus superinfection increases mortality in patients with cirrhosis. BMC Infect Dis 22(1):62, 2022

Centers for Disease Control and Prevention: Viral Hepatitis: Testing Recommendations for Hepatitis C Virus Infection. Atlanta, GA, Centers for Disease Control and Prevention, 2020. Available at: https://www.cdc.gov/hepatitis/hcv/guidelinesc.htm. Accessed February 2022.

Hepatitis, viral *(continued)*

Centers for Disease Control and Prevention: Viral Hepatitis: Hepatitis B Questions and Answers for Health Professionals. Atlanta, GA, Centers for Disease Control and Prevention, 2022. Available at: https://www.cdc.gov/hepatitis/hbv/hbvfaq.htm. Accessed February 2022.

Fontana RJ, Engle RE, Gottfried M, et al: Role of hepatitis E virus infection in North American patients with severe acute liver injury. Clin Transl Gastroenterol 11(11):e00273, 2020

Jha AK, Kumar G, Dayal VM, et al: Neurological manifestations of hepatitis E virus infection: an overview. World J Gastroenterol 27(18):2090–2104, 2021

Langan RC, Goodbred AJ: Hepatitis A. Am Fam Physician 104(4):368–374, 2021

Linder KA, Malani PN: Hepatitis A. JAMA 318(23):2393, 2017

HIV and AIDS

Clinical findings	AIDS continues to be a global public health problem with no cure, but now there is effective prevention, diagnosis, and treatment that enables affected people to lead long and healthy lives. In the United States, about 1.2 million people live with HIV, and ~13% of them are not aware of this fact and need testing. New cases disproportionately affect racial and ethnic minorities and gay, bisexual, and other men who have sex with men. Psychiatrists need to be aware of the rate of HIV infection in their catchment areas and that homeless and drug-abusing populations have greatly increased risk. Because patients with chronic mental illness may use their mental health professionals as primary care providers, becoming knowledgeable about testing and follow-up in these cases is essential for these providers. Most HIV infections in the United States are HIV-1; HIV-2 is endemic to West Africa. With infection, the virus localizes to lymphoid tissues, infecting CD4+ helper cells. An acute retroviral syndrome typically occurs within 2–4 weeks of infection, although some patients are asymptomatic during this phase. Signs and symptoms of the acute retroviral syndrome include headache, fatigue, sore throat, nausea, vomiting and/or diarrhea, night sweats and chills, myalgias and arthralgias, fever, lymphadenopathy, skin rash (red, non-pruritic, usually on torso), and ulcers (mouth, esophagus, anus, genitals). The symptoms of the acute syndrome resolve within days to weeks. When viremia clears, the patient enters a latent stage without clinical symptoms that can last a decade or longer. With progression, the number of functioning CD4+ cells declines to <200/mm^3, the threshold for diagnosing AIDS. This number is no longer used to decide when to start antiretroviral treatment because treatment is initiated as soon as HIV infection is confirmed. It is at this point, however, that opportunistic infections supervene. Malignancies such as non-Hodgkin's lymphoma, invasive cervical cancer, lung cancer, or Kaposi sarcoma can develop. Over time, HIV-associated neurocognitive disorder, HIV-associated distal sensory polyneuropathy, myocarditis, and chronic metabolic derangements (impaired glucose tolerance, dyslipidemia, lipodystrophy) can be seen. COVID-19 resources are available for individuals living with HIV. In general, the same precautions against infection are recommended, and vaccines are known to be safe. Specific vaccine recommendations can be found at www.cdc.gov/hiv/basics/covid-19.html.
Laboratory testing	HIV testing is recommended as follows: • At least once for all patients ages 13–64 years as part of routine medical care • Yearly for those at higher risk (see below) • Every 3–6 months for sexually active homosexual and bisexual males • Routinely for prenatal screening Factors that increase risk include the following: • Having vaginal or anal sex with someone who is HIV positive or whose HIV status is unknown

HIV and AIDS *(continued)*

Laboratory testing *(continued)*	• Injecting drugs using nonsterile needles, syringes, or other drug equipment
	• Exchanging sex for money or drugs
	• Having a sexually transmitted disease such as syphilis
	• Having hepatitis or tuberculosis
	• Having sex with anyone who has any of the above risk factors
	Three types of tests are used to diagnose HIV:
	• Antibody tests—use blood or oral fluid. Most rapid tests and home use tests are of this type.
	• Antigen/Antibody tests—detect parts of the virus and body's response to the virus
	• Nucleic acid tests—detect HIV virus in blood
	Initial testing uses either an antibody test or antigen/antibody test. Nucleic acid tests are costly and are not used for screening except for high-risk exposure or possible exposure with early HIV symptoms. If the initial test is positive, a follow-up test is conducted. A second positive test confirms HIV.
	AIDS is diagnosed when the CD4+ cell count is <200/mm^3. Treatment is monitored using quantitative viral load, CD4+ count, and drug resistance testing (genotyping). See **HIV Testing** in the *Laboratory Tests* chapter for further information.
	Patient counseling is mandatory for HIV testing. The following information should be provided to patients, whether for office- or lab-based testing: information about the HIV test, its benefits and consequences, ways HIV is transmitted and how it can be prevented, meaning of test results, and where to obtain further information and other services, including treatment. Those tested with rapid tests should be informed that results will be available during the visit and that confirmatory testing will be needed if the rapid test is positive. In this case, a return visit should be scheduled to discuss confirmatory test results.

Centers for Disease Control and Prevention: Types of HIV tests. Atlanta, GA, Centers for Disease Control and Prevention, 2021. Available at: https://www.cdc.gov/hiv/basics/hiv-testing/test-types.html. Accessed July 2021.

Centers for Disease Control and Prevention: HIV and COVID-19 basics. Atlanta, GA, Centers for Disease Control and Prevention, 2022. Available at: https://www.cdc.gov/hiv/basics/covid-19.html. Accessed February 2022.

HIV.gov: U.S. statistics. Available at: https://www.hiv.gov/hiv-basics/overview/data-and-trends/statistics. Accessed July 2021.

National Institutes of Health: HIV overview: HIV testing. Bethesda, MD, National Institutes of Health, 2021. Available at: https://hivinfo.nih.gov/understanding-hiv/fact-sheets/hiv-testing. Accessed July 2021.

Ntusi NAB: HIV and myocarditis. Curr Opin HIV AIDS 12(6):561–565, 2017

Parashar S, Collins AB, Montaner JS, et al: Reducing rates of preventable HIV/AIDS-associated mortality among people living with HIV who inject drugs. Curr Opin HIV AIDS 11(5):507–513, 2016

Post JJ, Benfield T, Woolley I: When pandemics collide: measuring the impact of coronavirus disease 2019 on people with HIV. AIDS 36(3):473–474, 2022

Sigel K, Makinson A, Thaler J. Lung cancer in persons with HIV. Curr Opin HIV AIDS 12(1):31–38, 2017

Thakur KT, Boubour A, Saylor D, et al: Global HIV neurology: a comprehensive review. AIDS 33(2):163–184, 2019

Huntington's disease (HD)

Clinical findings	HD is a rare hereditary brain disorder that begins with abnormal early brain development and is characterized by inexorable neural degeneration that usually becomes clinically apparent around age 40 years. Motor, cognitive, and psychiatric symptoms are then progressive over subsequent decades. Both sexes are affected equally.
	Typically, patients present with chorea, with depression present in almost half of patients in the first year. Personality changes are seen in two-thirds of patients within 2–3 years. Psychosis then occurs in about 10% of patients within 3–5 years. Dementia ultimately develops in almost all patients after about 5 years. Structural and functional brain changes visible on neuroimaging may predate symptoms by more than a decade, with the earliest changes seen in the striatum. Over time, the neocortex is affected, beginning anteriorly and moving to occipital areas in later stages.
	HD is caused by a mutation in the huntingtin gene (*HTT*), which codes for a protein with a critical role in prenatal brain development. One area of the gene contains a segment of DNA known as a CAG (cytosine-adenine-guanine) trinucleotide repeat that appears several times in a row. A normal number of CAG repeats is 10–26. When more repeats are present, the CAG segment becomes unusually long. This elongated protein is processed into smaller fragments that are neurotoxic, resulting in dysfunction and death of neurons. The more repeats, the earlier the onset of clinical HD, although age at onset is modified by environmental factors and variants elsewhere in the genome. As the mutation is passed to the next generation, the size of the CAG repeat segment often increases, a phenomenon known as "anticipation." The clinical effect of anticipation is that the disease presents earlier in life and in many cases is also more severe.
	Specific neuropsychiatric symptoms of HD include irritability, depression, psychosis, personality changes, apathy, and cognitive impairment. Depression and irritability can precede motor symptoms by many years, whereas apathy and cognitive impairment tend to occur after motor symptoms. Suicidal ideation, suicide attempt, and completed suicide are more common in HD patients than in the general population. In some patients, involuntary movements may be subtle until later stages of the disease. Motor abnormalities include chorea, dystonia, ataxia, parkinsonism, oculomotor problems, dysarthria, dysphagia, incoordination, and clumsiness. Seizures can be seen.
Laboratory testing	In a patient with suggestive clinical symptoms, testing of *HTT* can be performed to show the number of CAG repeats: • 10–26 repeats—normal • 27–35 repeats—will not develop HD, but children are at risk because CAG repeat size may increase into HD range as gene is transmitted from parent to child • 36–39 repeats—may or may not develop HD • 40 or more repeats—HD will develop • 60 or more repeats—early onset HD Structural imaging shows significant volume loss in gray and white matter, particularly in subcortical areas. Functional imaging shows altered functional connectivity between regions.

Huntington's disease (HD) *(continued)*

American Psychiatric Association: Diagnostic and Statistical Manual of Mental Disorders, 5th Edition, Text Revision. Washington, DC, American Psychiatric Association, 2022

Ghosh R, Tabrizi SJ: Clinical features of Huntington's disease. Adv Exp Med Biol 1049:1–28, 2018

Gregory S, Scahill RI: Functional magnetic resonance imaging in Huntington's disease. Int Rev Neurobiol 142:381–408, 2018

Johnson EB, Gregory S: Huntington's disease: brain imaging in Huntington's disease. Prog Mol Biol Transl Sci 165:321–369, 2019

Johnson EB, Ziegler G, Penny W, et al: Dynamics of cortical degeneration over a decade in Huntington's disease. Biol Psychiatry 89(8):807–816, 2021 [published correction appears in Biol Psychiatry 90(4):275 and 90(7):505, 2021]

Kachian ZR, Cohen-Zimerman S, Bega D, et al: Suicidal ideation and behavior in Huntington's disease: systematic review and recommendations. J Affect Disord 250:319–329, 2019

McAllister B, Gusella JF, Landwehrmeyer GB, et al: Timing and impact of psychiatric, cognitive, and motor abnormalities in Huntington disease. Neurology 96(19):e2395–e2406, 2021

McColgan P, Tabrizi SJ: Huntington's disease: a clinical review. Eur J Neurol 25(1):24–34, 2018

van der Plas E, Langbehn DR, Conrad AL, et al: Abnormal brain development in child and adolescent carriers of mutant huntingtin. Neurology 93(10):e1021–e1030, 2019

Hydrocephalus

Clinical findings	Hydrocephalus refers to the abnormal accumulation of CSF in the ventricles of the brain, caused by obstruction of the flow of CSF, problems with absorption of CSF into the venous system, or overproduction. Several systems of hydrocephalus classification exist, one of which divides this condition into two types, based on anatomy:
	• *Communicating hydrocephalus*, in which CSF flow is blocked after it leaves the ventricles. This type is also called nonobstructive because there is still CSF flow within the ventricular system.
	• *Noncommunicating hydrocephalus*, in which CSF flow is blocked within the ventricular system, usually in one of the narrow connecting passages. This type is also called obstructive hydrocephalus.
	Communicating hydrocephalus has two subtypes: NPH and hydrocephalus ex vacuo. NPH, which typically affects individuals age 50 years or older, develops slowly, with gradual buildup of CSF that enlarges the ventricles and exerts pressure on adjacent brain structures. NPH symptoms that result include the classic triad of urinary incontinence, memory problems, and gait unsteadiness. Although NPH can be a consequence of stroke, subarachnoid hemorrhage, tumor, TBI, meningitis, or brain surgery, in most cases it is idiopathic. In hydrocephalus ex vacuo, the ventricles enlarge to fill space created by the loss of brain tissue from conditions such as Alzheimer's disease, multiple strokes, leukodystrophies, multiple sclerosis, and Huntington's disease.
	Signs and symptoms of hydrocephalus typically include the following:
	• In non-elderly adults: headache, visual problems, nausea/vomiting, incoordination, balance problems, decline in school or work performance, difficulty waking up, sleepiness, irritability, personality changes, cognitive problems, and frequent urination or loss of bladder control.
	• In elderly patients: magnetic gait (feet appear stuck to the floor), memory impairment, motor and cognitive slowing, depression, apathy, and urinary urgency, frequency, or incontinence. Hyperreflexia, extensor plantar responses, and primitive reflexes (grasp and snout) may be present.
	Patients with acute hydrocephalus present *in extremis* with headache, vomiting, and stupor. Papilledema may be noted. These patients are at risk of rapid progression to coma and death. This form of hydrocephalus is usually a noncommunicating form, with complete or nearly complete obstruction of CSF flow.
Laboratory testing	Brain MRI can be used to evaluate size of ventricles, assess CSF flow to identify the site of obstruction, and detect changes in the tissue surrounding the lateral ventricles suggestive of transependymal CSF extravasation. Head CT can be used only to determine ventricular size and detect tissue changes of extravasation.
	In hydrocephalus ex vacuo, sulcal enlargement is seen in tandem with ventricular enlargement, and changes of transependymal CSF extravasation are not seen.
	Lumbar puncture may be performed to check CSF pressure and to obtain a CSF sample to identify blood and infectious causes of hydrocephalus.
	Funduscopic examination can also identify elevated CSF pressure.

Hydrocephalus *(continued)*

Factora R, Luciano M: When to consider normal pressure hydrocephalus in the patient with gait disturbance. Geriatrics 63:32–37, 2008

Filis AK, Aghayev K, Vrionis FD: Cerebrospinal fluid and hydrocephalus: physiology, diagnosis, and treatment. Cancer Control 24(1):6–8, 2017

Kameda M, Kajimoto Y, Kambara A, et al: Evaluation of the effectiveness of the tap test by combining the use of functional gait assessment and global rating of change. Front Neurol 13:846429, 2022

Nakajima M, Yamada S, Miyajima M, et al: Guidelines for Management of Idiopathic Normal Pressure Hydrocephalus (Third Edition): endorsed by the Japanese Society of Normal Pressure Hydrocephalus. Neurol Med Chir (Tokyo) 61(2):63–97, 2021

Said HM, Kaya D, Yavuz I, et al: A comparison of cerebrospinal fluid beta-amyloid and tau in idiopathic normal pressure hydrocephalus and neurodegenerative dementias. Clin Interv Aging 17:467–477, 2022

Theologou M, Natsis K, Kouskouras K, et al: Cerebrospinal fluid homeostasis and hydrodynamics: a review of facts and theories. Eur Neurol 85(4):313–325, 2022

Yusim A, Anbarasan D, Bernstein C, et al: Normal pressure hydrocephalus presenting as Othello syndrome: case presentation and review of the literature. Am J Psychiatry 165:1119–1125, 2008

Hypercalcemia

Clinical findings	Calcium, the most abundant extracellular cation in the body, has essential roles in neurotransmission, cardiac function, muscle contraction, blood clotting, and bone formation. Only 1% of calcium is found in the circulation, with the remainder residing in the bones and teeth. The level of calcium is kept within a physiological range through the actions of PTH and vitamin D. The most common causes of calcium elevation are primary hyperparathyroidism (slight to moderate elevation) and malignancy-associated hypercalcemia (high elevation). The latter is seen with more advanced cancers and carries a poor prognosis.
	Other causes of hypercalcemia include drugs (lithium, thiazides, excessive intake of antacids or calcium supplements, toxicity with vitamins A or D), granulomatous disease such as sarcoidosis or coccidioidomycosis, adrenal insufficiency, and chronic kidney disease. The mechanism by which lithium can induce hypercalcemia is by way of primary hyperparathyroidism.
	Most patients with hypercalcemia are asymptomatic, particularly with gradual onset of calcium elevation, and the condition is found only on routine testing. Symptoms are not usually seen until the total calcium level exceeds 12 mg/dL, although patients with a low albumin level may show symptoms at a lower (uncorrected) calcium level. Free or ionized calcium correlates more closely with symptoms, but this test is usually only available in hospital settings. Total calcium can be corrected for low albumin as described in the **Albumin** entry in the *Laboratory Tests* chapter.
	Signs and symptoms associated with elevated calcium level include irritability, anxiety, depression, fatigue, lethargy, weakness, apathy, decreased muscle tone, muscle pain, flat deep tendon reflexes, headache, increased thirst, increased urine output or urinary frequency, nausea, vomiting, constipation, loss of appetite, and flank or abdominal pain that may be colicky in nature. With more severe elevations, delirium, cardiac toxicity (including dysrhythmias), seizures, and coma occur. With extreme elevation, death may ensue.
Laboratory testing	Because most patients with hypercalcemia are asymptomatic even though the condition can cause end-organ damage, it is important to identify patients who should be screened. These include those with kidney stones, osteopenia/osteoporosis, or intestinal diseases and those taking the drugs listed above.
	The initial step in testing is to measure the patient's serum calcium level. This can be total calcium or ionized calcium; the latter is recommended for patients with abnormally high or low serum protein levels, multiple myeloma, macroglobulinemia, or thrombocytosis. The ionized calcium test is not widely available. The total calcium value can be corrected for low albumin levels using the equation noted in the **Calcium** entry in the *Laboratory Tests* chapter.
	The reference range for total serum calcium in adults is roughly 8.6–10.4 mg/dL.
	The reference range for ionized calcium in adults is 4.64–5.28 mg/dL.
	Hypercalcemia is defined by a total serum calcium level >10.5 mg/dL.
	• Mild hypercalcemia: 10.5–12 mg/dL
	• Moderate hypercalcemia: 12.1–14 mg/dL

Hypercalcemia *(continued)*

Laboratory testing *(continued)*	• Severe hypercalcemia: >14 mg/dL • Total calcium >13 mg/dL: cardiac toxicity, dysrhythmias, delirium, seizures, and coma • Total calcium >18 mg/dL: may be fatal • Free (ionized) calcium >7.0 mg/dL: coma The second step in the evaluation of hypercalcemia is to measure the serum level of PTH. A high or inadequately suppressed PTH level indicates hyperparathyroidism as the cause. Other laboratory tests include assay of vitamin D, total protein, albumin, phosphate, creatinine, and ECG. The latter may show characteristic changes such as shortened QTc interval, widened QRS, and prolonged PR interval.

Guise TA, Wysolmerski JJ: Cancer-associated hypercalcemia. N Engl J Med 386(15):1443–1451, 2022

Ioachimescu AG: Hypercalcemia and its multiple facets. Endocrinol Metab Clin North Am 50(4):xiii–xiv, 2021

Minisola S, Pepe J, Piemonte S, Cipriani C: The diagnosis and management of hypercalcaemia. BMJ 350:h2723, 2015

Sell J, Ramirez S, Partin M: Parathyroid disorders. Am Fam Physician 105(3):289–298, 2022

Tonon CR, Silva TAAL, Pereira FWL, et al: A review of current clinical concepts in the pathophysiology, etiology, diagnosis, and management of hypercalcemia. Med Sci Monit 28:e935821, 2022

Turner JJO: Hypercalcaemia: presentation and management. Clin Med (Lond) 17(3):270–273, 2017

Hyperglycemia

Clinical findings	Hyperglycemia is defined by the following blood glucose levels: • >125 mg/dL in the fasting state • >180 mg/dL 2 hours after eating Diabetes—the most common cause of persistent hyperglycemia—is discussed separately in the **Diabetes Mellitus** entry. Other causes of hyperglycemia include the following: • Acute stress response (e.g., in critical illness or postoperative state) • Pregnancy • Pancreatic tissue destruction from chronic pancreatitis, cystic fibrosis, cancer, or hemochromatosis • Endocrine disorders causing insulin resistance, such as Cushing's syndrome, acromegaly, and pheochromocytoma • Use of drugs such as diuretics, corticosteroids, phenytoin, TCAs, β-blockers, dextrothyroxine, epinephrine, estrogens, glucagon, isoniazid, lithium, or phenothiazines • Chronic renal failure • Glucagonoma • Total parenteral nutrition with dextrose infusion Signs and symptoms of hyperglycemia include polydipsia, polyuria, hypotension, tachycardia, headache, and blurred vision. With persistence and further elevation, altered mental status, lethargy, and focal neurological signs may be observed.
Laboratory testing	The panic value for glucose in both males and females is >400 mg/dL. Dipstick urinalysis can return quick results for glucose and ketones in urine. Other laboratory tests include serum electrolytes, BUN, creatinine, and CBC. Blood gases may be required if serum bicarbonate is significantly reduced. Serum and urine osmolality help diagnose diabetic ketoacidosis and hyperglycemic hyperosmolar nonketotic state.

Marik PE, Bellomo R: Stress hyperglycemia: an essential survival response! Crit Care 17(2):305, 2013

Mouri M, Badireddy M: Hyperglycemia, in StatPearls. Treasure Island, FL, StatPearls Publishing, 2022. Available at: https://www.ncbi.nlm.nih.gov/books/NBK430900. Accessed April 2022.

Perez A, Jansen-Chaparro S, Saigi I, et al: Glucocorticoid-induced hyperglycemia. J Diabetes 6(1):9–20, 2014

Pratiwi C, Zulkifly S, Dahlan TF, et al: Hospital related hyperglycemia as a predictor of mortality in non-diabetes patients: a systematic review. Diabetes Metab Syndr 15(6):102309, 2021

Roszali MA, Zakaria AN, Mohd Tahir NA: Parenteral nutrition-associated hyperglycemia: prevalence, predictors and management. Clin Nutr ESPEN 41:275–280, 2021

Scheen M, Giraud R, Bendjelid K: Stress hyperglycemia, cardiac glucotoxicity, and critically ill patient outcomes current clinical and pathophysiological evidence. Physiol Rep 9(2):e14713, 2021

Hyperkalemia

Clinical findings	Hyperkalemia is defined by a serum potassium level >5 mEq/L. Calcium elevation occurs because of reduced renal excretion (persistent elevation) and/or a shift of intracellular potassium to the extracellular space (transient elevation).
	Causes of hyperkalemia include the following:
	• Chronic renal failure/insufficiency
	• Systemic illness, dehydration, or the introduction of potassium-elevating drugs
	• Increased potassium intake in patients with renal insufficiency
	• Tissue injury: trauma, burns, tumor lysis, massive hemolysis, or rhabdomyolysis
	• Insulin deficiency
	• Exercise in the presence of β-blockers
	• Hyperchloremic metabolic acidosis with a normal anion gap
	• Hypertonic states such as hyperglycemia
	• Endocrine disease such as Addison's disease or primary hypoaldosteronism
	• SLE
	• *Drugs:* ACE inhibitors, angiotensin receptor blockers, potassium-sparing diuretics, potassium salts, succinylcholine, NSAIDs, and certain laxatives
	Signs and symptoms of hyperkalemia include bradycardia, weakness, ileus or diarrhea, low urine output, muscular irritability, tremors, fasciculations, paresthesias, and flaccid paralysis. The latter is an ascending paralysis leading to flaccid quadriplegia with sparing of the trunk, head, and respiratory muscles. Characteristic ECG changes are listed in the *Laboratory Testing* section below.
	Hyperkalemia can represent a medical emergency. Factors determining severity include not only the level of elevation but also the rapidity with which it develops and the duration of elevation. Patients with a rapid rise in serum potassium, ECG changes, reduced renal function, or significant acidosis must be treated urgently.
Laboratory testing	Spurious elevation of potassium can occur, mostly related to specimen handling and transport problems, as noted in the **Potassium** entry in the *Laboratory Tests* chapter. Spurious elevation can be suspected when a patient has normal renal function, normal serum bicarbonate, and/or a normal ECG. Spurious elevation can be confirmed by repeating potassium measurements in both serum and plasma; in this case, the serum potassium will be elevated but the plasma potassium will be normal.
	In addition to close monitoring of the potassium level, laboratory tests include the following:
	• ECG
	• BUN and creatinine
	• Electrolytes
	• Spot urine testing for potassium, creatinine, and osmoles

Hyperkalemia *(continued)*

Laboratory testing *(continued)*	ECG changes emerge when the potassium level is ≥6.0 mEq/L, although threshold depends in part on the rate of rise. Progression of ECG changes is as follows:
	• Tall, peaked T waves (higher than R waves)
	• ST segment depression
	• Prolonged PR interval
	• QRS widening
	• Reduced or absent P waves
	• Sine wave pattern: impending ventricular fibrillation and asystole

Ben Salem C, Badreddine A, Fathallah N, et al: Drug-induced hyperkalemia. Drug Saf 37(9):677–692, 2014

Hollander-Rodriguez JC, Calvert JF Jr: Hyperkalemia. Am Fam Physician 73(2):283–290, 2006

Littmann L, Gibbs MA: Electrocardiographic manifestations of severe hyperkalemia. J Electrocardiol 51(5):814–817, 2018

Montford JR, Linas S: How dangerous is hyperkalemia? J Am Soc Nephrol 28(11):3155–3165, 2017

Palmer BF, Clegg DJ: Diagnosis and treatment of hyperkalemia. Cleve Clin J Med 84(12):934–942, 2017

Hypermagnesemia

Clinical findings	Hypermagnesemia is defined by a serum magnesium level >2.6 mg/dL. It usually occurs in the presence of renal insufficiency or failure, often in an elderly patient with recent ingestion of magnesium-containing laxatives or antacids. Although it is not a common derangement, it can be fatal if it remains untreated.
	Causes of hypermagnesemia include the following:
	• Decreased renal excretion (acute or chronic renal insufficiency or failure)
	• Hyperparathyroidism
	• *Drugs*: lithium, certain antacids, certain laxatives
	• Increased intake of laxatives, antacids, bowel preps
	• Milk-alkali syndrome
	• Treatment of eclampsia with IV magnesium sulfate
	• Compartment shift: hemolysis, tumor lysis, rhabdomyolysis, acidosis
	The risk of developing hypermagnesemia is heightened in the presence of alcohol use disorder, malnutrition, hypothyroidism, and adrenal insufficiency.
	Signs and symptoms of hypermagnesemia include the following:
	• Mild elevation (<7 mg/dL): asymptomatic or nonspecific symptoms of nausea, dizziness, weakness, and confusion
	• Moderate elevation (7–12 mg/dL): hypotension, bradycardia, blurred vision, psychomotor retardation, hyporeflexia, sleepiness, worsening confusion, headache, flushing, constipation, and bladder dysfunction
	• Severe elevation (>12 mg/dL): worsening hypotension and bradycardia, arrhythmias, ECG changes, flaccid paralysis, respiratory depression, and lethargy
	• Very severe elevation (>15 mg/dL): cardiorespiratory arrest and coma
Laboratory testing	Normal serum magnesium levels:
	• <60 years: 1.6–2.6 mg/dL
	• 60–90 years: 1.6–2.4 mg/dL
	• >90 years: 1.7–2.3 mg/dL
	Laboratory evaluation for suspected hypermagnesemia includes the following:
	• Serum magnesium level
	• ECG
	• Renal evaluation: BUN, creatinine, eGFR, urine specific gravity
	• Arterial blood gases
	• Urine output quantification
	• Potassium, phosphate, and calcium levels (serum and urine)

Barra A, Camardese G, Tonioni F, et al: Plasma magnesium level and psychomotor retardation in major depressed patients. Magnes Res 20(4):245–249, 2007

Bokhari SR, Siriki R, Teran FJ, Batuman V: Fatal hypermagnesemia due to laxative use. Am J Med Sci 355(4):390–395, 2018

Hypermagnesemia *(continued)*

Brackenridge CJ, Jones IH: Relation of hypermagnesaemia to activity and neuroleptic drug therapy in schizophrenic states. J Neurol Neurosurg Psychiatry 34(2):195–199, 1971

Felsenfeld AJ, Levine BS, Rodriguez M: Pathophysiology of calcium, phosphorus, and magnesium dysregulation in chronic kidney disease. Semin Dial 28(6):564–577, 2015

Sawalha K, Kakkera K: Acute respiratory failure from hypermagnesemia requiring prolonged mechanical ventilation. J Investig Med High Impact Case Rep 8:2324709620984898, 2020

Stevens JS, Moses AA, Nickolas TL, et al: Increased mortality associated with hypermagnesemia in severe COVID-19 illness. Kidney360 2(7):1087–1094, 2021

Takahashi M, Uchino N: Risk factors of hypermagnesemia in end-stage cancer patients hospitalized in a palliative care unit. Ann Palliat Med 9(6):4308–4314, 2020

Van Laecke S: Hypomagnesemia and hypermagnesemia. Acta Clin Belg 74(1):41–47, 2019

Walker P, Parnell S, Dillon RC: Epsom salt ingestion leading to severe hypermagnesemia necessitating dialysis. J Emerg Med 58(5):767–770, 2020

Yamaguchi H, Shimada H, Yoshita K, et al: Severe hypermagnesemia induced by magnesium oxide ingestion: a case series. CEN Case Rep 8(1):31–37, 2019

Hypernatremia

Clinical findings	Hypernatremia is defined by a serum sodium concentration >145 mEq/L. It represents a state of total body water deficiency, either absolute or relative to total body sodium (and potassium). It is a consequence of water loss, hypotonic fluid loss, or hypertonic fluid gain. It is more common in elderly patients, those lacking the ability to monitor their thirst and drinking behavior, and in those who are critically ill. This is a potentially serious condition, particularly when the sodium elevation is large or occurs rapidly. The short-term mortality rate is as high as 60%.
	Usually, the cause of hypernatremia becomes apparent with the history and physical exam. Most cases result from water loss, either through the kidneys (diabetes insipidus), GI tract (vomiting or osmotic diarrhea), lungs (hyperventilation), or skin (diaphoresis). Cases resulting from hypertonic fluid gain are usually iatrogenic. On psychiatry services, hypernatremia occurs with lithium use (nephrogenic diabetes insipidus), excessive fluid loss (significant vomiting or diarrhea), and the use of restraints or seclusion rooms where access to water is restricted.
	Adult patients may be asymptomatic or may exhibit signs of CNS dysfunction such as irritability, somnolence, restlessness, weakness, nausea, chorea, myoclonus, myalgia, muscle cramps, altered mental status, delirium, or coma. The level of consciousness is correlated with the degree of hypernatremia. Hypovolemia is associated with orthostatic hypotension and tachycardia. Cellular dehydration causes brain shrinkage, with complications such as subdural hematoma and intracerebral hemorrhage that may cause permanent brain injury or death. Further complications include seizures and rhabdomyolysis.
Laboratory testing	In the evaluation of the patient who presents with hypernatremia (sodium >145 mEq/L), the first question to ask is why the patient is not drinking water. Nursing home patients with cognitive impairment, for example, might be relying on others to provide fluids.
	An algorithm for the workup of hypernatremia is as follows:
	• If the physical exam demonstrates hypovolemia or euvolemia, assess urine flow rate.
	• A urine flow rate ≥30 mL/hour indicates renal loss of hypotonic fluid.
	• A urine flow rate <30 mL/hour indicates hypotonic fluid loss from outside the kidney.
	• With renal loss, check urine osmolality.
	• Urine osmolality >300 mOsm/kg H_2O indicates osmotic diuresis.
	• Urine osmolality <300 mOsm/kg H_2O indicates water diuresis.
	• In the case of water diuresis, check either the copeptin level or plasma osmolality to compare with urine osmolality in order to distinguish central from nephrogenic diabetes insipidus.

Adrogué HJ, Madias NE: Hypernatremia. N Engl J Med 342(20):1493–1499, 2000

Braun MM, Barstow CH, Pyzocha NJ: Diagnosis and management of sodium disorders: hyponatremia and hypernatremia. Am Fam Physician 91(5):299–307, 2015

Kamel KS, Schreiber M, Harel Z: Hypernatremia. JAMA 327(8):774–775, 2022

Liamis G, Filippatos TD, Elisaf MS: Evaluation and treatment of hypernatremia: a practical guide for physicians. Postgrad Med 128(3):299–306, 2016

Muhsin SA, Mount DB: Diagnosis and treatment of hypernatremia. Best Pract Res Clin Endocrinol Metab 30(2):189–203, 2016

Qian Q: Hypernatremia. Clin J Am Soc Nephrol 14(3):432–434, 2019

Reynolds RM, Padfield PL, Seckl JR: Disorders of sodium balance. BMJ 332:702–705, 2006

Hyperparathyroidism

Clinical findings	Primary hyperparathyroidism (PHPT), characterized by mild to moderate elevation of serum calcium levels with non-suppressed or high levels of PTH, is most often caused by a single parathyroid adenoma. The disease primarily targets the kidneys and the skeleton, causing kidney stones and cortical bone loss with increased risk of fracture. It is also associated with an increased risk of hypertension and cardiac changes that may have a fatal outcome. Neuropsychiatric symptoms including anxiety, depression, poor concentration, and memory impairment are often reported. PHPT is relatively common, particularly in females older than 50 years. It is usually discovered when slightly elevated calcium is found on routine chemistry testing. At this stage, the patient is usually asymptomatic but may present with kidney stones, bone pain, or fracture. Long-term treatment with lithium can mimic PHPT laboratory values.
Laboratory testing	Laboratory evaluation for PHPT includes the following: • Ionized or corrected serum calcium (elevated) • Intact PTH level (normal or elevated) • 25-hydroxyvitamin D level (normal or low-normal) • GFR (normal) • 24-hour urine calcium excretion (elevated) • Bone density evaluation including the distal third of the radius • Renal ultrasound to detect stones

Bilezikian JP, Bandeira L, Khan A, Cusano NE: Hyperparathyroidism. Lancet 391(10116):168–178, 2018

Clarke BL: Asymptomatic primary hyperparathyroidism. Front Horm Res 51:13–22, 2019

Insogna KL: Primary hyperparathyroidism. N Engl J Med 379(11):1050–1059, 2018

Khan AA, Hanley DA, Rizzoli R, et al: Primary hyperparathyroidism: review and recommendations on evaluation, diagnosis, and management: a Canadian and international consensus. Osteoporos Int 28(1):1–19, 2017

Masi L: Primary hyperparathyroidism. Front Horm Res 51:1–12, 2019

Walker MD, Bilezikian JP: Primary hyperparathyroidism: recent advances. Curr Opin Rheumatol 30(4):427–439, 2018

Hypertensive encephalopathy

Clinical findings	Hypertensive encephalopathy is a clinical syndrome associated with the subacute onset of extreme hypertension, with a systolic blood pressure often >220 mmHg or a diastolic blood pressure >130 mmHg. The degree of hypertension required to develop the syndrome in a given patient depends on their premorbid blood pressure; for example, a previously normotensive person could develop encephalopathy at blood pressures of 160/100 mmHg. Hypertensive encephalopathy is a medical emergency requiring immediate treatment to lower blood pressure in all patients.
	The mechanism by which hypertension causes encephalopathy is thought to be a failure of autoregulation in the cerebral vasculature when the upper limit of autoregulation is exceeded, usually when the diastolic blood pressure exceeds 120 mmHg. At that point, massive constriction and reflex vasodilation of cerebral arterioles occur, giving rise to vasogenic edema that can be seen on neuroimaging.
	This syndrome overlaps with posterior reversible encephalopathy syndrome (PRES), which has more region-specific pathology either in the posterior supratentorial structures or the brainstem. PRES can also be identified in normotensive individuals in whom autoimmune disease, sepsis, renal disease, preeclampsia, or the use of cytotoxic drugs has caused vascular injury.
	Clinical presentation often involves a patient with chronically uncontrolled hypertension who recently stopped antihypertensive therapy. Underlying causes include acute or chronic kidney disease, autoimmune disorders, endocrine disorders, porphyria, thermal injury, TBI, autonomic hyperactivity, scorpion envenomation, cocaine or amphetamine abuse, tyramine reactions with MAOI treatment, and use of stimulants such as ephedrine, pseudoephedrine, or caffeine.
	Signs and symptoms of hypertensive encephalopathy typically include gradual onset of headache, nausea, and vomiting followed by neuropsychiatric symptoms of restlessness, confusion, delirium, stupor, seizures, and, in some cases, coma. Papilledema and visual changes may be noted. When neurological deficits are seen, they are not localized in the same manner as with PRES or a space-occupying lesion but instead indicate global cerebral dysfunction. End-organ injury from hypertension may also be seen in the kidneys, heart, and retinas, the latter showing retinal hemorrhages and exudates.
Laboratory testing	The diagnosis of hypertensive encephalopathy is based on clinical findings, but neuroimaging can be helpful by demonstrating the presence of vasogenic cerebral edema. MRI with T2-weighted and FLAIR sequences is preferred to CT for this purpose.
	Lumbar puncture may be performed to assist in the differential diagnosis of encephalopathy. Mild to modestly elevated protein levels without pleocytosis can be seen. Elevated intracranial pressure may be noted.
	Other diagnostic procedures may be needed to evaluate end-organ injury and identify potential causes of secondary hypertension, including ECG, chest X-ray or CT, urinalysis, cardiac enzymes, and BMP or CMP. Serum or urine pregnancy testing should be performed for patients of childbearing age. Urine drug screening should be considered if there is concern about stimulant use, but this will not detect over-the-counter drugs.

Hypertensive encephalopathy *(continued)*

Christopoulou F, Rizos EC, Kosta P, et al: Does this patient have hypertensive encephalopathy? J Am Soc Hypertens 10(5):399–403, 2016

Dunphy L, Kothari T, Ford J: Posterior reversible encephalopathy syndrome in the puerperium: a case report. BMJ Case Rep 15(1):e246570, 2022

Fischer M, Schmutzhard E: Posterior reversible encephalopathy syndrome. J Neurol 264(8):1608–1616, 2017

Gewirtz AN, Gao V, Parauda SC, Robbins MS: Posterior reversible encephalopathy syndrome. Curr Pain Headache Rep 25(3):19, 2021

Gifford RW Jr, Westbrook E: Hypertensive encephalopathy: mechanisms, clinical features, and treatment. Prog Cardiovasc Dis 17:115–124, 1974

Miller JB, Suchdev K, Jayaprakash N, et al: New developments in hypertensive encephalopathy. Curr Hypertens Rep 20(2):13, 2018

Tan YY, Tan K: Hypertensive brainstem encephalopathy: a diagnosis often overlooked. Clin Med (Lond) 19(6):511–513, 2019

Thambisetty M, Biousse V, Newman NJ: Hypertensive brainstem encephalopathy: clinical and radiographic features. J Neurol Sci 208:93–99, 2003

Hypocalcemia

Clinical findings	Calcium is an essential micronutrient with important roles in neuro-transmission, cardiac function, muscle contraction, blood clotting, and bone formation. The calcium level is maintained within a physiological range through the actions of PTH and vitamin D. Only ~1% of the body's calcium is in circulation, half bound to albumin and half in the free or ionized form. When the albumin level drops, the total calcium level drops as well, but the concentration of free calcium is unaffected. For this reason, the total calcium value is corrected when the albumin level is low, using the formula *corrected calcium* = [4 g/dL − plasma albumin] × 0.8 + total serum calcium. Alternatively, free calcium can be measured directly, but in this case, the specimen requires special handling and expedited processing.
	Hypocalcemia is defined by a corrected total calcium level ≤8 mg/dL and/or the presence of symptoms. The primary causes of hypocalcemia can be divided into PTH-mediated and non-PTH-mediated, the former represented by parathyroid deficiency after thyroid or parathyroid surgery and the latter by vitamin D deficiency. Risk factors for deficiency of vitamin D include limited sun exposure, skin pigmentation, and age-related thinning of the skin.
	Other causes of hypocalcemia include acute pancreatitis, renal failure, malnutrition, malabsorption due to GI disease, elevated phosphate levels (e.g., from laxative abuse), severe osteomalacia, and the use of drugs such as bisphosphonates, cisplatin, antiepileptics, diuretics, aminoglycosides, or proton pump inhibitors.
	The signs and symptoms of hypocalcemia depend on the rapidity of its development and the severity of the calcium reduction. Acutely developing hypocalcemia can be a medical emergency, with delirium, seizures, cardiac arrhythmias, QT prolongation, heart failure, laryngospasm, and bronchospasm. Almost any organ system can be affected, and the condition can be life-threatening.
	In contrast, gradually developing hypocalcemia can be asymptomatic, discovered only on routine health screening, or can be characterized by signs of neuromuscular irritability such as paresthesias, muscle twitching and spasm, and tetany. Carpopedal spasm is a classic sign. When neuromuscular signs are not apparent, they can sometimes be elicited by provocations such as tapping on the facial nerve just in front of the tragus to induce twitching of the mouth (Chvostek's sign) or inflating a blood pressure cuff above the systolic pressure for ≤3 minutes to induce carpal spasm (Trousseau's sign). Other signs and symptoms include anxiety, depression, irritability, fatigue, apathy, lethargy, weakness, anorexia, nausea, vomiting, constipation, polyuria, polydipsia, bone pain, and seizures. Chronic hypocalcemia can be associated with calcification in the lens of the eye, basal ganglia, cerebellum, and cerebral cortex.
Laboratory testing	An acute drop in total serum calcium to 8 mg/dL may cause symptoms, whereas gradual decline to 7 mg/dL may be asymptomatic. Most patients show symptoms when total calcium is at or around 6 mg/dL (ionized calcium <2 mg/dL). At this level and below, tetany and seizures are seen.

Hypocalcemia *(continued)*

Laboratory testing *(continued)*	To diagnose the cause of hypocalcemia, initial laboratory testing includes the following:
	• Serum calcium (corrected)
	• Electrolyte panel
	• Phosphate
	• Magnesium
	• Creatinine
	• ALP
	• PTH
	• 25-hydroxy vitamin D
	• Serum pH
	• CBC
	Cooper and Gittoes (2008; see below) offered a useful chart to help identify the cause of hypocalcemia with the results of these initial tests.
	Further investigations may include ionized calcium, renal ultrasound, 1,25-dihydroxy vitamin D, and 24-hour urinary measures of phosphate, calcium, magnesium, and creatinine. Testing for genetic mutations and evaluation of first-degree relatives may be indicated.

Calpena Martínez S, Arapiles Muñoz A: The value of the classic signs: hypocalcemia. Med Clin (Barc) 157(11):554, 2021

Cooper MS, Gittoes NJ: Diagnosis and management of hypocalcaemia. BMJ 336(7656):1298–1302, 2008 [published correction appears in BMJ 336(7659), 2008]

Fong J, Khan A: Hypocalcemia: updates in diagnosis and management for primary care. Can Fam Physician 58(2):158–162, 2012

Giusti F, Brandi ML: Clinical presentation of hypoparathyroidism. Front Horm Res 51:139–146, 2019

Hakami Y, Khan A: Hypoparathyroidism. Front Horm Res 51:109–126, 2019

Lawlor BA: Hypocalcemia, hypoparathyroidism, and organic anxiety syndrome. J Clin Psychiatry 49(8):317–318, 1988

Pepe J, Colangelo L, Biamonte F, et al: Diagnosis and management of hypocalcemia. Endocrine 69(3):485–495, 2020

Sapountzi P, Emanuele NV, Loutrianakis E, et al: Visual vignette. Diagnosis: hypocalcemia due to primary hypoparathyroidism. Endocr Pract 12:233, 2006

Teisseyre M, Moranne O, Renaud S: Late diagnosis of chronic hypocalcemia due to autoimmune hypoparathyroidism. BMJ Case Rep 14(6):e243299, 2021

Hypoglycemia

Clinical findings	Hypoglycemia is most often seen in patients treated for diabetes. Initial autonomic symptoms include hunger, sweating, palpitations, tremor, anxiety, and paresthesias. Without intervention, a further decline in glucose may result in brain glucose deprivation, with symptoms such as the following:
	• Behavioral changes, including agitation and aggression
	• Irritability
	• Depersonalization
	• Panic attacks
	• Confusion
	• Blurred vision
	• Slurred speech
	• Dizziness
	• Fatigue, lethargy
	• Headache
	• Transient focal neurological deficits
	• Seizures
	• Loss of consciousness, coma
	Because these symptoms are not specific to hypoglycemia, it is important to establish and document a link between the two before initiating a workup to determine the underlying cause. Not only should characteristic symptoms and low blood glucose values be present, but symptoms should resolve with correction of glucose. It may be necessary to simulate the conditions under which hypoglycemia is said to have occurred. For example, if the problem is postprandial, a meal should be provided, followed by glucose testing. The general rule of thumb, however, is that any person with diabetes who is taking antidiabetic medication and whose behavior is in any way odd is considered hypoglycemic until proven otherwise.
	Among insulin-treated diabetics, the annual incidence of hypoglycemia is up to 40% of those with type 1 diabetes and up to 30% of those with type 2 diabetes. Oral drugs for diabetes can also cause hypoglycemia, as can anabolic steroids, propranolol, and MAOIs. Non-drug causes include the following:
	• Insulinoma
	• Hypothyroidism
	• Hypopituitarism
	• Addison's disease
	• Autoimmune disease
	• Alcohol use disorder
	• Severe liver disease
	• End-stage renal disease
	• Post–bariatric surgery state
	• Starvation, fasting, anorexia nervosa

Hypoglycemia *(continued)*

Clinical findings *(continued)*	The risk of developing hypoglycemia is highest in elderly patients and in those with multiple comorbidities, a long duration of diabetes, or a prior history of hypoglycemia, even if mild. Dietary factors such as delaying or skipping meals or inadequate consumption of carbohydrates contribute to risk.
	The sequelae of hypoglycemia depend on the severity and duration of the deficiency. Severe hypoglycemia can cause brain injury, coma, and death if not treated emergently. Mild hypoglycemia, when prolonged, can cause peripheral nerve injury. Recurrent hypoglycemia is associated with cognitive deficits, particularly in executive function, and current hypoglycemia with attentional and memory impairment. Nocturnal hypoglycemia may increase the risk of cardiac events because blood sugar values at night can be very low and of long duration and may not easily be detected.
Laboratory testing	Glucose values requiring urgent intervention: • Males: <50 mg/dL • Females: <40 mg/dL The lower limit of normal for fasting glucose is ~70 mg/dL, but lower levels can occur normally after meals. Various definitions of hypoglycemia set the glucose threshold at slightly different levels. One reasonable definition is as follows: glucose level <55 mg/dL (by a reliable method) with characteristic symptoms that are relieved when glucose level is raised. Glucose monitors are not considered reliable gauges at low glucose levels. While the patient is symptomatic, check • Blood glucose (<55 mg/dL) • Insulin level (considered increased if >6 µL/mL) If factitious disorder is suspected, C peptide level can be checked. Both insulin level and C peptide level are increased in surreptitious use of oral hypoglycemic drugs (as well as with insulinomas). C peptide level is decreased with exogenous insulin use. Endocrinology consultation is recommended to determine what other tests are needed to investigate the underlying cause of hypoglycemia.

Benton D: Hypoglycemia and aggression: a review. Int J Neurosci 41:163–168, 1988

Galati SJ, Rayfield EJ: Approach to the patient with postprandial hypoglycemia. Endocr Pract 20(4):331–340, 2014

Grunberger G, Weiner JL, Silverman R, et al: Factitious hypoglycemia due to surreptitious administration of insulin: diagnosis, treatment, and long-term follow-up. Ann Intern Med 108:252–257, 1988

Languren G, Montiel T, Julio-Amilpas A, Massieu L: Neuronal damage and cognitive impairment associated with hypoglycemia: an integrated view. Neurochem Int 63(4):331–343, 2013

McNay EC, Cotero VE: Mini-review: impact of recurrent hypoglycemia on cognitive and brain function. Physiol Behav 100:234–238, 2010

Mohseni S: Neurologic damage in hypoglycemia. Handb Clin Neurol 126:513–532, 2014

Muneer M: Hypoglycaemia. Adv Exp Med Biol 1307:43–69, 2021

Murad MH, Coto-Yglesias F, Wang AT, et al: Clinical review: drug-induced hypoglycemia: a systematic review. J Clin Endocrinol Metab 94:741–745, 2009

Scarlett JA, Mako ME, Rubenstein AH, et al: Factitious hypoglycemia: diagnosis by measurement of serum C-peptide immunoreactivity and insulin-binding antibodies. N Engl J Med 297:1029–1032, 1977

Umpierrez G, Korytkowski M: Diabetic emergencies: ketoacidosis, hyperglycaemic hyperosmolar state and hypoglycaemia. Nat Rev Endocrinol 12(4):222–232, 2016

Hypogonadism

Clinical findings	Hypogonadism is a syndrome of sex hormone deficiency affecting both males and females. Menopause (and its counterpart in males) is the most common cause of this condition.
	Pathological causes are classified as primary or secondary. In primary hypogonadism, the problem resides with the testes or ovaries. In secondary (central) hypogonadism, the problem resides with the hypothalamus or pituitary gland. Primary hypogonadism can be genetic or can be the consequence of autoimmune disease, infection, liver disease, kidney disease, radiation to the gonads, surgery, or trauma. The most common genetic causes are Turner's syndrome in females and Klinefelter syndrome in males. Secondary hypogonadism causes include anorexia nervosa, pituitary hemorrhage, infection, malnutrition, hemochromatosis, radiation to the pituitary or hypothalamus, rapid significant weight loss, surgery adjacent to the pituitary gland, tumors, trauma, and drugs such as cortisol and opioids. Stopping high doses of anabolic steroids can result in very low testosterone levels. Kallmann syndrome is a genetic cause of secondary hypogonadism.
	Children with hypogonadism do not develop normally in terms of primary and secondary sexual characteristics. When hypogonadism develops after puberty, symptoms include the following:
	• In females: hot flashes, energy and mood changes, insomnia, irregular or absent menstruation, infertility
	• In males: hot flashes, lethargy, depression, low libido, erectile dysfunction, gynecomastia, loss of muscle mass, loss of body hair, testicular atrophy, oligospermia, and reduced bone density
	Other signs and symptoms may be seen with secondary hypogonadism, including visual loss, headaches, breast discharge (from prolactinoma), and symptoms of other hormonal deficiencies such as hypothyroidism.
Laboratory testing	In females age 45 years and older, symptoms typical of menopause are not an indication for laboratory testing. Estradiol levels are checked for symptoms occurring in females younger than 45 years, in undernourished patients with unexplained amenorrhea, and in the workup for infertility. In these cases, FSH and LH are checked along with estradiol. Primary hypogonadism is diagnosed when estradiol (and progesterone) levels are low but FSH and LH levels are normal or high. Secondary hypogonadism is diagnosed when estradiol (and progesterone) levels as well as FSH and LH levels are low.
	In males with symptoms of testosterone deficiency, testosterone level is checked (between 8:00 A.M. and 11:00 A.M.) along with LH and FSH. If the testosterone level is <200 ng/dL, the level is rechecked. If the level is 200–400 ng/dL, free testosterone level is checked. If the level is ≥400 ng/dL, the result is normal. Primary hypogonadism is diagnosed by low testosterone, elevated LH, and elevated FSH. Secondary hypogonadism is diagnosed by low testosterone, normal or low LH, and normal or low FSH.
	Additional tests may be indicated depending on results, including CBC and iron studies, prolactin level, thyroid function tests, ACTH, sperm count, sex hormone binding globulin, ultrasound of the ovaries, and brain MRI or head CT.

Hypogonadism *(continued)*

Alwani M, Yassin A, Talib R, et al: Cardiovascular disease, hypogonadism and erectile dysfunction: early detection, prevention and the positive effects of long-term testosterone treatment: prospective observational, real-life data. Vasc Health Risk Manag 17:497–508, 2021

Dobs AS: The role of accurate testosterone testing in the treatment and management of male hypogonadism. Steroids 73:1305–1310, 2008

Hall SA, Esche GR, Araujo AB, et al: Correlates of low testosterone and symptomatic androgen deficiency in a population-based sample. J Clin Endocrinol Metab 93:3870–3877, 2008

Khera M, Broderick GA, Carson CC III, et al: Adult-onset hypogonadism. Mayo Clin Proc 91(7):908–926, 2016

Livingston M, Kalansooriya A, Hartland AJ, et al: Serum testosterone levels in male hypogonadism: why and when to check—a review. Int J Clin Pract 71(11):e12995, 2017

Richard-Eaglin A: Male and female hypogonadism. Nurs Clin North Am 53(3):395–405, 2018

Salonia A, Rastrelli G, Hackett G, et al: Paediatric and adult-onset male hypogonadism. Nat Rev Dis Primers 5(1):38, 2019

Hypokalemia

Clinical findings	Potassium is an electrolyte present in all body fluids but concentrated inside cells, where it helps regulate water and acid-base balance, participates in nerve conduction, and stimulates contraction of muscle cells. Along with calcium and magnesium, potassium controls cardiac output (heart rate and force of contraction). Potassium is taken in from dietary sources and excreted primarily through the kidneys. A serum potassium level <3.5 mEq/L defines hypokalemia.
	Diuretic drugs are the most common cause of potassium deficiency, with the reduction being dose-dependent and usually mild. Other conditions implicated in hypokalemia include chronic starvation, prolonged IV hydration without potassium replacement, prolonged vomiting or diarrhea, hyperaldosteronism, fluid loss from intestinal fistula, excessive loss of potassium in urine, loss from draining wounds, chronic heavy alcohol use, treatment of megaloblastic anemia with vitamin B_{12} or folate, and cystic fibrosis. Other medications associated with hypokalemia include corticosteroids, β-adrenergic agonists such as isoproterenol, β-adrenergic antagonists such as clonidine, antibiotics such as gentamicin and carbenicillin, and the antifungal agent amphotericin B.
	Hypokalemia is often asymptomatic. Clinical signs and symptoms are more likely in elderly patients, including the following:
	• Malaise, fatigue, lethargy
	• Weakness, rhabdomyolysis
	• Hyporeflexia
	• Muscle cramps, myalgias
	• Loss of appetite
	• Increased thirst
	• Urinary frequency or polyuria
	• Vomiting, constipation
	• Weak pulse
	• Irregular heart rhythm
	• Hypotension
	• Delirium or confusion
	Severe untreated hypokalemia can be fatal.
Laboratory testing	Potassium levels at the low end of the normal range are usually associated with potassium deficiency, as is a trend downward of as little as 0.1–0.2 mEq/day. Often, the cause is apparent (e.g., diuretic use). Levels below the reference range are stratified as follows:
	• Mild: 3.1–3.5 mEq/L
	• Moderate: 2.6–3.0 mEq/L
	• Severe: ≤2.5 mEq/L
	Diagnosis is more urgent and treatment algorithms more aggressive for moderate to severe hypokalemia. For patients with an elevated risk of cardiac dysrhythmias, even mild hypokalemia can be serious. These include elderly patients, those with preexisting cardiac disease, those receiving digoxin, and post-MI patients. In the latter population, potassium levels should be maintained at ≥4.0 mEq/L.

Hypokalemia *(continued)*

Laboratory testing *(continued)*	The following laboratory tests are recommended in the workup for hypokalemia:
	• ECG
	• Serum potassium (recheck)
	• Serum magnesium
	• Serum glucose
	• Urine electrolytes, urine creatinine (urine potassium–to-creatinine ratio >1.5 mEq/mmol suggests urinary potassium wasting)
	• Arterial blood gas to evaluate acid-base balance
	If no cause is identified, further workup would include thyroid and adrenal function testing.
	ECG changes of hypokalemia include the following:
	• Flattened T waves
	• ST interval depression
	• T wave inversion
	• PR interval prolongation
	• Appearance of U waves, with increasing amplitude
	• Premature atrial contractions
	• Prolonged QTc interval
	• Premature ventricular contractions
	• Ventricular tachycardia
	• *Torsades de pointes*
	• Ventricular fibrillation (K^+ <2 mEq/L)

Alfano G, Ferrari A, Fontana F, et al: Hypokalemia in patients with COVID-19. Clin Exp Nephrol 25(4):401–409, 2021

Ballantyne F III, Vander Ark C: The difficult diagnosis of hypokalemia. Am Fam Physician 33:256–258, 1986

Elliott TL, Braun M: Electrolytes: potassium disorders. FP Essent 459:21–28, 2017

Viera AJ, Wouk N: Potassium disorders: hypokalemia and hyperkalemia. Am Fam Physician 92(6):487–495, 2015

Wang X, Han D, Li G: Electrocardiographic manifestations in severe hypokalemia. J Int Med Res 48(1):300060518811058, 2020

Hypomagnesemia

Clinical findings	Magnesium is an essential nutrient that serves as a cofactor for hundreds of enzymatic processes involved in DNA replication, bone formation, blood sugar regulation, blood pressure control, and heart, nerve, and muscle function. An adequate level of magnesium is maintained primarily via its reabsorption in the kidney. Risk factors for hypomagnesemia include advanced age, inadequate dietary intake, alcohol use disorder, significant diarrhea, malabsorption in the small intestine, the presence of type 2 diabetes mellitus, and the use of medications such as proton pump inhibitors, diuretics, antibiotics, bisphosphonates, certain monoclonal antibodies (e.g., denosumab), and antineoplastics. In addition, more than a dozen genetic mutations associated with renal magnesium wasting have been described. Signs and symptoms of magnesium deficiency include the following: • Fatigue, weakness • Poor appetite • Nausea, vomiting • Cardiac rate and rhythm disturbances • Neuromuscular irritability (e.g., cramps, tetany) • Paresthesias • Seizures • Delirium Consequences of hypomagnesemia include the following: • Hypertension • ECG changes: widened QRS, prolonged PR, prolonged QT, tall peaked T waves or inverted T waves, U waves • Arrhythmias: supraventricular tachycardia, ventricular arrhythmias, *torsades de pointes* • Sudden cardiac death • Risk of digitalis toxicity • Impaired release of and skeletal resistance to PTH • Vertigo, ataxia • Depression, psychosis • Other electrolyte disorders: hypokalemia, hypocalcemia, hypophosphatemia Low magnesium also significantly increases morbidity in patients with comorbid diseases such as type 2 diabetes who exhibit a more rapid progression of disease and a higher risk of diabetic complications. Patients with primary hyperparathyroidism who become magnesium deficient not only have more severe disease but also have a higher risk of osteoporosis, anemia, and hypercalcemic crisis. Because magnesium modulates vasomotor tone, blood pressure, and peripheral blood flow, deficiency can have significant cardiovascular effects, including worsening hypertension, onset of cardiovascular disease, and the appearance of serious arrhythmias including *torsades de pointes*.

Hypomagnesemia *(continued)*

Laboratory testing	Magnesium is sometimes overlooked as a cause of presenting symptoms because it is not part of the BMP or CMP. The magnesium level should be checked when unexplained hypocalcemia or hypokalemia is noted, in the presence of a ventricular arrhythmia, when drugs implicated in hypomagnesemia are administered, or when any other risk factor is present.
	Magnesium levels <1.6 mg/dL are common. Clinical symptoms do not usually appear until the level is <1.2 mg/dL. Analogous to the situation with calcium, a spurious result for magnesium can be obtained when hypoalbuminemia is present, such that a published correction formula should be used.

Bosman W, Hoenderop JGJ, de Baaij JHF: Genetic and drug-induced hypomagnesemia: different cause, same mechanism. Proc Nutr Soc 80(3):327–338, 2021

Chrysant SG, Chrysant GS: Adverse cardiovascular and blood pressure effects of drug-induced hypomagnesemia. Expert Opin Drug Saf 19(1):59–67, 2020

Na D, Tao G, Shu-Ying L, et al: Association between hypomagnesemia and severity of primary hyperparathyroidism: a retrospective study. BMC Endocr Disord 21(1):170, 2021

Srinutta T, Chewcharat A, Takkavatakarn K, et al: Proton pump inhibitors and hypomagnesemia: a meta-analysis of observational studies. Medicine (Baltimore) 98(44):e17788, 2019

van Kempen TATG, Deixler E: SARS-CoV-2: influence of phosphate and magnesium, moderated by vitamin D, on energy (ATP) metabolism and on severity of COVID-19. Am J Physiol Endocrinol Metab 320(1):E2-E6, 2021

Viering DHHM, de Baaij JHF, Walsh SB, et al: Genetic causes of hypomagnesemia, a clinical overview. Pediatr Nephrol 32(7):1123–1135, 2017

Hyponatremia

Clinical findings	Hyponatremia is defined by a serum sodium level <136 mEq/L, reflecting excess water relative to sodium. In this situation, water shifts into cells, causing them to swell and giving rise to a range of primarily neuropsychiatric symptoms, including the following:
	• Lethargy
	• Weakness
	• Restlessness
	• Headache
	• Disorientation
	• Delirium, confusion
	• Nausea, vomiting
	• Muscle cramps
	• Myoclonus
	• Asterixis
	• Seizures
	• Papilledema
	• Coma and death
	Hyponatremia is associated with several conditions encountered in psychiatric practice, including psychogenic polydipsia, SIAD, beer potomania, postsurgical pain, and use of drugs of abuse such as amphetamines, Ecstasy, and bath salts, as well as a long list of psychotropic drugs (especially antipsychotics and antidepressants). Common causes in the general medical population include use of diuretics, diarrhea, heart failure, liver disease, and kidney disease. In elderly patients, adrenal insufficiency secondary to pituitary disease should be considered. See also the discussion in the **Sodium** entry in the *Laboratory Tests* chapter for further details.
Laboratory testing	The lower limit of normal for sodium is 136 mEq/L in adults (132 mEq/L in those older than 90 years). The critical value for hyponatremia is <120 mEq/L, for which urgent intervention is required.
	Other tests used in the initial workup of hyponatremia include serum osmolality, urine osmolality, and urine sodium. In compulsive water drinking, psychogenic polydipsia (associated with schizophrenia), or beer potomania (in heavy beer drinkers), serum sodium, serum osmolality, and urine osmolality are all low. In SIAD, serum sodium and serum osmolality are low, but urine osmolality is not low.

Adrogue HJ, Madias NE: Hyponatremia. N Engl J Med 342:1581–1589, 2000

Braun MM, Barstow CH, Pyzocha NJ: Diagnosis and management of sodium disorders: hyponatremia and hypernatremia. Am Fam Physician 91(5):299–307, 2015

Buffington MA, Abreo K: Hyponatremia: a review. J Intensive Care Med 31(4):223–236, 2016

Hoorn EJ, Zietse R: Diagnosis and treatment of hyponatremia: compilation of the guidelines. J Am Soc Nephrol 28(5):1340–1349, 2017

Kugler JP, Hustead T: Hyponatremia and hypernatremia in the elderly. Am Fam Physician 61:3623–3630, 2000

Lien YH, Shapiro JI: Hyponatremia: clinical diagnosis and management. Am J Med 120:653–658, 2007

Palmer BF, Clegg DJ: Electrolyte disturbances in patients with chronic alcohol-use disorder. N Engl J Med 377(14):1368–1377, 2017

Sterns RH: Disorders of plasma sodium: causes, consequences, and correction. N Engl J Med 372(1):55–65, 2015

Hypoparathyroidism

Clinical findings	Hypoparathyroidism is a rare condition characterized by low calcium levels and inappropriately low or undetectable levels of PTH. It occurs most often in older females with parathyroid injury or accidental removal as complications of thyroid surgery. Other causes include genetic and autoimmune diseases. PTH regulates calcium and phosphate levels through its actions on the bones, kidneys, and intestines, and some of the clinical symptoms of hypoparathyroidism stem from the absence of physiological actions of PTH on the skeleton and kidneys. The skeleton adds bone, but bone turnover is low so that bone mass increases. The kidneys are unable to conserve calcium and thus excrete a greater amount in urine. Other biochemical abnormalities of hypoparathyroidism include elevated phosphate levels and low levels of 1,25-dihydroxy vitamin D.
	The most prominent symptoms of hypoparathyroidism are related to neuromuscular irritability and include paresthesias, muscle cramps, carpopedal spasm, seizures, and laryngospasm. Calcifications in the kidneys, basal ganglia, and soft tissues are common. The incidence of depression is increased, and there is some evidence of cognitive impairment referred to as "brain fog" that is proportional to calcium concentration and duration of disease. Cardiac signs include prolongation of the corrected QT interval and cardiac arrhythmias. Cataracts, dental abnormalities, increased rates of infection, and skin changes are seen, the latter including dry, scaly skin; brittle nails; and coarse or thin hair.
Laboratory testing	Laboratory tests used in the workup of suspected hypoparathyroidism include the following: • Ionized (free) calcium level or albumin-corrected total calcium level (low) • PTH level (inappropriately low or undetectable) • Phosphate (high)

Bilezikian JP: Hypoparathyroidism. J Clin Endocrinol Metab 105(6):1722–1736, 2020

Clarke BL, Brown EM, Collins MT, et al: Epidemiology and diagnosis of hypoparathyroidism. J Clin Endocrinol Metab 101(6):2284–2299, 2016

Gafni RI, Collins MT: Hypoparathyroidism. N Engl J Med 380(18):1738–1747, 2019

Mannstadt M, Bilezikian JP, Thakker RV, et al: Hypoparathyroidism. Nat Rev Dis Primers 3:17055, 2017 [published correction appears in Nat Rev Dis Primers 3:17080, 2017]

Hypothyroidism

Clinical findings	In areas of the world where iodine intake is sufficient, the most common cause of hypothyroidism is autoimmune disease. The prevalence of this condition increases with age and is more common in females. Certain medications are also associated with hypothyroidism through various mechanisms, including amiodarone, gonadal steroid hormones, glucocorticoids, furosemide, lithium, levodopa, antipsychotics, phenytoin, and propranolol, among others.
	The onset of hypothyroidism can be insidious. Signs and symptoms include the following:
	• Bradycardia
	• Weight gain
	• Fatigue
	• Cold intolerance
	• Dry skin
	• Alopecia
	• Myxedema (skin thickening) often apparent on face, legs, and dorsum of hands and feet
	• Carpal tunnel syndrome
	• Menstrual irregularities
	• Depression
	• Psychosis ("myxedema madness")
	• Cognitive impairment: poor concentration, memory difficulties, dullness
	• Coma when severe and untreated
	Hypothyroidism disrupts all aspects of metabolism and contributes to hypertension, dyslipidemia, infertility, and neuromuscular dysfunction. Importantly, it increases the risk of cardiovascular disease even in treated patients when treatment is inadequate. The effects in pregnancy can be serious, including bradycardia, goiter, inappropriate weight gain, and adverse effects on the fetus.
	Although the management of subclinical hypothyroidism (high TSH, normal free T4 [FT4]) has been controversial in the past, it is now recognized that patients with a TSH level >10 mIU/L with or without an elevated TPOAb are at risk of dyslipidemia and cardiovascular disease, and treatment is recommended. Treatment-refractory depression may also be related to subclinical thyroid disease. Even among patients with TSH values in the high-normal range, there is a higher frequency of depressive episodes, symptoms are more severe, and antidepressant treatment response can be suboptimal. Thyroid replacement with target TSH levels <2.5 mIU/L may be required to achieve remission, and this is true for patients with bipolar as well as unipolar disease. In fact, patients with treatment-resistant depression may benefit from thyroid supplementation titrated to a target TSH level as low as <2.0 mIU/L.
Laboratory testing	The testing laboratory's reference range should be consulted for determining the upper limit of normal for TSH, which varies with age.
	For screening purposes, TSH alone is considered sufficient testing.
	FT4 is needed in addition to TSH to diagnose subclinical thyroid dysfunction, central hypothyroidism (due to hypothalamic or pituitary disease), and drug effects and to monitor treatment.

Hypothyroidism *(continued)*

Laboratory testing *(continued)*	The FT4 level is measured in preference to the total T4 because its measurement is not affected by serum protein levels. TSH and FT4 together suggest the following diagnoses: • TSH high, FT4 low: hypothyroidism • TSH high, FT4 normal: subclinical hypothyroidism If the FT4 is normal in the context of high TSH, further workup should include thyroid antibodies to diagnose possible autoimmune disease. Recent reviews suggest that subclinical hypothyroidism in non-elderly patients should be treated when the TSH level is >4.0 mIU/L. Because subclinical hyperthyroidism is more injurious to elderly patients than subclinical hypothyroidism, treatment for these patients is individualized and based on symptoms. The treatment threshold in this population is a TSH level ≥10 mIU/L. The schedule for checking TSH in patients treated with thyroid hormone replacement is as follows: • 4–8 weeks after initiating treatment • 4–8 weeks after a change in dosage • 6 months after adequate replacement dosage is achieved • Every 12 months thereafter or as dictated by clinical situation

American Psychiatric Association: Diagnostic and Statistical Manual of Mental Disorders, 5th Edition, Text Revision. Washington, DC, American Psychiatric Association, 2022

Barbesino G: Thyroid function changes in the elderly and their relationship to cardiovascular health: a mini-review. Gerontology 65(1):1–8, 2019

Calissendorff J, Falhammar H: To treat or not to treat subclinical hypothyroidism, what is the evidence? Medicina (Kaunas) 56(1):40, 2020

Chiovato L, Magri F, Carlé A: Hypothyroidism in context: where we've been and where we're going. Adv Ther 36(Suppl 2):47–58, 2019

Chrysant SG: The current debate over treatment of subclinical hypothyroidism to prevent cardiovascular complications. Int J Clin Pract 74(7):e13499, 2020

Cohen BM, Sommer BR, Vuckovic A: Antidepressant-resistant depression in patients with comorbid subclinical hypothyroidism or high-normal TSH levels. Am J Psychiatry 175(7):598–604, 2018

Duntas LH, Yen PM: Diagnosis and treatment of hypothyroidism in the elderly. Endocrine 66(1):63–69, 2019

Garber JR, Cobin RH, Gharib H, et al: Clinical practice guidelines for hypothyroidism in adults: cosponsored by the American Association of Clinical Endocrinologists and the American Thyroid Association. Endocr Pract 18(6):988–1028, 2012 [published correction appears in Endocr Pract 19(1):175, 2013]

Redford C, Vaidya B: Subclinical hypothyroidism: should we treat? Post Reprod Health 23(2):55–62, 2017

Treister-Goltzman Y, Yarza S, Peleg R: Lipid profile in mild subclinical hypothyroidism: systematic review and meta-analysis. Minerva Endocrinol (Torino) 46(4):428–440, 2021

Infectious mononucleosis (IM)

Clinical findings	IM is a viral syndrome caused in most cases by the Epstein-Barr virus (EBV), a herpesvirus spread primarily by intimate oral contact. Seen mostly in adolescents and young adults, it also can occur in older adults and may have a more severe presentation in this population. Like other herpesviruses, EBV establishes an asymptomatic, lifelong latent infection of immune system B cells with occasional reactivation.
	The acute IM syndrome is characterized by fever, malaise, fatigue, headache, sore throat, pharyngeal inflammation with exudates, palatal petechiae, tonsillar enlargement, periorbital and eyelid edema, and symmetrical lymphadenopathy (especially cervical and postauricular, but also axial and inguinal). Splenomegaly and hepatomegaly may be observed, and an erythematous maculopapular rash may develop with or without the use of antimicrobials.
	Early complications include splenic rupture and hepatitis. Splenic rupture is uncommon but can occur spontaneously; this risk is increased by abdominal trauma, which is why athletes in contact sports are advised to refrain from playing for a period of ~3 weeks from the time symptoms resolve. Hepatitis is common and usually self-limiting.
	Importantly, IM has well-established associations with later development of multiple sclerosis, Hodgkin's lymphoma, nasopharyngeal carcinoma, and gastric cancer. There is also evidence that the risk of a depressive episode is increased in the 1- to 4-year period after IM is diagnosed. A tentative link has been established to later development of chronic fatigue syndrome, at least in a subset of patients.
Laboratory testing	Testing of blood for EBV-specific antibodies is the gold standard of diagnosis for IM, but turnaround time for this testing may be unacceptably long. For this reason, many clinicians use the rapid heterophile antibody test Monospot, a point-of-care test that yields results within 5–10 minutes. Specificity of this test is high, but sensitivity is low, particularly in first week of illness and for very young children. In these cases, testing by EBV-specific serology can be used.
	EBV-specific antibody testing for IgM and IgG antibodies to viral capsid antigen (VCA) and Epstein-Barr nuclear antigen (EBNA) can be used to follow up on Monospot testing, whether positive or negative. These tests have higher sensitivity than Monospot.
	Lymphocytosis ($>5\times10^9$/L) is seen in peripheral blood, and atypical lymphocytes are seen on blood smear. A combination of lymphocytes >50% and atypical lymphocytes >10% is useful in confirming the diagnosis.

Akiyama Y, Ishikane M, Ohmagari N: Epstein-Barr virus induced skin rash in infectious mononucleosis. IDCases 26:e01298, 2021

Cai X, Ebell MH, Haines L: Accuracy of signs, symptoms, and hematologic parameters for the diagnosis of infectious mononucleosis: a systematic review and meta-analysis. J Am Board Fam Med 34(6):1141–1156, 2021

Fevang B, Wyller VBB, Mollnes TE, et al: Lasting immunological imprint of primary Epstein-Barr virus infection with associations to chronic low-grade inflammation and fatigue. Front Immunol 12:715102, 2021

Murata T, Sugimoto A, Inagaki T, et al: Molecular basis of Epstein-Barr virus latency establishment and lytic reactivation. Viruses 13(12):2344, 2021

Vindegaard N, Petersen LV, Lyng-Rasmussen BI, et al: Infectious mononucleosis as a risk factor for depression: a nationwide cohort study. Brain Behav Immun 94:259–265, 2021

Womack J, Jimenez M: Common questions about infectious mononucleosis. Am Fam Physician 91(6):372–376, 2015

Insomnia disorder

Clinical findings	Insomnia disorder is diagnosed when the patient reports dissatisfaction with sleep quality or quantity associated with difficulty initiating or maintaining sleep or early morning awakening. The sleep disturbance causes significant impairment or distress and occurs at least 3 nights per week for at least 3 months. The problem can be isolated or can be associated with another mental disorder or medical condition. Risk factors for insomnia disorder include female sex, advancing age, being unmarried, and habits such as smoking, alcohol use, and sedentary lifestyle, although these factors by no means identify all individuals at risk. Precipitants include stressful events, worsening medical conditions such as cardiac or pulmonary disease or chronic pain, new-onset depression or anxiety disorder, or treatment with medications such as β-blockers, steroids, NSAIDs, decongestants, and antiandrogens. When a poor sleep pattern emerges, it can become chronic because of behavioral factors such as spending too much time in bed or taking too many naps, or due to classical conditioning in which the bed and bedroom have become feared stimuli because of past sleeplessness.
	About half of those reporting insomnia meet criteria for a psychiatric disorder, and this risk is heightened in both directions; psychiatric disorders increase the risk of insomnia, and insomnia increases the risk of psychiatric disorders. Insomnia may also be a risk factor for suicide, independent of depression. Insomnia is associated with cognitive deficits in working memory and attentional switching. Furthermore, chronic insomnia increases the risk of medical conditions such as hypertension, diabetes, coronary heart disease, heart failure, acute MI, and death. Although insomnia was once dismissed as a nuisance complaint among patients, it is now considered a serious problem requiring attention.
	Recent research has implicated brain circuits regulating arousal and emotion in the pathophysiology of insomnia, rather than circuits involved in circadian rhythms. Insomnia is increasingly understood as a state of constant hyperarousal during wake and sleep cycles in which metabolic rate is increased. During sleep, cortisol and ACTH are elevated (in the first part of the sleep cycle) and the normal relationship between parasympathetic tone and heart rate variability is disrupted.
	In most cases, the diagnosis of insomnia disorder is made clinically. The most important diagnostic tool is a complete history detailing medical and psychiatric problems, medications, and specific sleep issues. A sleep diary is highly recommended to capture data regarding the nature of sleep disruption. Various published insomnia scales can be used to determine the severity of insomnia and monitor the effects of treatment.
Laboratory testing	Polysomnography is indicated in the workup for insomnia only if sleep apnea, periodic limb movements, or parasomnias such as REM sleep behavior disorder are suspected.
	Wrist actigraphy is a noninvasive, low-cost means to obtain information about day-night cycles and to monitor the effects of treatment for insomnia.
	Although neuroimaging is not required for the diagnosis of insomnia disorder, if it is obtained for another indication in a patient with chronic insomnia, it may show reduced hippocampal volume and reduced gray matter in the frontal lobes.

Insomnia disorder *(continued)*

American Psychiatric Association: Diagnostic and Statistical Manual of Mental Disorders, 5th Edition, Text Revision. Washington, DC, American Psychiatric Association, 2022

Burman D: Sleep disorders: insomnia. FP Essent 460:22–28, 2017

Buysse DJ: Insomnia. JAMA 309(7):706–716, 2013

Patel D, Steinberg J, Patel P: Insomnia in the elderly: a review. J Clin Sleep Med 14(6):1017–1024, 2018

Perez MN, Salas RME: Insomnia. Continuum (Minneap Minn) 26(4):1003–1015, 2020

Riemann D, Nissen C, Palagini L, et al: The neurobiology, investigation, and treatment of chronic insomnia. Lancet Neurol 14(5):547–558, 2015

Sutton EL: Insomnia. Ann Intern Med 174(3):ITC33–ITC48, 2021

Van Someren EJW: Brain mechanisms of insomnia: new perspectives on causes and consequences. Physiol Rev 101(3):995–1046, 2021

Winkelman JW: Clinical practice: insomnia disorder. N Engl J Med 373(15):1437–1444, 2015

Klinefelter's syndrome

Clinical findings	Klinefelter's syndrome is a genetic disorder found in males that results from sex chromosome nondisjunction leading in most cases to a 47,XXY karyotype. In this classic form, the extra X chromosome gives rise to characteristic features of small testes, hypergonadotropic hypogonadism, and language processing difficulties. A wide range of clinical phenotypes is seen because of mosaic forms (e.g., 47,XXY/46,XY) and higher-grade forms (e.g., 48,XXXY or 48,XXYY) as well as variation in downstream effects, severity of hypogonadism, and duration of untreated disease. Only about 25% of cases are ever diagnosed, and those mostly in adulthood because symptoms worsen with age. The condition is not heritable.
	In its fully developed form, 47,XXY Klinefelter's syndrome may include any of the following signs and symptoms: small, firm testes, gynecomastia, broad hips, decreased facial and axillary hair, tall stature with long legs, underdeveloped musculature, incoordination, infertility, erectile dysfunction, decreased libido in some cases, speech and language impairment, and susceptibility to anxiety, depression, bipolar disorder, autism spectrum disorder, and schizophrenia, as well as various social and behavioral problems.
	In most cases, boys with this phenotype enter puberty as usual so that secondary sex characteristics are relatively unaffected. Serum testosterone levels then begin to decline in young adulthood. Infertility becomes an issue, and metabolic abnormalities develop, including obesity, insulin resistance, dyslipidemia, and hypertension. The risk of cardiovascular disease, autoimmune disease (e.g., lupus, Hashimoto's thyroiditis), osteoporosis, certain cancers (e.g., breast cancer, germ cell tumors), and dental caries is elevated and continues to increase with age.
	Psychological consequences of Klinefelter's syndrome are relatively under-researched and not well understood. The possibility of gender incongruence should be addressed as early as possible and appropriate referrals made. In addition, screening for psychiatric disorders should be undertaken routinely throughout life.
Laboratory testing	Chromosomal analysis (karyotyping) of peripheral blood cells is used to diagnose Klinefelter's syndrome.
	Karyotyping is recommended:
	• In males with primary hypogonadism (low serum testosterone levels and elevated gonadotropins [LH and FSH] along with small testicular volumes (<5 mL per testis)
	• In males with nonobstructive azoospermia or severe oligozoospermia (total sperm count $<10 \times 10^6$/ejaculate or sperm concentration $<5 \times 10^6$/mL)
	Other laboratory testing is recommended for patients diagnosed with Klinefelter's syndrome, as follows:
	• Metabolic profile at least annually
	• Testosterone and LH at least annually
	• Vitamin D and calcium levels at first visit and then as indicated
	• ECG to evaluate QTc at first visit and then as indicated
	• Bone mineral density (DEXA) scan at first visit and then as indicated

Klinefelter's syndrome *(continued)*

Bearelly P, Oates R: Recent advances in managing and understanding Klinefelter syndrome. F1000Res 8:F1000 Faculty Rev-112, 2019

Bonomi M, Rochira V, Pasquali D, et al: Klinefelter syndrome (KS): genetics, clinical phenotype and hypogonadism. J Endocrinol Invest 40(2):123–134, 2017

Giagulli VA, Campone B, Castellana M, et al: Neuropsychiatric aspects in men with Klinefelter's syndrome. Endocr Metab Immune Disord Drug Targets 19(2):109–115, 2019

Gravholt CH, Chang S, Wallentin M, et al: Klinefelter's syndrome: integrating genetics, neuropsychology, and endocrinology. Endocr Rev 39(4):389–423, 2018

Groth KA, Skakkebæk A, Høst C, et al: Clinical review—Klinefelter's syndrome: a clinical update. J Clin Endocrinol Metab 98(1):20–30, 2013

Kanakis GA, Nieschlag E: Klinefelter's syndrome: more than hypogonadism. Metabolism 86:135–144, 2018

Skakkebæk A, Wallentin M, Gravholt CH: Klinefelter's syndrome or testicular dysgenesis: genetics, endocrinology, and neuropsychology. Handb Clin Neurol 181:445–462, 2021

Zitzmann M, Aksglaede L, Corona G, et al: European Academy of Andrology guidelines on Klinefelter's syndrome. Andrology 9(1):145–167, 2021

Lead poisoning

Clinical findings	Lead poisoning is a well-recognized problem in children but can also affect adults, either acutely or from chronic exposure. In addition, there is evidence that childhood exposure can lead to neurodegenerative changes later in life consistent with Alzheimer's disease and Parkinson's disease. Lead is a neurotoxin that competes with calcium at binding sites, with serious nervous system, kidney, and bone effects. Until the early 1990s, lead was ubiquitous in the world, including the United States and other developed countries. Exposure from paints, pipes, gasoline additives, and a broad array of everyday products resulted in very high blood lead levels in the world's populations. In the United States, children born from the 1960s to the early 1980s are known to have had the highest exposure, and it is expected that this cohort will demonstrate the lasting effects of lead exposure when its members reach the age at which neurodegenerative disease usually appears.
	Lead mitigation efforts have had demonstrable effects on lead levels in developed countries, but risk remains for those in developing countries, those living near airports (within 1 km), consumers of Ayurvedic and other folk medicines, those who frequent firing ranges, those living in older homes with lead pipes, users of certain coated cookware, and those with PVC children's toys in the home. The most common sources of exposure in the United States are gunshot wounds and Ayurvedic and folk medicines.
	Acute ingestion of a large amount of lead (e.g., a patient with pica eating lead chips) is associated with colicky abdominal pain, a metallic taste, and a florid delirium termed *lead encephalopathy*. Acute lead poisoning can be fatal. Those who survive acute poisoning are usually left with cognitive and motor deficits.
	Adults with chronic low-level lead exposure may be asymptomatic or may present with mild cognitive impairment and a peripheral motor neuropathy with wrist and foot drop. Affected patients may or may not report abdominal pain or metallic taste. Chronic low-level exposure has cumulative effects and may go unnoticed until the patient presents with dementia, clear motor deficits, or kidney failure. All organ systems can be affected.
	With either acute or chronic toxicity, signs/symptoms may include anemia, fatigue, weakness, dyspnea, hypertension, hearing loss, osteopenia/osteoporosis, cognitive deficits, infertility, miscarriage, immune dysfunction, vitamin D deficiency, mood and personality changes, headaches, paresthesias, tremors, seizures, coma, weight loss, poor appetite, nausea and vomiting, and constipation or diarrhea.
Laboratory testing	The lead level can be measured in blood or 24-hour urine, but blood is the specimen of choice. In 2021, the CDC revised the reference levels for children as follows:
	• 0–5 years: ≤3.4 μg/dL
	• 6 years and older: ≤4.9 μg/dL
	Because even lower levels have been found to be associated with cognitive impairment and maladaptive behaviors, some experts maintain that no measurable lead level is safe. These values should be interpreted with this fact in mind.

Lead poisoning *(continued)*

Laboratory testing *(continued)*	Critical values of lead in blood:
	• Pregnant females: ≥10 µg/dL
	• Children: >20 µg/dL
	• Adults: >45 µg/dL
	• Medical emergency (any age): >70 µg/dL
	Reference interval for 24-hour urine lead: 0–31 µg/dL
	Other laboratory tests useful in the workup of suspected lead poisoning include the following:
	• CBC with platelets
	• Serum iron studies
	• Electrolytes
	• LFTs
	• ESR
	• Blood sugar
	• EMG/Nerve conduction studies (focused on extensor muscles of the wrist and fingers and abductor muscle of the thumb)

ARUP Laboratories: Lead, blood (venous), in Laboratory Test Directory. Salt Lake City, UT, ARUP Laboratories, 2022. Available at: https://ltd.aruplab.com/Tests/Pub/0020098. Accessed February 2022.

Ciocan C, Mansour I, Beneduce A, et al: Lead poisoning from Ayurvedic treatment: a further case. Med Lav 112(2):162–167, 2021

Hung DZ, Yang KW, Wu CC, Hung YH: Lead poisoning due to incense burning: an outbreak in a family. Clin Toxicol (Phila) 59(8):756–759, 2021

Mitra P, Sharma S, Purohit P, Sharma P: Clinical and molecular aspects of lead toxicity: an update. Crit Rev Clin Lab Sci 54(7–8):506–528, 2017

Nicolli A, Mina GG, De Nuzzo D, et al: Unusual domestic source of lead poisoning. Int J Environ Res Public Health 17(12):4374, 2020

Njati SY, Maguta MM: Lead-based paints and children's PVC toys are potential sources of domestic lead poisoning: a review. Environ Pollut 249:1091–1105, 2019

Reuben A: Childhood lead exposure and adult neurodegenerative disease. J Alzheimers Dis 64(1):17–42, 2018

Rocha A, Trujillo KA: Neurotoxicity of low-level lead exposure: history, mechanisms of action, and behavioral effects in humans and preclinical models. Neurotoxicology 73:58–80, 2019

Samarghandian S, Shirazi FM, Saeedi F, et al: A systematic review of clinical and laboratory findings of lead poisoning: lessons from case reports. Toxicol Appl Pharmacol 429:115681, 2021

Shabani M, Hadeiy SK, Parhizgar P, et al: Lead poisoning; a neglected potential diagnosis in abdominal pain. BMC Gastroenterol 20(1):134, 2020 [published correction appears in BMC Gastroenterol 21(1):411, 2021]

Štepánek L, Nakládalová M, Klementa V, Ferencíková V: Acute lead poisoning in an indoor firing range. Med Pr 71(3):375–379, 2020

Limbic encephalitis (LE)

Clinical findings	LE is an autoimmune disorder characterized by the acute to subacute development of psychiatric, cognitive, and/or epileptic symptoms attributed to inflammation in the brain's limbic system (hippocampus, amygdala, parahippocampal gyrus, cingulate gyrus, subcallosal gyri, and related structures). Typical symptoms include severe impairment in short-term memory, altered mental status (delirium, confusion, psychosis), anxiety, depression, irritability, personality changes, and seizures. Faciobrachial dystonic seizures are pathognomonic of leucine-rich glioma-inactivated 1 (LGI1) encephalitis. Other signs/symptoms reported in LE include autonomic disturbances, sleep problems, ataxia, dystonia, myoclonus, aphasia, apraxia, obsessiveness, and endocrine dysfunction. LE is caused by a reaction of the immune system to cancer, non-cancerous tumors, infections, and other autoimmune disorders. When LE represents a paraneoplastic syndrome, it usually appears before the diagnosis of malignancy is made. The most commonly associated cancer is small cell lung cancer, but breast, testicular, and other cancers can be implicated. According to published guidelines, the diagnosis of LE requires that the following criteria be met: • Subacute onset (rapid progression over <3 months) of working memory deficits, seizures, or psychiatric symptoms suggesting limbic system involvement • Bilateral brain abnormalities on T2-weighted or FLAIR MRI restricted to the medial temporal lobes • Either CSF pleocytosis (WBC count >5/mm^3) or EEG with epileptic or slow-wave activity involving temporal lobes • Reasonable exclusion of alternative causes
Laboratory testing	MRI is performed (T2 and FLAIR) to evaluate medial temporal lobe structures. MRI may be repeated or FDG-PET performed to evaluate medial temporal lobe metabolism. EEG is performed to screen for temporal lobe epileptiform or slow-wave activity. CSF is examined for pleocytosis. Usual CSF inflammatory markers such as WBC and protein are not sensitive or specific for LE. Oligoclonal bands, if present, can increase the sensitivity for diagnosis. Neuronal antibody detection is improved if both CSF and serum are examined. Each laboratory has an encephalitis panel and algorithm for reflex testing based on immunofluorescence patterns. Antibodies tested include LGI1, α-amino-3-hydroxy-5-methyl-4-isoxazolepropionic acid receptor (AMPAR), GABA-B receptor (GABA-BR), contactin-associated protein-like 2 (Caspr2), metabotropic glutamate receptor subtype 5 (mGluR5), dipeptidyl-peptidase-like protein-6 (DPPx), NMDAR, glutamic acid decarboxylase (GAD), Hu, Ma, Ri, collapsin response mediator protein 5 (CRMP5), Sry-like high-mobility group box (SOX1), amphiphysin, and adenylate kinase 5 (AK5). If the patient is antibody-positive, a tumor survey is undertaken.

Abboud H, Probasco JC, Irani S, et al: Autoimmune encephalitis: proposed best practice recommendations for diagnosis and acute management. J Neurol Neurosurg Psychiatry 92(7):757–768, 2021

Budhram A, Leung A, Nicolle MW, Burneo JG: Diagnosing autoimmune limbic encephalitis. CMAJ 191(19):E529–E534, 2019

Chiveri L, Verrengia E, Muscia F, et al: Limbic encephalitis in a COVID-19 patient? J Neurovirol 27(3):498–500, 2021

Limbic encephalitis (LE) *(continued)*

Graus F, Titulaer MJ, Balu R, et al: A clinical approach to diagnosis of autoimmune encephalitis. Lancet Neurol 15(4):391–404, 2016

Kao YC, Lin MI, Weng WC, Lee WT: Neuropsychiatric disorders due to limbic encephalitis: immunologic aspect. Int J Mol Sci 22(1):389, 2020

Li X, Yuan J, Liu L, Hu W: Antibody-LGI 1 autoimmune encephalitis manifesting as rapidly progressive dementia and hyponatremia: a case report and literature review. BMC Neurol. 19(1):19, 2019

Mahawish K, Teinert L, Cavanagh K, Brennan J: Limbic encephalitis. BMJ Case Rep 2014:bcr2014204591, 2014

Nissen MS, Ryding M, Meyer M, Blaabjerg M: Autoimmune encephalitis: current knowledge on subtypes, disease mechanisms and treatment. CNS Neurol Disord Drug Targets 19(8):584–598, 2020

Lyme disease

Clinical findings	Lyme disease, caused by the spirochete *Borrelia burgdorferi*, is the most common tick-borne illness in the United States and is endemic in the Northeastern states (Virginia to Maine), the upper Midwest (particularly Wisconsin and Minnesota), and Northern California, although sporadic cases occur elsewhere. Lyme disease is transmitted only by deer ticks, not by dog or wood ticks. The disease often begins with the characteristic skin lesion known as *erythema migrans* at the site of the tick bite. Within days to weeks, the spirochete may disseminate so that the patient is at risk of developing cardiac, neurological, and/or rheumatological symptoms. Treatment with an antibiotic accelerates resolution of the disease. If no treatment is given, the disease may resolve spontaneously but can then recur.
	The risk of contracting Lyme disease is highest in endemic areas when the bite involves the tick genus *Ixodes* and the tick remains attached for 36 or more hours. The tick should therefore be removed promptly and carefully with tweezers and should be saved for identification purposes. The tick itself should not be tested.
	Signs, symptoms, and sequelae of Lyme disease:
	• Constitutional symptoms that may be seen on presentation include fever, chills, myalgias, fatigue, headache, and swollen lymph nodes.
	• Lyme disease affects the nervous system in 10%–15% of cases, with manifestations including lymphocytic meningitis, cranial neuritis, painful radiculoneuritis, and mononeuropathy multiplex. During active systemic infection, encephalopathy can be seen.
	• Individuals diagnosed with Lyme disease also have a greatly increased risk of psychiatric disorders including mood disorders, suicidality, and completed suicide that is highest during the first 1–3 years after diagnosis. It should be noted that the converse is not true; individuals diagnosed with psychiatric disorders do not necessarily have an increased risk of Lyme disease, and testing in the general psychiatric population has given rise to a great deal of controversy.
	• Symptoms that have been attributed to *chronic* Lyme disease may in some cases be due to *posttreatment* Lyme disease, a syndrome characterized by symptoms seen within 6 months of treatment that persist for 6 months or longer. This posttreatment syndrome is thought to arise from persistent immune activation, a hypothesis bolstered by recent ^{11}C-DPA-713 PET studies of TSPO in affected patients versus healthy control subjects.
	• Cardiac effects of Lyme disease include pericarditis, myocarditis, and cardiac conduction disease that sometimes requires permanent pacemaker implantation. Presenting symptoms in cardiac involvement include dyspnea, chest pain, lightheadedness, syncope, palpitations, and/or edema.
	• In late-stage infection in which earlier stages were asymptomatic, the presenting problem can be Lyme arthritis. In these cases, joint pain and swelling can be persistent or intermittent and involve one or a few large joints (particularly the knees). This syndrome may persist for several years even in the absence of systemic symptoms.

Lyme disease *(continued)*

Laboratory testing	Diagnosis of Lyme disease is made by serum antibody testing. In patients with CNS symptoms, CSF antibodies are also tested. Antigen testing by PCR or culture is not recommended because of low sensitivity. Testing is recommended for patients presenting with characteristic neurological, cardiac, or rheumatological symptoms and in at-risk patients exhibiting a rash that is not typical of erythema migrans. Routine testing is not recommended for patients with known neurological conditions, cognitive decline, dementia, or psychiatric, behavioral, or developmental disorders.
	Guidelines for testing are as follows:
	• The tick should be saved for identification of species, but the tick itself should not be tested.
	• Asymptomatic patients with a tick-bite history do not require testing.
	• Patients presenting with an erythema migrans rash should be treated immediately; confirmatory testing is not needed.
	• Testing methods for the diagnosis of Lyme disease are of two types: antigen testing for *B. burgdorferi* and antibody testing to detect immune response. As of this writing, antigen testing is not recommended, in part because of the low sensitivity of existing assays.
	• Antibody testing uses a two-tiered approach, with an initial enzyme immunoassay (EIA) followed by either a second EIA or Western blot if the first EIA test is positive or borderline. This approach works well for later stages of infection but has low sensitivity for early infection. These assays do not distinguish active from inactive infection, and seropositivity may persist for years, even after treatment and resolution of the clinical disease.
	• Culture of *B. burgdorferi* has low sensitivity and requires lengthy incubation and special media and expertise. It is not routinely used.
	• For patients with skin lesions that suggest but are not typical of erythema migrans, Lyme antibody testing is recommended on both acute and convalescent serum samples (drawn 2–3 weeks later).
	• To test for nervous system involvement (Lyme neuroborreliosis), simultaneous sampling of serum and CSF for antibodies is recommended because sampling only CSF could yield spurious results due to the passive transfer of antibodies from the blood to the CSF. The two-tiered approach described above is used.
	• At-risk patients with acute myocarditis or pericarditis of unknown cause should undergo serum antibody testing for Lyme disease.
	• In addition to serum antibody testing, an ECG should be performed in patients evaluated for Lyme disease who have signs or symptoms of carditis: dyspnea, edema, palpitations, lightheadedness, chest pain, and/or syncope.
	• Serum antibody testing is also used for possible Lyme arthritis. PCR assay for *B. burgdorferi* can be used for evaluation of synovial fluid samples in untreated patients with suspected Lyme arthritis but cannot be used to show eradication of spirochetes after treatment.
	• In patients who have persistent constitutional symptoms such as high fever while being treated for Lyme disease, testing for co-infection with other organisms should be considered in consultation with an infectious disease specialist.

Lyme disease *(continued)*

Arvikar SL, Steere AC: Diagnosis and treatment of Lyme arthritis. Infect Dis Clin North Am 29(2):269–280, 2015

Chaconas G, Castellanos M, Verhey TB: Changing of the guard: how the Lyme disease spirochete subverts the host immune response. J Biol Chem 295(2):301–313, 2020

Coughlin JM, Yang T, Rebman AW, et al: Imaging glial activation in patients with post-treatment Lyme disease symptoms: a pilot study using [11C]DPA-713 PET. J Neuroinflammation 15(1):346, 2018

Dumes AA: Lyme disease and the epistemic tensions of "medically unexplained illnesses." Med Anthropol 39(6):441–456, 2020

Fallon BA, Madsen T, Erlangsen A, Benros ME: Lyme borreliosis and associations with mental disorders and suicidal behavior: a nationwide Danish cohort study. Am J Psychiatry 178(10):921–931, 2021

Hinds K, Sutcliffe K: Heterodox and orthodox discourses in the case of Lyme disease: a synthesis of arguments. Qual Health Res 29(11):1661–1673, 2019

John TM, Taege AJ: Appropriate laboratory testing in Lyme disease. Cleve Clin J Med 86(11):751–759, 2019

Lantos PM: Chronic Lyme disease. Infect Dis Clin North Am 29(2):325–340, 2015

Lantos PM, Rumbaugh J, Bockenstedt LK, et al: Clinical practice guidelines by the Infectious Diseases Society of America (IDSA), American Academy of Neurology (AAN), and American College of Rheumatology (ACR): 2020 Guidelines for the Prevention, Diagnosis, and Treatment of Lyme Disease. Arthritis Care Res (Hoboken) 73(1):1–9, 2021

Marques AR: Laboratory diagnosis of Lyme disease: advances and challenges. Infect Dis Clin North Am 29(2):295–307, 2015

Mead P, Petersen J, Hinckley A: Updated CDC recommendation for serologic diagnosis of Lyme disease. MMWR Morb Mortal Wkly Rep 68(32):703, 2019

Moore A, Nelson C, Molins C, et al: Current guidelines, common clinical pitfalls, and future directions for laboratory diagnosis of Lyme disease, United States. Emerg Infect Dis 22(7):1169–1177, 2016

Nigrovic LE, Lewander DP, Balamuth F, et al: The Lyme disease polymerase chain reaction test has low sensitivity. Vector Borne Zoonotic Dis 20(4):310–313, 2020

Pitrak D, Nguyen CT, Cifu AS: Diagnosis of Lyme disease. JAMA 327(7):676–677, 2022

Schriefer ME: Lyme disease diagnosis: serology. Clin Lab Med 35(4):797–814, 2015

Schutzer SE, Body BA, Boyle J, et al: Direct diagnostic tests for Lyme disease. Clin Infect Dis 68(6):1052–1057, 2019

Shapiro ED: Clinical practice: Lyme disease. N Engl J Med 370(18):1724–1731, 2014

Tetens MM, Haahr R, Dessau RB, et al: Assessment of the risk of psychiatric disorders, use of psychiatric hospitals, and receipt of psychiatric medication among patients with Lyme neuroborreliosis in Denmark. JAMA Psychiatry 78(2):177–186, 2021

Uzomah UA, Rozen G, Mohammadreza Hosseini S, et al: Incidence of carditis and predictors of pacemaker implantation in patients hospitalized with Lyme disease. PLoS One 16(11):e0259123, 2021

Waddell LA, Greig J, Mascarenhas M, et al: The accuracy of diagnostic tests for Lyme disease in humans, a systematic review and meta-analysis of North American research. PLoS One 11(12):e0168613, 2016

Williams AL, Bevan J, Arnold MJ: Lyme disease: updated recommendations from the IDSA, AAN, and ACR. Am Fam Physician 104(6):652–654, 2021

Major depressive disorder (MDD)

Clinical findings	According to DSM-5, MDD is characterized by five or more of the following symptoms present during the same 2-week period and representing a change from previous function: • Depressed mood • Marked loss of interest or pleasure in activities • Change in appetite or weight • Insomnia or hypersomnia • Psychomotor agitation or retardation • Fatigue or loss of energy • Feelings of worthlessness or excessive/inappropriate guilt • Reduced ability to think, concentrate, or make decisions • Recurrent thoughts of death, suicidal ideation, or suicide attempt or plan At least one of the symptoms above must be either depressed mood or loss of interest or pleasure. DSM-5 offers alternative diagnoses for depressive disorder due to another medical condition or substance/medication-induced depressive disorder, characterized only by a prominent and persistent period of depressed mood or markedly diminished interest or pleasure in activities. The importance of demonstrating a link between the depressive episode and the medical condition or substance use is emphasized. In practice, the abbreviated criteria for these secondary syndromes are easy to meet, but the temporal link is not so easily established. Moreover, it is self-evident that all patients presenting with depression must be evaluated for symptoms such as suicidality and for contributing factors including undiscovered medical illness. Depression commonly occurs in the context of established medical illnesses such as diabetes, coronary artery disease, cerebrovascular insufficiency, cancer, epilepsy, multiple sclerosis, alcohol use disorder, SLE, HIV infection, Huntington's disease, and neurodegenerative diseases such as Parkinson's disease, Alzheimer's disease, and FTD. Depression also commonly follows stroke, heart attack, and TBI and is associated with medications including glucocorticoids, β-blockers, calcium channel blockers, statins, antiviral drugs, benzodiazepines, opioids, birth control pills, isotretinoin, varenicline, reserpine, and methyldopa.
Laboratory testing	Laboratory abnormalities may facilitate diagnosis of as-yet undiscovered medical conditions that cause or contribute to depression or predict later development of depression. These include anemia, macrocytosis, neutrophilia, abnormalities of liver function (elevated AST, ALT, and GGT), abnormalities of renal function, various endocrine derangements (involving thyroid, parathyroid, and adrenal glands), elevated HbA1C, hypoglycemia, testosterone deficiency, adult growth hormone deficiency, viral and bacterial infections, pancreatic cancer, and vitamin B_{12} or folate deficiency. Certain of these abnormalities are sufficiently common that routine testing is indicated in patients presenting with depression. Basic screening tests for MDD include the following: • CMP • CBC with differential and platelets

Major depressive disorder (MDD) *(continued)*

Laboratory testing *(continued)*	• Vitamin B$_{12}$ and folate levels • TSH Based on the patient's demographics, medical history, physical exam, and specific signs and symptoms, the following tests should also be considered: • Urinalysis • Urine toxicology screen • RPR • HIV testing • Blood alcohol level • Therapeutic medication levels (for TCAs or mood stabilizers) • Urine pregnancy testing, if indicated • ECG • Brain MRI or head CT • EEG

American Psychiatric Association: Diagnostic and Statistical Manual of Mental Disorders, 5th Edition, Text Revision. Washington, DC, American Psychiatric Association, 2022

Hsu WY, Chang TG, Chang CC, et al: Suicide ideation among outpatients with alcohol use disorder. Behav Neurol 2022:4138629, 2022

Sealock JM, Lee YH, Moscati A, et al: Use of the PsycheMERGE network to investigate the association between depression polygenic scores and white blood cell count. JAMA Psychiatry 78(12):1365–1374, 2021

Wainberg M, Kloiber S, Diniz B, et al: Clinical laboratory tests and five-year incidence of major depressive disorder: a prospective cohort study of 433,890 participants from the UK Biobank. Transl Psychiatry 11(1):380, 2021

Manganese poisoning

Clinical findings	Manganese is an essential micronutrient that serves as a cofactor in enzymatic reactions involved in metabolism, bone formation, reproduction, immune response, scavenging of reactive oxygen species, and blood clotting. The mineral is present in foods such as whole grains, certain shellfish, legumes, and nuts and is also available as a dietary supplement. It is absorbed in the small intestine and circulates in the blood, to be taken up by tissues including the liver, pancreas, kidney, and brain, with the highest concentrations in the globus pallidus and striatum. Manganese is eliminated mainly in the feces via biliary excretion.
	Because food is the primary source of manganese exposure in the general population, toxicity is uncommon except in countries where pesticide laws are lax. The most important source of toxic exposure is the inhalation of air contaminated with particulate matter containing manganese. Those who are at highest risk include miners, arc welders, steelworkers, and dry-battery manufacturers and those living and working in proximity to these industries. The potential toxicity of manganese-containing gasoline additives such as MMT (methylcyclopentadienyl manganese tricarbonyl, which replaced lead as an anti-knock agent) is unclear. Cases of manganese toxicity have been reported among patients receiving long-term total parenteral nutrition, in those injecting methcathinone ("cat") intravenously due to poor purification procedures, and among individuals ingesting manganese-contaminated well water. The U.S. Environmental Protection Agency has set a "health advisory level" for manganese in drinking water of 0.3 mg/L.
	Constitutional symptoms of manganese poisoning include apathy, malaise, lethargy, weakness, headache, poor appetite, and sexual dysfunction. Although cardiovascular and pulmonary systems are affected by toxicity, the most prominent symptoms are neuropsychiatric.
	Psychiatric signs and symptoms include the following:
	• Mood and personality changes: anxiety, irritability, euphoria, lability of mood
	• Psychosis ("manganese madness"): agitation, hallucinations, delusions with intact reality testing
	• Behavioral changes: compulsive behaviors, pseudobulbar affect, inappropriate jocularity, apathy, aggression, social withdrawal
	• Cognitive impairment (usually mild) involving memory and judgment domains
	• Sleep disturbance (insomnia or daytime somnolence)
	Specific motor signs and symptoms include the following:
	• Parkinsonism
	• Cogwheel rigidity
	• Akinesia/bradykinesia
	• Masked facies
	• Tremor (intention type)
	• Dysarthria
	• Hypophonia
	• Postural instability, retropulsion
	• Hyperreflexia

Manganese poisoning *(continued)*

Clinical findings *(continued)*	• Dystonia (face, neck, and distal lower extremities) • Characteristic gait disorder ("cock walk," a forward-tilting stance, on tiptoes) • Poor response to dopaminergic drugs
Laboratory testing	Brain MRI can be used along with manganese levels and clinical signs and symptoms to diagnose toxicity. MRI shows characteristic T1 hyperintensities in the basal ganglia reflecting manganese accumulation. The ratio of the signal observed in the globus pallidus to the signal observed in the frontal white matter multiplied by 100 yields the pallidal index, which is a reliable marker of manganese load. Reference levels for manganese: • Serum: 0.0–2.0 µg/L • Whole blood: 4.2–16.5 µg/L • RBCs: by report Serum levels are useful to indicate recent, active exposure. Whole blood levels are useful for monitoring manganese accumulation with total parenteral nutrition. RBC levels are useful to indicate recent, active exposure and may be useful in confirming long-term, low-dose exposure. Values between 1 and 2 times the upper limit of normal (ULN) may be due to normal biological variation and should be interpreted with caution. Values >2 times the ULN correspond to toxicity. For monitoring over time, samples should be taken no more frequently than the half-life of manganese, which is 40 days.

Abdel-Naby S, Hassanein M: Neuropsychiatric manifestations of chronic manganese poisoning. J Neurol Neurosurg Psychiatry 28:282–288, 1965

ARUP Laboratories: Manganese, RBC, in Laboratory Test Directory. Salt Lake City, UT, ARUP Laboratories, 2022. Available at: https://ltd.aruplab.com/Tests/Pub/2007254. Accessed February 2022.

ARUP Laboratories: Manganese, serum, in Laboratory Test Directory. Salt Lake City, UT, ARUP Laboratories, 2022. Available at: https://ltd.aruplab.com/Tests/Pub/0099265. Accessed February 2022.

ARUP Laboratories: Manganese, whole blood, in Laboratory Test Directory. Salt Lake City, UT, ARUP Laboratories, 2022. Available at: https://ltd.aruplab.com/Tests/Pub/0099272. Accessed February 2022.

Balani SG, Umarji GM, Bellare RA, et al: Chronic manganese poisoning. J Postgrad Med 13:116–121, 1967

Chandra SV: Psychiatric illness due to manganese poisoning. Acta Psychiatr Scand Suppl 303:49–54, 1983

Crossgrove J, Zheng W: Manganese toxicity upon overexposure. NMR Biomed 17:544–553, 2004

Fitzgerald K, Mikalunas V, Rubin H, et al: Hypermanganesemia in patients receiving total parenteral nutrition. JPEN J Parenter Enteral Nutr 23(6):333–336, 1999

Manic episode

Clinical findings	A manic episode is characterized by a distinct period of abnormally and persistently elevated, expansive, or irritable mood and abnormally and persistently increased activity or energy, lasting at least 1 week and present most of the day, nearly every day (or for any duration if hospitalization is necessary). During this period, three or more of the following symptoms are present (four or more symptoms if the mood is only irritable): grandiosity, decreased need for sleep, pressured speech or increased talkativeness, flight of ideas or racing thoughts, distractibility, increase in goal-directed activity or agitation, or excessive involvement in activities that have a high potential for painful consequences.
	As with other secondary syndromes, the criteria for diagnosing a manic episode due to another medical disorder are abbreviated, including only the following (along with the usual exclusions and severity criterion):
	• Prominent and persistent period of abnormally elevated, expansive, or irritable mood and abnormally increased activity or energy that predominates in the clinical picture
	• Evidence from the history, physical examination, or laboratory findings that the disturbance is the direct pathophysiological consequence of another medical condition
	Medical conditions known to cause mania or hypomania include the following:
	• Cerebral neoplasm
	• Cushing's disease
	• Encephalitis/meningitis
	• Epilepsy
	• Multiple sclerosis
	• Stroke
	• SLE
	• TBI
	• Wilson's disease
	Numerous other endocrine, metabolic, and infectious conditions can also be associated with mania/ hypomania. A first manic episode appearing in late life is particularly likely to be secondary to a neurological condition. Medications associated with mania include corticosteroids, anabolic steroids, antidepressants, dopaminergic drugs, tumor necrosis factor-α inhibitors, sympathomimetics, bronchodilators, amphetamines, and certain herbal preparations. Abuse of alcohol and many illicit drugs is also well known to be associated with mania.
Laboratory testing	Laboratory testing is performed to exclude underlying medical conditions that could be causing or contributing to the manic episode and to help guide treatment. The following tests should be considered:
	• CMP
	• CBC with differential and platelets
	• Urinalysis
	• TSH
	• RPR

Manic episode *(continued)*

Laboratory testing *(continued)*	In the presence of risk factors or suggestive history, the following tests should also be considered:
	• Urine toxicology
	• HIV testing
	• Blood alcohol level
	• ESR or CRP
	• Vitamin B_{12} or folate levels
	• Urine pregnancy testing
	• EEG (to exclude epileptiform activity)
	• Brain MRI or head CT
	If any of the medical conditions listed in the *Clinical Findings* section above as a cause of mania is suspected, further laboratory workup should be performed as detailed in the entries for those conditions.

American Psychiatric Association: Diagnostic and Statistical Manual of Mental Disorders, 5th Edition, Text Revision. Washington, DC, American Psychiatric Association, 2022

Bhatt K, Yoo J, Bridges A: Ketamine-induced manic episode. Prim Care Companion CNS Disord 23(3):20l02811, 2021

Jiménez-Fernández S, Solis MO, Martínez-Reyes I, et al: Secondary mania in an elderly patient during SARS-CoV-2 infection with complete remission: a 1-year follow-up. Psychiatr Danub 33(3):418–420, 2021

Miola A, Dal Porto V, Meda N, et al: Secondary mania induced by TNF-alpha inhibitors: a systematic review. Psychiatry Clin Neurosci 76(1):15–21, 2022

Park JH, Kummerlowe M, Gardea Resendez M, et al: First manic episode following COVID-19 infection. Bipolar Disord 23(8):847–849, 2021

Ramírez-Bermúdez J, Marrufo-Melendez O, Berlanga-Flores C, et al: White matter abnormalities in late onset first episode mania: a diffusion tensor imaging study. Am J Geriatr Psychiatry 29(12):1225–1236, 2021

Rao S, Sunkara A, Ashwath A, et al: Lupus cerebritis refractory to guideline-directed therapy: a case report. J Investig Med High Impact Case Rep 9:23247096211008708, 2021

Sami M, Khan H, Nilforooshan R: Late onset mania as an organic syndrome: a review of case reports in the literature. J Affect Disord 188:226–231, 2015

Sloan S, Dosumu-Johnson RT: A New onset of mania in a 49-year-old man: an interesting case of Wilson disease. J Psychiatr Pract 26(6):510–517, 2020

Tohen M, Shulman KI, Satlin A: First-episode mania in late life. Am J Psychiatry 151(1):130–132, 1994

Marchiafava-Bignami disease (MBD)

Clinical findings	MBD is an uncommon disorder characterized by demyelination and necrosis of the corpus callosum that has been identified mainly among males with chronic alcoholism and malnutrition. Callosal involvement can be partial or complete and may or may not be reversible with treatment. Cortical structures may also be involved (Morel's laminar sclerosis). The pathophysiology of MBD is thought to involve alcohol toxicity, B vitamin deficiencies (particularly thiamine), and possibly other factors. MRI findings suggest that cytotoxic edema is present early in the disease course, with demyelination and necrosis following.
	Prominent signs and symptoms of MBD include the following:
	• Delirium, stupor, coma
	• Disorientation, amnesia
	• Mutism
	• Callosal disconnection syndrome
	• Behavioral abnormalities (apathy, depression, psychosis)
	• Seizures
	• Gait disturbance
	• Pyramidal tract signs
	• Rigidity
	• Dysarthria
	• Primitive reflexes
	• Visual disturbances (diplopia or gaze palsy)
	Disruption of commissural fibers results in a characteristic callosal disconnection syndrome. Because language is processed mostly in the left hemisphere, the right hemisphere becomes isolated from language information, causing left hand anomia, left hand agraphia, and left ear extinction. In addition, knowledge required to perform learned/skilled motor acts is also processed mostly in the left hemisphere, so the right hemisphere becomes isolated from praxis information, causing left hand apraxia and difficulty in performing purposeful actions with the left hand. Other disconnection syndromes include alien hand, wayward hand, and intermanual conflict.
Laboratory testing	Because several other conditions affecting the same patient population—delirium tremens, Wernicke's encephalopathy, and osmotic demyelination—may present with similar symptoms, laboratory evaluation using MRI has proven a critical component of early diagnosis in MBD. Diffusion-weighted MRI shows the earliest evidence of lesions compatible with MBD, at the stage at which treatment may forestall progression to coma and death. This window is within 2 weeks of the onset of symptoms.
	• The study of choice for diagnosing MBD is diffusion-weighted MRI, which shows hyperintensities in affected areas.
	• Recovery may best be monitored using diffusion tensor imaging and fiber tracking.
	• Early phase edema of the corpus callosum and other involved areas may appear as hypointense areas on T1-weighted images and hyperintense areas on T2-weighted FLAIR images.

Marchiafava-Bignami disease (MBD) *(continued)*

Laboratory testing *(continued)*	• The "sandwich sign" on sagittal T1-weighted and FLAIR images indicates involvement of the central portion of the corpus callosum with sparing of the dorsal and ventral layers.
	• Lesions characteristic of MBD seen on admission are frequently persistent.

DeDios-Stern S, Gotra MY, Soble JR: Comprehensive neuropsychological findings in a case of Marchiafava-Bignami disease. Clin Neuropsychol 35(6):1191–1202, 2021

Dong X, Bai C, Nao J: Clinical and radiological features of Marchiafava-Bignami disease. Medicine (Baltimore) 97(5):e9626, 2018

Hillbom M, Saloheimo P, Fujioka S, et al: Diagnosis and management of Marchiafava-Bignami disease: a review of CT/MRI confirmed cases. J Neurol Neurosurg Psychiatry 85(2):168–173, 2014

Kakkar C, Prakashini K, Polnaya A: Acute Marchiafava-Bignami disease: clinical and serial MRI correlation. BMJ Case Rep 2014:bcr2013203442, 2014

Kinsley S, Giovane RA, Daly S, Shulman D: Rare case of Marchiafava-Bignami disease due to thiamine deficiency and malnutrition. BMJ Case Rep 13(12):e238187, 2020

Li W, Ran C, Ma J: Diverse MRI findings and clinical outcomes of acute Marchiafava-Bignami disease. Acta Radiol 62(7):904–908, 2021

Namekawa M, Nakamura Y, Nakano I: Cortical involvement in Marchiafava-Bignami disease can be a predictor of a poor prognosis: a case report and review of the literature. Intern Med 52(7):811–813, 2013

Tung CS, Wu SL, Tsou JC, et al: Marchiafava-Bignami disease with widespread lesions and complete recovery. AJNR Am J Neuroradiol 31:1506–1507, 2010

Meningitis

Clinical findings	Meningitis refers to an inflammation of the layers of tissue surrounding the brain and spinal cord and the enclosed subarachnoid space that is caused by infectious or non-infectious pathologies. Meningeal infections include bacterial, viral, mycobacterial, spirochetal, parasitic, and fungal diseases that reach the CNS by crossing the blood-brain barrier directly or by infecting immune cells that then cross the blood-brain barrier. Aseptic meningitis refers to inflammation caused by pathogens other than pus-producing bacteria (most commonly viruses) or by non-infectious conditions. Except for viral meningitis, mortality rates in infectious meningitis remain high, particularly for tuberculous and cryptococcal pathogens in immunocompromised individuals. Prompt diagnosis and treatment of all cases is essential.
	Non-infectious causes of meningitis include neoplastic, autoimmune, and chemical pathologies. Neoplastic meningitis can be a complication of either hematological malignancies or solid tumors (most commonly breast cancer, non-small-cell lung cancer, or malignant melanoma). Autoimmune meningitis can be associated with diseases such as rheumatoid arthritis and SLE. Chemical- or drug-induced meningitis can result from direct meningeal irritation (with intrathecally administered drugs) or hypersensitivity reactions.
	Signs and symptoms of meningitis depend on the cause and chronicity of symptoms.
	Bacterial meningitis is characterized by the following:
	• Fulminant to subacute onset
	• Classic triad for meningitis: fever, headache, and neck rigidity (may be severe)
	• Delirium, lethargy, coma
	• Nausea and vomiting
	• Photophobia
	• Seizures (partial or generalized)
	• Evidence of increased intracranial pressure: stupor, papilledema, dilated and poorly reactive pupils, sixth nerve palsy, decerebrate posturing, bradycardia, hypertension, and irregular respiration
	• Skin rash with meningococcemia
	Viral meningitis is characterized by the following:
	• Classic triad for meningitis: fever, headache, and neck rigidity (mild)
	• Constitutional symptoms: malaise, myalgia, anorexia, nausea, vomiting, diarrhea, abdominal pain
	• Lethargy or drowsiness (stupor or delirium suggests another diagnosis)
	Chronic meningitis is diagnosed when signs and symptoms are present for ≥4 weeks. In chronic disease, signs and symptoms include the following:
	• Fever
	• Headache
	• Lethargy
	• Mental status changes
	• Hearing loss

Meningitis *(continued)*

Clinical findings *(continued)*	• Diplopia
	• Cognitive impairment
	• Hydrocephalus, elevated intracranial pressure (especially with cryptococcus)
	• Seizures
	• Stroke-like episodes
	• Radiculopathies (spinal cord involvement)
	• Less common: signs of meningeal irritation or neck rigidity
Laboratory testing	*CSF testing*
	The mainstay of testing for infectious meningitis involves lumbar puncture (LP) with CSF sampling. Before an LP, a CT scan should be performed in certain patients to identify those at risk of brain herniation, including the immunocompromised, those with a history of CNS disease (e.g., mass, stroke, or focal infection), those with a seizure within the past week, or those with papilledema, abnormal level of consciousness, or focal neurological deficit (e.g., dilated nonreactive pupil, gaze palsy, or arm/leg drift).
	When an LP is performed, the opening pressure is measured and fluid sent for the following:
	• Chemistries (total protein and glucose)
	• Cell count (and differential)
	• Microbiology (Gram stain and culture)
	About 6 mL of fluid is sufficient for routine testing, but if tuberculosis or fungal meningitis is suspected, a large-volume sample of 10–20 mL should be sent to the laboratory. Some CSF should be saved for further studies.
	In general, meningitis caused by bacteria or mycobacteria is associated with higher total protein, lower CSF glucose, and greater elevation in WBC count than that caused by viral disease.
	The diagnosis of bacterial meningitis is made by Gram stain and culture of CSF. PCR testing panels for multiple pathogens should be performed where available. Technologies such as matrix-assisted laser desorption/ionization–time of flight (MALDI-TOF) mass spectrometry testing for multiple pathogens should be considered.
	For tuberculous meningitis, acid-fast bacillus smear and culture may still be used but are insensitive, and culture takes weeks to return. Automated PCR could also be used, but the commercially available test Xpert MTB/RIF Ultra (*Mycobacterium tuberculosis* and rifampicin) is now a first-line recommendation for detection of tuberculosis, with information on drug sensitivity and drug resistance included. The result is returned within hours.
	The diagnosis of cryptococcal meningitis is based on the detection of cryptococcal antigen in CSF via lateral flow immunoassay. Culture may also be helpful.
	For viral meningitis, the focus of testing is PCR amplification of viral DNA.
	For chronic meningitis, serial LP (up to 3 times) may be indicated for fungal and mycobacterial cultures if the initial results are negative. Repeat testing of CSF cytology may also be indicated if initially negative.

Meningitis *(continued)*

Laboratory testing *(continued)*	Metagenomic next-generation sequencing (NGS) allows screening for a range of bacterial, fungal, parasitic, and viral pathogens in a single assay. Because this area of research is rapidly evolving, inquiry should be made to the laboratory to determine what is available for CSF testing. At this writing, NGS is used in tandem with traditional microbiological testing.
	Neuroimaging
	In general, neuroimaging does not facilitate the diagnosis of meningitis but may be useful in identifying parameningeal causes of CSF abnormalities or complications of meningitis such as hydrocephalus, brain abscess, or subdural empyema. In addition, neuroimaging should be performed in patients with seizures, focal neurological signs, altered consciousness, or an atypical CSF profile. In bacterial meningitis, MRI is preferred to CT because of its ability to detect edema and ischemia.

Abussuud ZA, Geneta VP: Rheumatoid meningitis. World Neurosurg 137:98–101, 2020

Aksamit AJ: Chronic meningitis. N Engl J Med 385(10):930–936, 2021

de Oliveira L, Melhem MSC, Buccheri R, et al: Early clinical and microbiological predictors of outcome in hospitalized patients with cryptococcal meningitis. BMC Infect Dis 22(1):138, 2022

Guziejko K, Czupryna P, Zielenkiewicz-Madejska EK, Moniuszko-Malinowska A: Pneumococcal meningitis and COVID-19: dangerous coexistence: a case report. BMC Infect Dis 22(1):182, 2022

Heller HM, Gonzalez RG, Edlow BL, et al: Case 40–2020: a 24-year-old man with headache and COVID-19. N Engl J Med 383(26):2572–2580, 2020

Kohil A, Jemmieh S, Smatti MK, Yassine HM: Viral meningitis: an overview. Arch Virol 166(2):335–345, 2021

Méchaï F, Bouchaud O: Tuberculous meningitis: challenges in diagnosis and management. Rev Neurol (Paris) 175(7–8):451–457, 2019

Poplin V, Boulware DR, Bahr NC: Methods for rapid diagnosis of meningitis etiology in adults. Biomark Med 14(6):459–479, 2020

Rigakos G, Liakou CI, Felipe N, et al: Clinical presentation, diagnosis, and radiological findings of neoplastic meningitis. Cancer Control 24(1):9–21, 2017

Straus SE, Thorpe KE, Holroyd-Leduc J: How do I perform a lumbar puncture and analyze the results to diagnose bacterial meningitis? JAMA 296:2012–2022, 2006

Vasudeva SS: Meningitis workup, in Medscape: Drugs and Diseases: Infectious Diseases, 2022. Available at: https://emedicine.medscape.com/article/232915-workup. Accessed March 2022.

Wilson MR, Sample HA, Zorn KC, et al: Clinical metagenomic sequencing for diagnosis of meningitis and encephalitis. N Engl J Med 380(24):2327–2340, 2019

Xing XW, Zhang JT, Ma YB, et al: Metagenomic next-generation sequencing for diagnosis of infectious encephalitis and meningitis: a large, prospective case series of 213 patients. Front Cell Infect Microbiol 10:88, 2020

Yelehe-Okouma M, Czmil-Garon J, Pape E, et al: Drug-induced aseptic meningitis: a mini-review. Fundam Clin Pharmacol 32(3):252–260, 2018

Mercury poisoning

Clinical findings	The chemical element mercury is known to be toxic to humans and other animals, and although mercury exposure occurs from a variety of everyday activities, the long-term and cumulative effects of exposure have been inadequately characterized. Mercury occurs in three forms: elemental, organic, and inorganic.
	• *Elemental mercury* exposure occurs primarily from dental amalgam and in occupations such as dentistry, electroplating, metallurgy, mining, and a long list of others in which mercury is used in processing. Toxicity arises from breathing mercury vapor, which can easily be generated from something as simple as drilling a "silver" filling or when mercury is removed from an enclosed container such as a thermometer. The vapor is lipid-soluble and readily crosses the blood-brain barrier.
	• *Inorganic mercury* has been used in cosmetics and medicines and as a topical antiseptic. Industrial exposure occurs in the tanning industry, in taxidermy, in the manufacturing of fireworks, and in dye production. This form can be found in patent medicines, Asian herbal preparations, and certain skin creams manufactured outside the United States. Toxicity arises from inhalation, ingestion, or absorption through the skin.
	• *Organic mercury* exposure occurs primarily through fish consumption because other uses of this form have been banned or severely curtailed. This form is highly toxic and a known teratogen. Accordingly, recommendations to limit fish intake (to three or fewer servings per week) and to stay informed as to current data regarding fish species have been published. One excellent source of information is the Environmental Working Group's *Consumer Guide to Seafood* cited in the reference list below.
	Exposure to mercury likely poses a greater risk among specific subpopulations, including pregnant females and their developing fetuses, nursing females and their infants, children, people with preexisting neurological or renal disease, those with known sensitivity to metals, and possibly those with certain susceptibility genes, not all of which are known. This latter possibility has generated concern that dental amalgam may not be safe for some individuals.
	Neuropsychiatric signs and symptoms of mercury poisoning include fatigue, headache, apathy, irritability, emotional instability, psychosis, amnestic mild cognitive impairment, paresthesias, parkinsonism, ataxia, postural and action tremor, myoclonus, neuromyotonia, choreoathetosis, deafness, dysarthria, dysphagia, visual field constriction, and coma. Some cases have a fatal outcome.
	With inhalation of elemental mercury, pulmonary symptoms are seen, including burning in the mouth and lungs, cough, difficulty breathing, and chest tightness. With ingestion of mercury salts or organic mercury, GI symptoms are seen, including nausea, vomiting, and diarrhea. Decreased urine output and renal toxicity may also be seen. High mercury load is a risk factor for ischemic heart disease and may be a risk factor for neurodegenerative disease.

Mercury poisoning *(continued)*

Laboratory testing	*Reference values*
	• Whole blood mercury, inorganic: ≤10.0 µg/L
	Urine:
	• Urine mercury/24 hours: 0.0–20.0 µg/day
	• Urine mercury/volume: 0.0–5.0 µg/L
	• Mercury-to-creatinine ratio: 0.0–20 µg/gCR
	The mercury level in whole blood is used for evaluation of acute exposure to inorganic forms because blood levels rise and fall quickly over several days. Exposure to organic mercury may contribute to elevated total mercury levels, with blood concentrations of 20–50 µg/L. Dietary and other restrictions are required before testing; see ARUP Laboratories reference cited below.
	Urine mercury levels are used for evaluating acute or chronic elemental or inorganic mercury exposure and for monitoring treatment. Dietary and other restrictions are required before testing (see ARUP Laboratories reference). Twenty-four-hour urine levels of 30–100 µg/L are associated with tremor and subclinical neuropsychiatric symptoms, while levels >100 µg/L are associated with overt neuropsychiatric impairment.
	Testing of other samples (e.g., blood, hair, toenails) for chronic mercury poisoning is less useful because the samples are not likely to reflect distant neuronal injury.

ARUP Laboratories: Mercury, urine, in Laboratory Test Directory. Salt Lake City, UT, ARUP Laboratories, 2022. Available at: https://ltd.aruplab.com/Tests/Pub/0025050. Accessed March 2022.

ARUP Laboratories: Mercury, whole blood, in Laboratory Test Directory. Salt Lake City, UT, ARUP Laboratories, 2022. Available at: https://ltd.aruplab.com/Tests/Pub/0099305. Accessed March 2022.

Cariccio VL, Samà A, Bramanti P, Mazzon E: Mercury involvement in neuronal damage and in neurodegenerative diseases. Biol Trace Elem Res 187(2):341–356, 2019

Ekino S, Susa M, Ninomiya T, et al: Minamata disease revisited: an update on the acute and chronic manifestations of methyl mercury poisoning. J Neurol Sci 262:131–144, 2007

Environmental Working Group: EWG's Consumer Guide to Seafood. Washington, DC, Environmental Working Group, 2014. Available at: https://www.ewg.org/consumer-guides/ewgs-consumer-guide-seafood. Accessed March 2022.

Homme KG, Kern JK, Haley BE, et al: New science challenges old notion that mercury dental amalgam is safe. Biometals 27(1):19–24, 2014

Hu XF, Lowe M, Chan HM: Mercury exposure, cardiovascular disease, and mortality: a systematic review and dose-response meta-analysis. Environ Res 193:110538, 2021

Jackson AC: Chronic neurological disease due to methylmercury poisoning. Can J Neurol Sci 45(6):620–623, 2018

Johnson-Arbor K, Schultz B: Effective decontamination and remediation after elemental mercury exposure: a case report in the United States. J Prev Med Public Health 54(5):376–379, 2021

Kolipinski M, Subramanian M, Kristen K, et al: Sources and toxicity of mercury in the San Francisco Bay Area, spanning California and beyond. J Environ Public Health 2020:8184614, 2020

Ran E, Wang M, Yi Y, et al: Mercury poisoning complicated by acquired neuromyotonia syndrome: a case report. Medicine (Baltimore) 100(32):e26910, 2021

Rice KM, Walker EM Jr, Wu M, et al: Environmental mercury and its toxic effects. J Prev Med Public Health 47(2):74–83, 2014

Siblerud R, Mutter J, Moore E, et al: A hypothesis and evidence that mercury may be an etiological factor in Alzheimer's disease. Int J Environ Res Public Health 16(24):5152, 2019

Stratakis N, Conti DV, Borras E, et al: Association of fish consumption and mercury exposure during pregnancy with metabolic health and inflammatory biomarkers in children. JAMA Netw Open 3(3):e201007, 2020

U.S. Food and Drug Administration: Dental amalgam fillings, in Medical Devices: Products and Medical Procedures: Dental Devices. Washington, DC, U.S. Food and Drug Administration, 2021. Available at: https://www.fda.gov/medical-devices/dental-devices/dental-amalgam-fillings#fish. Accessed March 2022.

Metabolic syndrome

Clinical findings	The metabolic syndrome is a group of risk factors that increase the risk of diabetes mellitus, heart disease, and stroke. These risk factors include hypertension, hyperlipidemia, hyperglycemia, and truncal obesity (excess body fat around the waist). There is substantial evidence that patients with psychiatric disorders are at increased risk of developing the syndrome. This elevated risk is seen with major depressive disorder, bipolar disorder, schizophrenia, alcohol use disorder, anxiety disorders, PTSD, and ADHD. The extent to which psychiatric illness itself is responsible for the increased risk independent of medication use remains unclear.
	It is well established that certain psychotropic medications contribute significantly to the risk of the metabolic syndrome. This is particularly true for atypical antipsychotics (especially olanzapine and clozapine) and, to a lesser extent, mood stabilizers and antidepressants (except bupropion). Unlike other atypical antipsychotics, aripiprazole and ziprasidone do not increase the risk, and there is evidence that aripiprazole may have protective effects.
	Psychiatrists and other behavioral medicine specialists are on the front lines of management for these at-risk populations, so it is critical that clinicians become fully aware of the need to initiate preventive measures, to closely monitor the syndrome parameters in the course of treatment with psychotropic drugs, and to ensure adequate treatment of metabolic abnormalities.
Laboratory testing	The metabolic syndrome is defined by three or more of the following: • Abdominal obesity: increased waist circumference; >38–41 inches in males and >32 inches in females • Impaired glycemic control: fasting blood sugar 100–125 mg/dL or HbA1C 5.7%–6.4% • Hypertension: blood pressure ≥130/85 or taking medication for hypertension • Hyperlipidemia: fasting triglycerides >150–180 mg/dL or fasting high-density lipoprotein cholesterol <40 mg/dL for males or <50 mg/dL for females, or taking medication for high triglycerides or low HDL cholesterol

Dregan A, Rayner L, Davis KAS, et al: Associations between depression, arterial stiffness, and metabolic syndrome among adults in the UK Biobank Population Study: a mediation analysis. JAMA Psychiatry 77(6):598–606, 2020

Ijaz S, Bolea B, Davies S, et al: Antipsychotic polypharmacy and metabolic syndrome in schizophrenia: a review of systematic reviews. BMC Psychiatry 18(1):275, 2018

Jeon SW, Kim YK: Unresolved issues for utilization of atypical antipsychotics in schizophrenia: antipsychotic polypharmacy and metabolic syndrome. Int J Mol Sci 18(10):2174, 2017

Mazereel V, Detraux J, Vancampfort D, et al: Impact of psychotropic medication effects on obesity and the metabolic syndrome in people with serious mental illness. Front Endocrinol (Lausanne) 11:573479, 2020

Penninx BWJH, Lange SMM: Metabolic syndrome in psychiatric patients: overview, mechanisms, and implications. Dialogues Clin Neurosci 20(1):63–73, 2018

Schuster MP, Borkent J, Chrispijn M, et al: Increased prevalence of metabolic syndrome in patients with bipolar disorder compared to a selected control group: a Northern Netherlands LifeLines population cohort study. J Affect Disord 295:1161–1168, 2021

Zhang M, Chen J, Yin Z, et al: The association between depression and metabolic syndrome and its components: a bidirectional two-sample Mendelian randomization study. Transl Psychiatry 11(1):633, 2021

Metachromatic leukodystrophy (MLD)

Clinical findings	MLD is a rare autosomal recessive genetic disorder arising from the accumulation of toxic metabolites known as sulfatides inside cells of the nervous system that appear as differently colored granules under the microscope. This toxic accumulation results in demyelination and destruction of white matter. The condition is the result of deficient activity of the lysosomal enzyme arylsulfatase A caused by a mutation in the arylsulfatase A gene (*ARSA*) or (in a minority of cases) in the saposin B gene (*PSAP*).
	Most cases of MLD come to clinical attention in early life, but up to 20% are adult-onset, presenting from adolescence to the seventh decade and representing a less severe form. Symptoms can progress slowly with this form, with periods of relative stability interspersed with rapid decline. Patients have been reported to survive up to 30 years after diagnosis.
	In adult-onset MLD, the initial symptoms are predominantly neuropsychiatric, with motor symptoms emerging only in later stages. For this reason, the condition is likely to be mistaken for dementia or a primary psychiatric disorder.
	Signs and symptoms include the following:
	• Decreased performance at work or school
	• Behavioral and personality changes—impulsiveness, irritability, disinhibition, socially inappropriate behaviors, neglect of personal affairs
	• Cognitive impairment—dementia with prominent frontal lobe features, memory impairment
	• Depression, mood swings
	• Psychosis—hallucinations (especially auditory) and delusions (may be bizarre)
	• Peripheral neuropathy
	• Cerebellar ataxia
	• Spasticity
	• Seizures
	• Optic atrophy
	• Gradual loss of motor skills
	The diagnosis is made based on clinical findings along with the lab studies noted below. One possibly helpful non-neurological sign is cholecystitis arising from sulfatide accumulation in the wall of the gallbladder.
Laboratory testing	The following tests are used to aid in diagnosis of MLD:
	• Genetic testing for mutations in *ARSA* and/or *PSAP*. This testing can also be used to identify carriers and for prenatal diagnosis.
	• Biochemical testing for arylsulfatase A enzyme activity in leukocytes or cultured skin fibroblasts. In MLD, values usually range from undetectable to <10% of normal. A pseudo-deficiency syndrome exists in which values range from 5% to 20% of normal, and clinical and MRI evidence of MLD is absent. These entities can be distinguished with further testing such as urine sulfatide levels, which are elevated in MLD and normal in the pseudo-deficiency syndrome.

Metachromatic leukodystrophy (MLD) *(continued)*

Laboratory testing *(continued)*	• Brain MRI: findings include symmetric, confluent hyperintensities in frontal more than parietal periventricular white matter on T2-weighted imaging with sparing of subcortical U fibers. In later disease stages, atrophy due to loss of white matter volume is seen. MLD is not excluded based on a normal MRI.

Beerepoot S, Nierkens S, Boelens JJ, et al: Peripheral neuropathy in metachromatic leukodystrophy: current status and future perspective. Orphanet J Rare Dis 14(1):240, 2019

Ben Ammar H, Hakiri A, Khelifa E, et al: Metachromatic leukodystrophy presenting as a bipolar disorder: a case report. Encephale 48(1):108–109, 2022

Benzoni C, Moscatelli M, Fenu S, et al: Metachromatic leukodystrophy with late adult-onset: diagnostic clues and differences from other genetic leukoencephalopathies with dementia. J Neurol 268(5):1972–1976, 2021 [published correction appears in J Neurol 268(5):1977–1979, 2021]

Etemadifar M, Ashourizadeh H, Nouri H, et al: MRI signs of CNS demyelinating diseases. Mult Scler Relat Disord 47:102665, 2021

Fumagalli F, Zambon AA, Rancoita PMV, et al: Metachromatic leukodystrophy: a single-center longitudinal study of 45 patients. J Inherit Metab Dis 44(5):1151–1164, 2021

Köhler W, Curiel J, Vanderver A: Adulthood leukodystrophies. Nat Rev Neurol 14(2):94–105, 2018

Resende LL, de Paiva ARB, Kok F, et al: Adult leukodystrophies: a step-by-step diagnostic approach. Radiographics 39(1):153–168, 2019

van Rappard DF, Boelens JJ, Wolf NI: Metachromatic leukodystrophy: disease spectrum and approaches for treatment. Best Pract Res Clin Endocrinol Metab 29(2):261–273, 2015

van Rappard DF, Bugiani M, Boelens JJ, et al: Gallbladder and the risk of polyps and carcinoma in metachromatic leukodystrophy. Neurology 87(1):103–111, 2016

Methanol poisoning

Clinical findings	Methanol, also known as methyl alcohol or wood alcohol, is a highly toxic substance found in windshield washer fluid, gas line antifreeze, carburetor cleaner, copy machine fluid, perfumes, food warming fuel, and other types of fuels. In the past, exposure to methanol occurred accidentally from contaminated home-distilled and fermented beverages, or intentionally, with ingestion of products such as windshield washer fluid as a means of suicide, use of food-warming fuel as a substitute for ethanol when the latter was unavailable, and abuse of carburetor cleaner via inhalation ("huffing"). More recently, worldwide exposures occurred starting in 2020 with the COVID-19 pandemic, when false rumors appeared on social media that the virus could be prevented or treated by drinking or gargling hand sanitizer. A significant number of those hand sanitizers, notably those from Mexico, contained methanol rather than ethyl alcohol or isopropanol.
	As little as 2 tbsp of methanol can be lethal for a child and 2 fl oz for an adult. The prognosis with poisoning depends on the amount ingested and how soon treatment is administered. Once ingested, methanol is rapidly absorbed and oxidized by alcohol dehydrogenase to formaldehyde, and then by aldehyde dehydrogenase to formic acid. An initial high osmolal gap decreases and an anion gap increases as metabolism proceeds. Formic acid is the primary toxic metabolite, causing retinal toxicity and later parkinsonism. Treatment consists of supportive care, correction of acidosis, use of an alcohol dehydrogenase inhibitor (fomepizole, or ethanol orally or intravenously if fomepizole is not available), and hemodialysis. Left untreated, methanol poisoning can be fatal.
	Psychiatrists may encounter methanol poisoning in patients who are suicidal, in those with alcohol use disorder who lack access to ethanol, in patients using solvents for huffing, and in misguided patients ingesting hand sanitizer. Acute poisoning causes optic neuropathy and necrotic lesions of the basal ganglia and subcortical white matter.
	On presentation, patients might initially appear normal or inebriated. Onset of clinical and laboratory features can be delayed for days with co-ingestion of ethanol. Initial symptoms are gastrointestinal, followed by CNS depression and hyperventilation. Visual changes such as blurred vision, decreased acuity, photophobia, and "halo vision" are associated with an abnormal funduscopic exam. Seizures can occur. Several weeks after exposure, parkinsonian signs can be seen, with tremor, cogwheel rigidity, hypokinesia, stooped posture, and shuffling gait. Necrosis of the putamen and globus pallidus are associated with these findings.
Laboratory testing	Methanol is not detectable at levels <5 mg/dL.

Toxicity is associated with levels >20 mg/dL.

Plasma level may be below the assay's limit of detection even though the patient shows signs of toxicity. Laboratory findings may be delayed up to 3–4 days when ethanol is co-ingested.

A newly developed handheld device to detect and quantify methanol in spiked breath can help to distinguish methanol from ethanol intoxication. |

Methanol poisoning *(continued)*

ARUP Laboratories: Methanol, in Laboratory Test Directory. Salt Lake City, UT, ARUP Laboratories, 2021. Available at: https://ltd.aruplab.com/Tests/Pub/0090165. Accessed August 2021.

Liu YS, Lin KY, Masur J, et al: Outcomes after recurrent intentional methanol exposures not treated with alcohol dehydrogenase inhibitors or hemodialysis. J Emerg Med 58(6):910–916, 2020

Mana J, Vaneckova M, Klempír J, et al: Methanol poisoning as an acute toxicological basal ganglia lesion model: evidence from brain volumetry and cognition. Alcohol Clin Exp Res 43(7):1486–1497, 2019

Mehrpour O, Sadeghi M: Toll of acute methanol poisoning for preventing COVID-19. Arch Toxicol 94(6):2259–2260, 2020

Sefidbakht S, Lotfi M, Jalli R, et al: Methanol toxicity outbreak: when fear of COVID-19 goes viral. Emerg Med J 37(7):416, 2020

van den Broek J, Bischof D, Derron N, et al: Screening methanol poisoning with a portable breath detector. Anal Chem 93(2):1170–1178, 2021

Yip L, Bixler D, Brooks DE, et al: Serious adverse health events, including death, associated with ingesting alcohol-based hand sanitizers containing methanol—Arizona and New Mexico, May–June 2020. MMWR Morb Mortal Wkly Rep 69(32):1070–1073, 2020

Zakharov S, Pelclova D, Navratil T, et al: Fomepizole versus ethanol in the treatment of acute methanol poisoning: comparison of clinical effectiveness in a mass poisoning outbreak. Clin Toxicol (Phila) 53(8):797–806, 2015

Mild neurocognitive disorder

Clinical findings	Mild neurocognitive disorder (also known as mild cognitive impairment or MCI) is characterized by 1) modest cognitive decline from a previous level of performance in one or more cognitive domains based on concern of the patient, informant, or clinician and 2) a modest impairment in cognitive performance documented by cognitive testing. Domains of cognition that may be affected include complex attention, executive function, learning and memory, language, perceptual motor, and social cognition. By definition, the decline does not interfere with the patient's capacity for independent living, but greater effort or accommodation may be required to complete activities. The deficits are not better explained by another mental disorder such as schizophrenia or major depressive disorder.
	In the evaluation of the patient presenting with cognitive concerns, it is important to determine which domains are affected. To this end, an instrument such as the Montreal Cognitive Assessment (MoCA) can be used, with neuropsychological testing providing a more comprehensive and detailed account. In addition, specific questions about daily function should be addressed to exclude the diagnosis of major neurocognitive disorder (dementia).
	If memory impairment is established, a preliminary diagnosis of amnestic MCI is made. This can involve memory only (single domain) or several domains (multiple-domain amnestic MCI). Single-domain amnestic MCI can be seen in depression or presage the development of dementia due to Alzheimer's disease (AD) or other conditions. Multiple-domain amnestic MCI can be seen in depression and/or vascular cognitive impairment or may presage the development of dementia due to AD or other conditions.
	If memory impairment is not present but other domains are affected, non-amnestic MCI (single or multiple domain) is diagnosed. Single-domain non-amnestic MCI may presage the development of FTD or dementia due to AD or other conditions. Multiple-domain non-amnestic MCI can be seen in vascular cognitive impairment or can presage the development of dementia with Lewy bodies (DLB) or dementia due to AD, among other conditions.
	In general, a gradually progressive course of impairment suggests the presence of a neurodegenerative disease, whereas a "stepwise" course is more consistent with cerebrovascular disease. The presence of amnestic MCI in an older patient may suggest AD. The presence of attention, concentration, and visuospatial impairment may suggest DLB. The presence of apathy, poor insight, inappropriate behaviors, and problems with attention and concentration may suggest FTD. In addition, other symptoms of primary psychiatric or medical disease must be considered because these conditions dictate different pathways for workup and treatment.
Laboratory testing	Workup for reversible causes of cognitive impairment includes the following blood lab tests: CBC, CMP, TSH, vitamin B_{12}, folate, and syphilis testing (may require FTA-ABS if tertiary syphilis is suspected).
	CT scan can be used to exclude a limited number of disease entities that could give rise to cognitive decline such as tumor, hydrocephalus, or hemorrhage.

Mild neurocognitive disorder *(continued)*

Laboratory testing *(continued)*	Brain MRI can be used to exclude a variety of conditions that could give rise to cognitive decline (including cerebrovascular disease) and provides detailed regional volumetric information helpful in differentiating dementia etiologies.
	FDG-PET shows abnormal patterns of metabolism in different etiologies of dementia. It is often used in differentiating AD from FTD.
	Amyloid PET scanning provides quantitative data regarding the presence of amyloid plaques, which is helpful in the diagnosis of AD. Tau PET scanning provides useful information on the degree of neurodegeneration, with the results closely associated with the degree of cognitive impairment.
	CSF studies are used to detect a variety of abnormalities corresponding to different etiologies of dementia. In AD, CSF levels of amyloid-β_{42} are reduced, while CSF tau and phosphorylated tau are elevated.
	Newer research has demonstrated that blood plasma levels of amyloid-β and phosphorylated tau can distinguish AD from other dementia etiologies. As of this writing, these tests are not widely commercially available.
	Although apolipoprotein E epsilon genetic testing in patients with underlying AD may show 4/4 homozygosity or 4/* heterozygosity, representing a risk factor for progression to clinical dementia, the test is less useful than others in distinguishing etiology.

American Psychiatric Association: Diagnostic and Statistical Manual of Mental Disorders, 5th Edition, Text Revision. Washington, DC, American Psychiatric Association, 2022

Anderson ND: State of the science on mild cognitive impairment (MCI). CNS Spectr 24(1):78–87, 2019

Breton A, Casey D, Arnaoutoglou NA: Cognitive tests for the detection of mild cognitive impairment (MCI), the prodromal stage of dementia: meta-analysis of diagnostic accuracy studies. Int J Geriatr Psychiatry 34(2):233–242, 2019

Campbell NL, Unverzagt F, LaMantia MA, et al: Risk factors for the progression of mild cognitive impairment to dementia. Clin Geriatr Med 29(4):873–893, 2013

Giau VV, Bagyinszky E, An SSA: Potential fluid biomarkers for the diagnosis of mild cognitive impairment. Int J Mol Sci 20(17):4149, 20109

Jongsiriyanyong S, Limpawattana P: Mild cognitive impairment in clinical practice: a review article. Am J Alzheimers Dis Other Demen 33(8):500–507, 2018

Morozova A, Zorkina Y, Abramova O, et al: Neurobiological highlights of cognitive impairment in psychiatric disorders. Int J Mol Sci 23(3):1217, 2022

Petersen RC. Mild cognitive impairment. Continuum (Minneap Minn) 22(2):404–418, 2016

Multiple sclerosis (MS)

Clinical findings	MS is a degenerative disorder characterized by inflammatory demyelination and axonal degeneration in the white matter of the brain and spinal cord. Some lesions undergo repair of myelin, while others evolve into chronic plaques. Both genetic and environmental factors are believed to contribute to the development of MS, which typically affects individuals between 20 and 40 years of age and is most common in Whites of northern European ancestry.
	For many patients, the first evidence of MS appears as a clinically isolated syndrome (CIS), which involves one or more neurological symptoms lasting ~24 hours. Common symptoms of CIS are optic neuritis (with blurred vision, color distortion, and eye pain), usually affecting only one eye, and paresthesias, usually involving the legs or neck (Lhermitte's sign). At this stage, the presence of gadolinium-enhancing lesions on MRI and oligoclonal bands on CSF analysis predict the progression from CIS to MS.
	Signs and symptoms of MS include fatigue, depression, hearing or visual loss, weakness, muscle spasm, tremor, bowel/bladder dysfunction, sexual dysfunction, increased tone, pain, dizziness, incoordination, and ataxia. Each symptomatic episode of MS lasts from days to weeks. About half of affected patients develop some degree of cognitive impairment (which may be mild) involving attention, concentration, memory, and judgment. Suicide risk may be high.
	In addition to CIS, three patterns of clinical disease are recognized:
	• *Relapsing-remitting MS*: symptoms worsen and then remit episodically. This is the most common form of MS, with a varying frequency of relapse but usually not more than one or two per year. Infection is a common trigger of relapse. About half of relapses lead to residual deficits so that stepwise deterioration is seen.
	• *Primary progressive MS*: symptoms worsen slowly and steadily.
	• *Secondary progressive MS*: begins as the relapsing-remitting form, then develops into progressive disease. Most untreated patients with relapsing-remitting MS develop secondary progressive MS after a median interval of 19 years.
	Early diagnosis of MS is critical because aggressive intervention with disease-modifying and anti-inflammatory treatments reduces the rate of relapse, slows the formation of new lesions, and reduces the risk of brain atrophy, all resulting in a reduction of disability.
Laboratory testing	*Magnetic resonance imaging*
	MRI with gadolinium contrast is the testing modality of choice for diagnosis of MS, used in conjunction with clinical findings. Conventional MRI using T1- and T2-weighted sequences and FLAIR imaging can identify lesions in the brain, brainstem, and spinal cord for initial diagnosis and to monitor the effects of treatment, although there may be discordance between lesion burden and location and clinical examination. T1-weighted images show cerebral atrophy and hypointense areas reflecting axonal death, while T2-weighted images show edema and chronic lesions (plaques). Advanced MRI techniques such as diffusion tensor imaging can detect lesions that are missed by conventional MRI.

Multiple sclerosis (MS) *(continued)*

Laboratory testing *(continued)*	*CSF analysis*
	In cases in which insufficient clinical and MRI evidence is available to diagnose MS or atypical demographic or presenting signs are seen, CSF analysis for oligoclonal bands (OCBs) and IgG index is recommended. OCBs are present in ~95% of MS cases; the presence of two or more OCBs in the CSF that are not also present in the serum constitutes a positive test. An IgG index >0.66 suggests the presence of MS and is seen in 70%–95% of MS cases. Other CSF findings include mild lymphocytic pleocytosis and mildly elevated protein.
	Evoked potentials
	Evoked potentials—visual, somatosensory, and brainstem auditory—can be used to identify subclinical lesions of MS. Marked delay in latency of waveforms in one or more of these modalities can demonstrate where demyelination has occurred. There is no specific indication for visual evoked potentials in patients with clear evidence of optic neuritis.
	Blood
	As of this writing, blood tests are not used in the diagnosis of MS except to exclude other diseases. For example, neuromyelitis optica can be distinguished from MS by the presence of serum antibodies to aquaporin 4 receptor in the former condition. New research involving serum neurofilament light chain (NfL) suggests that elevation in NfL might be useful as a biomarker of axonal and myelin damage as well as inflammation in MS.

ARUP Consult: Multiple sclerosis, in ARUP Consult: The Physician's Guide to Laboratory Test Selection and Interpretation. Salt Lake City, UT, 2022. Available at: https://arupconsult.com/content/multiple-sclerosis. Accessed March 2022.

Axisa PP, Hafler DA: Multiple sclerosis: genetics, biomarkers, treatments. Curr Opin Neurol 29(3):345–353, 2016

Etemadifar M, Abhari AP, Nouri H, et al: Does COVID-19 increase the long-term relapsing-remitting multiple sclerosis clinical activity? A cohort study. BMC Neurol 22(1):64, 2022

Hori M, Maekawa T, Kamiya K, et al: Advanced diffusion MR imaging for multiple sclerosis in the brain and spinal cord. Magn Reson Med Sci 21(1):58–70, 2022

Klineova S, Lublin FD: Clinical course of multiple sclerosis. Cold Spring Harb Perspect Med 8(9):a028928, 2018

Michelena G, Casas M, Eizaguirre MB, et al: Can COVID-19 exacerbate multiple sclerosis symptoms? A case series analysis. Mult Scler Relat Disord 57:103368, 2022

Olek MJ: Multiple sclerosis. Ann Intern Med 174(6):ITC81–ITC96, 2021

Wattjes MP, Ciccarelli O, Reich DS, et al: 2021 MAGNIMS-CMSC-NAIMS consensus recommendations on the use of MRI in patients with multiple sclerosis. Lancet Neurol 20(8):653–670, 2021

Yik JT, Becquart P, Gill J, et al: Serum neurofilament light chain correlates with myelin and axonal magnetic resonance imaging markers in multiple sclerosis. Mult Scler Relat Disord 7:103366, 2022

Myocardial infarction (MI)

Clinical findings	Acute MI refers to acute myocardial injury in the presence of clinical evidence of myocardial ischemia and with detection of a significant rise and/or fall of cardiac troponin values and at least one of the following: symptoms of myocardial ischemia, new ischemic ECG changes, development of pathological Q waves on ECG, imaging evidence of loss of viable myocardium or new regional wall motion abnormality, or identification of a coronary thrombus by angiography. A thrombus totally occluding the vessel causes ST segment elevation MI (STEMI), while a thrombus partially occluding the vessel or with collateral circulation causes non-STEMI or unstable angina. Infarction due to atherothrombosis is labeled type 1 and infarction due to a mismatch of perfusion supply and demand is labeled type 2.
	Typical STEMI occurs in some patients suddenly, without warning. In others, prodromal symptoms such as fatigue, malaise, and chest discomfort may be seen in the days or weeks preceding the attack. When the attack occurs, the typical episode of chest pain is characterized by substernal pressure (or squeezing, aching, burning, or sharp pain) often radiating to the neck, shoulder, back, and jaw and down the left arm. The pain is intense and unremitting for 30–60 minutes. In some patients, the pain is felt in the epigastrium and described as fullness, gas, or indigestion. Vital signs may show tachycardia, irregular pulse or various arrhythmias (including bradyarrhythmias), hypertension, and/or increased respiratory rate. Dyspnea, nausea, vomiting, weakness, flu-like symptoms, dizziness, diaphoresis, coughing, wheezing, and frothy sputum may be seen. Anxiety and a sense of dread may be prominent. In general, females present with more symptoms but less severe chest pain that is less often central. In addition, females appear to have a higher frequency of type 2 MI, which carries a higher mortality rate.
	A collaborative model of care involving cardiology/primary care and behavioral medicine is particularly important for patients with coronary heart disease (CHD). Not only do patients with serious mental illness have a higher risk of MI and complications, but patients with CHD are adversely affected by psychiatric conditions in complex ways. Among patients with CHD, for example, mental stress can induce ischemia associated with MI or cardiovascular death. This may be particularly true for females. In addition, post-MI patients have high rates of depression, anxiety, insomnia, and PTSD, all possibly mediated by inflammation, sympathetic overactivity, and/or HPA axis dysfunction. These factors could be expected to contribute to illness burden and to hinder recovery.
Laboratory testing	The two most important laboratory tests used to diagnose MI are ECG and plasma troponin I.
	• Electrocardiography: a 12-lead ECG is evaluated within 10 minutes of arrival in the emergency setting. The event is then classified as STEMI, non-STEMI, or non-ischemic chest pain. ECG elements consistent with ischemia include T wave changes, pathological Q waves, ST segment elevation, pathological R waves, ST segment depression, new bundle branch block, and others in patterns indicating location of infarction. Serial or continuous electrocardiographic monitoring is used for persistent or recurrent symptoms or with an initial non-diagnostic ECG.

Myocardial infarction (MI) *(continued)*

Laboratory testing *(continued)*	• The blood biomarker troponin I has replaced other tests as an indicator of myocardial injury. The reference range for troponin I is 0.0–0.03 ng/mL, with a level of ≥0.30 ng/mL consistent with myocardial injury. Troponin I levels may be obtained on presentation and after 6 and 12 hours, although more frequent testing can be used. Peak levels are seen 12 hours after initial symptoms.

Anderson JL, Morrow DA: Acute myocardial infarction. N Engl J Med 376(21):2053–2064, 2017

ARUP Laboratories: Troponin I, in Laboratory Test Directory. Salt Lake City, UT, ARUP Laboratories, 2022. Available at: https://ltd.aruplab.com/Tests/Pub/0090613. Accessed March 2022.

Kumar M, Nayak PK: Psychological sequelae of myocardial infarction. Biomed Pharmacother 95:487–496, 2017

Lala A, Johnson KW, Januzzi JL, et al: Prevalence and impact of myocardial injury in patients hospitalized with COVID-19 infection. J Am Coll Cardiol 76(5):533–546, 2020

Mehta LS, Beckie TM, DeVon HA, et al: Acute myocardial infarction in women: a scientific statement from the American Heart Association. Circulation 133(9):916–947, 2016

Nielsen RE, Banner J, Jensen SE: Cardiovascular disease in patients with severe mental illness. Nat Rev Cardiol 18(2):136–145, 2021

Roest AM, Zuidersma M, de Jonge P: Myocardial infarction and generalised anxiety disorder: 10-year follow-up. Br J Psychiatry 200(4):324–329, 2012

Shapiro PA: Management of depression after myocardial infarction. Curr Cardiol Rep 17(10):80, 2015

Thygesen K, Alpert JS, Jaffe AS, et al: Fourth universal definition of myocardial infarction (2018). Circulation 138(20):e618–e651, 2018 [published correction appears in Circulation 138(20):e652, 2018]

Vaccarino V, Almuwaqqat Z, Kim JH, et al: Association of mental stress-induced myocardial ischemia with cardiovascular events in patients with coronary heart disease. JAMA 326(18):1818–1828, 2021

Narcolepsy

Clinical findings	Narcolepsy is a chronic sleep disorder characterized by overwhelming daytime drowsiness and sleep attacks, cataplexy, REM sleep dysregulation, hallucinations, and sleep paralysis. Two types of narcolepsy are recognized that have similar symptoms, but with type 1 (NT1) being more severe and more fully described in terms of pathophysiology. In NT1, sleep-onset REM periods are found on multiple sleep latency testing (MSLT), a deficiency of orexin-A (hypocretin-1) is seen in the CSF, and the HLA-DQB1*06:02 allele is identified in >98% of those affected. In type 2 narcolepsy (NT2), cataplexy is not seen, and the level of orexin in CSF is normal.
	Orexin neuropeptides stimulate target neurons in wakefulness-promoting brain regions, so that deficiency results in inconstant signaling with unpredictable sleepiness. In addition, orexins increase activity in brain regions that suppress REM sleep, resulting in paralysis or hallucinations during wakefulness. Cataplexy is defined as the sudden onset of partial or complete paralysis of voluntary muscles triggered by strong emotions (usually positive) without loss of consciousness. The paralysis begins usually in the face and neck and then spreads to involve the trunk and limbs, with immobility lasting ≤2 minutes. With narcolepsy of recent onset, cataplexy can take the form of spontaneous grimaces or jaw-opening episodes with tongue-thrusting or a global hypotonia with no apparent emotional triggers.
	Narcolepsy typically begins in the second decade of life with the sudden onset of daytime sleepiness that can be quite marked, causing problems such as falling asleep in class or while stopped at a red light. It can be distinguished from sleep deprivation by the observation that patients with narcolepsy are excessively sleepy every day, regardless of whether they have had adequate nighttime sleep. In fact, individuals with narcolepsy typically sleep a normal amount of time in a 24-hour period and report feeling rested after a 20-minute nap.
	Evidence to date suggests that narcolepsy is an autoimmune disease. In addition to the HLA association noted above, the condition has been observed to follow closely certain upper airway infections such as influenza-A and streptococcus, which may serve as triggers. In support of this, elevated titers of antibodies to antistreptolysin O are common soon after the onset of narcolepsy.
	Comorbid neuropsychiatric conditions in narcolepsy include depression, anxiety, psychosis, obstructive sleep apnea, periodic limb movement disorder, sleepwalking, and REM sleep behavior disorder. Subjective reports of "brain fog" in patients with narcolepsy may be attributable to the excessive cognitive resources that must be devoted to maintaining attention during testing rather than to true deficits.
Laboratory testing	Even when clinical evaluation provides clear evidence of narcolepsy, the diagnosis is confirmed with an overnight sleep study followed the next day by MSLT. The overnight study excludes alternative diagnoses such as severe sleep apnea, provides documentation of the quality of sleep preceding the MSLT, and reveals presence of sleep-onset REM periods (SOREMPs). Given the opportunity to nap during MSLT, individuals with narcolepsy will usually fall asleep in <8 minutes (normal ≥15 minutes) and show SOREMPs—defined as REM sleep within 15 minutes (normal ≥90 minutes)—on two or more naps.

Narcolepsy *(continued)*

Laboratory testing *(continued)*	In addition to clinical features and REM sleep abnormalities, CSF hypocretin levels can be used to aid in the diagnosis of NT1. A CSF hypocretin-1 (orexin-A) level ≤110 pg/mL that is not attributable to another cause such as brain infection, injury, or inflammation is considered a positive test.
	HLA-DQB1*06:02 genotyping has excellent negative predictive value and is useful in ruling out narcolepsy.

American Psychiatric Association: Diagnostic and Statistical Manual of Mental Disorders, 5th Edition, Text Revision. Washington, DC, American Psychiatric Association, 2022

ARUP Consult: Narcolepsy, in ARUP Consult: The Physician's Guide to Laboratory Test Selection and Interpretation. Salt Lake City, UT, ARUP Laboratories, 2020. Available at: https://arupconsult.com/content/narcolepsy.

ARUP Laboratories: Narcolepsy (HLA-DQB1*06:02) genotyping, in Laboratory Test Directory. Salt Lake City, UT, ARUP Laboratories, 2022. Available at: https://ltd.aruplab.com/Tests/Pub/2005023. Accessed March 2022.

BaHammam AS, Alnakshabandi K, Pandi-Perumal SR: Neuropsychiatric correlates of narcolepsy. Curr Psychiatry Rep 22(8):36, 2020

Bassetti CLA, Adamantidis A, Burdakov D, et al: Narcolepsy: clinical spectrum, aetiopathophysiology, diagnosis and treatment. Nat Rev Neurol 15(9):519–539, 2019

Golden EC, Lipford MC: Narcolepsy: diagnosis and management. Cleve Clin J Med 85(12):959–969, 2018

Hanin C, Arnulf I, Maranci JB, et al: Narcolepsy and psychosis: a systematic review. Acta Psychiatr Scand 144(1):28–41, 2021

Kornum BR: Narcolepsy type I as an autoimmune disorder. Handb Clin Neurol 181:161–172, 2021

Krahn LE, Zee PC, Thorpy MJ: Current understanding of narcolepsy 1 and its comorbidities: what clinicians need to know. Adv Ther 39(1):221–243, 2022

Mahoney CE, Cogswell A, Koralnik IJ, Scammell TE: The neurobiological basis of narcolepsy. Nat Rev Neurosci 20(2):83–93, 2019

Mignot E, Black S: Narcolepsy risk and COVID-19. J Clin Sleep Med 16(10):1831–1833, 2020

Ollila HM: Narcolepsy type 1: what have we learned from genetics? Sleep 43(11):zsaa099, 2020

Scammell TE: Narcolepsy. N Engl J Med 373(27):2654–2662, 2015

Neuroleptic malignant syndrome (NMS)

Clinical findings	NMS is an idiosyncratic adverse effect of dopamine antagonism characterized by fever, altered mental status, muscle rigidity, and autonomic dysfunction. The syndrome is most often caused by antipsychotic drugs but can also be caused by withdrawal of dopamine agonists used to treat parkinsonism, TCAs, and other drugs with neuroleptic effects. The syndrome can be severe, particularly in the presence of high fever and hemodynamic instability. Risk factors include changes to the antipsychotic regimen (especially adding an antipsychotic), higher antipsychotic dosage, and co-treatment with lithium, benzodiazepines, or anticholinergic drugs. Long-acting injectable drugs pose no higher risk than oral drugs. The literature is in disagreement as to whether first-generation antipsychotics pose a greater risk than second-generation drugs. Certain polymorphisms in the CYP2D6 gene may increase vulnerability to NMS. Overall, mortality rates of 10%–20% are reported, with higher risk in older patients and in those with very high fever and respiratory alterations. Features of NMS include the following: • Exposure to a dopamine blocking agent or related drug preceding the onset of symptoms • Altered mental status (delirium, stupor, coma, catatonia) • Severe muscle rigidity—lead pipe rigidity or diffuse rigidity at onset • Fever >100.4°F (>38°C) measured orally on two occasions • Tachypnea, dyspnea • Tachycardia • Hypertension or labile blood pressure • Cardiac dysrhythmia • Diaphoresis • Skin pallor, flushing • Tremor • Dystonia • Chorea • Oral-buccal dyskinesias • Urinary incontinence • Dysphagia • Mutism • Leukocytosis • Elevation of creatine kinase The differential diagnosis of NMS includes serotonin syndrome, which is characterized by marked hyperreflexia and clonus and involves a different drug exposure. Fever is less severe in serotonin syndrome, but shivering is more prominent and persistent. Laboratory findings also assist in distinguishing the two conditions.
Laboratory testing	Laboratory abnormalities in NMS include the following: • Elevated creatine kinase ≥4 times the upper limit of normal • Leukocytosis, often with a left shift

Neuroleptic malignant syndrome (NMS) *(continued)*

Laboratory testing *(continued)*	• Metabolic acidosis identified by blood gas analysis and serum electrolytes • Myoglobinuria in the presence of rhabdomyolysis

American Psychiatric Association: Diagnostic and Statistical Manual of Mental Disorders, 5th Edition, Text Revision. Washington, DC, American Psychiatric Association, 2022

Dos Santos DT, Imthon AK, Strelow MZ, et al: Parkinsonism-hyperpyrexia syndrome after amantadine withdrawal: case report and review of the literature. Neurologist 26(4):149–152, 2021

Guinart D, Misawa F, Rubio JM, et al: Outcomes of neuroleptic malignant syndrome with depot versus oral antipsychotics: a systematic review and pooled, patient-level analysis of 662 case reports. J Clin Psychiatry 82(1):20r13272, 2020

Guinart D, Misawa F, Rubio JM, et al: A systematic review and pooled, patient-level analysis of predictors of mortality in neuroleptic malignant syndrome. Acta Psychiatr Scand 144(4):329–341, 2021

Guinart D, Taipale H, Rubio JM, et al: Risk factors, incidence, and outcomes of neuroleptic malignant syndrome on long-acting injectable vs oral antipsychotics in a nationwide schizophrenia cohort. Schizophr Bull 47(6):1621–1630, 2021

Misawa F, Okumura Y, Takeuchi Y, et al: Neuroleptic malignant syndrome associated with long-acting injectable versus oral second-generation antipsychotics: analyses based on a spontaneous reporting system database in Japan. Schizophr Res 231:42–46, 2021

Nagamine T: Beware of neuroleptic malignant syndrome in COVID-19 pandemic. Innov Clin Neurosci 18(7–9):9–10, 2021

Tse L, Barr AM, Scarapicchia V, Vila-Rodriguez F: Neuroleptic malignant syndrome: a review from a clinically oriented perspective. Curr Neuropharmacol 13(3):395–406, 2015

Neuromyelitis optica spectrum disorder (NMOSD)

Clinical findings	Neuromyelitis optica (NMO) is a chronic autoimmune inflammatory disease targeting astrocytes of the CNS and leading to secondary oligodendrocyte loss that presents clinically as relapsing episodes of optic neuritis and transverse myelitis. In most cases, serum IgG autoantibodies to the aquaporin-4 (AQP4) receptor (a CNS water channel protein) are present. In some cases that are negative for AQP4 IgG, autoantibodies are seen to myelin oligodendrocyte glycoprotein (MOG) residing in the myelin sheath of CNS neurons. Rarely, the condition is triggered by paraneoplastic syndromes, neurosarcoidosis, or vaccination. Brain involvement in NMO is now recognized with the identification of lesions in the area postrema, brainstem, and diencephalon. Due to the range of pathologies described, the condition has been renamed *neuromyelitis optica spectrum disorder* (NMOSD). The prevalence of NMOSD is much higher in females than males, with the average age at onset between 30 and 40 years. Those of Asian and African ancestry are at higher risk than Whites. Individuals with existing autoimmune disease are also at higher risk.
	The onset of NMOSD is abrupt but may feature a prodrome of headache and low-grade fever. Upper respiratory or GI symptoms often precede the neurological presentation. Core clinical characteristics are neurological and depend on the location of CNS lesions:
	• In most cases, the first neurological symptom is severe optic neuritis (ON) with visual loss. Bilateral or rapidly sequential ON is highly suggestive of NMOSD.
	• Transverse myelitis with paralysis follows ON by an interval of days to years. Myelitis is symmetrical and involves three or more vertebral segments. Residual deficits are seen, and pathology is cumulative with each exacerbation.
	• The area postrema syndrome (involving the dorsal surface of the medulla oblongata) is characterized by nausea and vomiting or by intractable hiccups.
	• Signs of brainstem involvement include oculomotor dysfunction, ataxia, and long tract signs (e.g., spasticity, hyperreflexia, positive Babinski reflex).
	• Diencephalic involvement has various manifestations, including narcolepsy, anorexia, inappropriate diuresis, hypothermia, and hypersomnia.
	• Acute disseminated encephalomyelitis is more common in children and is associated with MOG.
	In most patients, NMOSD has a relapsing course with a relapse rate double that of multiple sclerosis (MS) despite maintenance treatment. The interval between relapses is shorter and the duration of relapse is longer than in MS. The negative impact on quality of life in patients with NMOSD is greater in those with pain, bowel/bladder dysfunction, sexual dysfunction, and/or an inability to work. More than one-quarter of patients report moderate to severe depression, which is associated with pain (neuropathic pain and headache). Cognitive impairment is identified in ≤70% of patients with NMOSD, involving domains of attention, language, processing speed, and executive function.

Neuromyelitis optica spectrum disorder (NMOSD) *(continued)*

Clinical findings *(continued)*	In the past, NMOSD was often mistaken for MS given the abrupt onset of similar symptoms. Distinguishing between the two conditions is critical because treatments differ and some treatments for MS exacerbate NMOSD. In addition, early intervention for NMOSD has substantially improved the prognosis for this condition.
Laboratory testing	*AQP4 IgG antibody* testing is performed on serum, preferably using cell-based assay. If negative, MOG IgG antibody testing is performed. The presence of either antibody confirms NMOSD when clinical symptoms are seen.
	MRI with gadolinium shows long corticospinal tract lesions in three or more contiguous vertebral segments; enhancing ON lesions that are longitudinally extensive with preference for the posterior optic pathway; hemispheric cerebral white matter lesions; and peri-ependymal lesions in the diencephalon, dorsal brainstem, and white matter adjacent to the lateral ventricles. Lumbosacral myelitis is more typical of MOG-associated disease. Cerebellar peduncle lesions are frequent in children with MOG-associated disease.
	Optical coherence tomography (OCT) is an imaging technique that uses low-coherence light to capture high-resolution images of the retina in two and three dimensions. Measurement of retinal peripapillary nerve fiber layer thickness by OCT provides a reliable biomarker for the diagnosis and progression of ON pathology.
	NMOSD usually occurs sporadically but appears to be associated with HLA-DRB1*03 and negatively associated with HLA-DRB*1501 (which is associated with MS).

Anamnart C, Tisavipat N, Owattanapanich W, et al: Newly diagnosed neuromyelitis optica spectrum disorders following vaccination: case report and systematic review. Mult Scler Relat Disord 58:103414, 2022

Barzegar M, Mirmosayyeb O, Ebrahimi N, et al: COVID-19 susceptibility and outcomes among patients with neuromyelitis optica spectrum disorder (NMOSD): a systematic review and meta-analysis. Mult Scler Relat Disord 57:103359, 2022

Dutra BG, da Rocha AJ, Nunes RH, Maia ACM Jr: Neuromyelitis optica spectrum disorders: spectrum of MR imaging findings and their differential diagnosis. Radiographics 38(1):169–193, 2018 [published correction appears in Radiographics 38(2):662, 2018]

Hamaguchi M, Fujita H, Suzuki T, Suzuki K: Sick sinus syndrome as the initial manifestation of neuromyelitis optica spectrum disorder: a case report. BMC Neurol 22(1):56, 2022

Holroyd KB, Manzano GS, Levy M: Update on neuromyelitis optica spectrum disorder. Curr Opin Ophthalmol 31(6):462–468, 2020

Huda S, Whittam D, Bhojak M, et al: Neuromyelitis optica spectrum disorders. Clin Med (Lond) 19(2):169–176, 2019

Jarius S, Paul F, Weinshenker BG, et al: Neuromyelitis optica. Nat Rev Dis Primers 6(1):85, 2020

Jovicevic V, Ivanovic J, Andabaka M, et al: COVID-19 and vaccination against SARS-CoV-2 in patients with neuromyelitis optica spectrum disorders. Mult Scler Relat Disord 57:103320, 2022

Paul S, Mondal GP, Bhattacharyya R, et al: Neuromyelitis optica spectrum disorders. J Neurol Sci 420:117225, 2021

Obsessive-compulsive disorder

Clinical findings	OCD is characterized by obsessions and/or compulsions:
	• *Obsessions* are recurrent and persistent thoughts, urges, or images that are experienced at some time during the disturbance as intrusive and unwanted and that usually cause marked anxiety or distress. The person attempts to ignore or suppress such thoughts, urges, or images or to neutralize them with some other thought or action (i.e., by performing a compulsion).
	• *Compulsions* are repetitive behaviors (e.g., hand washing, ordering, checking) or mental acts (e.g., praying, counting, repeating words silently) that the person feels driven to perform in response to an obsession or according to rules that must be applied rigidly. The behaviors or mental acts are aimed at preventing or reducing anxiety or distress or preventing some dreaded event or situation; however, these behaviors or mental acts either are not connected in a realistic way with what they are designed to neutralize or prevent or are clearly excessive.
	The obsessions or compulsions are time-consuming (e.g., take more than 1 hour/day) or cause clinically significant distress or impairment in functioning. The content of the obsessions or compulsions is not restricted to the symptoms of another mental disorder. Insight is variable.
	Most individuals with OCD are diagnosed by about age 19 years, although adult-onset cases have been reported. Males typically have an earlier onset than females. The risk of OCD is higher in those with an affected first-degree relative. Comorbid tic disorders are more common in males. Suicidal ideation is reported in half of patients with OCD, and suicide attempt in one-quarter. Related disorders such as body dysmorphic disorder, trichotillomania, and excoriation disorder occur more frequently in patients with OCD than in the general population.
	A confluence of research findings from imaging, neuropsychology, and pharmacology suggest that OCD arises from dysfunction in the cortico-striato-thalamo-cortical circuit. The serotonin hypothesis that emerged from the observed efficacy of serotonin reuptake inhibitor drugs to treat OCD is now being supplemented with a glutamate hypothesis based on multiple lines of research. The latter might help to explain why some patients' OCD is refractory to serotonergic treatments.
	A compelling case has been made for the establishment of autoimmune OCD as distinct from idiopathic OCD. Autoimmune OCD develops weeks to months after an infection such as group A streptococcus and is characterized by atypical age at onset (early childhood or later adulthood), atypical presentation (with cognitive deficits or severe hypersomnia), treatment resistance, neurological signs (focal deficits, new-onset seizures or headaches), autonomic dysfunction, adverse reaction to antipsychotic drugs, and comorbid autoimmune disease or malignancy (e.g., ovarian teratoma). Various laboratory abnormalities are found, as noted below.

Obsessive-compulsive disorder *(continued)*

Laboratory testing	There are no known laboratory abnormalities specific to idiopathic OCD. Clinicians may screen for metabolic abnormalities with a CMP, hematological issues with a CBC, covert drug use with a urine toxicology screen, and thyroid dysfunction with a TSH level. Patients starting psychotropic medication to treat OCD may require screening and monitoring lab tests as outlined in the *Psychotropic Medications* chapter.
	Laboratory abnormalities found on evaluation of patients with suspected autoimmune OCD have included the following:
	• Serum neuronal autoantibodies (e.g., against NMDAR, basal ganglia, dopamine receptors), antinuclear antibodies against double-strand DNA, streptococcal antibodies
	• CSF pleocytosis, oligoclonal bands, detection of neuronal autoantibodies, markers of injury such as neurofilament light and glial fibrillary acid protein (GFAP)
	• MRI showing basal ganglia and mesiotemporal hyperintensities and inflammatory lesions
	• FDG-PET showing encephalitic patterns
	• EEG showing spike-wave activity or intermittent slowing consistent with encephalopathy

American Psychiatric Association: Diagnostic and Statistical Manual of Mental Disorders, 5th Edition, Text Revision. Washington, DC, American Psychiatric Association, 2022

Endres D, Pollak TA, Bechter K, et al: Immunological causes of obsessive-compulsive disorder: is it time for the concept of an "autoimmune OCD" subtype? Transl Psychiatry 12(1):5, 2022

Goodman WK, Grice DE, Lapidus KA, Coffey BJ: Obsessive-compulsive disorder. Psychiatr Clin North Am 37(3):257–267, 2014

Moreira-de-Oliveira ME, de Menezes GB, Loureiro CP, et al: The impact of COVID-19 on patients with OCD: a one-year follow-up study. J Psychiatr Res 147:307–312, 2022

Richter PMA, Ramos RT: Obsessive-compulsive disorder. Continuum (Minneap Minn) 24(3):828–844, 2018

Robbins TW, Vaghi MM, Banca P: Obsessive-compulsive disorder: puzzles and prospects. Neuron 102(1):27–47, 2019

Zai G: Pharmacogenetics of obsessive-compulsive disorder: an evidence update. Curr Top Behav Neurosci 49:385–398, 2021

Obstructive sleep apnea (OSA)

Clinical findings	OSA is a syndrome characterized by episodes of upper airway collapse during sleep that cause reduced or absent ventilation, resulting in hypoxia, hypercapnia, and arousal from sleep. The condition is grossly underrecognized, even in developed countries; in the United States, it is estimated that 82% of males and 93% of females with OSA remain undiagnosed. Moderate to severe OSA with consequent daytime sleepiness is a recognized cause of motor vehicle and work-related accidents and significantly affects quality of life. Timely diagnosis and treatment can dramatically improve the related cardiovascular conditions listed below.
	The most significant risk factor for OSA is obesity, mostly due to excess adipose tissue in the tongue and pharynx that reduce upper airway dimensions. OSA affects >40% of individuals with a BMI >30 and 60% of those with the metabolic syndrome. The use of drugs associated with muscle relaxation (e.g., opioids, benzodiazepines, and alcohol) also increases risk by increasing collapsibility of the airway. Other risk factors include endocrine disorders (hypothyroidism, acromegaly), deviated nasal septum, smoking, male sex, older age, family history of OSA, and a habit of sleeping in a supine position. Individuals with Down syndrome are at risk as well.
	Among females, the risk of developing OSA is low until menopause, when it increases to match that of males of similar age and BMI. This protective effect is thought to be due to progesterone stimulation of upper airway muscles and ventilation. Higher androgen levels from hormone supplementation or with polycystic ovary syndrome are thought to increase muscle mass in the tongue and thereby increase OSA risk.
	Symptoms of OSA include the following:
	• Loud or irregular snoring
	• Gasping, choking, or breath-holding during sleep
	• Fragmented sleep
	• Unrefreshing sleep regardless of sleep duration
	• Daytime sleepiness, particularly when sedentary
	• Fatigue
	• Nocturia (two or more episodes per night)
	• Enuresis
	• Night sweats
	• Dry mouth or headache upon awakening
	• Cognitive issues: inattention, poor concentration, decreased psychomotor speed, and memory impairment that may be confirmed by testing
	• Mood changes: depression, irritability, anxiety
	• Erectile dysfunction, reduced libido
	Physical exam may show the following:
	• BMI often >30
	• Increased neck circumference (males >17 inches; females >16 inches)
	• Crowded oropharynx with macroglossia and/or enlarged tonsils or uvula

Obstructive sleep apnea (OSA) *(continued)*

Clinical findings *(continued)*	• Jaw misalignment (e.g., retrognathia) • Deviated nasal septum or turbinate hypertrophy Medical conditions often comorbid with OSA include coronary artery disease, hypertension, hyperlipidemia, stroke, MI, congestive heart failure, atrial fibrillation, nocturnal dysrhythmias, pulmonary hypertension, diabetes, the metabolic syndrome, and depression. A causal relationship has not been established between OSA and these conditions, and their association may reflect common risk factors, but timely diagnosis and treatment of OSA results in their improvement and reduces the rate of fatal and nonfatal cardiovascular events. In addition to the elements of the history and physical examination listed above, a validated screening instrument such as the Epworth Sleepiness Scale or the STOP-BANG can help to identify patients who should be referred for sleep study. The STOP-BANG includes eight yes/no questions with the following items: **S**nore, **T**ired, **O**bserved stopped breathing, high blood **P**ressure, **B**MI>35 kg/m^2, **A**ge>50, **N**eck>15.75, **G**ender=male. A score of 0–2 indicates low risk and a score of 5–8 indicates high risk for moderate to severe OSA.
Laboratory testing	The gold standard for diagnosis of OSA is a PSG, an all-night laboratory sleep study described in the ***Diagnostic Tests*** chapter. Home sleep apnea testing is now possible using a subset of criteria (not electroencephalography) that can support the diagnosis for symptomatic patients with a high pretest probability of moderate to severe OSA in the absence of significant cardiopulmonary comorbidity. Home testing cannot exclude the diagnosis of OSA, however; a negative test must be followed up with a PSG. Home testing is not recommended for patients with a history of stroke, pulmonary disorder with hypoventilation, neuromuscular disease, or congestive heart failure or for those treated with opioid medication. On a PSG study, obstructive respiratory events during sleep are classified as 1) apneas—nearly complete ($>90\%$) obstruction of airflow lasting ≥10 seconds despite ventilatory effort, or 2) hypopneas—reduction of airflow by $\geq30\%$ for ≥10 seconds with reduction in oxygen saturation of $\geq3\%$ or arousal from sleep. The sum of apneas and hypopneas per hour of sleep is termed the apnea-hypopnea index (AHI). This index is used to stratify OSA severity, with an AHI ≥30 classified as severe OSA, an AHI of 15 to <30 classified as moderate, and an AHI of 5 to <15 classified as mild. In the latter case, the diagnosis of OSA must also include clinical evidence of the syndrome. Home sleep apnea testing does not record sleep, so this modality cannot calculate an AHI. Instead, home testing replaces sleep time with monitored time and measures the frequency of breathing events to arrive at a respiratory event index (REI). The REI is equal to apneas plus hypopneas divided by total monitoring time.

American Psychiatric Association: Diagnostic and Statistical Manual of Mental Disorders, 5th Edition, Text Revision. Washington, DC, American Psychiatric Association, 2022

Chung F, Abdullah HR, Liao P: STOP-BANG questionnaire: a practical approach to screen for obstructive sleep apnea. Chest 149(3):631–638, 2016

Iannella G, Magliulo G, Greco A, et al: Obstructive sleep apnea syndrome: from symptoms to treatment. Int J Environ Res Public Health 19(4):2459, 2022

Jordan AS, McSharry DG, Malhotra A: Adult obstructive sleep apnoea. Lancet 383(9918):736–747, 2014

Laratta CR, Ayas NT, Povitz M, Pendharkar SR: Diagnosis and treatment of obstructive sleep apnea in adults. CMAJ 189(48):E1481–E1488, 2017

Obstructive sleep apnea (OSA) *(continued)*

Miller MA, Cappuccio FP: A systematic review of COVID-19 and obstructive sleep apnoea. Sleep Med Rev 55:101382, 2021

Patel SR: Obstructive sleep apnea. Ann Intern Med 171(11):ITC81–ITC96, 2019

Rundo JV: Obstructive sleep apnea basics. Cleve Clin J Med 86(9 Suppl 1):2–9, 2019

Semelka M, Wilson J, Floyd R: Diagnosis and treatment of obstructive sleep apnea in adults. Am Fam Physician 94(5):355–360, 2016

Veasey SC, Rosen IM: Obstructive sleep apnea in adults. N Engl J Med 380(15):1442–1449, 2019

Organophosphate poisoning

Clinical findings	Organophosphate compounds are still widely used in the United States and globally despite what is known about their harmful effects on human health. These chemicals are found in insecticides (e.g., malathion and parathion), nerve gases (e.g., soman and sarin), nerve agents such as Novichok, and other herbicides, pesticides, fungicides, and antihelminthics and are used in the manufacture of products such as plastics and solvents. Individuals at particular risk of exposure include farmworkers, gardeners, manufacturers, fumigators, military personnel, and children. Exposure from "fume events" in which the cabin air of a commercial aircraft is contaminated with heated engine oil fumes containing organophosphate compounds has been reported, but the frequency of this exposure is unknown. In developing countries, ingestion of organophosphate compounds as a means of attempting suicide occurs regularly. These compounds readily leak into the environment and are now detected in rivers, lakes, groundwater, soil, air, and plants. Residues are found in fruits, vegetables, and small grains (e.g., wheat, barley, oats) sold in grocery stores. Outbreaks of organophosphate poisoning from local drinking water have been reported.
	Organophosphates act by irreversibly inhibiting acetylcholinesterase, an enzyme responsible for the breakdown of acetylcholine found at synapses, autonomic ganglia, and neuromuscular junctions. Accumulation of acetylcholine at these sites results in overstimulation of nicotinic and muscarinic receptors, leading to clinical symptoms. Routes of organophosphate exposure include inhalation, ingestion, and direct dermal contact, with inhalation giving rise to the most severe and most rapid onset of symptoms.
	Three phases of acute organophosphate poisoning have been described: acute cholinergic crisis, intermediate syndrome, and organophosphate-induced delayed neuropathy.
	• *Acute cholinergic crisis* develops within minutes to hours of exposure and includes hypersalivation, lacrimation, bronchorrhea, nausea, vomiting, abdominal cramping, urinary incontinence, bronchospasm, miosis, hypotension, bradycardia, muscle fasciculations, paralysis, irritability, restlessness, confusion, and generalized tonic-clonic seizures. Respiratory failure, coma and death may ensue.
	• *Intermediate syndrome* arises within 1–4 days and is characterized by paralysis affecting proximal limb muscles, respiratory muscles, and muscles innervated by cranial nerves. This phase occurs in conscious patients after atropine treatment of cholinergic crisis.
	• *Organophosphate-induced delayed neuropathy* develops 2–5 weeks after exposure, with symptoms of peripheral motor and sensory neuropathy including weakness, paresthesias, and numbness. In some cases, paraplegia, quadriplegia, or impotence can develop and persist for years.
	Complications of acute organophosphate poisoning include aspiration pneumonia, noncardiogenic pulmonary edema, cardiac dysrhythmias (bradycardia, ventricular tachycardia), prolonged QT, pancreatitis, electrolyte derangements, acute kidney injury, depression, and suicidality.

Organophosphate poisoning *(continued)*

Clinical findings *(continued)*	Chronic low-dose exposure such as that affecting farmworkers is associated with chronic organophosphate-induced neuropsychiatric disorder (COPIND), which may be seen by behavioral health professionals.
	
	Suggested diagnostic criteria for COPIND include the following:
	
	• Repeated exposure to organophosphates
	   • At least four of the following:
	   • Personality change and destabilization of mood
	   • Impairment of concentration and memory
	   • Impaired exercise tolerance
	   • Reduced tolerance to alcohol (assume positive for teetotalers)
	   • Heightened sensitivity to organophosphates
	   • At least three of the following:
	   • Exacerbation of "dippers' flu"*
	   • Impulsive suicidal thinking
	   • Language disorder
	   • Heightened sense of smell
	   • Deterioration of handwriting
	
	Other signs and symptoms of chronic organophosphate exposure include the following:
	
	• Cognitive deficits—impairments in attention, concentration, judgment, learning, memory, information processing, eye-hand coordination, reaction time
	• Psychiatric issues— emotional lability, anxiety, depression, psychosis, chronic fatigue, suicidality, alcohol intolerance
	• Neurological symptoms—dystonia, rigidity (facial muscles), resting tremor, bradykinesia, postural instability, autonomic dysfunction, peripheral neuropathy

Laboratory testing	Plasma or RBC cholinesterase levels can be tested to determine organophosphate exposure. RBC cholinesterase is more accurate, but plasma cholinesterase is easier to perform and more widely available. Cholinesterase levels are used to evaluate acute poisoning but normalize within 10–14 days of the last significant exposure, so they cannot be used to evaluate chronic exposure. Sample reference levels: • Plasma cholinesterase: 2.9–7.1 U/mL • RBC cholinesterase: 7.9–17.1 U/mL RBC • RBC cholinesterase-to-hemoglobin ratio: 25–52 U/g hemoglobin Urinary dialkyl phosphate metabolites can be used to evaluate chronic organophosphate exposure. Autonomic function testing and peripheral NCT can be used to evaluate nerve injury from chronic exposure. MRI of the brain with T2, FLAIR, and diffusion-weighted sequences may show bilaterally symmetric basal ganglia hyperintensities.

*Dippers' flu is a syndrome named for sheep handlers who are exposed to organophosphates and related compounds in sheep dip.

Organophosphate poisoning *(continued)*

ARUP Laboratories: Insecticide exposure panel, in Laboratory Test Directory. Salt Lake City, UT, ARUP Laboratories, 2022. Available at: https://ltd.aruplab.com/Tests/Pub/0020175. Accessed March 2022.

Dassanayake TL, Weerasinghe VS, Gawarammana I, Buckley NA: Subacute and chronic neuropsychological sequalae of acute organophosphate pesticide self-poisoning: a prospective cohort study from Sri Lanka. Clin Toxicol (Phila) 59(2):118–130, 2021

Davies R, Ahmed G, Freer T: Psychiatric aspects of chronic exposure to organophosphates: diagnosis and management. Adv Psychiatr Treat 6(5): 356–361, 2000

Jokanovic M: Neurotoxic effects of organophosphorus pesticides and possible association with neurodegenerative diseases in man: a review. Toxicology 410:125–131, 2018

Muñoz-Quezada MT, Lucero BA, Iglesias VP, et al: Chronic exposure to organophosphate (OP) pesticides and neuropsychological functioning in farm workers: a review. Int J Occup Environ Health 22(1):68–79, 2016

Naughton SX, Terry AV Jr: Neurotoxicity in acute and repeated organophosphate exposure. Toxicology 408:101–112, 2018

Pannu AK, Bhalla A, Vishnu RI, et al: Organophosphate induced delayed neuropathy after an acute cholinergic crisis in self-poisoning. Clin Toxicol (Phila) 59(6):488–492, 2021

Stallones L, Beseler CL: Assessing the connection between organophosphate pesticide poisoning and mental health: a comparison of neuropsychological symptoms from clinical observations, animal models and epidemiological studies. Cortex 74:405–416, 2016

Osteoporosis

Clinical findings	*Osteoporosis* is a condition of thinning and weakening of the bones with changes in bone microarchitecture that particularly affects postmenopausal females. An earlier stage of osteoporosis, when bone loss is less significant, is termed *osteopenia*. In addition to age, female sex, and postmenopausal status, risk factors for primary osteoporosis include White or Asian ancestry, low BMI, personal or family history of fracture, rheumatoid arthritis, current smoking status, use of glucocorticoids, and low bone density on testing. Secondary osteoporosis may develop in patients with hyperparathyroidism, multiple myeloma, malabsorption, diabetes mellitus, or inflammatory bowel disease.
	Osteoporosis increases the risk of fractures, especially of the hip, spine, and wrist. Other signs of the disease include kyphosis, loss of height, and bone pain. The Fracture Risk Assessment Tool (FRAX) developed by the World Health Organization predicts the individual 10-year risk of hip or major osteoporotic fracture based on demographic and bone density data. It can be accessed at www.sheffield.ac.uk/FRAX.
	Osteoporosis is underdiagnosed in the general population, even among individuals with a history of fracture in older age. The condition can be treated, in some cases with at least partial reversal of bone loss. Progression of bone loss can be slowed through a healthy diet (enriched with fruits, vegetables, seafood, fish oil supplements, and dairy products) along with regular physical activity that includes strength training.
Laboratory testing	The diagnosis of osteoporosis is confirmed by a DEXA scan of the hip and spine, which compares the patient's bone density to that of the healthy population to generate a T-score.
	• T-score of -2.5 or lower confirms osteoporosis.
	• T-score of -1.0 to -2.4 confirms osteopenia.
	Laboratory testing may also be useful to evaluate the potential causes of secondary osteoporosis:
	• Calcium—elevation could suggest hyperparathyroidism, multiple myeloma, cancer, and other conditions.
	• CBC—anemia could suggest cancer, multiple myeloma.
	• ALP—to exclude Paget's disease
	• Vitamin D (25-hydroxy vitamin D)—performed even for those taking vitamin D supplements
	• TSH—to exclude hyperthyroidism

Black DM, Rosen CJ: Clinical practice: postmenopausal osteoporosis. N Engl J Med 374(3):254–262, 2016 [published correction appears in N Engl J Med 374(18):1797, 2016]

Camacho PM, Petak SM, Binkley N, et al: American Association of Clinical Endocrinologists/American College of Endocrinology clinical practice guidelines for the diagnosis and treatment of postmenopausal osteoporosis: 2020 update. Endocr Pract 26(Suppl 1):1–46, 2020

Ensrud KE, Crandall CJ: Osteoporosis. Ann Intern Med 167(3):ITC17–ITC32, 2017 [published correction appears in Ann Intern Med 167(7):528, 2017]

Holubiac IS, Leuciuc FV, Craciun DM, Dobrescu T: Effect of strength training protocol on bone mineral density for postmenopausal women with osteopenia/osteoporosis assessed by dual-energy X-ray absorptiometry (DEXA). Sensors (Basel) 22(5):1904, 2022

Johnston CB, Dagar M: Osteoporosis in older adults. Med Clin North Am 104(5):873–884, 2020

Martiniakova M, Babikova M, Mondockova V, et al: The role of macronutrients, micronutrients and flavonoid polyphenols in the prevention and treatment of osteoporosis. Nutrients 14(3):523, 2022

Pancreatitis, acute

Clinical findings	Acute pancreatitis refers to inflammation of the pancreas sometimes accompanied by a systemic inflammatory response that causes dysfunction in other organs. The most common cause is gallstones, followed by chronic alcohol overuse. Severity of the syndrome varies from mild (with resolution over several days) to severe (with a prolonged hospital stay, critical care, and up to 20% mortality). Chronic alcohol overuse is defined as four or more drinks daily for males and three or more drinks daily for females over 5 years or longer. Rare causes of pancreatitis include drugs such as valproate, estrogen, corticosteroids, ACE inhibitors, metronidazole, and mesalamine, as well as several immunosuppressant and antiviral drugs. Pancreatitis caused by medication is usually mild. In some cases, the risk of developing pancreatitis is partly genetic, with mutations or polymorphisms serving as cofactors that interact with triggers such as drinking.
	Acute pancreatitis is a medical emergency requiring hospital admission. In most patients, it is characterized by a severe, constant abdominal pain with vomiting. The pain radiates to the back in half of patients. The pain from alcoholic pancreatitis may develop over several days, while the pain from gallstone-associated pancreatitis develops suddenly. Patients appear acutely ill, with fever, tachycardia, tachypnea, unstable blood pressure, and altered level of consciousness. Ileus with decreased bowel sounds and abdominal distention may be seen. Signs of hemorrhage may be seen in the flank and umbilical areas, indicating a poor prognosis.
	Acute pancreatitis is diagnosed when at least two of the following three features are present:
	• Characteristic abdominal pain
	• Serum lipase or amylase level ≥3 times the upper limit of normal (ULN)
	• Acute pancreatitis identified by CT or MRI on cross-sectional imaging
	Inflammation usually subsides after several days to a few weeks. Subsequently, the patient is at risk of developing recurrent attacks or chronic pancreatitis. The risk is particularly great for patients who continue to smoke or to drink alcohol.
Laboratory testing	Basic tests to diagnose acute pancreatitis include the following:
	• Serum lipase is the test of choice to diagnose acute pancreatitis because it is more specific than amylase. Lipase becomes elevated within 4–8 hours and remains elevated up to 14 days longer than amylase. Lipase levels ≥3 times the ULN are diagnostic, while levels ≥7 times the ULN predict a severe course.
	• An abdominal ultrasound is recommended for all patients to identify gallstones and bile duct dilatation.
	• If the diagnosis remains unclear, contrast-enhanced CT scan is performed.
	Other tests often performed include the following:
	• CMP
	• CBC with differential and platelets
	• Chest X-ray to identify pleural effusions indicating more severe disease

Pancreatitis, acute *(continued)*

Laboratory testing *(continued)*	• CT in patients who fail to improve or who worsen over 48 hours despite fluid resuscitation, to identify pancreatic necrosis
	• Endoscopic ultrasonography or magnetic resonance cholangio-pancreatography for non-resolving or recurrent pancreatitis

Forsmark CE, Vege SS, Wilcox CM: Acute pancreatitis. N Engl J Med 375(20):1972–1981, 2016

Johnson CD, Besselink MG, Carter R: Acute pancreatitis. BMJ 349:g4859, 2014

Porter KK, Cason DE, Morgan DE: Acute pancreatitis: how can MR imaging help. Magn Reson Imaging Clin N Am 26(3):439–450, 2018

Pancreatitis, chronic

Clinical findings	Chronic pancreatitis refers to a progressive inflammation of the pancreas that ultimately leads to irreversible fibrosis and atrophy affecting both endocrine and exocrine functions. At this end stage, pancreatogenic diabetes (type 3c) develops because insufficient insulin is secreted, and symptoms of pancreatic insufficiency (steatorrhea, flatulence, and weight loss) are seen because of the reduced secretion of digestive enzymes. The two most important causes of chronic pancreatitis are heavy drinking and cigarette smoking. Less common causes include genetic disorders such as cystic fibrosis, autoimmune disease, gallstones, and malignancy.
	Most patients present with episodic upper abdominal pain, nausea, and vomiting. Three pain patterns are seen:
	• Type A: Intermittent severe attacks
	• Type B: Persistent pain between intermittent severe attacks
	• Type C: Chronic severe pain without attacks
	Pain is worse after eating and can sometimes be reduced by sitting upright or leaning forward.
	The pain pattern may begin as Type A but then progress to persistent pain associated with visceral sensitivity, allodynia, and hyperalgesia because of sensitization.
	Endocrine insufficiency develops when insulin-secreting cells are lost, resulting in diabetes. Exocrine insufficiency with persistent steatorrhea is associated with malabsorption, weight loss, sarcopenia, and deficiencies of fat-soluble vitamins as well as vitamin B_{12}, zinc, magnesium, and other micronutrients. Vitamin D deficiency leads to osteopenia and osteoporosis with bone pain and susceptibility to fracture. Other complications of chronic pancreatitis include pseudocysts, biliary strictures, and pancreatic cancer. Pseudocysts—incompletely walled-off cysts containing leaked pancreatic fluids—may expand to block the bile ducts or duodenum, bleed, or rupture into the peritoneal cavity.
	The diagnosis of chronic pancreatitis is based on the presenting symptoms, clinical history (including alcohol use and smoking), and cross-sectional imaging, with pancreatic function testing having a secondary role. Of necessity, the evaluation includes an assessment of nutritional status, disability, and motivation for change to contributing lifestyle factors.
Laboratory testing	Cross-sectional imaging with CT or MRI is the primary diagnostic tool. Imaging findings include pancreatic ductal calcifications, ductal dilatation, pseudocysts, and parenchymal atrophy. If these tests are inconclusive, endoscopic ultrasound can be used. Alternatively, magnetic resonance cholangiopancreatography can be used to identify subtle morphological changes, particularly when secretin stimulation is used. Endoscopic retrograde cholangiopancreatography (ERCP) is no longer used for diagnosis.
	Exocrine insufficiency can be assessed by the level of the digestive enzyme fecal elastase-1 measured in a single random stool sample. Values ≥200 µg/g are considered normal. Very low values ≤50 µg/g are consistent with insufficiency. Values between 50 µg/g and 200 µg/g are found with other conditions, such as inflammatory bowel disease, renal failure, and water diarrhea from any cause.

Pancreatitis, chronic *(continued)*

Laboratory testing *(continued)*	The gold standard for evaluation of exocrine insufficiency is a 48- or 72-hour fecal fat test, which requires a 100-g fat diet for 2 days before and throughout the stool collection period. Fecal fat values >7 g/day are diagnostic of abnormal absorption and digestion of fat.
	Diagnosis of pancreatogenic diabetes (type 3c diabetes) is made when pancreatic pathology is identified by imaging, exocrine insufficiency is present, and autoimmune markers of type 1 diabetes are absent.
	Blood tests are less useful in the workup of chronic than of acute pancreatitis. Some clinicians request a CMP, CBC with differential, lipase and amylase levels, and a lipid panel. In the assessment of nutritional status, levels of fat-soluble vitamins, vitamin B_{12}, and micronutrients may be used.

Beyer G, Habtezion A, Werner J, et al: Chronic pancreatitis. Lancet 396(10249):499–512, 2020

Gardner TB, Adler DG, Forsmark CE, et al: ACG clinical guideline: chronic pancreatitis. Am J Gastroenterol 115(3):322–339, 2020

Kleeff J, Whitcomb DC, Shimosegawa T, et al: Chronic pancreatitis. Nat Rev Dis Primers 3:17060, 2017

Singh VK, Yadav D, Garg PK: Diagnosis and management of chronic pancreatitis: a review. JAMA 322(24):2422–2434, 2019

Vege SS, Chari ST: Chronic pancreatitis. N Engl J Med 386(9):869–878, 2022

Panic attack and panic disorder

Clinical findings	A *panic attack* is an abrupt surge of intense fear or intense discomfort that reaches a peak within minutes, during which time four or more of the following symptoms occur:
	• Palpitations, pounding heart, or accelerated heart rate
	• Sweating
	• Trembling or shaking
	• Sensations of shortness of breath or smothering
	• Feeling of choking
	• Chest pain or discomfort
	• Nausea or abdominal distress
	• Feeling dizzy, unsteady, lightheaded, or faint
	• Chills or heat sensations
	• Paresthesias (numbness or tingling sensations)
	• Derealization (feelings of unreality) or depersonalization (feeling detached from oneself)
	• Fear of losing control or going crazy
	• Fear of dying
	Panic disorder is defined by recurrent, unexpected panic attacks that are accompanied by persistent anticipatory concern or worry and/or maladaptive behaviors such as avoidance. Panic disorder is a primary condition, meaning that the panic attacks are not due to substance abuse or a medical disorder and are not restricted to the symptoms of another mental disorder. Attacks with fewer than four symptoms—limited-symptom attacks—can occur in those with full-symptom panic attacks or in isolation. Panic disorder should not be diagnosed when only limited-symptom attacks occur.
	There is a wide variation in the frequency and severity of panic attacks in those with panic disorder. Some individuals have nocturnal as well as daytime attacks, and this likely represents a more severe form of the disorder. More general worry often accompanies panic disorder. The mean age at onset of panic disorder is in the mid-30s, and onset after age 55 years is uncommon. Most affected individuals report stressful life events before their first panic attack, and chronic stress is associated with a more severe disorder over time. Suicidal ideation and behaviors are more common in panic disorder than in the general population.
	Challenge tests using agents such as sodium lactate, isoproterenol, carbon dioxide, cholecystokinin, and yohimbine provoke panic attacks in patients with panic disorder to a greater extent than in unaffected individuals, but these tests have not been used clinically. Caffeine at a dose equivalent to five cups of coffee similarly provokes panic, and this dose can discriminate panic disorder patients from healthy control subjects.
Laboratory testing	Isolated panic attacks may not require laboratory workup. For recurrent panic attacks, a metabolic panel (BMP or CMP) to check calcium and glucose levels and thyroid function testing to check TSH are recommended.

Panic attack and panic disorder *(continued)*

Laboratory testing *(continued)*	Depending on patient characteristics and history, other elements of the evaluation might include one or more of the following:
	• ECG, Holter monitoring, cardiac stress testing, and/or echocardiogram
	• Chest X-ray, pulmonary function tests, and/or arterial blood gases
	• Urine drug screening (especially for cannabis and hallucinogens)
	• GGT with or without CDT for suspicion of covert drinking
	• Plasma free metanephrines to exclude pheochromocytoma
	• Urine porphyrin precursors
	• Pulmonary CT scan
	• EEG to exclude seizures

American Psychiatric Association: Diagnostic and Statistical Manual of Mental Disorders, 5th Edition, Text Revision. Washington, DC, American Psychiatric Association, 2022

Javelot H, Weiner L: Panic and pandemic: Narrative review of the literature on the links and risks of panic disorder as a consequence of the SARS-CoV-2 pandemic. Encephale 47(1):38–42, 2021

Klevebrant L, Frick A: Effects of caffeine on anxiety and panic attacks in patients with panic disorder: a systematic review and meta-analysis. Gen Hosp Psychiatry 74:22–31, 2022

Machado S, Sancassiani F, Paes F, et al: Panic disorder and cardiovascular diseases: an overview. Int Rev Psychiatry 29(5):436–444, 2017

Meuret AE, Kroll J, Ritz T: Panic disorder comorbidity with medical conditions and treatment implications. Annu Rev Clin Psychol 13:209–240, 2017

Micoulaud-Franchi JA, Kotwas I, Arthuis M, et al: Screening for epilepsy-specific anxiety symptoms: French validation of the EASI. Epilepsy Behav 128:108585, 2022

Smith NS, Bauer BW, Capron DW: Comparing symptom networks of daytime and nocturnal panic attacks in a community-based sample. J Anxiety Disord 85:102514, 2022

Parkinson's disease (PD)

Clinical findings	PD is a neurodegenerative disorder arising from the loss of dopaminergic neurons, misfolding of α-synuclein protein, and neuroinflammation. Clinically, it is characterized by bradykinesia, muscular rigidity, resting tremor, and postural instability. A spectrum of disease ranging from mild, motor-predominant to diffuse malignant forms is recognized. Both motor and non-motor symptoms are seen.
	Bradykinesia has various manifestations, including decreased blink rate, mask-like expression, difficulty arising from a chair, micrographia, and reduced finger dexterity. It may be understood by patients as tiredness or weakness. Rigidity is a nearly universal finding, often taking the form of cogwheeling, which is a combination of rigidity and tremor. Like tremor, rigidity usually appears unilaterally, but it eventually progresses to involve both sides of the body. Rigidity can significantly interfere with sleep. The resting tremor of PD—often described as a "pill rolling" movement—is most apparent when the body part is not engaged in any purposeful activity. Postural instability with an increased risk of falling is a symptom of later disease stages; when it occurs early, this suggests the presence of a different disorder, such as progressive supranuclear palsy. Festinating gait, with quick, short steps and a running forward posture, is a manifestation of gait instability. Other motor manifestations include dystonia, stooped posture, a sudden inability to move termed "freezing," hypophonia, and retropulsion.
	Non-motor manifestations of PD include neuropsychiatric, autonomic, sleep, and sensory disturbances. A subset of these symptoms can occur as a prodrome, years before the onset of motor symptoms. These prodromal symptoms can include REM sleep behavior disorder, erectile dysfunction, orthostatic hypotension, constipation, urge urinary incontinence, hyposmia, and depression. Cognitive dysfunction commonly develops over time, with impairment in decision-making, multitasking, memory retrieval, and visuospatial perception leading to a subcortical dementia syndrome. An early onset of dementia raises the possibility of the alternative diagnosis of dementia with Lewy bodies.
	Significant depression is seen in approximately half of patients with PD and has a substantial impact on the course of PD itself, with greater functional disability, more rapid physical and cognitive decline, poorer quality of life, increased mortality, and more significant caregiver distress. Other common psychiatric symptoms include anxiety, fatigue, apathy, anhedonia, psychosis (illusions, visual and nonvisual hallucinations, and delusions), insomnia, daytime sleepiness, and sleep attacks. Some of these symptoms may be attributable to the dopaminergic drugs that are used to treat PD. Manic symptoms can occur, usually as adverse effects of dopaminergic drugs. Other common autonomic symptoms include dysphagia, gastroparesis, sialorrhea, rhinorrhea, and temperature dysregulation. Fecal incontinence can develop in advanced disease.
	Older age is the most important risk factor for PD; average age at onset is 50–60 years. Other important risk factors include male sex, a positive family history of PD, and past exposure to pesticides.

Parkinson's disease (PD) *(continued)*

Laboratory testing	Clinical diagnosis is based on the signs and symptoms discussed above. In cases in which the diagnosis is uncertain, dopamine transporter SPECT or PET imaging can be helpful if it shows reduced binding in the striatum consistent with the loss or dysfunction of dopaminergic neurons. In early PD, these studies may be normal. Other advanced neuroimaging techniques may be helpful in the differential diagnosis of PD but are not recommended for routine use.

American Psychiatric Association: Diagnostic and Statistical Manual of Mental Disorders, 5th Edition, Text Revision. Washington, DC, American Psychiatric Association, 2022

Armstrong MJ, Okun MS: Diagnosis and treatment of Parkinson disease: a review. JAMA 323(6):548–560, 2020

Bloem BR, Okun MS, Klein C: Parkinson's disease. Lancet 397(10291):2284–2303, 2021

Hayes MT: Parkinson's disease and parkinsonism. Am J Med 132(7):802–807, 2019

Lintel H, Corpuz T, Paracha SU, Grossberg GT: Mood disorders and anxiety in Parkinson's disease: current concepts. J Geriatr Psychiatry Neurol 34(4):280–288, 2021

Marsh L: Depression and Parkinson's disease: current knowledge. Curr Neurol Neurosci Rep 13(12):409, 2013

Ray S, Agarwal P: Depression and anxiety in Parkinson disease. Clin Geriatr Med 36(1):93–104, 2020

Reich SG, Savitt JM: Parkinson's disease. Med Clin North Am 103(2):337–350, 2019

Tolosa E, Garrido A, Scholz SW, Poewe W: Challenges in the diagnosis of Parkinson's disease. Lancet Neurol 20(5):385–397, 2021

Pellagra

Clinical findings	Pellagra is a disease caused by a deficiency of niacin (vitamin B$_3$) and tryptophan (a precursor to niacin) and characterized by the "4Ds" of diarrhea, dermatitis, dementia, and death when untreated. The condition is still common in countries with limited food resources and occurs sporadically in developed countries among individuals with alcohol overuse, eating disorders, HIV infection, carcinoid syndrome, highly restrictive diets, and malabsorption syndromes or who are post–bariatric surgery. Historically, pellagra was associated with subsistence diets that included only corn, millet, or sorghum. Case reports indicate that several medications in current use can cause pellagra, including certain chemotherapeutic and anti-tuberculosis drugs, anticonvulsants (phenytoin, carbamazepine, phenobarbital), and chloramphenicol.
	Signs and symptoms of pellagra include the following:
	• Diarrhea—often the first symptom, stool is typically watery but can contain blood and mucus. Diarrhea can be continuous or episodic. The entire GI tract is affected, with symptoms including sialorrhea, angular cheilitis, beefy red tongue, gingivitis, epigastric discomfort, nausea, and loss of appetite, all of which lead to further malnutrition.
	• Dermatitis—the rash of pellagra is the hallmark of the disease and is so distinctive that it indicates the diagnosis in many cases. In early stages, the rash resembles a bad sunburn. It is bilaterally symmetrical and appears on sun-exposed areas with sharp demarcations. It can appear as a band or collar around the neck, known as the *Casal necklace*. Subsequently, an exudative skin eruption develops, with severe pruritus and burning. The skin of the hands, arms, feet, face, and neck becomes rough, hard, cracked, and brittle on dorsal surfaces.
	• Neuropsychiatric—symptoms include irritability, headache, dizziness, photophobia, fatigue, insomnia, apathy, anxiety, depression, suicidal ideation and behavior, inattentiveness, memory impairment, disorientation, confusion, delirium, mania, psychosis (delusions, auditory and visual hallucinations), dysarthria, spasticity, tremor, extensor plantar reflexes, gegenhalten, startle myoclonus, ataxia, polyneuropathy, and seizures. Untreated, the condition can progress to stupor, coma, and death.
Laboratory testing	The diagnosis of pellagra relies on a high index of suspicion for at-risk patients presenting with diarrhea, dermatitis, and dementia (including cognitive and other neuropsychiatric symptoms) and relief of symptoms with niacin supplementation. In most cases, lab testing is not required.
	Blood levels are not reliable as indicators of niacin status. Combined excretion of two urinary metabolites of niacin—*N*-methylnicotinamide and pyridone—is consistent with niacin deficiency when levels are <1.5 mg/24 hours. Other tests include a "niacin index," the ratio of RBC nicotinamide adenine dinucleotide (NAD) to nicotinamide adenine dinucleotide phosphate (NADP) concentration, which suggests a risk of niacin deficiency when the ratio is <1.

Pellagra *(continued)*

Alagesan M, Chidambaram Y: Pellagra. N Engl J Med 386(10):e24, 2022

Cao S, Wang X, Cestodio K: Pellagra, an almost-forgotten differential diagnosis of chronic diarrhea: more prevalent than we think. Nutr Clin Pract 35(5):860–863, 2020

Gama Marques J: Pellagra with Casal necklace causing secondary schizophrenia with Capgras syndrome in a homeless man. Prim Care Companion CNS Disord 24(2):21cr03014, 2022

Gasperi V, Sibilano M, Savini I, Catani MV: Niacin in the central nervous system: an update of biological aspects and clinical applications. Int J Mol Sci 20(4):974, 2019

Luthe SK, Sato R: Alcoholic pellagra as a cause of altered mental status in the emergency department. J Emerg Med 53(4):554–557, 2017

Mills K, Akintayo O, Egbosiuba L, et al: Chronic diarrhea in a drinker: a breakthrough case of pellagra in the US south. J Investig Med High Impact Case Rep 8:2324709620941305, 2020

Moro C, Nunes C, Onzi G, et al: Gastrointestinal: life-threatening diarrhea due to pellagra in an elderly patient. J Gastroenterol Hepatol 35(9):1465, 2020

National Institutes of Health Office of Dietary Supplements: Niacin, in Dietary Supplement Fact Sheets. Bethesda, MD, National Institutes of Health, 2021. Available at: https://ods.od.nih.gov/factsheets/Niacin-HealthProfessional. Accessed March 2022.

Ng E, Neff M: Recognising the return of nutritional deficiencies: a modern pellagra puzzle. BMJ Case Rep 11(1):e227454, 2018

Periyasamy S, John S, Padmavati R, et al: Association of schizophrenia risk with disordered niacin metabolism in an Indian genome-wide association study. JAMA Psychiatry 76(10):1026–1034, 2019

Portale S, Sculati M, Stanford FC, Cena H: Pellagra and anorexia nervosa: a case report. Eat Weight Disord 25(5):1493–1496, 2020

Peripheral neuropathy

Clinical findings	Peripheral neuropathy refers to dysfunction of one or more nerves outside the brain and spinal cord. It can involve the axon, the myelin sheath, or both. Function can be affected in large, myelinated fibers or small, unmyelinated fibers. Syndromes are characterized by different combinations of sensory symptoms, pain, weakness, muscle atrophy, flattened deep tendon reflexes, and vasomotor symptoms. Peripheral neuropathy is usefully classified as mononeuropathy (involving one nerve), multiple mononeuropathy (involving two or more nerves in different areas of the body), or polyneuropathy (involving many nerves simultaneously).
	• *Mononeuropathy*—characterized by pain, weakness, and paresthesias in the distribution of the involved nerve. Trauma is the most common cause, and this can involve acute injury, repetitive injury from grasping tools, compression injury such as from a bicycle seat, or entrapment injury such as that in carpal tunnel syndrome.
	• *Multiple mononeuropathy*—characterized by pain, weakness, and paresthesias in the distributions of the involved nerves. It can be caused by connective tissue diseases (e.g., SLE, rheumatoid arthritis) or infectious diseases (e.g., Lyme disease, HIV/AIDS) and other systemic illnesses. It is often asymmetric at onset.
	• *Polyneuropathy*—a diffuse peripheral nerve disorder not confined to single nerve distributions and usually bilaterally symmetric. Polyneuropathies can be primarily motor (e.g., Guillain-Barré syndrome, lead toxicity, porphyria) or primarily sensory (e.g., diabetes, HIV/AIDS, leprosy).
	Patients at risk of peripheral neuropathy include those with diabetes, the metabolic syndrome, a history of trauma, infection (e.g., herpes zoster, Lyme disease, HIV/AIDS), vascular insufficiency, alcohol use disorder, nutritional deficiencies (e.g., thiamine, vitamin B_{12}), kidney failure, tumors, toxin exposure, exposure to certain drugs, autoimmune disease (e.g., Guillain-Barré syndrome), or inherited neuropathies. Drugs implicated in peripheral neuropathy include chemotherapeutic agents, antimicrobials, cardiovascular drugs, statins, amiodarone, levodopa, and the anticonvulsants carbamazepine, phenytoin, and phenobarbital. Onset of symptoms is usually weeks to months after exposure, when drug levels have reached a threshold value.
	Signs and symptoms of motor neuropathies include the following:
	• Weakness
	• Muscle cramps
	• Fasciculations (visible twitching)
	• Muscle atrophy
	• Bone degeneration
	• Skin, hair, and nail changes (e.g., hair loss, shiny skin)
	Signs and symptoms of sensory neuropathies depend on whether the affected nerves are large, myelinated fibers or small, unmyelinated fibers.
	Large-fiber sensory neuropathies cause the following signs and symptoms:
	• Numbness and/or tingling
	• Loss of vibration sense

Peripheral neuropathy *(continued)*

Clinical findings *(continued)*	• Loss of position sense • Graphesthesia (inability to recognize objects by touch) • Pain that worsens at night Small-fiber sensory neuropathies cause the following symptoms: • Sharp pains, shooting pains, aching • Burning sensation • Allodynia (pain from a usually nonpainful stimulus) • Loss of sensation to painful stimuli • Loss of temperature sensation Autonomic nerves may also be affected in peripheral neuropathies generally, with signs and symptoms such as the following: • Heat intolerance • Loss of bladder control • Labile blood pressure • Orthostatic hypotension • GI symptoms, including dysphagia, diarrhea, constipation, or fecal incontinence
Laboratory testing	EMG/NCT is the most important tool in the diagnosis of peripheral neuropathy. The EMG examines the muscle itself, at rest and with contraction, and helps to distinguish muscle from nerve disorders. NCT evaluates the degree of injury in large nerve fibers and reveals whether the problem is primarily axonal, primarily demyelinating, or both. Slow impulse transmission rates indicate myelin involvement, whereas reduction of strength of impulses indicates axonal involvement. The limitation of EMG/NCT is that it cannot evaluate small nerve fibers. These are assessed with other tests, such as the heart rate response to tilt, heart rate variability with respiration and Valsalva maneuver, and sweat testing, among others. Blood tests routinely used to identify the cause of neuropathy include the following: • CBC • CMP—includes renal function tests and LFTs, fasting glucose • ESR • TSH • Vitamin B_{12} and MMA, folate • Tests for infection such as Lyme disease or HIV • Serum protein electrophoresis Other tests that may be useful in individual cases: • MRI for muscle quality and size, fatty infiltration, and nerve compression • CT for bone and vascular abnormalities that may contribute to symptoms • CSF analysis for paraneoplastic and inflammatory conditions • Biopsy (skin preferred to muscle) to examine small fibers • Genetic testing for suspected hereditary neuropathy

Peripheral neuropathy *(continued)*

Barrell K, Smith AG: Peripheral neuropathy. Med Clin North Am 103(2):383–397, 2019

Castelli G, Desai KM, Cantone RE: Peripheral neuropathy: evaluation and differential diagnosis. Am Fam Physician 102(12):732–739, 2020

Jones MR, Urits I, Wolf J, et al: Drug-induced peripheral neuropathy: a narrative review. Curr Clin Pharmacol 15(1):38–48, 2020

Julian T, Glascow N, Syeed R, Zis P: Alcohol-related peripheral neuropathy: a systematic review and meta-analysis. J Neurol 266(12):2907–2919, 2019

Kazamel M, Stino AM, Smith AG: Metabolic syndrome and peripheral neuropathy. Muscle Nerve 63(3):285–293, 2021

Lau KHV: Laboratory evaluation of peripheral neuropathy. Semin Neurol 39(5):531–541, 2019

Selvarajah D, Kar D, Khunti K, et al: Diabetic peripheral neuropathy: advances in diagnosis and strategies for screening and early intervention. Lancet Diabetes Endocrinol 7(12):938–948, 2019

Siao P, Kakxu M: A clinician's approach to peripheral neuropathy. Semin Neurol 39(5):519–530, 2019

Watson JC, Dyck PJ: Peripheral neuropathy: a practical approach to diagnosis and symptom management. Mayo Clin Proc 90(7):940–951, 2015

Pheochromocytoma

Clinical findings	Pheochromocytomas are rare catecholamine-secreting tumors that arise in the adrenal glands and paraganglionic chromaffin tissues and come to psychiatric attention because of symptoms of anxiety and recurrent panic attacks. Outside the adrenal glands, the tumors are termed *paragangliomas*, and these can form anywhere from the base of the brain to the urinary bladder. Ninety-eight percent are within the abdomen. About 10% of pheochromocytomas and 35% of paragangliomas are malignant, and these can metastasize to the lymph nodes, liver, and bone. About one-third occur as components of hereditary syndromes.
	Paroxysmal symptoms of pheochromocytoma are caused by secreted epinephrine, norepinephrine, dopamine, and dopa. Episodic attacks can be associated with severe hypertension and cardiac dysrhythmias that can prove fatal. Attacks can arise unexpectedly or be triggered by postural changes, abdominal compression, tumor palpation, emotional trauma, induction of anesthesia, unopposed beta blockade, or urination (with bladder tumors).
	Drugs that can trigger attacks include dopamine D_2-blocking antipsychotics, TCAs, SNRIs, MAOIs, ketamine, cocaine, sympathomimetics, non-selective β-blockers, and certain hormones and anesthetic agents. False-positive results on catecholamine testing may occur when these drugs are used, meaning that both the blood pressure and catecholamine levels are elevated, but no tumor is identified. For this reason, these drugs must be discontinued at least 2 weeks before testing. More importantly, the diagnosis of pheochromocytoma requires both proof of excessive catecholamine release and anatomical documentation of the tumor.
	The classic presentation of pheochromocytoma is paroxysmal hypertension accompanied by the triad of headache, palpitations, and excessive sweating. The paroxysms are associated with significant anxiety symptoms that often meet criteria for panic attacks. Tremor, nausea, weakness, and epigastric and flank pain may be present. The episodes last from seconds to hours, and their frequency varies from monthly to several times daily. With growth of the underlying tumor, the episodes can become more frequent and severe.
Laboratory testing	Diagnosis is confirmed by the finding of elevated catecholamine products in the blood or urine in the presence of a tumor. Imaging is used to localize tumors. Tests for catecholamines include plasma free metanephrines and fractionated 24-hour urine metanephrines. Because metanephrines are secreted continuously by the tumor, it is not necessary to draw samples during a panic attack or hypertensive episode. Generally, plasma testing is used for patients at high risk, including those with genetic syndromes or a personal/family history of pheochromocytoma, and urine testing is used for patients at lower risk.
	Free plasma metanephrine levels consistent with pheochromocytoma:
	• Normetanephrine>2.2 nmol/L
	• Metanephrine>1.1 nmol/L
	Patients with essential hypertension with normetanephrine <0.9 nmol/L and metanephrine <0.5 nmol/L do not require further testing. If clinical suspicion remains, 24-hour urine testing should be considered.

Pheochromocytoma *(continued)*

Laboratory testing *(continued)*	Urine 24-hour metanephrine reference levels: • Males ≥18 years: 55–320 μg/24 hours • Females ≥18 years: 36–229 μg/24 hours Urine 24-hour normetanephrine reference levels: • Males ≥30 years: 114–865 μg/24 hours • Females ≥18 years: 95–650 μg/24 hours One or both urine metanephrine levels ≥3 times the upper reference limit is consistent with pheochromocytoma. Smaller elevations of <2 times the upper reference limit can result from intense physical activity, drug interference, or other factors. Imaging studies are performed after metanephrine testing has confirmed the presence of a tumor, to localize the mass and determine its size, consistency, and shape. For this purpose, CT or MRI can be used to evaluate the retroperitoneum and other structures. In many centers, CT is the modality of choice because it is cheaper, is more widely available, and has better spatial resolution. MRI is used for children and pregnant females because it does not involve radiation exposure. It is also an option for those who are unable to tolerate iodinated contrast media. Further evaluation with nuclear medicine scanning (^{123}I-MIBG scintigraphy) or PET scanning may be needed in selected cases.

Anderson NE, Chung K, Willoughby E, Croxson MS: Neurological manifestations of phaeochromocytomas and secretory paragangliomas: a reappraisal. J Neurol Neurosurg Psychiatry 84(4):452–457, 2013

ARUP Laboratories: Metanephrines fractionated by HPLC-MS/MS, urine, in Laboratory Test Directory. Salt Lake City, UT, ARUP Laboratories, 2022. Available at: https://ltd.aruplab.com/Tests/Pub/2007996. Accessed March 2022.

ARUP Laboratories: Metanephrines, plasma (free), in Laboratory Test Directory. Salt Lake City, UT, ARUP Laboratories, 2022. Available at: https://ltd.aruplab.com/Tests/Pub/0050184. Accessed March 2022.

Carrasquillo JA, Chen CC, Jha A, et al: Imaging of pheochromocytoma and paraganglioma. J Nucl Med 62(8):1033–1042, 2021

Farrugia FA, Charalampopoulos A: Pheochromocytoma. Endocr Regul 53(3):191–212, 2019

Neary NM, King KS, Pacak K: Drugs and pheochromocytoma: don't be fooled by every elevated metanephrine. N Engl J Med 364(23):2268–2270, 2011

Neumann HPH, Young WF Jr, Eng C: Pheochromocytoma and paraganglioma. N Engl J Med 381(6):552–565, 2019

Sbardella E, Grossman AB: Pheochromocytoma: an approach to diagnosis. Best Pract Res Clin Endocrinol Metab 34(2):101346, 2020

Pica

Clinical findings	Pica is characterized by persistent eating of nonnutritive, nonfood substances over a period of at least 1 month that is inappropriate to the developmental level of the individual and is not part of a culturally supported or socially normative practice. If it occurs in the context of another mental disorder or medical condition, it is sufficiently severe to warrant additional clinical attention. Mental disorders associated with pica in adults include intellectual developmental disorder, autism spectrum disorder, and schizophrenia. Triggers of pica appear to include boredom, curiosity, and psychological tension. Relief is commonly reported after ingestion.
	Specific food cravings in pregnancy are common. Pica is only diagnosed when nonfood items are ingested to the extent that medical risks are introduced. Among pregnant Hispanic females in the United States, pica is prevalent and is strongly linked to iron deficiency and food insecurity. Among pregnant females in parts of Africa, the eating of soil is known to increase the rate of helminth infection.
	In general, pica can be a protracted problem, with serious sequelae such as esophageal perforation, intestinal obstruction, bezoar formation, poisoning, and acute weight loss. Bezoars are tightly packed masses of undigested material that commonly form in the stomach.
Laboratory testing	Laboratory testing for pica may include the following: • CBC to diagnose anemia • Serum iron level (often low) • Serum zinc level (often low) • Lead level in cases in which the ingested material includes paint or other lead-containing substances • In cases in which clay was ingested, chemistries such as potassium and phosphate (may be low) • To identify swallowed objects, abdominal flat plate X-ray, ultrasound, or esophagram • Endoscopy to identify and remove swallowed objects

American Psychiatric Association: Diagnostic and Statistical Manual of Mental Disorders, 5th Edition, Text Revision. Washington, DC, American Psychiatric Association, 2022

Busch JR, Löchte L, Lindh AS, Jacobsen C: Lethal small bowel obstruction due to pica. J Forensic Sci 67(1):374–376, 2022

Getachew M, Yeshigeta R, Tiruneh A, et al: Soil-transmitted helminthic infections and geophagia among pregnant women in Jimma Town health institutions, Southwest Ethiopia. Ethiop J Health Sci 31(5):1033–1042, 2021

Hartmann AS: Pica behaviors in a German community-based online adolescent and adult sample: an examination of substances, triggers, and associated pathology. Eat Weight Disord 25(3):811–815, 2020

Nakiyemba O, Obore S, Musaba M, et al: Covariates of pica among pregnant women attending antenatal care at Kawempe Hospital, Kampala, Uganda: a cross-sectional study. Am J Trop Med Hyg 105(4):909–914, 2021

Roy A, Fuentes-Afflick E, Fernald LCH, Young SL: Pica is prevalent and strongly associated with iron deficiency among Hispanic pregnant women living in the United States. Appetite 120:163–170, 2018

Schmidt C, Oxley Oxland J, Freercks R: A rare case of hypokalaemia and hypophosphataemia secondary to geophagia. BMJ Case Rep 14(5):e239322, 2021

Thihalolipavan S, Candalla BM, Ehrlich J: Examining pica in NYC pregnant women with elevated blood lead levels. Matern Child Health J 17(1):49–55, 2013

Yocum AD, Dennison JL, Simon EL: Esophageal obstruction and death in a nonverbal patient. J Emerg Med 60(5):e109–e113, 2021

Porphyria

Clinical findings	Porphyria refers to a group of disorders arising from a deficiency of particular enzymes involved in the production of heme, a component of the oxygen transporter hemoglobin. Heme production requires eight steps, each catalyzed by a separate enzyme. When one enzyme is affected by a genetic mutation or environmental toxin, the process halts and intermediate products from earlier steps accumulate, depositing in the skin, liver, or bone marrow and other tissues and potentially causing injury before being eliminated in urine and feces.
	Acute intermittent porphyria (AIP) caused by a deficiency of porphobilinogen deaminase, the third enzyme of heme production, is the disorder most often encountered clinically and is noteworthy for its neuropsychiatric effects. This is a genetic disorder with an autosomal dominant inheritance but with low penetrance, meaning that <10% of affected individuals show symptoms. Symptoms can be triggered by environmental factors, however, as discussed below.
	AIP mostly affects females of reproductive age and can be catamenial, occurring during the progesterone surge between ovulation and menstruation. It is more common in those of Scandinavian or English descent. Symptoms occur episodically and can be triggered by specific medications, alcohol ingestion, infection, stress, menstruation, pregnancy, and caloric deprivation or low-carbohydrate diets. Medications considered unsafe in AIP include steroids, oral contraceptives, valproate, carbamazepine, lamotrigine, phenobarbital, phenytoin, primidone, hydroxyzine, carisoprodol, and spironolactone. Possibly unsafe medications include ketamine, imipramine, and various antibiotics. The American Porphyria Foundation maintains a searchable database for prescription and over-the-counter drugs at https://porphyriafoundation.org/drugdatabase/drug-safety-database-search.
	The classic presentation of AIP is that of a previously healthy young female reporting a prodrome of fatigue and difficulty concentrating followed by an acute attack of severe, progressive abdominal pain, nausea, and vomiting accompanied by autonomic symptoms of tachycardia and elevated blood pressure and neuropsychiatric symptoms of weakness, dysesthesia, anxiety, agitation, depression, and confusion. A benign abdominal exam and normal imaging results, in conjunction with a poor response to analgesics (even opioids), often leads to a diagnosis of psychosomatic disorder or drug addiction. This is particularly problematic because progression of the disease results in more serious problems, such as chronic hypertension, end-stage renal disease, and eventually hepatocellular carcinoma. The syndrome can be fatal.
	Other signs and symptoms of AIP include the following: • Delirium • Psychosis (hallucinations and delusions) • Acute development of peripheral neuropathy (predominantly motor), which can progress to quadriparesis • Encephalopathy • General hyporeflexia with preservation of Achilles reflex • Pain outside of the abdomen, affecting the back, limbs, head, neck, and/or chest • Constipation, abdominal distention

Porphyria *(continued)*

Clinical findings *(continued)*	• Urinary retention • Respiratory distress • SIAD • Seizures • Urine darkening upon exposure to light at ambient temperatures The triad of abdominal pain, seizures, and hyponatremia (see below) is highly suggestive of AIP. Spontaneous attacks vary in duration from months to years, significantly impacting the quality of life of affected individuals. The identification of relatives also affected by genetic mutations is important so that education can be provided regarding triggers of attacks.
Laboratory testing	Initial testing requires measurement of porphobilinogen levels in urine or plasma, which when elevated are specific for AIP. During an acute attack, elevations can be 10–150 times the upper limit of normal. Urine testing can be performed on a random sample, with the result normalized to grams of creatinine so a 24-hour sample is not needed. The tests take a minimum of 4 days to return results, introducing a problematic delay in confirming diagnosis. A negative result during an attack excludes the diagnosis of AIP. A negative result in a currently asymptomatic patient requires repeat testing during an attack. Once a diagnosis of AIP has been made, stool is tested for porphyrins to differentiate among the types of porphyria. Genetic testing is performed to identify known mutations for the patient and first-degree relatives. Other laboratory abnormalities that may be returned include hyponatremia, mild elevation in liver enzymes, elevation of serum T_4 and thyroxine-binding globulin in the absence of hyperthyroidism, and elevated serum cholesterol and low-density lipoprotein. WBC count may be elevated in the presence of infection or stress. Brain imaging (CT or MRI) in some cases shows symmetrical white matter abnormalities suggestive of edema in the posterior parieto-occipital areas that is consistent with posterior reversible encephalopathy syndrome. Because of the greatly elevated risk of hepatocellular carcinoma after age 50 years in patients with AIP, annual screening of the abdomen using ultrasound or other imaging modality and annual measurement of α-fetoprotein are recommended.

Bissell DM, Anderson KE, Bonkovsky HL: Porphyria. N Engl J Med 377(9):862–872, 2017

Duque-Serrano L, Patarroyo-Rodriguez L, Gotlib D, Molano-Eslava JC: Psychiatric aspects of acute porphyria: a comprehensive review. Curr Psychiatry Rep 20(1):5, 2018

Ramanujam VS, Anderson KE: Porphyria diagnostics, part 1: a brief overview of the porphyrias. Curr Protoc Hum Genet 86:17.20.1–17.20.26, 2015

Stölzel U, Doss MO, Schuppan D: Clinical guide and update on porphyrias. Gastroenterology 157(2):365–381, 2019

Suh Y, Gandhi J, Seyam O, et al: Neurological and neuropsychiatric manifestations of porphyria. Int J Neurosci 129(12):1226–1233, 2019

Tracy JA, Dyck PJ: Porphyria and its neurologic manifestations. Handb Clin Neurol 120:839–849, 2014

Yasuda M, Chen B, Desnick RJ: Recent advances on porphyria genetics: inheritance, penetrance and molecular heterogeneity, including new modifying/causative genes. Mol Genet Metab 128(3):320–331, 2019

Prader-Willi syndrome (PWS)

Clinical findings	PWS is a rare genetic disorder characterized by intellectual disability, dysmorphic features, psychiatric and behavioral problems, and hypothalamic dysfunction associated with obesity, growth hormone deficiency, hypogonadism, adrenal insufficiency, hypothyroidism, and reduced bone mineral density. PWS is a genomic imprinting disorder usually involving a lack of gene expression from the paternal chromosome 15q11-q13 region. Most cases occur sporadically. The disorder is often apparent at birth or in early childhood, but affected individuals can live into adulthood and sometimes come to medical attention as adults.
	Psychopathologies in PWS include intellectual disability, hyperphagia, autistic behaviors, anxiety, obsessions, temper outbursts, impulsivity, self-injury, and others. Psychiatric comorbidities include pica, mood disorders, autism spectrum disorders, anxiety disorders, OCD, psychosis, and others. Hyperphagia resulting in obesity is likely related to a defect in the satiety system.
	Beyond childhood, individuals with PWS have a range of health problems, including growth hormone deficiency with short stature, hypogonadism, hypertension, type 2 diabetes, hypercholesterolemia, hypothyroidism, heart failure, water intoxication, fatty liver, sleep apnea, narcolepsy, reduced pain sensitivity, seizures, GI hypomotility, stasis ulcers, cellulitis, scoliosis, and vitamin D deficiency. Most males with PWS are infertile. Dysmorphic features include narrowed temples, almond-shaped eyes, mild strabismus, thin upper lip, downturned mouth, small hands with tapered fingers, and small feet. Life expectancy for affected individuals is reduced unless strict weight control is maintained.
Laboratory testing	In an undiagnosed patient with suspected PWS, genetic testing on a blood sample is required. The first step is to confirm the diagnosis using DNA methylation analysis. The second step is to determine the specific genetic lesion involving chromosome 15.
	Evaluation of growth hormone deficiency is required. See **Human Growth Hormone** entry in the *Laboratory Tests* chapter.
	Assessment of adrenal hormone reserves is recommended. Initial testing involves measurement of morning cortisol and ACTH levels from a venous blood sample.
	Assessment of thyroid status is recommended. See the entries on **Thyroid Function Testing** in the *Laboratory Tests* chapter.
	Other recommended tests include the following: • Creatinine and creatinine clearance • Vitamin D and calcium levels • Fasting glucose • Lipid profile A low threshold should be maintained for obtaining the following tests, depending on presenting signs/symptoms: • Polysomnography • DEXA scan for bone density • Spine X-ray for kyphosis • Cardiac evaluation

Prader-Willi syndrome (PWS) *(continued)*

Alves C, Franco RR: Prader-Willi syndrome: endocrine manifestations and management. Arch Endocrinol Metab 64(3):223–234, 2020

Bellis SA, Kuhn I, Adams S, et al: The consequences of hyperphagia in people with Prader-Willi syndrome: a systematic review of studies of morbidity and mortality. Eur J Med Genet 65(1):104379, 2022

Butler MG, Miller JL, Forster JL: Prader-Willi syndrome: clinical genetics, diagnosis and treatment approaches: an update. Curr Pediatr Rev 15(4):207–244, 2019

Godler DE, Butler MG: Special issue: genetics of Prader-Willi syndrome. Genes (Basel) 12(9):1429, 2021

Noordam C, Höybye C, Eiholzer U: Prader-Willi syndrome and hypogonadism: a review article. Int J Mol Sci 22(5):2705, 2021

Online Mendelian Inheritance in Man: Prader-Willi syndrome (#176270). Baltimore, MD, Johns Hopkins University, 2022. Available at: https://www.omim.org/entry/176270#clinicalFeatures. Accessed March 2022.

Ozsezen B, Emiralioglu N, Özön A, et al: Sleep disordered breathing in patients with Prader Willi syndrome: impact of underlying genetic mechanism. Respir Med 187:106567, 2021

Pellikaan K, Rosenberg AGW, Kattentidt-Mouravieva AA, et al: Missed diagnoses and health problems in adults with Prader-Willi syndrome: recommendations for screening and treatment. J Clin Endocrinol Metab 105(12):e4671–e4687, 2020

Schwartz L, Caixàs A, Dimitropoulos A, et al: Behavioral features in Prader-Willi syndrome (PWS): consensus paper from the International PWS Clinical Trial Consortium. J Neurodev Disord 13(1):25, 2021

Wieting J, Eberlein C, Bleich S, et al: Behavioural change in Prader-Willi syndrome during COVID-19 pandemic. J Intellect Disabil Res 65(7):609–616, 2021

Progressive multifocal leukoencephalopathy (PML)

Clinical findings	PML is an opportunistic brain infection caused by the John Cunningham virus (JCV), named after the patient in whom the virus was first identified and bearing no relation to CJD, another disease discussed in an earlier entry. Initial JCV infection typically occurs in childhood through person-to-person contact or contaminated surfaces, food, or water. Seroconversion increases with age, reaching almost 80% by age 70 years. Contaminated sewage is thought to be the major source of environmental exposure. Not unlike a herpesvirus, JCV establishes an asymptomatic and persistent lifelong infection, in this case remaining latent in the kidneys and lymphoid organs. Under circumstances of prolonged compromise of cellular immunity, however, the virus can reactivate and undergo sequential genomic rearrangement. These mutations enable the virus to become neurotropic, infecting oligodendrocytes and other CNS cell populations and causing lytic infection that leads to expanding areas of demyelination.
	Patients at risk of developing PML include those with HIV/AIDS, cancer, tuberculosis, sarcoidosis, autoimmune disease, chronic inflammatory disease, or drug-induced immunosuppression or immunomodulation. HIV/AIDS, lymphoproliferative disease, and multiple sclerosis now account for most cases of the disease. PML exists on a spectrum of immune response, with an absence of antiviral immune activity at one end (classic PML) and an extensive inflammatory reaction at the other. The latter, known as PML-associated immune reconstitution inflammatory syndrome (PML-IRIS), is characterized by further clinical worsening due to immune-mediated injury.
	PML can progress rapidly, but symptoms vary depending on the location and extent of brain demyelination. The most common features are clumsiness, weakness, cognitive dysfunction, behavioral and personality changes, speech/language impairment, ataxia, and visual field defects. Paresthesias, headaches, and seizures can be seen. When the virus infects other cell populations, encephalopathy or meningitis can occur. Notably, the peripheral nervous system is not involved. When the cause of immunosuppression can be addressed—for example, when an implicated drug can be stopped—recovery is possible, although residual symptoms may be seen. When the underlying cause cannot be addressed, the outcome can be fatal; death commonly occurs within 1–9 months.
	The diagnosis of PML is established by typical clinical symptoms, characteristic findings on MRI scanning, and detection of JCV DNA in CSF using PCR assay. Alternatively, brain biopsy can establish the diagnosis directly, but this approach is not without associated morbidity.
Laboratory testing	*CSF*
	Sampling for JCV using PCR amplification is one cornerstone of diagnosis. In the presence of characteristic symptoms, this test has high sensitivity. False-negative results do occur; a negative test does not exclude PML. If clinical suspicion of PML remains high after a negative test is returned, an ultra-sensitive quantitative JCV PCR is available through the National Institutes of Health. CSF testing should also include cell count with differential, protein, and glucose measurements. Culture is not performed because JCV growth is too slow.

Progressive multifocal leukoencephalopathy (PML) *(continued)*

Laboratory testing *(continued)*	*Neuroimaging*
	Brain MRI is more sensitive to PML changes than head CT. MRI commonly demonstrates one or more hyperintense areas on T2 and FLAIR images and hypointense areas on T1 images involving subcortical and juxtacortical white matter. Often, lesions are sharply delineated at the cortical border. Except with PML-IRIS, there is no enhancement with gadolinium. Lesions can be multifocal or unifocal, often involving the frontal lobes and parieto-occipital areas. Isolated or associated involvement of the external capsule, basal ganglia, brainstem, and/or cerebellum can be seen. With cerebellar involvement, MRI may show the "shrimp sign," a T2/FLAIR hyperintense white matter lesion abutting but sparing the dentate nucleus. Both PML and inflammatory activity will cause dynamic changes on MRI images over weeks to months. If MRI is not available, CT can be performed. CT shows patchy or confluent hypodense areas in white matter. Lesions seen on MRI or CT do not respect anatomical boundaries or vascular territories. If the patient survives, neurodegenerative changes such as atrophy may develop over weeks to months.
	Histopathology
	Biopsy tissue demonstrates demyelination, large and bizarre astrocytes, and oligodendroglial nuclear inclusions. These findings are confirmed with molecular analysis or specific histopathology. Tissue PCR for JCV will be positive.

Adra N, Goodheart AE, Rapalino O, et al: MRI shrimp sign in cerebellar progressive multifocal leukoencephalopathy: description and validation of a novel observation. AJNR Am J Neuroradiol 42(6):1073–1079, 2021

ARUP Consult: JC virus: progressive multifocal leukoencephalopathy, in ARUP Consult: The Physician's Guide to Laboratory Test Selection and Interpretation. Salt Lake City, UT, ARUP Laboratories, 2022. Available at: https://arupconsult.com/content/jc-virus. Accessed March 2022.

Bartsch T, Rempe T, Leypoldt F, et al: The spectrum of progressive multifocal leukoencephalopathy: a practical approach. Eur J Neurol 26(4):566-e41, 2019

Berger JR, Aksamit AJ, Clifford DB, et al: PML diagnostic criteria: consensus statement from the AAN Neuroinfectious Disease Section. Neurology 80(15):1430–1438, 2013

Cortese I, Reich DS, Nath A: Progressive multifocal leukoencephalopathy and the spectrum of JC virus-related disease. Nat Rev Neurol 17(1):37–51, 2021

Grebenciucova E, Berger JR: Progressive multifocal leukoencephalopathy. Neurol Clin 36(4):739–750, 2018

Khan F, Sharma N, Ud Din M, Akabalu IG: Clinically isolated brainstem progressive multifocal leukoencephalopathy: diagnostic challenges. Am J Case Rep 23:e935019, 2022

Kromm JA, Power C, Blevins G, et al: Rapid multifocal neurologic decline in an immunocompromised patient. JAMA Neurol 73(2):226–231, 2016

Patel A, Sul J, Gordon ML, et al: Progressive multifocal leukoencephalopathy in a patient with progressive multiple sclerosis treated with ocrelizumab monotherapy. JAMA Neurol 278(6):736–740, 2021

Psychogenic polydipsia

Clinical findings	Psychogenic polydipsia—also known as primary polydipsia or poto-mania—is characterized by compulsive water drinking in the absence of a physical cause of overdrinking. In this disorder, water intake exceeds the capacity of the kidney to excrete water, leading to hypo-osmolar hyponatremia. The secretion of arginine vasopressin (also known as antidiuretic hormone) is reduced in response to low osmolality, and urine output is increased. Polygenic polydipsia is seen in up to 20% of patients hospitalized with serious mental illness and can have a grave or even fatal outcome. Typical volumes ingested average 8 L/day.
	Polygenic polydipsia most often affects patients diagnosed with schizophrenia, mood disorders, and addiction but also is seen in those with anxiety disorders, dementia, anorexia, developmental disabilities, and personality disorders. It is highly recurrent because of recrudescence of drinking behavior and so requires long-term follow-up. Triggers of excessive drinking are not well described, although the sensation of a dry mouth is often reported, and anxious feelings are likely implicated. In some cases, delusions drive the drinking behavior. Restriction of fluid is often not successful in treating the condition because patients may find other sources such as toilet water. Antipsychotic, mood-stabilizing, antidepressant, and other drugs can exacerbate the condition.
	Signs and symptoms of water intoxication depend on the severity and chronicity of hyponatremia. These include the following, arranged from mildest to most severe:
	• Polyuria
	• Nausea without vomiting
	• Headache
	• Dizziness
	• Ataxia
	• Somnolence, stupor
	• Confusion
	• Delirium
	• Vomiting
	• Seizures
	• Cardiorespiratory distress
	• Cardiac arrest
	• Coma
	• Death due to cerebral edema with brain herniation
Laboratory testing	The following laboratory abnormalities are seen:
	• Hyponatremia
	• Low serum and urine osmolality
	• Low serum arginine vasopressin (also known as antidiuretic hormone)
	Water deprivation tests may be of limited value in differentiating polygenic polydipsia from diabetes insipidus. Urine arginine vasopressin may be superior to serum for testing but is not widely available.

Psychogenic polydipsia *(continued)*

Ahmadi L, Goldman MB: Primary polydipsia: update. Best Pract Res Clin Endocrinol Metab 34(5):101469, 2020

Benítez-Mejía JF, Morales-Cuellar J, Restrepo-López JS, et al: Psycogenic polydipsia and severe hyponatremia in bipolar affective disorder. Actas Esp Psiquiatr 49(6):288–290, 2021

Rangan GK, Dorani N, Zhang MM, et al: Clinical characteristics and outcomes of hyponatraemia associated with oral water intake in adults: a systematic review. BMJ Open 11(12):e046539

Sailer CO, Winzeler B, Nigro N, et al: Characteristics and outcomes of patients with profound hyponatraemia due to primary polydipsia. Clin Endocrinol (Oxf) 87(5):492–499, 2017

Torosyan N, Spencer D, Penev S, Bota RG: Psychogenic polydipsia in a woman with anorexia nervosa: case report and recommendations. Prim Care Companion CNS Disord 20(1):17l02120, 2018

Trimpou P, Olsson DS, Ehn O, Ragnarsson O: Diagnostic value of the water deprivation test in the polyuria-polydipsia syndrome. Hormones (Athens) 16(4):414–422, 2017

Psychotic disorder due to another medical condition

Clinical findings	This syndrome is one of prominent hallucinations and/or delusions occurring in a patient with a clear sensorium (i.e., not delirious). The symptoms are not psychologically mediated but instead are the direct pathophysiological effects of a medical condition. Reality testing is not intact. Modality of hallucinations may suggest the area of the brain affected (e.g., olfactory with complex partial seizures arising from the temporal lobes, or visual with occipital lobe tumors), but this is less true for delusions.
	Patients at highest risk of developing secondary psychosis include those with untreated endocrine, metabolic, or autoimmune disease and those with epilepsy. Specific examples include anti-NMDAR encephalitis, acute intermittent porphyria, SLE, multiple sclerosis, thyroid dysfunction, brain tumor, Parkinson's disease, and TBI. In late life, neurodegenerative diseases such as Alzheimer's disease and dementia with Lewy bodies are often implicated. The list of specific medical causes is extensive, and it is often necessary to rely on associated features of the presentation to suggest the direction of the workup (e.g., abdominal pain with acute intermittent porphyria or malar rash with SLE).
	Postictal psychosis is a syndrome that may follow a cluster of seizures (generalized or complex partial) in patients with long-standing epilepsy. Typically, the patient has a lucid interval of hours to days, followed by abrupt onset of psychosis. The episode usually resolves in days to weeks, but the psychosis can recur after subsequent seizure episodes, and with each recurrence it tends to lengthen in duration. Chronic interictal psychosis closely resembles the psychosis of schizophrenia, with prominent delusions and auditory hallucinations. This syndrome is more common among patients with complex partial seizures, left temporal lobe foci, and/or left medial temporal sclerosis.
	When the underlying medical condition is successfully treated, psychotic symptoms often remit. For chronic conditions, long-term treatment of psychosis may be necessary.
Laboratory testing	The patient's presentation and demographics will determine the direction of the laboratory workup, but basic screening tests include the following: • CMP • CBC with differential and platelets • Urinalysis • TSH • ESR or CRP • Head CT with contrast or MRI with gadolinium Other tests to be considered include the following: • EEG • ECG • Lumbar puncture for CSF analysis (routine studies and anti-NMDAR antibodies) • Antithyroid antibodies • Urine pregnancy testing • Antinuclear antibody testing • Syphilis serology

Psychotic disorder due to another medical condition *(continued)*

Laboratory testing *(continued)*	• HIV testing
	• Urine toxicology screen
	• Cortisol (blood and 24-hour urine)
	• Spot urine for porphyrin precursors
	• Heavy metal screening
	• Vitamin B_{12} level
	• Ceruloplasmin and free serum copper levels
	• Serum testosterone level

Abrol E, Coutinho E, Chou M, et al: Psychosis in systemic lupus erythematosus (SLE): 40-year experience of a specialist centre. Rheumatology (Oxford) 60(12):5620–5629, 2021

American Psychiatric Association: Diagnostic and Statistical Manual of Mental Disorders, 5th Edition, Text Revision. Washington, DC, American Psychiatric Association, 2022

Andrews JP, Taylor J, Saunders D, Qayyum Z: Peduncular psychosis. BMJ Case Rep 2016:bcr2016216165, 2016

Dalmau J, Armangué T, Planagumà J, et al: An update on anti-NMDA receptor encephalitis for neurologists and psychiatrists: mechanisms and models. Lancet Neurol 18(11):1045–1057, 2019

Keshavan MS, Kaneko Y: Secondary psychoses: an update. World Psychiatry 12(1):4–15, 2013

Kimoto S, Yamamuro K, Kishimoto T: Acute psychosis in patients with subclinical hyperthyroidism. Psychiatry Clin Neurosci 73(6):348–349, 2019

Murphy R, O'Donoghue S, Counihan T, et al: Neuropsychiatric syndromes of multiple sclerosis. J Neurol Neurosurg Psychiatry 88(8):697–708, 2017

Schneider RB, Iourinets J, Richard IH: Parkinson's disease psychosis: presentation, diagnosis and management. Neurodegener Dis Manag 7(6):365–376, 2017

Suh Y, Gandhi J, Seyam O, et al: Neurological and neuropsychiatric manifestations of porphyria. Int J Neurosc 129(12):1226–1233, 2019

Zgaljardic DJ, Seale GS, Schaefer LA, et al: Psychiatric disease and post-acute traumatic brain injury. J Neurotrauma 32(23):1911–1925, 2015

Pyridoxine deficiency

Clinical findings	Pyridoxine or vitamin B_6 is a dietary nutrient comprising a group of closely related compounds including pyridoxine itself, pyridoxal, and pyridoxamine. These compounds are transformed in the body to the active form pyridoxal 5'-phosphate (PLP), which serves as a coenzyme in more than 150 biochemical reactions involved in metabolism and in the synthesis of proteins, carbohydrates, lipids, heme, and various bioactive metabolites. Pyridoxine has a critical role in neurotransmitter metabolism (especially GABA synthesis), has antioxidant and anti-inflammatory functions, and helps to modulate gene expression and immunity.
	Dietary sources of pyridoxine include organ meats such as liver, whole grain cereals, fish, and legumes. Although frank deficiency is rare, subclinical deficiency is not, and there is some evidence that this state may contribute to inflammatory conditions involved in cardiovascular disease. Subclinical deficiency has been identified in up to 23% of individuals age 65–75 years and up to 40% of those 85 years and older.
	Other patients at risk of pyridoxine deficiency include strict vegetarians, those with chronic alcohol overuse, cirrhosis, hyperthyroidism, protein-energy undernutrition, malabsorption, congestive heart failure, hepatic or renal disease, HIV/AIDS, rheumatoid arthritis, sickle cell disease, pregnancy, preeclampsia, or lactation; those on dialysis; and those taking medications such as TCAs, anticonvulsants (valproate, carbamazepine, phenytoin), corticosteroids, cycloserine, isoniazid, rifampin, penicillamine, or hydralazine.
	Signs and symptoms of pyridoxine deficiency include peripheral neuropathy, microcytic anemia, a pellagra-like syndrome (seborrheic dermatitis, glossitis, and cheilosis), kidney stones, depression, confusion, EEG abnormalities, seizures, and status epilepticus. Treatment of pyridoxine deficiency with vitamin B_6 doses >50 mg/day can result in toxicity manifesting as a sensory neuropathy and other symptoms like those of deficiency.
Laboratory testing	Measures of pyridoxine status are of two types: direct biomarkers and functional biomarkers. Direct testing most commonly measures PLP in blood (plasma or serum) and reflects recent intake. A normal PLP level is >10 ng/mL. A level <5 ng/mL identifies deficiency. Albumin levels are measured in tandem for proper interpretation.
	Functional testing uses erythrocyte aspartate aminotransferase (EAST) and the EAST activation coefficient (EAST-AC) to provide information about longer-term functional pyridoxine status. Because the EAST-AC reduction lags the onset of pyridoxine deficiency, a low value confirms a subacute to chronic deficiency state. Newer function tests involve plasma levels of metabolites involved in PLP-dependent pathways such as the kynurenine pathway and one-carbon metabolism.

Berkins S, Schiöth HB, Rukh G: Depression and vegetarians: association between dietary vitamin B6, B12 and folate intake and global and subcortical brain volumes. Nutrients 13(6):1790, 2021

Bird RP: The emerging role of vitamin B6 in inflammation and carcinogenesis. Adv Food Nutr Res 83:151–194, 2018

Dave HN, Ramsay RE, Khan F, et al: Pyridoxine deficiency in adult patients with status epilepticus. Epilepsy Behav 52(Pt A):154–158, 2015

Galimberti F, Mesinkovska NA: Skin findings associated with nutritional deficiencies. Cleve Clin J Med 83(10):731–739, 2016

Ghavanini AA, Kimpinski K: Revisiting the evidence for neuropathy caused by pyridoxine deficiency and excess. J Clin Neuromuscul Dis 16(1):25–31, 2014

Pyridoxine deficiency *(continued)*

Hadtstein F, Vrolijk M: Vitamin B-6-induced neuropathy: exploring the mechanisms of pyridoxine toxicity. Adv Nutr 12(5):1911–1929, 2021

Kumrungsee T, Peipei Zhang, Yanaka N, et al: Emerging cardioprotective mechanisms of vitamin B6: a narrative review. Eur J Nutr 61(2):605–613, 2022

Stach K, Stach W, Augoff K: Vitamin B6 in health and disease. Nutrients 13(9):3229, 2021

Ueland PM, Ulvik A, Rios-Avila L, et al: Direct and functional biomarkers of vitamin B6 status. Annu Rev Nutr 35:33–70, 2015

Wilson MP, Plecko B, Mills PB, Clayton PT: Disorders affecting vitamin B6 metabolism. J Inherit Metab Dis 42(4):629–646, 2019

Restless legs syndrome (RLS)

Clinical findings	RLS is a sensorimotor condition characterized by an urge to move the legs, usually accompanied by or in response to uncomfortable and unpleasant sensations. Sensations begin or worsen during periods of rest or inactivity and are partially or totally relieved by movement. Symptoms either develop only during the evening/nighttime hours or become worse at those times. They occur at least 3 times weekly for at least 3 months and are not attributable to a mental disorder, medical condition, drug of abuse, or medication. RLS is associated with significant sleep disruption and in severe cases affects mood and quality of life.
	RLS is best understood as involving a gene-environment interaction in which individuals with high genetic loading experience early symptoms, and those with lesser loading become symptomatic only with the onset of triggers that appear later in life (e.g., iron deficiency, kidney disease). Family studies suggest an autosomal dominant pattern of inheritance with variable penetrance. Recent research suggests that neural pathways such as the hypothalamus-spinal dopaminergic circuit and possibly pathways including the basal ganglia and limbic structures are implicated and that a link exists between RLS and systemic inflammation.
	Conditions that increase the risk of developing RLS symptoms—the "triggers" in this model—include iron deficiency, renal insufficiency (especially end-stage renal disease), pregnancy, Parkinson's disease, stroke (especially in the basal ganglia, thalamus, or internal capsule), diabetes, vitamin B_{12} or folate deficiency, fibromyalgia, and possibly cardiovascular disease and chronic obstructive pulmonary disease. Medications such as antipsychotics and antidepressants can also be triggers, the latter including SSRIs, SNRIs, and mirtazapine. RLS of pregnancy mostly resolves after delivery, but affected females are at risk of later episodes. RLS in end-stage renal disease also resolves after kidney transplantation but recurs in the event of transplant failure.
	The differential diagnosis for RLS includes akathisia, neuropathy, nocturnal leg cramps, "painful legs and moving toes," and peripheral vascular disease. Patients with akathisia do not experience the paresthesias characteristic of RLS, their movements are not related to sleep, and movement does not relieve the urge of akathisia. Neuropathy is distinguished by the absence of motor restlessness, lack of association with sleep, and absence of relief by movement. Neuropathy can coexist with RLS. Nocturnal leg cramps are typically unilateral, painful muscle contractions that are palpable as a hard mass. Painful legs/moving toes are spontaneous flexions/extensions of the toes secondary to spinal cord injury or nerve root lesions. These movements are not associated with an urge to move and are not associated with sleep. Symptoms of peripheral vascular disease typically worsen with activity rather than with rest and are not associated particularly with sleep. In addition, in RLS, peripheral pulses are intact.
	The diagnosis of RLS is based on a history of typical symptoms and the physical examination. Laboratory tests are used to evaluate the contribution of diseases to the emergence of symptoms. A screening question formulated and validated by RLS specialists can be useful for initial evaluation: "When you try to relax in the evening or sleep at night, do you ever have unpleasant, restless feelings in your legs that can be relieved by walking or movement?" This question reportedly has 100% sensitivity and 96.8% specificity for the diagnosis.

Restless legs syndrome (RLS) *(continued)*

Laboratory testing	Laboratory tests recommended for the workup of RLS include the following:
	• Iron studies: serum iron, total iron-binding capacity, ferritin
	• CBC with red cell indices, reticulocyte index, and peripheral smear
	• CMP
	• Vitamin B_{12} and folate levels
	• TSH

American Psychiatric Association: Diagnostic and Statistical Manual of Mental Disorders, 5th Edition, Text Revision. Washington, DC, American Psychiatric Association, 2022

Dowsett J, Didriksen M, von Stemann JH, et al: Chronic inflammation markers and cytokine-specific autoantibodies in Danish blood donors with restless legs syndrome. Sci Rep 12(1):1672, 2022

Garcia-Malo C, Romero-Peralta S, Cano-Pumarega I: Restless legs syndrome: clinical features. Sleep Med Clin 16(2):233–247, 2021

Gossard TR, Trotti LM, Videnovic A, St Louis EK: Restless legs syndrome: contemporary diagnosis and treatment. Neurotherapeutics 18(1):140–155, 2021

Klingelhoefer L, Bhattacharya K, Reichmann H: Restless legs syndrome. Clin Med (Lond) 16(4):379–382, 2016

Manconi M, Garcia-Borreguero D, Schormair B, et al: Restless legs syndrome. Nat Rev Dis Primers 7(1):80, 2021

Mogavero MP, Mezzapesa DM, Savarese M, et al: Morphological analysis of the brain subcortical gray structures in restless legs syndrome. Sleep Med 88:74–80. 2021

Nardone R, Sebastianelli L, Versace V, et al: Involvement of central sensory pathways in subjects with restless legs syndrome: a neurophysiological study. Brain Res 1772:147673, 2021

Trenkwalder C, Allen R, Högl B, et al: Restless legs syndrome associated with major diseases: a systematic review and new concept. Neurology 86(14):1336–1343, 2016

Trenkwalder C, Allen R, Högl B, et al: Comorbidities, treatment, and pathophysiology in restless legs syndrome. Lancet Neurol 217(11):994–1005, 2018

Sarcoidosis

Clinical findings	Sarcoidosis is a multisystem inflammatory disease involving granuloma formation, most commonly in the lungs, liver, skin, and eyes. Nervous system involvement, termed *neurosarcoidosis*, occurs in 3%–10% of affected patients, most of whom also show signs of systemic disease. The most frequently affected sites in the nervous system are the cranial nerves, meninges, brain parenchyma, and spinal cord.
	The risk of developing sarcoidosis is highest among Scandinavians and Black Americans, and the disease most often presents in patients 30–50 years of age. The disease can be time-limited or chronic.
	The presenting symptoms of sarcoidosis are most often pulmonary, usually including cough and dyspnea. Constitutional symptoms include prominent fatigue, fever, night sweats, and weight loss. Liver involvement is identified in up to 80% of cases at autopsy, but the most common clinical presentation is of asymptomatic elevation of liver enzymes. A wide variety of skin lesions are seen, including multiple erythematous macules, papules, plaques, or subcutaneous nodules. Uveitis is the most common symptom of ocular disease. Cardiac involvement in the form of heart failure and ventricular dysrhythmia is an important cause of morbidity and mortality.
	Neurosarcoidosis may involve any of the following signs:
	• Sudden, transient paresis of the seventh cranial nerve (facial droop) or other cranial nerve involvement
	• Papilledema
	• Headache
	• Blindness, visual changes
	• Hearing loss
	• Anosmia
	• Dysgeusia
	• Hydrocephalus
	• Hypothalamic/pituitary-driven endocrine changes (most commonly causing hypogonadism, TSH deficiency, diabetes insipidus, or hyperprolactinemia)
	• Cognitive deficits of variable severity in ~50% of patients (e.g., concentration problems, amnestic syndrome, dementia)
	• Personality change (with frontal lobe features)
	• Depression
	• Psychosis (hallucinations and delusions)
	• Catatonia
	• Delirium
	• Seizures, with generalized tonic-clonic seizures conferring a poorer prognosis than partial seizures
	• Autonomic symptoms including dizziness, orthostasis
	• Limb weakness
	• Small fiber neuropathy with hyperalgesia and allodynia

Sarcoidosis *(continued)*

Clinical findings *(continued)*	The diagnosis of neurosarcoidosis is established by the clinical manifestations and laboratory findings from MRI, CSF, or EMG/NCT that are typical of granulomatous inflammation of the nervous system, and after rigorous exclusion of other causes. Diagnostic certainty increases with pathological confirmation of granulomatous disease outside the nervous system (e.g., skin lesions) and further increases with pathological confirmation of nervous system disease.
Laboratory testing	The neuroimaging test of choice is contrast-enhanced MRI. Multiple nonenhancing white matter hyperintensities on T2-weighted images are the most common MRI findings.
	MRI may show basal meningeal enhancement with lesions in the hypothalamus, pituitary stalk, and adjacent tissues.
	Spinal cord MRI may show "trident sign" on axial images, representing enhancement in the subpial and/or meningeal areas.
	If MRI is not available, contrast-enhanced CT can be used.
	CSF may show lymphocytic pleocytosis with mildly increased protein, decreased glucose, increased IgG index, and oligoclonal bands. Elevated levels of ACE are seen in CSF in about half of patients.
	Elevated levels of serum ACE are seen in two-thirds of patients with acute disease but only in one-fifth of those with chronic disease. Current use of an ACE inhibitor will cause a falsely low level.
	Diagnosis is confirmed by tissue biopsy, usually taken from affected skin, lymph node, or lung tissue.

Bradshaw MJ, Pawate S, Koth LL, et al: Neurosarcoidosis: pathophysiology, diagnosis, and treatment. Neurol Neuroimmunol Neuroinflamm 8(6):e1084, 2021

Epstein S, Xia Z, Lee AJ, et al: Vaccination against SARS-CoV-2 in neuroinflammatory disease: early safety/tolerability data. Mult Scler Relat Disord 57:103433, 2022

Gibbons E, Whittam D, Jacob A, Huda S: Images of the month 1: trident sign and neurosarcoidosis. Clin Med (Lond) 21(6):e667-e668, 2021

Ibitoye RT, Wilkins A, Scolding NJ: Neurosarcoidosis: a clinical approach to diagnosis and management. J Neurol 264(5):1023–1028, 2017

Pandey A, Stoker T, Adamczyk LA, Stacpoole S: Aseptic meningitis and hydrocephalus secondary to neurosarcoidosis. BMJ Case Rep 14(8):e242312, 2021

Perlman DM, Sudheendra MT, Furuya Y, et al: Clinical presentation and treatment of high-risk sarcoidosis. Ann Am Thorac Soc 18(12):1935–1947, 2021

Posada J, Mahan N, Abdel Meguid AS: Catatonia as a presenting symptom of isolated neurosarcoidosis in a woman with schizophrenia. J Acad Consult Liaison Psychiatry 62(5):546–550, 2021

Ramos-Casals M, Pérez-Alvarez R, Kostov B, et al: Clinical characterization and outcomes of 85 patients with neurosarcoidosis. Sci Rep 11(1):13735, 2021

Steriade C, Shumak SL, Feinstein A: A 54-year-old man with hallucinations and hearing loss. CMAJ 186(17):1315–1318, 2014 [published correction appears in CMAJ 187(6):439, 2015]

Stern BJ, Royal W III, Gelfand JM, et al: Definition and consensus diagnostic criteria for neurosarcoidosis: from the Neurosarcoidosis Consortium Consensus Group. JAMA Neurol 75(12):1546–1553, 2018

Ungprasert P, Matteson EL: Neurosarcoidosis. Rheum Dis Clin North Am 43(4):593–606, 2017

Schizophrenia

Clinical findings	Schizophrenia is a highly heterogeneous mental illness with core features including psychosis, cognitive dysfunction, and negative symptoms such as avolition, flattened affect, and anhedonia. The peak age at onset is in the third decade, although onset in childhood and later life does occur. Often, prodromal symptoms precede the active phase of the disease and residual symptoms follow, both of which are characterized by negative symptoms and milder expressions of delusions and hallucinations. The lifetime course of the illness varies, although most individuals go on to have a chronic series of exacerbations and remissions.
	Schizophrenia is diagnosed in its active phase by two or more of the following symptoms, each present for a significant portion of time during a 1-month period (less if treated): delusions, hallucinations, disorganized speech, grossly disorganized or catatonic behavior, or negative symptoms (diminished emotional expression or avolition). At least one symptom must be from the first three listed. Level of functioning in work, interpersonal relations, or self-care is impaired. Continuous signs of the disturbance persist for at least 6 months. The diagnosis is excluded when there is evidence for schizoaffective disorder or mood disorder or when the disturbance is due to a drug or a general medical condition. If there is a history of autistic disorder or another pervasive developmental disorder, the additional diagnosis of schizophrenia is made only if prominent delusions or hallucinations are also present for at least 1 month (less if treated).
	Mood symptoms may be present in schizophrenia but do not dominate the clinical picture. Features associated with the disease include inappropriate affect, dysphoria, disturbed sleep, food refusal, depersonalization, derealization, somatic concerns, anxiety, phobias, abnormal sensory processing, anosognosia, deficits in social cognition, and hostility. Most affected individuals are not prone to aggression or violence. Cognitive deficits include inattention and difficulties with declarative memory, working memory, language functions, executive functions, and processing speed. Neurological soft signs and minor physical anomalies are seen.
	Schizophrenia is not a neurodegenerative disorder, but persistent symptoms can lead to progressive dysfunction in severe cases. A number of biological abnormalities have been described, but none is pathognomonic for the disease. Based on twin and family studies, heritable factors are known to account for 80% of the risk of developing schizophrenia, but hundreds of genes have been implicated, each accounting for only a small part of the risk. In current thinking, complex environmental, physiological, and genetic factors interact to explain disease development.
	Comorbid psychiatric conditions include substance abuse, tobacco use disorder, anxiety disorders, and OCD. Comorbid medical conditions and factors—obesity, diabetes, the metabolic syndrome, cardiovascular and pulmonary disease, poor health maintenance, lack of exercise, and poor diet—are thought to explain the reduced life expectancy of affected patients. Suicide is also a significant risk.

Schizophrenia *(continued)*

Clinical findings *(continued)*	Treatment-resistant disease is defined by failure to respond to two or more adequate antipsychotic trials (involving two or more different drugs, preferably including one long-acting injectable, for up to 4 months). An adequate trial is defined by a dosage equivalence of up to 600 mg/day of chlorpromazine for 6 weeks or longer. So-called ultra treatment resistance is further defined by failure to respond to an adequate clozapine trial (with blood levels drawn) for at least 3 months.
Laboratory testing	For patients presenting with acute psychosis, laboratory investigation directed toward exclusion of potential medical causes or contributors is indicated. Choice of test(s) will be determined by specific symptoms and patient demographics.

Tests to be considered include the following:

- CMP
- CBC with differential and platelets
- TSH
- Syphilis serology
- HIV testing
- ESR or CRP
- Blood alcohol level
- Urine toxicology screen
- Levels of prescribed drugs (e.g., antipsychotic level for a treated patient)
- Urinalysis
- Head CT with contrast or MRI with gadolinium
- EEG
- ECG
- Urine pregnancy testing
- Lumbar puncture for CSF analysis
- Antinuclear antibody test
- Cortisol (blood and 24-hour urine)
- Spot urine for porphyrin precursors
- Heavy metal screening
- Vitamin B_{12} level
- Ceruloplasmin and free serum copper levels
- Antithyroid antibodies
- Serum testosterone level
- MRI with gadolinium (if CT done first)

Patients with schizophrenia treated with antipsychotics will require monitoring laboratory tests ("safety labs") as outlined in the *Psychotropic Medications* chapter. In addition, vigilance in monitoring for tardive dyskinesia (for conventional antipsychotics) and the metabolic syndrome (for atypical antipsychotics) is required. Laboratory tests used to diagnose the metabolic syndrome are covered under that entry. Depending on the patient's exposure history, tuberculosis testing may also be indicated.

Schizophrenia *(continued)*

American Psychiatric Association: Diagnostic and Statistical Manual of Mental Disorders, 5th Edition, Text Revision. Washington, DC, American Psychiatric Association, 2022

Gaebel W, Zielasek J: Schizophrenia in 2020: trends in diagnosis and therapy. Psychiatry Clin Neurosci 69(11):661–673, 2015

Jauhar S, Johnstone M, McKenna PJ: Schizophrenia. Lancet 399(10323):473–486, 2022

Kahn RS, Sommer IE, Murray RM, et al: Schizophrenia. Nat Rev Dis Primers 1:15067, 2015

Marder SR, Cannon TD: Schizophrenia. N Engl J Med 381(18):1753–1761, 2019

McCutcheon RA, Reis Marques T, Howes OD: Schizophrenia: an overview. JAMA Psychiatry 77(2):201–210, 2020

Nucifora FC Jr, Woznica E, Lee BJ, et al: Treatment resistant schizophrenia: clinical, biological, and therapeutic perspectives. Neurobiol Dis 131:104257, 2019

Pardamean E, Roan W, Iskandar KTA, et al: Mortality from coronavirus disease 2019 (COVID-19) in patients with schizophrenia: a systematic review, meta-analysis and meta-regression. Gen Hosp Psychiatry 75:61–67, 2022

Seizures

Clinical findings	Seizures of interest to behavioral health clinicians include partial and generalized epileptic seizures and functional nonepileptic seizures. Single seizures can occur in healthy individuals in response to stressors such as sleep deprivation. Patients with two or more such seizures are considered to have epilepsy. Epileptic seizures can be idiopathic/primary or symptomatic/secondary or due to toxic causes (e.g., clozapine), metabolic causes (e.g., hypoglycemia, hyponatremia), structural lesions (e.g., tumors, strokes), or alcohol/sedative withdrawal. Behavioral health patients at risk of epileptic seizures include those with a family history of epilepsy and those with autism spectrum disorder, cerebral palsy, alcoholism, lead poisoning, TBI, stroke, tumor, Alzheimer's disease, cerebrovascular disease, AIDS, meningitis, encephalitis, and other conditions. Epileptic seizures are classified as partial or generalized.
	Partial (focal) seizures
	Partial seizures are brief, lasting seconds to minutes. In a *simple partial seizure*, the patient is conscious but exhibits or experiences motor, sensory, autonomic, or psychic symptoms. Motor symptoms often appear as tonic or clonic movements in the hands, feet, or head that may "march" to adjacent body areas. Sensory symptoms include hallucinations (tactile, visual, auditory, or gustatory), most of which are simple (buzzing in the ears or seeing plain geometric forms) or unpleasant (smelling burning toast). Psychic symptoms are numerous and varied and include *déjà vu*, *jamais vu*, forced thinking, panic, mood changes, depersonalization, sexual arousal, complex hallucinations (whole scenes), and brief delusions.
	In a *complex partial seizure* (formerly known as psychomotor seizures or temporal lobe epilepsy), the patient experiences a loss or change in consciousness ranging from fogginess to confusion and is amnestic for the events of the seizure. The change in consciousness may be preceded by an aura, which represents a simple partial seizure heralding the complex event. During the seizure, the patient may have repetitive movements or behaviors called automatisms, such as bruxism or fumbling with buttons. More complex behaviors include pelvic thrusting, dancing, disrobing, or even driving a car. When the seizure has terminated, the patient is usually somnolent, confused, and/or dysphoric.
	Status seizure can occur with both simple partial and complex partial seizures. With simple partial status, symptoms can persist for months or years. With complex partial status, symptoms persist for hours to days. Partial seizures usually arise from an anatomical abnormality in the brain, with specific causes dependent on the age of the patient.
	Generalized seizures
	Generalized seizures involve both brain hemispheres from the outset and take one of many forms. The most recognized is that of *tonic-clonic seizures* (formerly known as grand mal seizures), in which there is loss of consciousness along with tonic stiffening of the limbs and neck and repetitive jerking (clonic) movements of the limbs. *Tonic seizures* can occur alone, as can *clonic seizures*. *Atonic seizures* involve abrupt loss of muscle tone, frequently with falls. *Absence seizures* (formerly known as petit mal), which primarily affect children, involve momentary lapses of consciousness. At times, these lapses are accompanied by stereotyped movements such as eyeblinks.

Seizures *(continued)*

Clinical findings *(continued)*	*Functional nonepileptic seizures* DSM-5 includes the functional nonepileptic seizure (FNES) category in conversion disorder (functional neurological symptom disorder), wherein symptoms are noted to be incompatible with known neurological diseases. Features that may help distinguish FNES from epileptic seizure include the following: • Closed eyes during the event, particularly with resistance to eye opening, suggest FNES. Most patients with epileptic seizures have their eyes open. • Out-of-phase shaking movements and side-to-side head shaking suggest FNES. • Wild thrashing and yelling suggest FNES. • Stuttering during the event suggests FNES. • A patient who exhibits movement of all four limbs should not be able to communicate because this would represent diffuse cortical involvement in an epileptic seizure. • A clenched mouth during a tonic spell suggests FNES. In the tonic phase of a generalized epileptic seizure, the mouth is usually open. • A startle response to a sudden loud noise suggests FNES. A patient with a generalized epileptic seizure would not respond to a stimulus during an event. • A postictal period of confusion or somnolence is often seen after a generalized epileptic seizure but may be absent in FNES. • Postictal deep, noisy breathing follows generalized epileptic seizures but not FNES. • Video EEG monitoring during a typical event that does not show epileptiform activity is the gold standard for diagnosis of FNES. The psychological mechanism thought to underlie FNES is that of conversion, in which a physical symptom is substituted for a repressed idea. The patient is not "faking" such symptoms and cannot control them, and the patient's distress is real. Individuals who develop FNES and other conversion disorders are mostly adult females with a history of sexual or physical abuse, and a large proportion have training in health care. Uncommonly, FNES arises in the context of malingering, but this is often obvious because of clear secondary gain.
Laboratory testing	Patients who are undergoing a workup for seizures for the first time require both a structural neuroimaging study (preferably MRI) and an EEG. Those with known epilepsy or a known cause of seizure often undergo only electroencephalography, to monitor the efficacy of anticonvulsant medication. Functional neuroimaging may be used in certain cases. If possible, an EEG should be performed within 24 hours of the first seizure. Ideally, the EEG should capture an ictal event. A sample of the patient's sleep (stage 2) should be obtained along with wakefulness during the EEG session, and standard stimulation procedures should be performed, including hyperventilation and photic stimulation. A complete EEG study will maximize the chance of eliciting ictal (seizure) or epileptiform (interictal) activity.

Seizures *(continued)*

Laboratory testing *(continued)*	In some cases, it may be desirable to have the patient deprived of sleep in preparation for the study because this not only elicits epileptiform activity but also helps ensure that a sample of sleep is obtained. (See **Electroencephalogram** entry in the *Laboratory Tests* chapter for instructions on sleep deprivation.)
	A single EEG is often normal, even in patients with witnessed generalized tonic-clonic seizures before the recording. The longer the interval between seizure and EEG, the more likely the EEG has normalized. In addition, many patients with seizures take some form of medication that dampens seizure activity (e.g., anticonvulsants, mood stabilizers, or benzodiazepines). Epileptiform activity is especially difficult to capture in partial seizures. Anterior temporal electrodes (T1 and T2) and ear electrodes are used to detect temporal lobe discharges; nasopharyngeal electrodes offer no advantage and are uncomfortable for the patient. Where the seizure focus is deep, depth electrodes may be needed.
	A prolactin level that is twice the baseline value or greater can help distinguish generalized tonic-clonic seizures or complex partial seizures from FNES. For this test, the sample should be drawn 10–20 minutes after a suspected ictal event, and a baseline sample should be drawn >6 hours later. Other tests that may be helpful include a neuron-specific enolase level drawn 1–2 days after the event and/or a creatine kinase level drawn 1.5 days after the event.

American Psychiatric Association: Diagnostic and Statistical Manual of Mental Disorders, 5th Edition, Text Revision. Washington, DC, American Psychiatric Association, 2022

Foster E, Carney P, Liew D, et al: First seizure presentations in adults: beyond assessment and treatment. J Neurol Neurosurg Psychiatry 90(9):1039–1045, 2019

Johnson EL: Seizures and epilepsy. Med Clin North Am 103(2):309–324, 2019

Leibetseder A, Eisermann M, LaFrance WC Jr, et al: How to distinguish seizures from non-epileptic manifestations. Epileptic Disord 22(6):716–738, 2020

Perez DL, LaFrance WC Jr: Nonepileptic seizures: an updated review. CNS Spectr 21(3):239–246, 2016

Popkirov S, Asadi-Pooya AA, Duncan R, et al: The aetiology of psychogenic non-epileptic seizures: risk factors and comorbidities. Epileptic Disord 21(6):529–547, 2019

Santos de Lima F, Issa N, Seibert K, et al: Epileptiform activity and seizures in patients with COVID-19. J Neurol Neurosurg Psychiatry 92(5):565–566, 2021

Stroke

Clinical findings	For several reasons, patients with stroke or at risk of stroke come to the attention of behavioral health clinicians. Stroke itself is associated with neuropsychiatric syndromes of depression, anxiety, and apathy. In addition, individuals with serious mental illness may have a greatly increased stroke risk because of the metabolic syndrome, smoking, and other factors. Although early studies found an association between lesion location and post-stroke depression, more recent investigations have called that finding into question. Patients at risk of stroke and TIA include those age 55 years or older and those with diabetes, hypertension, hyperlipidemia, high homocysteine levels, migraine, atrial fibrillation, obesity, and/or cardiovascular disease. Smokers, methamphetamine users, and patients who take oral contraceptives or other hormones are also at risk.
	There are two general types of stroke: ischemic stroke and intracerebral hemorrhage. Ischemic strokes—the most common type—are of two kinds: thrombotic and embolic. *Thrombotic* strokes are the result of a blood clot (thrombus) that usually forms where the vessel is damaged from atherosclerosis. This can occur in the carotid arteries, the vertebral arteries, or any of the intracranial arteries. *Embolic* strokes are the result of a particle traveling from some distant source and lodging in a brain artery. Emboli commonly originate from the heart, particularly in patients with atrial fibrillation, patent foramen ovale, or endocarditis. Intracerebral hemorrhages are usually due to the rupture of small blood vessels in patients with hypertension. Stroke may also occur secondary to subarachnoid hemorrhage, usually due to rupture of an aneurysm.
	Symptoms of acute stroke depend on the vessel affected, the rapidity with which occlusion develops, and the extent of collateral circulation.
	Internal carotid artery occlusion
	With occlusion of the internal carotid artery, if collateral circulation is good, the patient may be asymptomatic. In the absence of good collateral flow, the following signs and symptoms may be seen:
	• Recurrent TIAs as the artery is progressively occluded or as emboli continue to arise from the heart. These prodromal symptoms include amaurosis fugax and transient hemisensory or hemimotor deficit.
	• With complete occlusion, the patient experiences an acute deterioration in consciousness, contralateral motor and sensory deficits, and gaze palsy ("eyes look toward the lesion"). If the occlusion is on the side of the dominant hemisphere, global aphasia occurs.
	Anterior cerebral artery (ACA) occlusion
	With occlusion of the ACA, symptoms depend on the site of occlusion and the anatomy.
	• Occlusion distal to the anterior communicating artery: contralateral leg weakness, contralateral leg sensory loss, urinary incontinence.
	• Occlusion proximal to the anterior communicating artery when both ACAs arise from the same side: bilateral leg weakness, sensory loss, urinary incontinence, and frontal release signs (grasp, snout, palmomental).
	• Bilateral frontal lobe infarction is associated with alteration in consciousness or akinetic mutism.

Stroke *(continued)*

Clinical findings *(continued)*	*Middle cerebral artery (MCA) occlusion*
	With occlusion of the MCA, symptoms depend on the site of the occlusion and whether the dominant hemisphere is involved.
	• Occlusion in the stem of the MCA: contralateral hemiplegia (arm > leg), contralateral hemianopia, contralateral hemianesthesia, aphasia (dominant hemisphere), contralateral neglect and dressing difficulties (nondominant hemisphere).
	• More distal occlusion is associated with more limited motor or sensory symptoms.
	Vertebral artery stroke
	• Vertebral artery occlusion may present as a posterior inferior cerebellar artery syndrome, with cerebellar and brainstem signs: dysarthria, ipsilateral limb ataxia, vertigo, nystagmus, ipsilateral Horner syndrome, ipsilateral pain/temperature loss in the face, ipsilateral pharyngeal and laryngeal paralysis, contralateral pain, and temperature loss in the limbs and trunk.
	• When one vertebral artery is hypoplastic, occlusion of the other may be equivalent to basilar artery stroke, depending on retrograde flow in the posterior communicating arteries.
	• Vertebral artery compression during neck extension may result in symptoms of transient vertebrobasilar insufficiency.
	Basilar artery stroke
	• Prodromal symptoms are common: diplopia, visual loss, vertigo, ataxia, paresis, and paresthesias.
	• With complete occlusion, coma, bilateral motor and sensory signs, cerebellar signs, and cranial nerve signs are seen.
	Posterior cerebral artery stroke
	• With proximal occlusion involving perforating vessels, one may see a midbrain syndrome (third nerve palsy with contralateral hemiplegia, known as Weber syndrome) or a thalamic syndrome (chorea or hemiballismus with hemisensory disturbance).
	• With occlusion of cortical vessels, one may see visual field loss such as homonymous hemianopia with sparing of macular vision.
	• With posterior cortical infarction in the dominant hemisphere, one may see anomia for colors and objects.
	Lacunar strokes
	• Usually associated with hypertension.
	• Cause small subcortical infarctions (0.5–1.5 cm).
	• Distribution: 80% in periventricular white matter and basal ganglia, 20% in cerebellum and brainstem.
	• Classic lacunar syndromes include pure motor stroke, ataxic hemiparesis, dysarthria/clumsy hand syndrome, pure sensory stroke, and sensorimotor stroke.
	• Subcortical dementia due to small vessel disease is a major consequence of recurrent lacunar stroke.
	Transient ischemic attack
	A TIA has the same symptoms as a stroke, but the duration of symptoms is brief—no more than 1 hour. An event lasting longer than this will show positive results on diffusion-weighted imaging.

Stroke *(continued)*

Laboratory testing	For a patient with suspected acute stroke, urgent neuroimaging is required. For ischemic stroke—the most common type—thrombolytic therapy with recombinant tissue plasminogen activator (rTPA) must be administered within 4.5 hours. CT scanning can detect acute blood but may not detect changes of early anterior circulation ischemic stroke or small posterior circulation strokes. MRI can detect acute blood and can detect ischemic strokes missed by CT. Diffusion-weighted MRI detects early infarction and helps distinguish old from acute lesions.
	To determine general stroke risk, the following laboratory tests may be used: blood glucose, lipid profile, serum total homocysteine, high-sensitivity CRP, lipoprotein A, ECG and/or Holter monitoring (to evaluate atrial fibrillation and coronary heart disease), and echocardiogram (to exclude thrombus and valvular vegetations).
	To investigate the patency of cerebral vasculature, the following tests may be used: carotid duplex study (ultrasound and Doppler), angiography, CT angiography, and MR angiography.

Cai W, Mueller C, Li YJ, et al: Post stroke depression and risk of stroke recurrence and mortality: a systematic review and meta-analysis. Ageing Res Rev 50:102–109, 2019

Harciarek M, Mankowska A: Hemispheric stroke: mood disorders. Handb Clin Neurol 183:155–167, 2021

Knight-Greenfield A, Nario JJQ, Gupta A: Causes of acute stroke: a patterned approach. Radiol Clin North Am 57(6):1093–1108, 2019

Lappin JM, Darke S, Farrell M: Stroke and methamphetamine use in young adults: a review. J Neurol Neurosurg Psychiatry 88(12):1079–1091, 2017

Makin SD, Turpin S, Dennis MS, Wardlaw JM: Cognitive impairment after lacunar stroke: systematic review and meta-analysis of incidence, prevalence and comparison with other stroke subtypes. J Neurol Neurosurg Psychiatry 84(8):893–900, 2013

Montaño A, Hanley DF, Hemphill JC III: Hemorrhagic stroke. Handb Clin Neurol 176:229–248, 2021

Ntaios G, Michel P, Georgiopoulos G, et al: Characteristics and outcomes in patients with COVID-19 and acute ischemic stroke: the Global COVID-19 Stroke Registry. Stroke 51(9):e254–e258, 2020

Øie LR, Kurth T, Gulati S, Dodick DW: Migraine and risk of stroke. J Neurol Neurosurg Psychiatry 91(6):593–604, 2020

Robinson RG, Jorge RE: Post-stroke depression: a review. Am J Psychiatry 173(3):221–231, 2016

Swain S, Turner C, Tyrrell P, et al: Diagnosis and initial management of acute stroke and transient ischaemic attack: summary of NICE guidance. BMJ 337:a786, 2008

Yew KS, Cheng E: Acute stroke diagnosis. Am Fam Physician 80:33–40, 2009

Subdural hematoma (SDH)

Clinical findings	Injury to the veins underlying the dura mater—the outermost covering of the brain—causes bleeding into the subdural space, a condition known as subdural hematoma (SDH). This can occur acutely with serious TBI or develop chronically with minor head injury in patients with more fragile vessels. SDH is seen in up to 20% of patients with TBI. In about 95% of cases, the hematomas occur in the frontoparietal regions, and in about 10%–15% the hematomas are bilateral. Aside from TBI, risk factors for SDH include older age, chronic alcohol overuse, long-term anticoagulation or antiplatelet therapy, and prior surgical interventions such as ventricular shunting.
	Presenting signs and symptoms of SDH depend on the extent and rate of bleeding and the location of the hematoma. Acute SDH develops within minutes to hours, usually in the context of moderate to severe TBI involving a rapid increase in intracranial pressure. About one-third of patients experience a lucid interval lasting minutes to hours before the onset of coma. The other two-thirds are stuporous or comatose from the time of TBI. Other common signs include headache on one side, mild dilation of the pupil on the same side, and hemiparesis. This is a medical emergency with a high mortality rate. Subacute development of an SDH occurs over several hours to days after injury. Signs and symptoms include drowsiness, confusion, delirium, headache, and hemiparesis. Other signs of both acute and subacute SDH include behavioral changes, seizures, weakness, nausea, and vomiting. In the event of brain herniation, loss of brainstem reflexes, respiratory arrest, and pulseless cardiac arrest are seen.
	Chronic SDH develops over weeks to years with more indolent signs and symptoms. This condition does not involve a rapid increase in intracranial pressure, but the hematoma can be very large by the time of clinical presentation. Changes in personality, psychomotor slowing, and cognitive impairment suggest the presence of dementia, a particular hazard because elderly patients are the population most affected. Headache can be noted that is sometimes positional. Mild hemiparesis can be seen, and seizures can occur. When chronic SDH is bilateral, symptoms can include fluctuating focal neurological signs that are suggestive of TIAs. Chronic SDH is thought to arise from a mild to moderate TBI in association with chronic inflammation. With the passage of time before presentation, the patient may not recall the brain injury.
	Small hematomas can resolve spontaneously, but large hematomas can further compromise subdural veins, leading to continued bleeding and, in some cases, brain herniation. Chronic hematomas are less likely to resolve on their own, and in these cases, recurrent hemorrhage is an important complication that occurs in up to 20% of patients.
Laboratory testing	• CT can detect acute, subacute, and many chronic SDHs. • MRI is superior for characterizing a chronic SDH. MRI can determine the age of the hematoma and is better at detecting mild changes and imaging brainstem areas. • Other laboratory tests include CBC with red cell indices and platelets, clotting studies, and BMP to check for elevated potassium, which indicates breakdown of red cells in the subdural space.

Subdural hematoma (SDH) *(continued)*

Cousins Z, Forbes M, Coulson B: Chronic subdural haematoma in an elderly patient with a manic episode. Aust NZ J Psychiatry 55(6):632–633, 2021

Mehta V, Harward SC, Sankey EW, et al: Evidence based diagnosis and management of chronic subdural hematoma: a review of the literature. J Clin Neurosci 50:7–15, 2018

Sahyouni R, Goshtasbi K, Mahmoodi A, et al: Chronic subdural hematoma: a historical and clinical perspective. World Neurosurg 108:948–953, 2017

Singh RD, van Dijck JTJM, van Essen TA, et al: Randomized Evaluation of Surgery in Elderly with Traumatic Acute SubDural Hematoma (RESET-ASDH trial): study protocol for a pragmatic randomized controlled trial with multicenter parallel group design. Trials 23(1):242, 2022

Yuh EL, Jain S, Sun X, et al: Pathological computed tomography features associated with adverse outcomes after mild traumatic brain injury: a TRACK-TBI study with external validation in CENTER-TBI. JAMA Neurol 78(9):1137–1148, 2021

Syndrome of inappropriate antidiuresis (SIAD)

Clinical findings	The syndrome of inappropriate antidiuresis (SIAD or SIADH) is a condition in which antidiuretic hormone (ADH) is produced in excess of physiological needs. Water is retained and concentrated solutes are excreted, resulting in dilute blood with low osmolality and hyponatremia and concentrated urine with high osmolality and high urine sodium, all in the context of clinical euvolemia. A diagram of this process appears in Appendix E. Although the hyponatremia of SIAD can reach extreme levels, it often develops gradually over days to weeks, so symptoms are mild or absent. This is not the case, however, when severe hyponatremia develops rapidly, over 48 hours or less; this syndrome can be fatal.
	The risk of developing SIAD increases with age and is particularly high among nursing home residents. Medical risk factors generally fall into four categories: cancer, pulmonary disease, CNS disease, or medications/drugs.
	• *Cancer*—lung (especially small cell carcinoma), oropharynx, GI tract, genitourinary tract; lymphomas, sarcoma
	• *Pulmonary disease*—infection (including COVID-19, viral and bacterial pneumonia, abscess, tuberculosis), chronic obstructive pulmonary disease, asthma, cystic fibrosis, sarcoidosis, acute respiratory failure
	• *CNS disease*—infection (meningitis, encephalitis, abscess, Rocky Mountain spotted fever, AIDS), stroke, TBI, epilepsy, brain tumor, hydrocephalus, subdural hematoma, subarachnoid hemorrhage, cavernous sinus thrombosis, delirium tremens, acute intermittent porphyria, multiple sclerosis, lupus cerebritis, Guillain-Barré syndrome, Shy-Drager syndrome
	• *Medications/Drugs*—antidepressants (SSRIs, SNRIs, TCAs), antipsychotics (first- and second-generation), anticonvulsants (carbamazepine, valproate, lamotrigine, phenytoin, phenobarbital), analgesics (tramadol, opioids, pregabalin), NSAIDs, nicotine, 3,4-methylenedioxymethamphetamine (MDMA, Ecstasy), and cytotoxic and other drugs
	Rapid development of severe hyponatremia (<125 mEq/L) in SIAD may be associated with the following severe signs and symptoms:
	• Confusion
	• Hallucinations
	• Delirium
	• Seizures
	• Coma
	• Decerebrate posture
	• Respiratory arrest
	This syndrome can be fatal.
	Milder sodium reductions may be associated with the following:
	• Headache
	• Difficulty concentrating
	• Memory impairment
	• Weakness

Syndrome of inappropriate antidiuresis (SIAD) *(continued)*

Clinical findings *(continued)*	• Muscle cramps • Dysgeusia Chronic hyponatremia may be asymptomatic, although affected patients may have subtle neurological deficits that lead to falls.
Laboratory testing	Specific laboratory testing includes serum and urine osmolality, serum and urine sodium, and BUN. SIAD is diagnosed when the following criteria are met: • Decreased effective osmolality (<275 mOsm/kg); effective osmolality=[measured osmolality−the value of BUN]/2.8, where BUN is measured in mg/dL • Urine osmolality >100 mOsm/kg • Clinical euvolemia (absence of orthostasis, tachycardia, decreased skin turgor, dry mucous membranes, edema, and ascites) • Urinary sodium >40 mEq/L with normal dietary salt intake • Normal thyroid and adrenal function • No recent use of diuretics Hyponatremia is not included in the diagnostic criteria, although symptoms do not appear unless sodium is low, and sodium level is usually <130 mEq/L.

Ellison DH, Berl T: Clinical practice: the syndrome of inappropriate antidiuresis. N Engl J Med 356:2064–2072, 2007

Peri A, Grohé C, Berardi R, Runkle I: SIADH: differential diagnosis and clinical management. Endocrine 55(1):311–319, 2017

Pinkhasov A, Xiong G, Bourgeois JA, et al: Management of SIADH-related hyponatremia due to psychotropic medications: an expert consensus from the Association of Medicine and Psychiatry. J Psychosom Res 151:110654, 2021

Salathe C, Blanc AL, Tagan D: SIADH and water intoxication related to ecstasy. BMJ Case Rep 2018:bcr2018224731, 2018

Shepshelovich D, Schechter A, Calvarysky B, et al: Medication-induced SIADH: distribution and characterization according to medication class. Br J Clin Pharmacol 83(8):1801–1807, 2017

Yousaf Z, Al-Shokri SD, Al-Soub H, Mohamed MFH: COVID-19-associated SIADH: a clue in the times of pandemic! Am J Physiol Endocrinol Metab 318(6):E882–E885, 2020

Syphilis

Clinical findings	Syphilis is a sexually transmitted disease caused by the organism *Treponema pallidum*, known for its invasiveness and ability to evade the immune system. It is emerging again as a public health problem globally, particularly among men who have sex with men, and is especially pathogenic in patients co-infected with HIV. The presence of syphilis increases the risk of HIV transmission and acquisition. CNS involvement can occur at any stage of the disease, with neuropsychiatric symptoms predominating. Syphilis can also be transmitted vertically, from mother to fetus.
	Primary syphilis, the first stage of the disease, begins within weeks to months of infection. At this time, a painless sore (chancre) is seen at the site of inoculation (e.g., penis, vagina, anus, rectum, mouth). The sore may go unnoticed, and it resolves after 4–6 weeks. In the stage of secondary syphilis, a macular skin rash is seen, often involving the palms and the soles of the feet. In addition, mucocutaneous lesions such as condylomata lata, diffuse lymphadenopathy, fever, and sore throat may occur. Even untreated, most infected patients will ultimately enter a latent stage in which they are asymptomatic. In the first 1–2 years of latency, they are still considered infectious because of a 25% risk of secondary syphilis-like relapses. Eventually, 15%–40% of untreated patients will subsequently develop tertiary syphilis, which can involve the heart, eyes, brain, spinal cord, bones, or skin.
	Neuropsychiatric manifestations of syphilis include the following syndromes:
	• *Meningovascular syphilis:* Symptoms appear within the first decade after infection. Meningitis can affect cranial nerves, resulting in symptoms such as ophthalmoplegia, diplopia, facial paralysis, and the Argyll Robertson pupil (which is reactive to accommodation but not to direct light and is a consequence of midbrain infection). Obstructive hydrocephalus may develop. Endarteritis can involve large vessels, resulting in stroke with lateralizing signs, or small vessels, resulting in slowly progressive dementia. Myelopathy is seen.
	• *Gummas:* These masses are of varying size and resemble tuberculomas seen in tuberculosis. They can occur in conjunction with meningovascular disease, also within the first decade. These space-occupying lesions can be associated with seizures.
	• *General paresis:* This is a late manifestation of syphilis that appears 10–20 years after infection. It most often presents as a dementia with prominent frontal lobe features, including change in personality, self-neglect, lack of judgment, disinhibition, inattention, amnesia, shifting delusions, and auditory or visual hallucinations. The Argyll Robertson pupil is invariably present. Alternative presentations include manic and depressive or melancholic syndromes with prominent delusional features and loss of insight and judgment. As general paresis progresses, severe amnesia develops, with confabulation in many cases. Speech and language are affected, facial muscles become flaccid, coarse tremor develops, gait becomes unsteady, mood becomes labile, and eventually, the patient is too weak (paretic) to get out of bed. Death often ensues within 2–3 years. It should be noted that atypical or *formes frustes* of this presentation occur in current clinical practice, in large part because of prior treatment with antibiotics.

Syphilis *(continued)*

Clinical findings *(continued)*	• *Tabes dorsalis:* This occurs 10–30 years after infection and involves demyelination of the posterior columns, dorsal roots, and dorsal root ganglia, with manifestations of weakness, ataxia with wide-based gait, diminished reflexes, urinary incontinence, and paresthesias. Intense paroxysmal pains (lightning pains and visceral crises) can occur. With late neurological involvement, trophic degeneration of joints can be seen (Charcot joints). In addition, the Argyll Robertson pupil is often seen in association with tabes dorsalis.
Laboratory testing	Laboratory testing is used to screen for disease in particular populations and to confirm disease in those with a positive screening test.
	For syphilis screening, the RPR test is used, with titers drawn if reactive. A VDRL test can be used as an alternative screen, with titers drawn if positive. The RPR is preferred because the VDRL test has a higher rate of false-positive results.
	If either of these tests is positive, treponemal testing is performed, using one of the following:
	• FTA-ABS
	• Microhemagglutination assay for antibodies to *T. pallidum*
	• IgM antibody detection by enzyme-linked immunosorbent assay (ELISA)
	If these tests are reactive, then syphilis is likely, and the disease should be staged and treated.
	For suspected cases of *neurosyphilis*, one of two approaches can be used:
	• RPR is performed on serum, and VDRL is performed on CSF.* If the serum RPR is negative but there remains a suspicion for neurosyphilis, FTA-ABS is performed on serum, because some patients with late syphilis have false-negative RPR tests. In HIV patients, the affected site is usually the CNS.
	• If the patient has dementia, FTA-ABS is performed on serum. If this test is negative, neurosyphilis is ruled out. If positive, VDRL is performed on CSF, and if that test is also positive, neurosyphilis is confirmed. If the VDRL is negative but suspicion remains high because of other CSF findings and clinical symptoms, FTA-ABS can be performed on CSF, although this is controversial due to the probability of false-positive results from blood contamination of the CSF sample.
	All patients with syphilis should undergo HIV testing (and vice versa).
	Routine CSF testing for syphilis in persons with dementia is indicated if there is a risk of syphilis.
	The organism *T. pallidum* cannot be cultured in vitro. If a skin lesion is present, a scraping from the lesion may be examined by darkfield microscopy to identify the bacterium.
	Contrast-enhanced MRI or CT can show meningitis, areas of infarction, gummas, and generalized atrophy in the case of general paresis.

*CSF studies also include protein, glucose, cell count and differential, antibodies, and oligoclonal bands. In neurosyphilis, CSF shows a mild lymphocytic pleocytosis and elevated protein (50–150 mg/dL). IgG index may be increased, and oligoclonal bands may be present.

Syphilis *(continued)*

Boog GHP, Lopes JVZ, Mahler JV, et al: Diagnostic tools for neurosyphilis: a systematic review. BMC Infect Dis 21(1):568, 2021

Clyne B, Jerrard DA: Syphilis testing. J Emerg Med 18:361–367, 2000

Gonzalez H, Koralnik IJ, Marra CM: Neurosyphilis. Semin Neurol 39(4):448–455, 2019

Hobbs E, Vera JH, Marks M, et al: Neurosyphilis in patients with HIV. Pract Neurol 18(3):211–218, 2018

Jeon C, Gough K: Neurosyphilis presenting as hypomania. CMAJ 193(30):E1177, 2021

Jum'ah A, Aboul Nour H, Alkhoujah M, et al: Neurosyphilis in disguise. Neuroradiology 64(3):433–441, 2022

Krishnan D, Zaini SS, Latif KA, Joseph JP: Neurosyphilis presenting as acute ischemic stroke. Clin Med (Lond) 20(1):95–97, 2020

Ropper AH: Neurosyphilis. N Engl J Med 381(14):1358–1363, 2019 [published correction appears in N Engl J Med 381(18):1789, 2019]

Satyaputra F, Hendry S, Braddick M, et al: The laboratory diagnosis of syphilis. J Clin Microbiol 59(10):e0010021, 2021

Young H: Guidelines for serological testing for syphilis. Sex Transm Infect 76:403–405, 2000

Systemic lupus erythematosus (SLE)

Clinical findings	SLE is an autoimmune disease with multisystem inflammatory involvement and organ damage. It is much more common in females than males and affects Blacks and other minority groups more than Whites. Both environmental and genetic factors contribute to disease expression. Despite familial segregation and high concordance in identical twins, however, no pattern of inheritance is known, and most affected patients have no family history of the disease. Epidemiological evidence exists for links to cigarette smoking, oral contraceptives, hormone therapy, endometriosis, and crystalline silica exposure. Although SLE can develop at any age and in either sex, it most commonly affects persons of childbearing age. Onset varies from acute to insidious.
	Systemic manifestations of SLE include the following:
	• Fever
	• Weight loss
	• Fatigue
	• Rash (malar "butterfly" rash or discoid rash)
	• Oral ulcers
	• Arthritis and/or arthralgia
	• Pleuritis (pleurisy)
	• Pericarditis
	• Nephritis
	• Anemia, leukopenia, or thrombocytopenia in the absence of offending drugs
	• Transverse myelitis
	• Optic neuritis
	• Cranial and peripheral neuropathies
	In addition, SLE is associated with antiphospholipid syndrome in up to 40% of cases.
	Neuropsychiatric manifestations are seen in most patients with SLE, with signs and symptoms including the following:
	• Intractable headaches in more than half of cases
	• Psychosis
	• Mood changes (depression or hypomania)
	• Anxiety
	• Delirium
	• Cognitive dysfunction including dementia
	• Seizures (mostly generalized tonic-clonic, but can be focal)
	• Ischemic stroke
	• Aseptic meningitis
	• Focal neurological deficits
	• Cerebellar symptoms
	• Abnormal movements (chorea, dystonia, hemiballismus)
	Drug-induced lupus is generally not associated with CNS manifestations. It is a less severe condition that resolves when the implicated drugs are stopped.

Systemic lupus erythematosus (SLE) *(continued)*

Clinical findings *(continued)*	Classification criteria have been developed that can help standardize SLE diagnosis. The criteria list 24 weighted items in 10 domains that should be useful in most cases despite the heterogeneity of presentations. Those criteria are included in the Aringer et al. (2019) publication in the reference list below.
Laboratory testing	Diagnosis requires the presence of antinuclear antibodies (ANAs) at a titer of ≥1:80 on HEp-2 cells or an equivalent positive test at some time during the illness. A negative ANA test makes SLE unlikely, although the test may need to be repeated because of the episodic nature of the disease.
	Positive ANA testing should be followed by IgG titers to double-stranded DNA antigen (anti-dsDNA) and/or to the Smith antigen (anti-Sm), which are more specific for SLE.
	Complement proteins C3 and/or C4 may be low.
	Antiphospholipid antibodies (anticardiolipin, anti-β2GP1, or lupus anticoagulant) may be present and may help identify those at risk of thromboembolism. Individuals of childbearing potential with SLE should be screened for antiphospholipid antibodies and anti-Ro antibodies (the latter because of increased risk of neonatal lupus).
	Lupus nephritis is detected by urinalysis, with proteinuria >0.5 g/day (≥3) or diagnosed by renal biopsy.
	Hematological abnormalities in SLE include hemolytic anemia, leukopenia (<4,000 cells/μL), lymphopenia (<1,500/μL) or thrombocytopenia (<100,000/μL).
	In patients with psychosis or depression, the serum antiribosomal P antibody may be elevated.
	A high ANA titer in combination with antihistone antibodies is consistent with drug-induced lupus.
	Serum VDRL results may be falsely positive in SLE.
	CSF may be normal or may show increased protein. The IgG index may be elevated, and oligoclonal bands and antineuronal antibodies may be seen.
	MRI may be normal or may show T2 hyperintensities corresponding to small- or large-vessel disease, particularly in cases with focal neurological findings.

Aringer M: Inflammatory markers in systemic lupus erythematosus. J Autoimmun 110:102374, 2020

Aringer M, Costenbader K, Daikh D, et al: 2019 European League Against Rheumatism/American College of Rheumatology classification criteria for systemic lupus erythematosus. Arthritis Rheumatol 71(9):1400–1412, 2019

Barbhaiya M, Costenbader KH: Environmental exposures and the development of systemic lupus erythematosus. Curr Opin Rheumatol 28(5):497–505, 2016

Dörner T, Furie R: Novel paradigms in systemic lupus erythematosus. Lancet 393(10188):2344–2358, 2019

Grasso EA, Cacciatore M, Gentile C, et al: Epilepsy in systemic lupus erythematosus. Clin Exp Rheumatol 39(3):651–659, 2021

Kiriakidou M, Ching CL: Systemic lupus erythematosus. Ann Intern Med 172(11):ITC81–ITC96, 2020

Shaban A, Leira EC: Neurological complications in patients with systemic lupus erythematosus. Curr Neurol Neurosci Rep 19(12):97, 2019

Wekking EM: Psychiatric symptoms in systemic lupus erythematosus: an update. Psychosom Med 55:219–228, 1993

Zhang L, Fu T, Yin R, et al: Prevalence of depression and anxiety in systemic lupus erythematosus: a systematic review and meta-analysis. BMC Psychiatry 17(1):70, 2017

Thiamine deficiency

Clinical findings	Thiamine (vitamin B_1) is a water-soluble vitamin and an essential micronutrient involved in the metabolism of carbohydrates to produce energy. Good dietary sources of thiamine include whole grains, cereals, seeds, yeasts, nuts, legumes, eggs, fish, poultry, and pork. Diets that are restricted to white flour, white sugar, and other highly processed carbohydrates can cause thiamine deficiency, as can foods that cause thiamine breakdown such as tea, coffee, raw fish, and shellfish. Only small amounts of thiamine are stored in the liver, so regular intake is required. As little as 1 week without thiamine is associated with tachycardia, weakness, and hyporeflexia, even in healthy individuals.
	Deficiency manifests as one or more of the following syndromes:
	• *Wet beriberi*—a cardiovascular syndrome with high-output heart failure
	• *Dry beriberi*—a neurological syndrome with symmetrical peripheral neuropathy
	• *Wernicke's encephalopathy (WE)*—a triad of ocular abnormalities, cerebellar ataxia, and altered mental status
	• *Wernicke-Korsakoff syndrome*—memory impairment with confabulation that develops in patients untreated for Wernicke's encephalopathy
	Thiamine treatment is very effective in reversing the symptoms of wet beriberi, which can begin to improve within 24 hours. Symptoms of dry beriberi are slower to resolve. Symptoms of WE improve more gradually and are generally resolved within 1 month. Once Korsakoff pathology develops, however, minimal improvement is seen. Because 80% of patients who are untreated for WE go on to develop Korsakoff's syndrome, clinical recognition of WE is critical. A high index of suspicion must be maintained for patients at risk, even when the complete triad of clinical signs is not present. Beyond the syndromes noted above, thiamine deficiency has other neurological effects. For example, Marchiafava-Bignami disease is at least partly due to this deficiency. There is evidence as well that this deficiency might be a factor in the pathogenesis of Alzheimer's disease.
	Thiamine deficiency can arise because of poor intake, poor absorption, increased loss, or increased physiological requirement or from genetic factors. In the United States and other developed countries, chronic alcohol overuse is the most common risk factor. Other risk factors include older age, eating disorders, prolonged fasting, gastric bypass surgery, malabsorption, AIDS, GI malignancy, chronic vomiting, chronic diarrhea, diuretic use, dialysis, hyperthyroidism, pregnancy, lactation, and use of drugs such as diuretics, antacids, anticonvulsants, contraceptives, antineoplastics, and others.
	The signs and symptoms of thiamine deficiency syndromes are as follows:
	• *Wet beriberi*—an overuse syndrome representing a medical emergency that without treatment can be fatal within days. Most patients require ICU support. High-output heart failure is associated with tachycardia, exertional dyspnea, orthopnea, peripheral edema, and ECG abnormalities.

Thiamine deficiency *(continued)*

Clinical findings *(continued)*	• *Dry beriberi*—mild to moderate long-term thiamine deficiency induces a peripheral neuropathy that manifests as acute or subacute onset of paresthesias, dysesthesias, and mild lower-extremity weakness; signs include stocking-glove sensory loss, distal leg and foot weakness, and absent ankle jerks. Neuropathy is worse distally than proximally and involves myelin more than axons. Other signs and symptoms include nonspecific mental status changes such as apathy, low energy, fatigue, slowness, memory and other cognitive impairments, and disturbance of consciousness ranging from inattention to coma. *Confusion* is the term most often applied, although some patients also exhibit hallucinations, delusions, and behavioral disturbances, suggesting the presence of delirium.
	• *WE*—severe acute thiamine deficiency syndrome characterized by the classic triad of triad of ocular abnormalities, cerebellar ataxia, and altered mental status (identified in only 20% of cases). First symptoms often include nausea and vomiting, followed by horizontal nystagmus and ocular nerve palsy, fever, ataxia, and progressive cognitive dysfunction.
	• *Korsakoff's syndrome*—usually develops after repeated episodes of WE. Prominent global amnesia that in severe cases may involve confabulation, apathy, mood disorders, perceptual disorders, and cognitive impairment in other domains.
Laboratory testing	Thiamine reference range: 70–180 nmol/L
	In adults, thiamine pyrophosphate levels<70 nmol/L in whole blood are consistent with deficiency.
	MRI findings in WE include symmetric changes in the thalamus, mamillary bodies, periaqueductal area, and tectal plate (superior and inferior colliculi).

Dhir S, Tarasenko M, Napoli E, Giulivi C: Neurological, psychiatric, and biochemical aspects of thiamine deficiency in children and adults. Front Psychiatry 10:207, 2019

DiNicolantonio JJ, Liu J, O'Keefe JH: Thiamine and cardiovascular disease: a literature review. Prog Cardiovasc Dis 61(1):27–32, 2018

Gibson GE, Hirsch JA, Fonzetti P, et al: Vitamin B$_1$ (thiamine) and dementia. Ann NY Acad Sci 1367(1):21–30, 2016

Gomes F, Bergeron G, Bourassa MW, Fischer PR: Thiamine deficiency unrelated to alcohol consumption in high-income countries: a literature review. Ann NY Acad Sci 1498(1):46–56, 2021

Mulholland PJ: Susceptibility of the cerebellum to thiamine deficiency. Cerebellum 5:55–63, 2006

O'Keeffe ST: Thiamine deficiency in elderly people. Age Ageing 29:99–101, 2000

Pacei F, Tesone A, Laudi N, et al: The relevance of thiamine evaluation in a practical setting. Nutrients 12(9):2810, 2020

Rao SN, Chandak GR: Cardiac beriberi: often a missed diagnosis. J Trop Pediatr 56:284–285, 2010

Sechi G, Serra A: Wernicke's encephalopathy: new clinical settings and recent advances in diagnosis and management. Lancet Neurol 6:442–455, 2007

Sinha S, Kataria A, Kolla BP, et al: Wernicke encephalopathy: clinical pearls. Mayo Clin Proc 94(6):1065–1072, 2019

Smith TJ, Johnson CR, Koshy R, et al: Thiamine deficiency disorders: a clinical perspective. Ann NY Acad Sci 1498(1):9–28, 2021

Thrombocytopenia

Clinical findings	*Platelets* are small disc-shaped cell fragments produced in the bone marrow that circulate in the blood to help stop bleeding and assist with wound healing. These fragments also have a role in inflammation, immunity, and cancer biology. A normal platelet count in the blood is ~150 to 450×10^9 cells/L. Some individuals maintain a lower count in the range of 100 to 150×10^9 cells/L without developing disease, but any value below the lower limit of normal requires investigation. Causes of low platelet count—thrombocytopenia—include decreased production, increased destruction, sequestration in the spleen, and dilution, which can result from fluid overload.
	Patients at risk of true thrombocytopenia include those with alcohol use disorder, cirrhosis, folate or vitamin B_{12} deficiency, autoimmune disease (e.g., SLE), disseminated intravascular coagulation, hypersplenism, aplastic anemia, myelodysplasia, and cancer or infection involving the bone marrow. Pregnancy and the use of certain drugs are also associated with this condition. Alcohol can cause myelotoxicity (suppression of bone marrow) without apparent toxicity to other organs. Thrombocytopenia can be seen in up to 43% of patients with alcohol use disorder in the community and up to 81% of those hospitalized. Drugs associated with thrombocytopenia include heparin, antidepressants, antipsychotics, anticonvulsants, prescribed stimulants, acetylcholinesterase inhibitors, commonly used analgesics (e.g., acetaminophen, aspirin, codeine, ibuprofen), β-blockers, and certain herbal medicines.
	Signs and symptoms of thrombocytopenia include bruising, ecchymoses, spontaneous nosebleeds, gum bleeding, petechiae (usually prominent in the lower legs), blood in the stool or urine, heavy menstrual bleeding, and prolonged bleeding after surgery or trauma. Mucocutaneous bleeding occurs when the platelet count is $<20 \times 10^9$ cells/L and intracranial hemorrhage occurs when the count is $<10 \times 10^9$ cells/L.
Laboratory testing	Platelet count and examination of a peripheral blood smear are the cornerstones of initial diagnosis.
	Normal platelet count is $150–450 \times 10^9$ cells/L.
	Low platelet count in a patient receiving heparin is an indication for urgent hematology consultation.
	If platelet count is $<30 \times 10^9$/L, confirm immediately by repeat testing, stop all antiplatelet drugs, and refer urgently to hematology.
	Platelets are replaced if the count is $<20 \times 10^9$/L or in certain cases of bleeding.
	One unit of platelets raises the count by 15×10^9/L.
	If alcohol or an implicated drug is stopped, platelet count recovers in 5–7 days.

Bakchoul T, Marini I: Drug-associated thrombocytopenia. Hematology Am Soc Hematol Educ Program 2018(1):576–583, 2018

Beckert BW, Concannon MJ, Henry SL, et al: The effect of herbal medicines on platelet function: an in vivo experiment and review of the literature. Plast Reconstr Surg 120:2044–2050, 2007

Kam T, Alexander M: Drug-induced immune thrombocytopenia. J Pharm Pract 27(5):430–439, 2014

Lee EJ, Lee AI: Thrombocytopenia. Prim Care 43(4):543–557, 2016

Murt A, Eskazan AE, Yılmaz U, et al: COVID-19 presenting with immune thrombocytopenia: a case report and review of the literature. J Med Virol 93(1):43–45, 2021

Smock KJ, Perkins SL: Thrombocytopenia: an update. Int J Lab Hematol 36(3):269–278, 2014

Swain F, Bird R: How I approach new onset thrombocytopenia. Platelets 31(3):285–290, 2020

Thrombocytosis

Clinical findings	*Platelets* are small disc-shaped cell fragments produced in the bone marrow that circulate in the blood to help stop bleeding and assist with wound healing. These fragments also have a role in inflammation, immunity, and cancer biology. A normal platelet count in the blood is ~150 to 450×10^9 cells/L.
	Most cases of elevated platelet count—thrombocytosis—are a reaction to underlying disease. Patients at risk of this type of reactive thrombocytosis include those with infection, inflammation, trauma, malignancy, iron deficiency, past splenectomy, pancreatitis, or renal failure and those who have been treated with drugs known to increase platelet count (e.g., amoxapine, clozapine, danazol, donepezil, steroids, immune globulin, lithium, megestrol, metoprolol, paroxetine, propranolol, venlafaxine, and zidovudine). In general, reactive thrombocytosis is not associated with thrombosis or hemorrhage, but it can provide a clue to a serious underlying disease. In the case of reactive thrombocytosis from acute disease, the platelet count usually normalizes when the disease resolves.
	The second most common cause of thrombocytosis is clonal, referring to myeloproliferative neoplasms such as essential thrombocythemia, polycythemia vera, primary myelofibrosis, chronic myeloid leukemia, and other primary marrow disorders. These cases can be complicated by thrombosis and bleeding events.
Laboratory testing	Platelet count $<450 \times 10^3$/mm^3—no action required.
	Platelet count $\geq 450 \times 10^3$/mm^3—refer to hematology.
	Platelet count $>1{,}000 \times 10^3$/mm^3—refer for urgent hematological consultation.
	Workup for platelet counts above the upper limit of normal comprises three initial tests:
	• Examination of peripheral blood smear—to exclude spurious results and examine other cells to aid differential diagnosis of both reactive and clonal thrombocytosis.
	• Acute-phase reactants—elevation in CRP or ESR supports the diagnosis of reactive thrombocytosis.
	• Iron studies—to identify iron deficiency anemia, a common condition in adults.
	When thrombocytosis is noted as an incidental finding, <10% of patients will demonstrate thrombocytosis on repeat testing 8 months later.

Appleby N, Angelov D: Clinical and laboratory assessment of a patient with thrombocytosis. Br J Hosp Med (Lond) 78(10):558–564, 2017

Mathur A, Samaranayake S, Storrar NP, Vickers MA: Investigating thrombocytosis. BMJ 366:l4183, 2019 [published correction appears in BMJ 367:l4569, 2019]

Schafer AI: Thrombocytosis. JAMA 314(11):1171–1172, 2015

Vo QT, Thompson DF: A review and assessment of drug-induced thrombocytosis. Ann Pharmacother 53(5):523–536, 2019

Thyrotoxicosis

Clinical findings	*Hyperthyroidism* refers to the excessive production and secretion of hormones from the thyroid gland that give rise to a hypermetabolic state known as thyrotoxicosis. These two terms are not interchangeable; hyperthyroidism is a process, whereas thyrotoxicosis is a clinical syndrome. In fact, thyrotoxicosis can develop due to external factors such as excessive intake of levothyroxine, not implicating the thyroid gland at all. The most common cause of hyperthyroidism leading to thyrotoxicosis is Graves' disease, an autoimmune disorder with often florid symptoms due to very high thyroid hormone levels (and very low or undetectable TSH levels). Other causes include toxic multinodular goiter, toxic adenoma, gestational trophoblastic disease, and thyroiditis, among others.
	Physical signs and symptoms of thyrotoxicosis include tachycardia, systolic hypertension with widened pulse pressure, palpitations, weight loss despite increased appetite and eating, widened palpebral fissures ("bug eyes"), lid lag, stare, eye irritation, heat intolerance, increased sweating, fine distal hand tremors, chorea, hyperactive deep tendon reflexes, weakness, diarrhea or increased frequency of bowel movements, alopecia, menstrual irregularity in females, and erectile dysfunction in males.
	Psychiatric signs and symptoms include depression, anxiety, mania/ hypomania, psychosis, delirium, irritability, restlessness, agitation, emotional lability, insomnia, and fatigue.
	The presentation of thyrotoxicosis is variable, with younger patients tending to have more symptoms of sympathetic activation and older patients more cardiovascular symptoms such as dyspnea and atrial fibrillation. Graves' disease is distinguished by the presence of ophthalmopathy (periorbital edema, proptosis, and diplopia) and pretibial myxedema.
	The syndrome of apathetic hyperthyroidism affects primarily geriatric patients and includes symptoms of lethargy, tachycardia, atrial fibrillation, heart failure, and cognitive impairment severe enough to warrant a diagnosis of dementia.
	Thyroid storm involves the hyperacute development of symptoms in a patient with untreated hyperthyroidism who becomes medically ill or undergoes surgery. Severe symptoms are seen, along with fever and delirium. If left untreated, the syndrome is almost always fatal.
	Thyrotoxicosis can lead to serious complications when not diagnosed and treated appropriately, including impaired renal function, osteoporosis, atrial fibrillation, congestive heart failure, thromboembolic disease, and cardiovascular collapse. Psychiatric symptoms may be persistent, even after successful treatment.
Laboratory testing	Laboratory workup for suspected hyperthyroidism is as follows:
	• Check TSH level. This is a very sensitive test because small changes in free T4 (FT4) result in large changes in TSH values.
	• If TSH level is low or if clinical suspicion is high despite normal TSH, check FT4.
	• If TSH is low and FT4 is high, patient has hyperthyroidism.

Thyrotoxicosis *(continued)*

Laboratory testing *(continued)*	Thyroid antibodies—TPO, TSH receptor antibody (TRAb), and thyroid-stimulating immunoglobulin (TSI)—help distinguish Graves' disease from other common causes of hyperthyroidism:
	• Graves' disease—significantly elevated TPO, elevated TSI
	• Toxic multinodular goiter, toxic adenoma, and subacute thyroiditis—low or absent TPO and negative TSI
	Further evaluation involves scintigraphy using iodine-123 or technetium-99m to scan the thyroid, looking for diffuse versus nodular uptake.
	An ECG is recommended for any patient with a heart rate >100 beats per minute or evidence of heart failure.
	For elderly patients, further cardiac evaluation may be needed, including an echocardiogram, Holter monitoring, or myocardial perfusion study.

American Psychiatric Association: Diagnostic and Statistical Manual of Mental Disorders, 5th Edition, Text Revision. Washington, DC, American Psychiatric Association, 2022

Bennett B, Mansingh A, Fenton C, Katz J: Graves' disease presenting with hypomania and paranoia to the acute psychiatry service. BMJ Case Rep 14(2):e236089, 2021

Bunevicius R, Prange AJ Jr: Psychiatric manifestations of Graves' hyperthyroidism: pathophysiology and treatment options. CNS Drugs 20(11):897–909, 2006

Hu LY, Shen CC, Hu YW, et al: Hyperthyroidism and risk for bipolar disorders: a nationwide population-based study. PLoS One 8(8):e73057, 2013

Iglesias P, Devora O, Garcia J, et al: Severe hyperthyroidism: aetiology, clinical features and treatment outcome. Clin Endocrinol (Oxf) 72:551–557, 2010

Jadresic DP: Psychiatric aspects of hyperthyroidism. J Psychosom Res 34(6):603–615, 1990

Ross DS, Burch HB, Cooper DS, et al: 2016 American Thyroid Association guidelines for diagnosis and management of hyperthyroidism and other causes of thyrotoxicosis. Thyroid 26(10):1343–1421, 2016 [published correction appears in Thyroid 27(11):1462, 2017]

Sönmez E, Bulur O, Ertugrul DT, et al: Hyperthyroidism influences renal function. Endocrine 65(1):144–148, 2019

Tuberculosis (TB)

Clinical findings	TB is a communicable disease resulting from infection with *Mycobacterium tuberculosis*, usually transmitted by cough aerosol and characterized by necrotizing granulomatous inflammation in the lung and other tissues, including the brain and meninges. Two types of infection are recognized: latent infection and active disease. Latent infection, which is known to affect one-quarter of the world's population, involves a persistent immune response to *M. tuberculosis* antigens in the absence of symptoms. Most individuals with latent infection never develop active disease, but the risk of progression depends on their degree of immunocompetence and the time since initial infection. Moreover, recent evidence suggests that new TB disease even in low-incidence settings is, in many cases, due to recent transmission rather than reactivation.
	In low-incidence countries such as the United States, individuals at risk of TB exposure include residents of correctional facilities, chronic mental health facilities, and nursing homes. At even higher risk are those who are homeless and those with alcoholism, IV drug abuse, HIV/AIDS, or chronic liver or kidney disease.
	Patients with active pulmonary TB exhibit cough (sometimes with bloody sputum), fever, chills, night sweats, fatigue, weakness, and weight loss. Those with spinal TB exhibit back pain and paralysis. Other sites of infection include the joints, bone marrow, urinary system, reproductive system, and heart. Miliary TB involves infection of the blood itself and can result in multiple TB emboli.
	In the CNS, TB typically involves the meninges, where it causes basilar meningitis, or the brain parenchyma, where it causes masses known as tuberculomas. Meningitis causes delirium, stiff neck, fever, and headache. SIAD can be seen, as can cranial nerve III, IV, and VI palsies. Less commonly, obstructive hydrocephalus is seen. Other sequelae include basal ganglia infarctions with tremor, chorea, and dystonia. Inflammation of both large pial and small penetrating arteries can occur, with consequent territorial or lacunar infarctions. With tuberculomas, symptoms depend on the brain area affected; these masses are usually multiple and can be supratentorial or infratentorial. Seizures may occur.
Laboratory testing	The first step in laboratory testing involves indirect assessment of infection through detection of cell-mediated immune responses to *M. tuberculosis*. The test of choice is the IGRA, a blood test analyzed in the laboratory. If the IGRA is not available, a TB skin test can be used. Neither of these tests can distinguish latent infection from active TB. False-negative skin tests using purified protein derivative tests are common in AIDS patients.
	If the IGRA or skin test is positive, a chest X-ray is performed, and the patient is evaluated for any evidence of active disease. HIV testing is also indicated at this point because HIV favors progression to active disease.
	If active disease is detected, further testing usually includes sputum culture, smear microscopy, and nucleic acid amplification testing. In addition, bronchoscopy and biopsy of infected tissue may be required.

Tuberculosis (TB) *(continued)*

Laboratory testing *(continued)*	CNS disease requires further testing as follows:
	• CSF in TB meningitis shows a pleocytosis (initially polymorphonuclear leukocytes; later, lymphocytes), low blood sugar, and elevated protein. Smears usually yield no results, but cultures are positive in more than half of cases. CSF cultures are positive in three-quarters of patients but may take weeks to return. PCR assay is also positive in three-quarters of patients and is returned the day of testing. In tuberculomas, CSF is normal or only mildly abnormal.
	• Meningitis and tuberculomas can be visualized on contrast-enhanced CT or MRI.

Brodie D, Schluger NW: The diagnosis of tuberculosis. Clin Chest Med 26:247–271, 2005

Cain KP, McCarthy KD, Heilig CM, et al: An algorithm for tuberculosis screening and diagnosis in people with HIV. N Engl J Med 362:707–716, 2010

Carranza C, Pedraza-Sanchez S, de Oyarzabal-Mendez E, Torres M: Diagnosis for latent tuberculosis infection: new alternatives. Front Immunol 11:2006, 2020

Dheda K, Barry CE III, Maartens G: Tuberculosis. Lancet 387(10024):1211–1226, 2016 [published corrections appear in Lancet 387(10024):1162 and 387(10033):2092, 2016]

Furin J, Cox H, Pai M: Tuberculosis. Lancet 393(10181):1642–1656, 2019

Phypers M, Harris T, Power C: CNS tuberculosis: a longitudinal analysis of epidemiological and clinical features. Int J Tuberc Lung Dis 10:99–103, 2006

Shah M, Dorman SE: Latent tuberculosis infection. N Engl J Med 385(24):2271–2280, 2021

Suárez I, Fünger SM, Kröger S, et al: The diagnosis and treatment of tuberculosis. Dtsch Arztebl Int 116(43):729–735, 2019

Uremic syndrome

Clinical findings	The uremic syndrome of chronic kidney disease refers to a range of signs and symptoms arising from the accumulation of toxic substances normally excreted in urine. The syndrome is now understood to involve alterations in the metabolic, hormonal, vascular, inflammatory, and other systems with progression of kidney dysfunction. Most organs are affected. The CNS is affected because of changes to the blood-brain barrier, with direct neuronal toxicity causing cognitive impairment, dementia, and uremic encephalopathy.
	Specific neuropsychiatric signs and symptoms of uremia include fatigue, lethargy, anorexia, nausea, cognitive impairment, sleep disturbance, delirium (encephalopathy), restless legs syndrome, reduced sense of smell and taste, and peripheral neuropathy. Cognitive impairment may be so mild that it is undetected by bedside mental status examination. Neuropsychological testing shows deficits in attention, memory, and higher-order intellectual processing. Sleep is often fragmented, with brief arousals and apneic episodes as well as repetitive leg movements. In uremic encephalopathy (delirium), a prodrome may be seen, with worsening fatigue, inattention, inability to concentrate, and somnolence. The delirium is often associated with dysarthria and asterixis, as seen in hepatic encephalopathy. Myoclonus can be seen and may herald the onset of seizures. The seizures can be nonconvulsive, mimicking encephalopathy. In untreated uremia, there may be progression to stupor and coma. The syndrome can be fatal.
	Other signs of uremia include amenorrhea, sexual dysfunction, hypothermia, bone disease, insulin resistance, catabolic state, serositis (pericarditis), pruritus, hiccups, anemia, immune system dysfunction, and platelet dysfunction. Cardiovascular disease mediated by inflammatory processes introduces significant morbidity and mortality, as does an increased rate of infections.
Laboratory testing	Patient well-being is reduced when the GFR is <60 mL/min. Cognitive impairment may develop with a GFR of 30–60 mL/min. In general, neuropsychiatric symptoms are thought to be caused by retained solutes that are not directly measured, including guanidines, amines, phenols, and indoles, among others.
	Severity of delirium is correlated with degree of elevation in BUN and the rapidity of its rise. In acute renal failure, symptoms appear at BUN levels >100 mg/dL. In chronic renal failure, BUN can be >200 mg/dL or more without symptoms.
	In cases in which encephalopathy is the first evidence that uremia is present, a CMP should be checked and a nephrology consultation obtained.
	In uremic encephalopathy, an EEG shows generalized slowing, and triphasic waves may be seen. Patients with myoclonus or seizures may show epileptiform or ictal activity.
	MRI may show cortical atrophy. In patients with uremia in the context of diabetes, cortical and subcortical hyperintensities on T2-weighted scans may be seen.

Battaglia F, Quartarone A, Bagnato S, et al: Brain dysfunction in uremia: a question of cortical hyperexcitability? Clin Neurophysiol 116:1507–1514, 2005

Bergstrom J: Toxicity of uremia: physiopathology and clinical signs. Contrib Nephrol 71:1–9, 1989

Hamed SA: Neurologic conditions and disorders of uremic syndrome of chronic kidney disease: presentations, causes, and treatment strategies. Expert Rev Clin Pharmacol 12(1):61–90, 2019

Uremic syndrome *(continued)*

Hamed S, Mohamed K, Abd Elhameed S, et al: Movement disorders due to selective basal ganglia lesions with uremia. Can J Neurol Sci 47(3):350–365, 2020

Hur W, Chung JY, Choi PK, Kang HG: Uremia presented as acute cranial neuropathy. Neurol Sci 40(7):1487–1489, 2019

Meyer TW, Hostetter TH: Uremia: N Engl J Med 357:1316–1325, 2007

Rosner MH, Husain-Syed F, Reis T, et al: Uremic encephalopathy. Kidney Int 101(2):227–241, 2022

Sanchez-Meza F, Torre A, Castillo-Martinez L, et al: Evaluation of cerebral dysfunction in patients with chronic kidney disease using neuropsychometric and neurophysiological tests. Ren Fail 43(1):577–584, 2021

Scherer JS, Combs SA, Brennan F: Sleep disorders, restless legs syndrome, and uremic pruritus: diagnosis and treatment of common symptoms in dialysis patients. Am J Kidney Dis 69(1):117–128, 2017

Títoff V, Moury HN, Títoff IB, Kelly KM: Seizures, antiepileptic drugs, and CKD. Am J Kidney Dis 73(1):90–101, 2019

Urinary tract infection (UTI)

Clinical findings	UTI can involve the bladder and related structures—termed *cystitis*—or the upper tract including the kidneys—termed *pyelonephritis*. Cystitis is a common condition and usually self-limiting, although it sometimes can be recurrent. Pyelonephritis is more serious and often presents with additional constitutional symptoms. The diagnosis of UTI depends on the presence of both clinical symptoms and laboratory confirmation. Asymptomatic patients can exhibit either bacteria in the urine (bacteriuria) or WBCs in the urine (pyuria), neither of which in isolation defines UTI. Syndromes of asymptomatic bacteriuria and sterile pyuria are also seen.
	Increased risk of UTI is found in females, elderly individuals, those with recent sexual activity, those who use diaphragms for birth control, patients with recent instrumentation, and kidney transplant patients. Recurrent symptomatic UTI risk factors include diabetes, functional disability, urinary retention, and urinary incontinence.
	Clinical signs and symptoms of UTI include dysuria, suprapubic tenderness, urinary frequency, urinary urgency, and hematuria. Additional signs of upper tract involvement include fever and costovertebral angle and flank pain.
Laboratory testing	Laboratory evaluation for UTI includes urine dipstick testing, urinalysis, and culture.
	Dipstick testing
	• Point of care test for leukocyte esterase (LE), nitrite, WBCs, and blood.
	• In a patient with symptoms consistent with lower UTI, a positive LE test on dipstick is sufficient to diagnose UTI.
	• If pretest probability of UTI is high, urine should be cultured even if the LE test is negative.
	• A positive nitrite test is specific but not sensitive for UTI.
	Urinalysis
	• Pyuria is best measured in unspun fresh urine using a hemocytometer chamber. More than 10 WBCs/mL is consistent with pyuria. *Sterile pyuria* refers to persistent WBCs in the absence of bacteria.
	• Microscopic hematuria is identified in half of cystitis cases.
	Urine culture
	• This is the gold standard of UTI diagnosis. A low threshold for obtaining a urine culture should be used for patients who are pregnant, immunosuppressed, or elderly; who have had recent exposure to antibiotics or urinary tract instrumentation; or who are having recurrent UTI infections.
	UTI is defined by the following culture results from clean-catch urine: Cystitis: $>10^3$ colony-forming units (CFU)/mL Pyelonephritis: $>10^5$ CFU/mL
	• Any uropathogens grown from a suprapubic aspirate sample provide evidence of UTI
	• Asymptomatic bacteriuria: $>10^5$ CFU/mL in an asymptomatic patient
	Urine susceptibility (sensitivity)
	• If pathogenic bacteria are found on culture, susceptibility to a panel of antibiotics is tested.

Urinary tract infection (UTI) *(continued)*

Bent S, Nallamothu BK, Simel DL, et al: Does this woman have an acute uncomplicated urinary tract infection? JAMA 287:2701–2710, 2002

Brusch JL: Medscape: urinary tract infection (UTI) and cystitis (bladder infection) in females, in Medscape: Drugs and Diseases: Infectious Diseases, January 2, 2020. Available at: https://emedicine.medscape.com/article/233101-overview. Accessed April 2022.

Fihn SD: Clinical practice: acute uncomplicated urinary tract infection in women. N Engl J Med 349:259–266, 2003

Hay AD, Fahey T: Clinical diagnosis of urinary tract infection. JAMA 288:1229, 2002

Mehnert-Kay SA: Diagnosis and management of uncomplicated urinary tract infections. Am Fam Physician 72:451–456, 2005

Mody L, Juthani-Mehta M: Urinary tract infections in older women: a clinical review. JAMA 311(8):844–854, 2014

Wise GJ, Schlegel PN: Sterile pyuria. N Engl J Med 372(11):1048–1054, 2015

Vitamin B$_{12}$ deficiency

Clinical findings	Vitamin B$_{12}$, or cobalamin, is a water-soluble vitamin required for protein synthesis, fat and carbohydrate metabolism, absorption and digestion of food, formation of RBCs, production of acetylcholine, maintenance of nerve cells, and fertility in females. This vitamin is obtained from dietary sources such as fish, meat, dairy products, and fortified cereals and can be taken as a supplement. Its absorption depends on the presence of intrinsic factor secreted by gastric parietal cells; reduced levels of this factor in elderly patients and individuals with gastric disease are known to cause deficiency. Others at risk for deficiency include strict vegetarians, malnourished individuals (e.g., with anorexia nervosa), patients who have undergone gastric or ileal resection, those with malabsorption syndromes, individuals with alcohol use disorder, and those who have been treated chronically with metformin, proton pump inhibitors, or histamine H$_2$ blockers. Among elderly individuals, the most common type of vitamin B$_{12}$ deficiency is pernicious anemia caused by chronic atrophic gastritis leading to intrinsic factor deficiency. Recreational nitrous oxide abuse has more recently been identified as a risk factor, and even use of nitrous oxide as a dental anesthetic can precipitate deficiency symptoms in a marginally deficient patient.
	The organ systems most affected by vitamin B$_{12}$ deficiency are the bone marrow, blood, and nervous system. A megaloblastic anemia is seen in which fewer and larger RBCs are produced. Leukopenia, thrombocytopenia or thrombocytosis, and pancytopenia can also be noted. In the nervous system, the degenerative process involves demyelination in the brain, spinal cord, and peripheral nerves. If the deficiency is left untreated, axonal loss is seen. The classic syndrome of subacute combined degeneration of the spinal cord involves demyelination in the posterior columns and lateral corticospinal tracts, with signs and symptoms that include spastic paraparesis, positive Romberg sign, ataxic gait, and loss of vibration sense, proprioception, and two-point discrimination.
	Cerebral signs and symptoms of vitamin B$_{12}$ deficiency include the following:
	<ul><li>Chronic cognitive impairment (dementia)</li><li>Confusion and/or delirium</li><li>Depression, apathy</li><li>Personality change</li><li>Mania, agitation</li><li>Psychosis: delusions, hallucinations, disorganization ("megaloblastic madness")</li></ul>
Laboratory testing	Screening for vitamin B$_{12}$ deficiency is indicated for patients with any of the risk factors noted above, including age >75 years.
	Initial testing includes a CBC with differential and platelets and a serum vitamin B$_{12}$ level.
	Macrocytic anemia is variably present. Blood smear may show hypersegmented neutrophils and macro-ovalocytes.
	Vitamin B$_{12}$ level may be falsely elevated in patients with alcohol use disorder, liver disease, or cancer.

Vitamin B$_{12}$ deficiency *(continued)*

Laboratory testing *(continued)*	Vitamin B$_{12}$ level interpretation:
	• ≥400 pg/mL: no deficiency
	• 150–399 pg/mL: low-normal
	• <150 pg/mL: deficiency
	For high-risk patients with low-normal B$_{12}$ levels, MMA testing is used. Elevation of MMA is more sensitive for B$_{12}$ deficiency and helps to distinguish it from folate deficiency, in which this level is normal.
	If MMA level is high and there is clinical suspicion of pernicious anemia, anti–parietal cell and anti–intrinsic factor antibodies are checked. If these tests are negative but suspicion of pernicious anemia remains, the serum gastrin level is checked. An elevated gastrin level is consistent with a diagnosis of pernicious anemia.
	A newer metabolic marker, the cobalamin transporter *holotranscobalamin* (holoTC), can also be measured in serum. This marker is a better measure of cobalamin deficiency than the B$_{12}$ level itself because it assays only the active part of the molecule. At this writing, the holoTC test is investigational only.
	In elderly patients, given the high pretest probability of deficiency in the presence of characteristic symptoms and the low risk of replacement, it is a common clinical practice to replace B$_{12}$ for any patient with a vitamin B$_{12}$ level <400 pg/mL.
	Other laboratory findings not part of the diagnostic algorithm include the following:
	• MRI may show patchy hyperintensities on T2-weighted images in the centrum semiovale, more prominent in frontal lobe areas.
	• EEG may show generalized slowing or slowing of the posterior dominant frequency.
	• CSF is usually unremarkable except for slightly increased protein.
	To monitor the effectiveness of vitamin B$_{12}$ replacement:
	• Perform CBC after 2 weeks to document increase in hemoglobin and decrease in MCV.
	• Perform CBC after 8 weeks to document resolution of anemia.
	• B$_{12}$ level does not need to be checked unless noncompliance is suspected with oral therapy.

Baig FA, Khan S, Rizwan A: Frequency of vitamin B12 deficiency in type 2 diabetic patients taking metformin. Cureus 14(3):e22924, 2022

Green R, Miller JW: Vitamin B12 deficiency. Vitam Horm 119:405–439, 2022

Hvas AM, Nexo E: Diagnosis and treatment of vitamin B12 deficiency: an update. Haematologica 91:1506–1512, 2006

Langan RC, Goodbred AJ: Vitamin B12 deficiency: recognition and management. Am Fam Physician 96(6):384–389, 2017

Maheshwari M, Athiraman H. Whippets causing vitamin B12 deficiency. Cureus 14(3):e23148, 2022

Sahu P, Thippeswamy H, Chaturvedi SK: Neuropsychiatric manifestations in vitamin B12 deficiency. Vitam Horm 119:457–470, 2022

Ueno A, Hamano T, Enomoto S, et al: Influences of vitamin B12 supplementation on cognition and homocysteine in patients with vitamin B$_{12}$ deficiency and cognitive impairment. Nutrients 14(7):1494, 2022

Wong C, Benyaminov F, Block L: Reversible dementia in the setting of multiple medical comorbidities due to B12 deficiency. BMJ Case Rep 15(3):e248440, 2022

Wernicke's encephalopathy (WE) and Wernicke-Korsakoff syndrome

Clinical findings	WE is a neuropsychiatric syndrome reflecting thiamine deficiency and classically characterized by the clinical triad of mental status changes, ataxia, and ophthalmoplegia. Because this fully developed triad is rarely seen, symptoms may be dismissed and the opportunity for treatment missed, an unfortunate situation because the syndrome can progress to permanent cognitive deficits or be fatal. The incidence of WE is much higher in necropsy series than in clinical practice. Individuals at risk of WE include those with alcohol use disorder, anorexia nervosa, severe malnutrition, hyperemesis gravidarum of pregnancy, vomiting in the context of inflammatory bowel disease, hyperthyroidism, liver disease, hemodialysis, prolonged parenteral nutrition, malignancy, and immunodeficiency syndromes. The index of clinical suspicion of WE should be particularly high in any of these patients with recent rapid weight loss, acute infection, or carbohydrate loading.
	The onset of WE is usually subacute, but by the time the patient presents for evaluation, urgent intervention is needed in the form of high doses of parenteral thiamine. This treatment must be given before parenteral glucose because glucose given before thiamine can precipitate WE acutely in a marginally deficient patient. One mnemonic for this is "Thank God I gave thiamine before glucose!"
	Mental status changes in WE include inattentiveness, apathy, paucity of speech, disorientation, and memory problems. Ataxia affects both stance and gait, with vestibular as well as cerebellar involvement, and can progress to inability to stand or walk. Ocular signs include nystagmus, diplopia, blurred vision, conjugate gaze palsies, pupillary sluggishness, ptosis, anisocoria, and, in end stages, complete ophthalmoplegia. Voice changes can be noted, as can general weakness. Seizures can occur. Often, vital signs are abnormal, with hypothermia, tachycardia, and postural hypotension.
	Patients with WE who remain untreated or undertreated with thiamine develop Korsakoff's syndrome, characterized by severe anterograde amnesia and, in many patients, confabulation. Some degree of retrograde amnesia may also be seen, with a temporal gradient (worst for the most recent events). Affected patients appear to be indifferent to this condition. Persistent ophthalmoplegia and ataxia can be seen. Typically, symptoms of Korsakoff's syndrome cannot be reversed, although success has been reported in isolated cases of aggressive thiamine repletion, even in treating memory deficits.
Laboratory testing	A thiamine level should be drawn before treatment commences, but treatment should not be withheld until the result is returned.
	MRI can assist in confirming the diagnosis after acute treatment has commenced.
	• Coronal sections through the mammillary bodies should be requested, with a clinical note "to evaluate Wernicke-Korsakoff syndrome."
	• In WE, abnormal signal intensity is seen in mammillary bodies on diffusion-weighted imaging, FLAIR, and T2-weighted scans.
	• In Korsakoff's syndrome, T2-weighted scans show atrophy of mammillary bodies.

Wernicke's encephalopathy (WE) and
Wernicke-Korsakoff syndrome *(continued)*

Laboratory testing *(continued)*	• Other brain areas that may be affected in Wernicke-Korsakoff syndrome include periaqueductal gray, midbrain tectum, dorsomedial nucleus of the thalamus, and mammillothalamic tract.

Alexandri M, Reynolds BZ, Smith H, et al: Wernicke's encephalopathy and cranial nerve VII palsy in a 24-year-old patient with COVID-19. Int J Emerg Med 15(1):6, 2022

Aomura D, Kurasawa Y, Harada M, et al: Brain MRI detection of early Wernicke's encephalopathy in a hemodialysis patient. Clin Case Rep 10(3):e05539, 2022

Bagash H, Marwat A, Marwat A, Kraus B: A case of chronic wernicke encephalopathy (WE): an underdiagnosed phenomena. Cureus 13(10):e19100, 2021

Kho J, Mandal AKJ, Geraldes R, et al: COVID-19 encephalitis and Wernicke's encephalopathy. J Med Virol 93(9):5248–5251, 2021

Kohnke S, Meek CL: Don't seek, don't find: the diagnostic challenge of Wernicke's encephalopathy. Ann Clin Biochem 58(1):38–46, 2021

Llansó L, Bartolomé-Solanas A, Renú A: Wernicke's encephalopathy following hyperemesis gravidarum. Pract Neurol 22:237–238, 2022

Novo-Veleiro I, Herrera-Flores J, Rosón-Hernández B, et al: Alcoholic liver disease among patients with Wernicke encephalopathy: a multicenter observational study. Drug Alcohol Depend 230:109186, 2022

Oudman E, Wijnia JW, Oey M, et al: Wernicke's encephalopathy in hyperemesis gravidarum: a systematic review. Eur J Obstet Gynecol Reprod Biol 236:84–93, 2019

Oudman E, Wijnia JW, Oey MJ, et al: Wernicke's encephalopathy in Crohn's disease and ulcerative colitis. Nutrition 86:111182, 2021

Sechi G, Serra A: Wernicke's encephalopathy: new clinical settings and recent advances in diagnosis and management. Lancet Neurol 6(5):442–455, 2007

Seto N, Ishida M, Hamano T, et al: A case of Wernicke encephalopathy arising in the early stage after the start of hemodialysis. CEN Case Rep 11(3):314–320, 2022

Wilson's disease

Clinical findings	Wilson's disease is an inherited disorder of copper excretion caused by mutations in the ATP7B gene (*ATP7B*) on chromosome 13. Slightly more copper is taken in from dietary sources than is needed, and the excess is normally excreted through the biliary tract. *ATP7B* encodes a copper-transporting enzyme in the liver that, when dysfunctional, leads to copper accumulation in the liver, brain, and other tissues. Clinical features can become apparent at any age, but peak incidence is around 17 years of age.
	The hallmarks of Wilson's disease are liver disease/cirrhosis, prominent neuropsychiatric signs and symptoms, acute episodes of hemolysis with acute liver failure, and Kayser-Fleischer rings in Descemet's membrane of the cornea. The disease can progress slowly over decades, with clinically apparent liver disease preceding neuropsychiatric symptoms by as much as a decade. If not recognized and treated early enough, serious neurological disability can develop, and the disease can be fatal. With treatment, on the other hand, affected patients have a normal life and life expectancy.
	The first signs of Wilson's disease can be psychiatric, commonly including personality changes, disinhibition, irritability, anxiety, and depression. As the disease progresses, catatonia and mania can be seen, and substance abuse may supervene. In older patients, paranoia and other psychotic symptoms suggestive of schizophrenia can be observed. Cognition is generally spared until later disease stages, when frontal-subcortical impairment is seen.
	When the first evidence of Wilson's disease is neurological, signs commonly include dysarthria, dystonia, abnormal gait, tremor, parkinsonism, and chorea/athetosis. Tremor may be of the characteristic "wing-beating" type involving the upper limbs, but in early stages it usually resembles essential tremor. As the disease progresses, dysphagia, drooling, bulbar and pseudobulbar palsies, pyramidal signs, myoclonus, and eye movement abnormalities are seen. Seizures can be seen at any stage, sometimes occurring when treatment is initiated.
	When the first signs of Wilson's disease are hepatic, the presentation can be one of acute hepatitis, chronic active hepatitis, cirrhosis, or fulminant hepatic failure.
	Kayser-Fleischer rings are copper and sulfur deposits in the limbic region of the cornea visible on slit-lamp examination, with an ophthalmoscope (at +40), or even by the naked eye when well developed. These rings are seen in all patients with neurological disease and in half of those with hepatic disease.
	Other clinical manifestations of Wilson's disease include renal tubular dysfunction (including Fanconi syndrome), kidney stones, gallstones, osteoporosis, osteomalacia, arthritis/arthralgias, myocarditis, interstitial fibrosis of the myocardium, amenorrhea/oligomenorrhea in females, pancreatic disease, parathyroid dysfunction, skin changes, orthostatic hypotension, and ECG changes.
Laboratory testing	The most common test used to screen for Wilson's disease is serum ceruloplasmin. Reference values for ceruloplasmin in adults age 18 years and older are as follows: • Males: 15–30 mg/dL • Females: 16–45 mg/dL

Wilson's disease *(continued)*

Laboratory testing *(continued)*	A value <5 mg/dL is diagnostic of Wilson's disease. A moderately low level requires further investigation, as does a normal level in patient with high pretest probability of disease. First-degree relatives should also be tested.
	Further testing can involve either a bundled Wilson's disease screening panel or individual tests (serum copper, free serum copper, and LFTs). The most reliable measure is a 24-hour urine copper test. In a symptomatic patient, the 24-hour urine copper measure value is always >100 µg/day (normal 3.0–45.0 µg/day). Any value >40 µg/day requires further evaluation. The specimen for urine screening requires special collection and handling; consult the laboratory for guidance.
	The gold standard for the diagnosis of Wilson's disease is measurement of copper in a sample of liver tissue obtained by percutaneous biopsy. A hepatic copper content >250 µg/g dry weight is diagnostic. Levels <40–50 µg/g dry weight usually exclude the diagnosis. Levels between these values require further investigation.
	Wilson's disease is an autosomal recessive disorder involving *ATP7B* mapped to chromosome 13 (13q14.3). Testing for *ATP7B* variants is routine for patients and their first-degree relatives. Whole-exome or whole-genome sequencing may be required in some cases.
	Imaging abnormalities are found in patients with neuropsychiatric signs but often are absent in those with only liver disease. High T2 signals in lentiform and caudate nuclei, thalamus, brainstem, and white matter are most common. In a minority of cases, the characteristic "face of the giant panda" is seen on axial view. Imaging abnormalities are seen to resolve with treatment.

Arora N, Wasti K, Suri V, Malhotra P: "Face of a giant panda" and "beating wings" in a young male. Cureus 14(2):e22429, 2022

ARUP Laboratories: Ceruloplasmin, in Laboratory Test Directory, Salt Lake City, UT, ARUP Laboratories, 2022. Available at: https://ltd.aruplab.com/Tests/Pub/0050160. Accessed April 2022.

Bandmann O, Weiss KH, Kaler SG: Wilson's disease and other neurological copper disorders. Lancet Neurol 14(1):103–113, 2015

European Association for the Study of the Liver: EASL clinical practice guidelines: Wilson's disease. J Hepatol 56(3):671–685, 2012

Hedera P: Wilson's disease: a master of disguise. Parkinsonism Relat Disord 59:140–145, 2019

Jackson GH, Meyer A, Lippmann S: Wilson's disease: psychiatric manifestations may be the clinical presentation. Postgrad Med 95:135–138, 1994

Lorincz MT: Neurologic Wilson's disease. Ann N Y Acad Sci 1184:173–187, 2010

Mak CM, Lam CW: Diagnosis of Wilson's disease: a comprehensive review. Crit Rev Clin Lab Sci 45:263–290, 2008

Shribman S, Marjot T, Sharif A, et al: Investigation and management of Wilson's disease: a practical guide from the British Association for the Study of the Liver. Gastroenterol Hepatol 7(6):560–575, 2022

CHAPTER 3

Psychotropic Medications

Laboratory Screening and Monitoring

Acamprosate

Screening laboratory tests	• BUN, creatinine, and eGFR to ensure that the drug is not contraindicated and to determine whether dosage reduction is needed.
	• Consider pregnancy testing in patients of childbearing potential.
Monitoring laboratory tests	• Periodic monitoring of BUN, creatinine, and eGFR to determine whether dosage reduction is needed.
	• ECG if angina or other cardiac signs/symptoms develop.
	• EEG if signs/symptoms of seizures develop.
	• Amylase, lipase, and other tests for suspected pancreatitis if relevant signs/symptoms are noted.

American Society of Health-System Pharmacists: AHFS Drug Information. Bethesda, MD, American Society of Health-System Pharmacists, 2016

U.S. National Library of Medicine: Acamprosate calcium: acamprosate calcium enteric-coated tablet, delayed release. DailyMed, July 17, 2019. Available at: https://dailymed.nlm.nih.gov/dailymed/drugInfo.cfm?setid=75ddfd10-55b2-426e-bc74-3413cd0d7c94. Accessed April 2022.

Amphetamines

Screening laboratory tests	• ECG and echocardiogram in patients with physical findings suggestive of cardiac disease or a family history of sudden death or ventricular arrhythmia.
	• TSH to exclude hyperthyroidism.
	• Pregnancy testing in patients of childbearing potential.
Monitoring laboratory tests	• Prompt cardiac evaluation (ECG, echocardiogram) if syncope, exertional chest pain, or other cardiac symptoms develop.
	• EEG if seizures develop.
	• Periodic check of TSH.

American Society of Health-System Pharmacists: AHFS Drug Information. Bethesda, MD, American Society of Health-System Pharmacists, 2016

U.S. National Library of Medicine: Dextroamphetamine saccharate, amphetamine aspartate, dextroamphetamine sulfate, amphetamine sulfate tablets. DailyMed, January 4, 2022. Available at: https://dailymed.nlm.nih.gov/dailymed/drugInfo.cfm?setid=c907301d-e24d-9609-5529-fed14f94549f. Accessed April 2022.

Antipsychotics, first generation

Screening laboratory tests	• BUN, creatinine, and eGFR. These drugs should be used with caution in patients with renal impairment. • LFTs (AST, ALT, total bilirubin). These drugs should be used with caution in patients with hepatic impairment. • CBC with differential to establish baseline values. Antipsychotics are associated with leukopenia and agranulocytosis, and this risk is greater for those with preexisting leukopenia/neutropenia. • ECG to establish baseline QTc value and exclude existing heart disease, arrhythmia, and recent MI. Thioridazine, chlorpromazine, haloperidol, and pimozide confer the highest risk of QT prolongation. • Electrolytes (potassium and magnesium). Low levels predispose to QT prolongation. • Prolactin level to establish baseline value. • Abnormal Involuntary Movement Scale (AIMS) evaluation to establish a baseline score. • Pregnancy testing in patients of childbearing potential. These drugs may cause fetal and neonatal harm. Metabolic syndrome screening: • Fasting glucose • Lipid profile • Weight, height, and BMI calculation • Waist circumference • Blood pressure
Monitoring laboratory tests	• Periodic checks of BUN, creatinine, eGFR, AST, ALT, total bilirubin, electrolytes, and CBC with differential. • Patients with preexisting or a history of drug-induced leukopenia/neutropenia should have their CBC monitored frequently during the first few months of treatment, and the drug should be discontinued at the first sign of decline in WBC count in the absence of other causative factors. • ECG at least yearly for patients treated with drugs that pose a high risk of QT prolongation. • Prolactin level for any symptoms of hyperprolactinemia. • AIMS evaluation every 6 months. Metabolic syndrome monitoring: • Fasting glucose at 12 weeks, then at least yearly • Lipid profile at 12 weeks, then at least yearly • Waist circumference yearly • Blood pressure at 12 weeks, then every 6 months • Weight and BMI at 4 weeks, 8 weeks, and 12 weeks, then quarterly

American Society of Health-System Pharmacists: AHFS Drug Information. Bethesda, MD, American Society of Health-System Pharmacists, 2016

U.S. National Library of Medicine: DailyMed. Available at: https://dailymed.nlm.nih.gov/dailymed. Accessed April 2022.

Aripiprazole

Screening laboratory tests	• Consider CBC with differential. Low initial values for WBCs or ANC or any history of drug-induced neutropenia increases the risk of more severe neutropenia.
	• Consider ECG. Drug should be used with caution in patients with known cardiovascular disease (history of MI or ischemic heart disease, heart failure, or conduction abnormalities).
Monitoring laboratory tests	Consider periodic check of CBC with differential.

American Society of Health-System Pharmacists: AHFS Drug Information. Bethesda, MD, American Society of Health-System Pharmacists, 2016

U.S. National Library of Medicine: Aripiprazole: aripiprazole tablet. DailyMed, June 18, 2021. Available at: https://dailymed.nlm.nih.gov/dailymed/drugInfo.cfm?setid=2d8d574b-fbf4-4d2c-a37c-25556ecbf1aa. Accessed April 2022.

Asenapine

Screening laboratory tests	• CMP (LFTs, potassium) and magnesium. Drug is contraindicated in severe hepatic impairment (Child-Pugh Class C).
	• Consider ECG for baseline QTc measurement, although the risk is lower with this drug compared to others in its class. Hypokalemia and hypomagnesemia magnify effects of QTc prolongation.
	• Consider pregnancy testing for patients of childbearing potential.
Monitoring laboratory tests	Routine laboratory testing is not required.

American Society of Health-System Pharmacists: AHFS Drug Information. Bethesda, MD, American Society of Health-System Pharmacists, 2016

U.S. National Library of Medicine: Asenapine: asenapine maleate tablet. DailyMed, July 8, 2021. Available at: https://dailymed.nlm.nih.gov/dailymed/drugInfo.cfm?setid=f5cd9abb-40e3-4cb5-a1b2-40cdba8a1c7e. Accessed April 2022.

Atomoxetine

Screening laboratory tests	• ECG and echocardiogram in patients with physical findings suggestive of cardiac disease or with a family history of sudden death or ventricular arrhythmia.
	• Blood pressure and pulse to establish baseline values.
	• LFTs to determine whether dosage adjustment is needed.
	• Consider CYP2D6 genotyping to determine whether the patient is a poor metabolizer; in this case, dosage adjustment is needed.
	• Pregnancy test for patients of childbearing potential.
Monitoring laboratory tests	• Blood pressure and pulse measurement soon after initiating treatment, after every dosage increase, and periodically during treatment.
	• Prompt cardiac evaluation (ECG, echocardiogram) if syncope, exertional chest pain, or other cardiac symptoms develop.
	• LFTs at first signs of hepatic dysfunction (jaundice, dark urine, pruritus, right upper quadrant tenderness, or flu-like symptoms). Drug should be discontinued and not reinstated in patients with jaundice or laboratory evidence of hepatic injury.

American Society of Health-System Pharmacists: AHFS Drug Information. Bethesda, MD, American Society of Health-System Pharmacists, 2016

U.S. National Library of Medicine: Atomoxetine: atomoxetine capsule. DailyMed, March 20, 2021. Available at: https://dailymed.nlm.nih.gov/dailymed/drugInfo.cfm?setid=f266ab7b-5a68-42b5-b204-e3249bea0aed. Accessed April 2022.

Benzodiazepines*

Screening laboratory tests	• LFTs (AST, ALT, total bilirubin) before drug initiation. In most cases of impaired liver function, dosage reduction is required.
	• BUN, creatinine, and eGFR. Caution should be used for patients with impaired renal function because some metabolites are excreted through the kidneys.
	• CBC with differential and platelets to establish baseline values.
	• Consider PSG in patients with suspected sleep apnea. Deaths have been reported shortly after benzodiazepines were initiated in undiagnosed patients.
	• Pregnancy testing in patients of childbearing potential. These drugs are known to harm the fetus and neonate.
Monitoring laboratory tests	• Periodic CBC with differential and platelets.
	• Periodic liver function testing.

*Summary includes alprazolam, chlordiazepoxide, clonazepam, diazepam, lorazepam, oxazepam, and temazepam.

American Society of Health-System Pharmacists: AHFS Drug Information. Bethesda, MD, American Society of Health-System Pharmacists, 2016

U.S. National Library of Medicine: DailyMed. Available at: https://dailymed.nlm.nih.gov/dailymed/index.cfm. Accessed April 2022.

Bremelanotide

Screening laboratory tests	• Assess cardiovascular risk (Appendix C) and determine baseline blood pressure. Drug is not recommended for patients at high risk for cardiovascular disease and is contraindicated in patients with uncontrolled hypertension or existing cardiovascular disease. • Consider baseline testing for renal and hepatic impairment. Drug must be used with caution in patients with severe impairment.
Monitoring laboratory tests	Periodic assessment of cardiovascular risk (see Appendix C) and blood pressure.

U.S. National Library of Medicine: Vyleesi: bremelanotide injection. DailyMed, January 12, 2021. Available at: https://dailymed.nlm.nih.gov/dailymed/drugInfo.cfm?setid=9146ae05-918b-483e-b86d-933485ce36eb. Accessed April 2022.

Brexpiprazole

Screening laboratory tests	• Evaluate baseline renal and hepatic function. Dosage adjustment is required for moderate to severe impairment. • Obtain baseline fasting glucose, lipid profile, and weight. Metabolic parameters may be affected by brexpiprazole. • Obtain baseline WBC count and differential. Preexisting leukopenia or neutropenia is a risk factor for significant decline in these values. If baseline values are low or the patient has a history of drug-induced leukopenia/neutropenia, obtain CBC with differential.
Monitoring laboratory tests	• Periodic monitoring of metabolic parameters: fasting glucose, lipid profile, and weight. • Obtain CBC with differential frequently during the first few months of therapy for patients with a low baseline WBC count or ANC or a history of drug-induced leukopenia/neutropenia. • If ANC is <1,000/mm^3, discontinue drug and follow WBC count until recovery.

U.S. Food and Drug Administration: Rexulti (brexpiprazole) package insert. Available at: https://www.accessdata.fda.gov/drugsatfda_docs/label/2018/205422s003lbl.pdf. Accessed April 2022.

Buprenorphine

Screening laboratory tests	• LFTs, including GGT • Urine drug screen
Monitoring laboratory tests	• Periodic check of LFTs, including GGT • Urine drug screen

American Society of Health-System Pharmacists: AHFS Drug Information. Bethesda, MD, American Society of Health-System Pharmacists, 2016

U.S. National Library of Medicine: Buprenorphine and naloxone: buprenorphine hydrochloride and naloxone hydrochloride tablet. DailyMed, March 31, 2021. Available at: https://dailymed.nlm.nih.gov/dailymed/drugInfo.cfm?setid=6cccf229-9611-4b6f-8f1b-acc8ff1ed3f8. Accessed April 2022.

Bupropion

Screening laboratory tests	• LFTs to establish baseline values. Dosage reductions are required in moderate to severe hepatic impairment and should be considered in mild impairment.
	• Renal function tests (BUN, creatinine) to establish baseline values.
	• Drug should be used with extreme caution in patients with renal disease or failure.
	• Consider EEG to evaluate for epileptiform activity.
	• Blood pressure baseline values
Monitoring laboratory tests	• LFTs, BUN, creatinine, and eGFR every 6–12 months
	• Periodic blood pressure checks
	• ECG for palpitations or other cardiac signs/symptoms
	• EEG for signs/symptoms suggestive of seizure

American Society of Health-System Pharmacists: AHFS Drug Information. Bethesda, MD, American Society of Health-System Pharmacists, 2016

U.S. National Library of Medicine: Bupropion hydrochloride extended release: bupropion hydrochloride tablet. DailyMed, August 16, 2021. Available at: https://dailymed.nlm.nih.gov/dailymed/drugInfo.cfm?setid=9d2c209b-248e-4e26-9cde-fe0abe4428c1. Accessed April 2022.

Buspirone

Screening laboratory tests	Laboratory screening is not required.
Monitoring laboratory tests	Laboratory testing is not required.

American Society of Health-System Pharmacists: AHFS Drug Information. Bethesda, MD, American Society of Health-System Pharmacists, 2016

U.S. National Library of Medicine: Buspirone hydrochlorate tablet. DailyMed, February 19, 2022. Available at: https://dailymed.nlm.nih.gov/dailymed/drugInfo.cfm?setid=07a789a9-c9e8-4737-a56d-7d5405fe8100. Accessed April 2022.

Carbamazepine

Screening laboratory tests	• CBC with differential and platelets to establish baseline values. Drug can cause aplastic anemia, agranulocytosis, and thrombocytopenia.
	• LFTs, including AST, ALT, bilirubin, ALP, and lactate dehydrogenase.
	• Serum sodium to determine baseline value. Drug is associated with hyponatremia and SIAD.
	• BUN, creatinine, and urinalysis. Drug can be toxic to the kidneys.
	• TSH to establish baseline value. Drug can reduce thyroid function.
	• Lipid profile to establish baseline values. Drug is associated with changes in lipid values.
	• ECG to identify preexisting conduction abnormalities. Drug should be avoided in patients with AV block, bundle-branch block, or other conduction abnormalities.
	• Pregnancy test for patients of childbearing potential. Drug is associated with neural tube defects.
Monitoring laboratory tests	• Drug level should be drawn 5 days after initiation of therapy and after any change in dosage.
	• CBC with differential and platelets, electrolytes, and LFTs should be checked every 2 weeks for the first 2 months of treatment. If neutropenia or thrombocytopenia develops, the patient should be monitored closely.
	• Thereafter, periodic checks should be made of the CBC with differential and platelets, LFTs, BUN, creatinine, urinalysis, electrolytes, lipid profile, and TSH.

American Society of Health-System Pharmacists: AHFS Drug Information. Bethesda, MD, American Society of Health-System Pharmacists, 2016

U.S. National Library of Medicine: Carbamazepine capsule, extended release. DailyMed, January 13, 2022. Available at: https://dailymed.nlm.nih.gov/dailymed/drugInfo.cfm?setid=e91f9de3-3fdd-0a6b-71ce-53a2cc142816. Accessed April 2022.

Cariprazine

Screening laboratory tests	• CBC with differential. Leukopenia and neutropenia have been reported with this drug, and low baseline values increase this risk.
	• Consider LFTs, BUN, and creatinine. Drug is not recommended in patients with severe hepatic or renal impairment.
	• Fasting glucose, lipid profile, and weight to establish baseline values.
Monitoring laboratory tests	• Periodic check of CBC with differential. In patients with low baseline WBC count or ANC, check CBC with differential frequently during the first few months of treatment. Discontinue the drug in patients with an ANC <1,000/mm^3 and follow the WBC count until recovery.
	• Soon after initiation of the drug and periodically during treatment, check patient's fasting glucose and lipid profile and obtain weight.

U.S. National Library of Medicine: DailyMed: Vraylar: cariprazine capsule, gelatin coated. DailyMed, July 15, 2021 Available at: https://dailymed.nlm.nih.gov/dailymed/drugInfo.cfm?setid=3435ec73-86ed-46d1-bd1f-ee6c30209123. Accessed April 2022.

Citalopram

Screening laboratory tests	• LFTs (AST, ALT, total bilirubin). Dosing is limited in patients with hepatic impairment.
	• Serum sodium to establish baseline value. Drug is associated with hyponatremia, in many cases as result of SIAD.
	• Consider CYP2C19 genotyping. Dosing is limited in patients who are poor metabolizers of CYP2C19.
	• Consider ECG to determine baseline QTc and evaluate for other abnormalities. Drug should be avoided in patients with congenital long QT syndrome, bradycardia, recent MI, and uncompensated heart failure.
	• Consider checking potassium and magnesium. Low values increase risk of QT prolongation.
	• Consider EEG in patients with uncertain seizure control. Drug is associated with seizures in susceptible individuals.
	• Pregnancy testing for patients of childbearing potential. Drug may cause fetal and neonatal harm.
Monitoring laboratory tests	• Periodic check of sodium, potassium, and magnesium levels. In patients with symptomatic hyponatremia, drug should be discontinued and appropriate medical intervention instituted.
	• Periodic ECG to evaluate QTc changes. Drug should be discontinued if QTc is persistently >500 msec or QTc changes >20 msec.

American Society of Health-System Pharmacists: AHFS Drug Information. Bethesda, MD, American Society of Health-System Pharmacists, 2016

U.S. National Library of Medicine: Citalopram: citalopram tablets. DailyMed, September 26, 2020. Available at: https://dailymed.nlm.nih.gov/dailymed/drugInfo.cfm?setid=cf7b6823-108b-ebff-8f41-91f8b8325e3a. Accessed April 2022.

Clozapine

Screening laboratory tests	• For patient to be eligible for treatment, ANC must be ≥1,500/μL for the general population or ≥1,000/μL for patients with benign ethnic neutropenia (BEN). For patients with diagnosed BEN, obtain at least two baseline ANC levels before initiating clozapine. • ECG in patients older than 50 years or those with preexisting cardiac disease. Metabolic syndrome screening: • Fasting glucose • Fasting lipid profile • Weight, height, and BMI calculation • Waist circumference • Blood pressure
Monitoring laboratory tests	• ANC monitoring: See the Clozapine REMS document in the reference list below for monitoring instructions and schedules. • ECG if cardiac symptoms develop (e.g., extreme tiredness, flu-like symptoms, difficulty breathing or fast breathing, fever, chest pain, or fast, irregular, or pounding heartbeat) Metabolic syndrome monitoring: • Weight and BMI at 4 weeks, 8 weeks, and 12 weeks, then quarterly • Waist circumference yearly • Blood pressure at 12 weeks, then at least yearly • Fasting glucose and lipid profile every 6 months during treatment

American Society of Health-System Pharmacists: AHFS Drug Information. Bethesda, MD, American Society of Health-System Pharmacists, 2016

Clozapine REMS: Clozapine and the Risk of Neutropenia: A Guide for Healthcare Providers. Rockville, MD, 2021. Available at: https://www.accessdata.fda.gov/drugsatfda_docs/rems/Clozapine_2021_07_29_Clozapine_and_the_Risk_of_Neutropenia_A_Guide_for_Healthcare_Providers.pdf. Accessed April 2022.

U.S. National Library of Medicine: Clozapine tablet. DailyMed, September 8, 2020 Available at: https://dailymed.nlm.nih.gov/dailymed/drugInfo.cfm?setid=25c0c6d5-f7b0-48e4-e054-00144ff8d46c. Accessed April 2022.

Desvenlafaxine

Screening laboratory tests	• BUN, creatinine, and eGFR: Dosage adjustment is required in patients with moderate to severe renal impairment. • LFTs (AST, ALT, total bilirubin): Dosage adjustment is required in patients with moderate to severe hepatic impairment. • Blood pressure: Hypertension should be controlled before the drug is initiated. • Consider serum sodium to establish baseline value. Drug is associated with hyponatremia, in many cases as a result of SIAD. • Consider an EEG in patients with uncertain seizure control. Drug is associated with seizures in susceptible individuals. • Pregnancy testing for patients of childbearing potential. Drug may cause fetal harm.
Monitoring laboratory tests	Blood pressure should be checked regularly.

American Society of Health-System Pharmacists: AHFS Drug Information. Bethesda, MD, American Society of Health-System Pharmacists, 2016

U.S. National Library of Medicine: Desvenlafaxine: desvenlafaxine succinate tablet, extended release. DailyMed, October 9, 2019. Available at: https://dailymed.nlm.nih.gov/dailymed/drugInfo.cfm?setid=5bd203d2-477e-4d12-a875-cb8009f42410. Accessed April 2022.

Donepezil

Screening laboratory tests	Consider ECG to exclude preexisting conduction abnormalities before initiating treatment. Cholinesterase inhibitors may have vagotonic effects on sinoatrial and atrioventricular nodes that could manifest as bradycardia or heart block.
Monitoring laboratory tests	Monitoring labs are not required.

American Society of Health-System Pharmacists: AHFS Drug Information. Bethesda, MD, American Society of Health-System Pharmacists, 2016

U.S. National Library of Medicine: Donepezil: donepezil hydrochloride tablet. DailyMed, December 27, 2019. Available at: https://dailymed.nlm.nih.gov/dailymed/drugInfo.cfm?setid=2b1b7b5f-2f20-418c-b1ac-794c2ef1ce5e. Accessed April 2022.

Duloxetine

Screening laboratory tests	• Blood pressure and fasting blood sugar to establish baseline values. • Serum sodium to establish baseline value. Drug is associated with hyponatremia and SIAD. • LFTs to establish baseline values. Drug may aggravate preexisting liver disease and should not be prescribed to patients with chronic liver disease or evidence of hepatic insufficiency. • BUN, creatinine, and eGFR to establish baseline values. Drug should not be prescribed for patients with severe renal impairment (GFR <30 mL/min).
Monitoring laboratory tests	• LFTs monthly for first 3 months of treatment, then every 6 months • Serum sodium if patient develops symptoms of SIAD or hyponatremia, including headache, difficulty concentrating, memory impairment, confusion, weakness, and unsteadiness that could lead to falls. More severe and/or acute cases can be associated with hallucinations, syncope, seizures, coma, respiratory arrest, and death. • Periodic checks of blood pressure and fasting blood sugar

American Society of Health-System Pharmacists: AHFS Drug Information. Bethesda, MD, American Society of Health-System Pharmacists, 2016

U.S. National Library of Medicine: Duloxetine capsule, delayed release. DailyMed, November 25, 2021. Available at: https://dailymed.nlm.nih.gov/dailymed/drugInfo.cfm?setid=2dde979d-b6f8-41d1-96fb-325c75ea3a74. Accessed April 2022.

Escitalopram

Screening laboratory tests	• LFTs (AST, ALT, total bilirubin). Dosing is limited in patients with hepatic impairment. • Serum sodium to establish baseline value. Drug is associated with hyponatremia, in many cases as a result of SIAD. • Consider an ECG to determine baseline QTc if dosages above those recommended are to be used. Drug is associated with QT prolongation at supratherapeutic dosages. Also consider checking potassium and magnesium because low values increase risk of QT prolongation. • Consider an EEG in patients with uncertain seizure control. Drug is associated with seizures in susceptible individuals. • Pregnancy testing for patients of childbearing potential. Drug may cause fetal and neonatal harm.
Monitoring laboratory tests	• Periodic check of sodium, potassium, and magnesium levels. In patients with symptomatic hyponatremia, drug should be discontinued and appropriate medical intervention instituted. • Periodic ECG to evaluate QTc changes if supratherapeutic dosages are used. Drug should be discontinued if QTc is persistently >500 msec or QTc changes >20 msec.

American Society of Health-System Pharmacists: AHFS Drug Information. Bethesda, MD, American Society of Health-System Pharmacists, 2016

U.S. National Library of Medicine: Escitalopram: escitalopram oxalate tablet, film coated. DailyMed, October 7, 2021. Available at: https://dailymed.nlm.nih.gov/dailymed/drugInfo.cfm?setid=d5fbc8ce-bd41-4bd0-b413-0dea97e596c3. Accessed April 2022.

Fluoxetine

Screening laboratory tests	• Serum sodium to establish baseline value. Drug is associated with hyponatremia, in many cases as a result of SIAD.
	• Consider LFTs (AST, ALT, total bilirubin). Dosing is limited in patients with severe hepatic impairment (cirrhosis).
	• Consider an ECG to determine baseline QTc and evaluate for other abnormalities. Drug should be used with caution in patients with congenital long QT syndrome, prior history of QT prolongation, a family history of long QT syndrome or sudden cardiac death, or other conditions that predispose to QT prolongation and ventricular arrhythmia (including hypokalemia, hypomagnesemia, and use of other drugs that prolong the QT interval).
	• Consider an EEG in patients with uncertain seizure control. Drug is associated with seizures in susceptible individuals.
	• Pregnancy testing for patients of childbearing potential. Drug may cause fetal and neonatal harm.
Monitoring laboratory tests	• Periodic check of sodium, potassium, and magnesium levels. In patients with symptomatic hyponatremia, drug should be discontinued and appropriate medical intervention instituted.
	• Periodic ECG to evaluate QTc changes. Drug should be discontinued if QTc is persistently >500 msec or QTc changes >20 msec.

American Society of Health-System Pharmacists: AHFS Drug Information. Bethesda, MD, American Society of Health-System Pharmacists, 2016

U.S. National Library of Medicine: Fluoxetine capsule. DailyMed, October 20, 2021. Available at: https://dailymed.nlm.nih.gov/dailymed/drugInfo.cfm?setid=9de65da4-73f8-4c88-8198-c92e63224ddb. Accessed April 2022.

Fluvoxamine

Screening laboratory tests	• Serum sodium to establish baseline value. Drug is associated with hyponatremia, in many cases as a result of SIAD.
	• Consider LFTs (AST, ALT, total bilirubin). Drug should be started at a low dosage and titrated slowly in patients with liver dysfunction.
	• Consider an EEG in patients with uncertain seizure control. Drug is associated with seizures in susceptible individuals.
	• Consider an ECG to determine baseline QTc. Drug potently inhibits CYP1A2 and has significant interactions with other substrates of that enzyme that prolong the QT interval.
	• Pregnancy testing in patients of childbearing potential. Although studies of potential harm have had mixed results for this drug, fetal and neonatal harm is a class effect with SSRIs.
Monitoring laboratory tests	• Check serum sodium if any clinical evidence of hyponatremia is found. In patients with symptomatic hyponatremia, drug should be discontinued and appropriate medical intervention instituted.
	• ECG if other drugs metabolized by CYP1A2 are initiated or the dosage is changed.

American Society of Health-System Pharmacists: AHFS Drug Information. Bethesda, MD, American Society of Health-System Pharmacists, 2016

U.S. National Library of Medicine: Fluvoxamine maleate tablet. DailyMed, November 30, 2021. Available at: https://dailymed.nlm.nih.gov/dailymed/drugInfo.cfm?setid=8bbd7e39-b9ab-4716-9522-aa8c4b92210e. Accessed April 2022.

Gabapentin

Screening laboratory tests	• BUN, creatinine, and eGFR. Dosage adjustment is required if GFR is <60 mL/min.
	• Pregnancy testing in patients of childbearing potential. Drug may cause fetal harm.
Monitoring laboratory tests	Routine laboratory monitoring is not required.

American Society of Health-System Pharmacists: AHFS Drug Information. Bethesda, MD, American Society of Health-System Pharmacists, 2016

U.S. National Library of Medicine: Gabapentin capsule. DailyMed, December 30, 2021. Available at: https://dailymed.nlm.nih.gov/dailymed/drugInfo.cfm?setid=f2d9c3de-4749-4265-a26e-50026ab46ee4. Accessed April 2022.

Galantamine

Screening laboratory tests	• Consider an ECG to exclude preexisting conduction abnormalities before initiating treatment. Cholinesterase inhibitors have vagotonic effects on the sinoatrial and atrioventricular nodes that could manifest as bradycardia or heart block. • BUN, creatinine, and eGFR to determine whether dosage adjustment is necessary. • LFTs (AST, ALT, total bilirubin) to determine whether dosage adjustment is necessary.
Monitoring laboratory tests	Monitoring labs are not required.

American Society of Health-System Pharmacists: AHFS Drug Information. Bethesda, MD, American Society of Health-System Pharmacists, 2016

U.S. National Library of Medicine: Galantamine tablet, film coated. DailyMed, August 16, 2021. Available at: https://dailymed.nlm.nih.gov/dailymed/search.cfm?labeltype=all&query=galantamine. Accessed April 2022.

Guanfacine

Screening laboratory tests	Consider LFTs (AST, ALT, total bilirubin), BUN, creatinine, and eGFR. Drug should be used with caution in patients with chronic renal or hepatic failure.
Monitoring laboratory tests	Monitoring labs are not required.

American Society of Health-System Pharmacists: AHFS Drug Information. Bethesda, MD, American Society of Health-System Pharmacists, 2016

U.S. National Library of Medicine: Guanfacine hydrochloride tablet. DailyMed, January 13, 2022. Available at: https://dailymed.nlm.nih.gov/dailymed/drugInfo.cfm?setid=1c492e87-3406-ddb8-aaf2-e609c2ded503. Accessed April 2022.

Iloperidone

Screening laboratory tests	• ECG to determine baseline QTc. Drug prolongs the QT interval and may be associated with arrhythmia and sudden death. If baseline QTc is >500 msec, consider risks/benefits.
	• Serum potassium and magnesium levels to determine baseline. Hypokalemia and/or hypomagnesemia increase the risk of QT prolongation and arrhythmia.
	• Fasting glucose, lipid profile, and weight to determine baseline values.
	• CBC with differential. Low initial values for WBC count or ANC or any history of drug-induced neutropenia increases the risk of more severe neutropenia.
Monitoring laboratory tests	• Periodic ECG to determine QTc. If QTc is persistently >500 msec or increases >20 msec, consult cardiology and consider discontinuing drug.
	• Periodic serum potassium and magnesium levels
	• Periodic fasting glucose, lipid profile, and weight checks
	• Periodic check of CBC with differential. In patients with low baseline WBC count or ANC or a history of drug-induced neutropenia, check CBC with differential frequently during the first few months of treatment. Discontinue drug in patients with an ANC <1,000/mm^3 and follow WBC count until recovery.

American Society of Health-System Pharmacists: AHFS Drug Information. Bethesda, MD, American Society of Health-System Pharmacists, 2016

U.S. National Library of Medicine: Iloperidone tablet. DailyMed, August 2, 2019. Available at: https://dailymed.nlm.nih.gov/dailymed/drugInfo.cfm?setid=6f17cc91-86b3-42e3-9bf2-935dd360c3eb. Accessed April 2022.

Ketamine and esketamine

Screening laboratory tests	• Ketamine (parenteral) and esketamine (intranasal) are contraindicated in patients with recent MI (within 6 weeks), New York Heart Association Class III heart failure, aneurysmal vascular disease, or arteriovenous malformation.
	• Blood pressure must be taken at baseline and monitored frequently.
	• Urine toxicology screen could be performed if drug use is suspected.
	• LFTs (AST, ALT, total bilirubin) should be taken at baseline. Patients with moderate hepatic impairment may require a longer period of monitoring after drug dosing. These drugs are is not recommended for patients with severe hepatic impairment.
	• Pregnancy testing for patients of childbearing potential. Drug(s) may cause fetal harm.
Monitoring laboratory tests	• Treatment protocols include ECG and oxygen saturation monitoring during treatment.
	• Blood pressure closely monitored.
	• Capnography (exhaled carbon dioxide monitoring) used for higher dosages.

U.S. Food and Drug Administration: Spravato (esketamine) package insert. Available at: https://www.accessdata.fda.gov/drugsatfda_docs/label/2019/211243lbl.pdf. Accessed April 2022.

Lamotrigine

Screening laboratory tests	• ECG for baseline analysis. Patients with clinically important structural or functional heart disease require cardiovascular investigation and consultation with a cardiologist prior to drug initiation. • LFTs (AST, ALT, total bilirubin). Dosage adjustment is required in patients with moderate to severe hepatic dysfunction. • BUN and creatinine, with eGFR. A reduced maintenance dosage may be effective in patients with significant renal impairment. • Pregnancy testing in patients of childbearing potential. Drug may cause fetal harm.
Monitoring laboratory tests	• Repeat ECG at target dosage for patients with structural or functional heart disease. • Periodic check of BUN, creatinine, GFR, and LFTs.

American Society of Health-System Pharmacists: AHFS Drug Information. Bethesda, MD, American Society of Health-System Pharmacists, 2016

U.S. National Library of Medicine: Lamotrigine extended release tablet. DailyMed, April 30, 2021. Available at: https://dailymed.nlm.nih.gov/dailymed/drugInfo.cfm?setid=fb59c76a-9b6f-40ea-ac3a-58c3195c4377. Accessed April 2022.

Lemborexant

Screening laboratory tests	• Drug is contraindicated in patients with narcolepsy. If the diagnosis is uncertain, a multiple sleep latency test could be performed. • LFTs (AST, ALT, total bilirubin) to determine whether dosage adjustment is needed (for moderate hepatic impairment) or if the drug should be avoided (severe hepatic impairment).
Monitoring laboratory tests	Laboratory monitoring is not required.

U.S. National Library of Medicine: Dayvigo: lemborexant tablet, film coated. DailyMed, March 21, 2022. Available at: https://dailymed.nlm.nih.gov/dailymed/drugInfo.cfm?setid=7074cb65-77b3-45d2-8e8d-da8dc0f70bfd. Accessed April 2022.

Levetiracetam

Screening laboratory tests	• BUN, creatinine, and eGFR. Dosage adjustment is required for creatinine clearance ≤80 mL/min/1.73 m².
	• CBC with differential and platelets. Drug is associated with a range of hematological abnormalities.
	• Pregnancy testing in patients of childbearing potential. Drug may cause fetal harm.
Monitoring laboratory tests	• Periodic check of CBC with differential and platelets.
	• Periodic check of BUN, creatinine, and eGFR.

American Society of Health-System Pharmacists: AHFS Drug Information. Bethesda, MD, American Society of Health-System Pharmacists, 2016

U.S. National Library of Medicine: Levetiracetam ER: levetiracetam tablet, film coated, extended release. DailyMed, October 6, 2021. Available at: https://dailymed.nlm.nih.gov/dailymed/drugInfo.cfm?setid=5d3ce612-94de-4ad3-b873-27cb09304d45. Accessed April 2022.

Levomilnacipran

Screening laboratory tests	• BUN, creatinine, and urinalysis. Drug is mostly excreted renally. Dosage adjustment is required in patients with moderate to severe renal impairment, and drug is not recommended in patients with end-stage renal disease.
	• Serum sodium for baseline value. Hyponatremia has been reported, in many cases as a result of SIAD.
	• Consider an EEG in patients with a history suggestive of seizure disorder.
	• Pregnancy testing in patients of childbearing potential. Drug may cause fetal harm.
Monitoring laboratory tests	Although routine laboratory testing is not required, consider periodic checks of BUN, creatinine, urinalysis, and serum sodium.

American Society of Health-System Pharmacists: AHFS Drug Information. Bethesda, MD, American Society of Health-System Pharmacists, 2016

U.S. National Library of Medicine: Levomilnacipran capsule, extended release. DailyMed, July 30, 2020. Available at: https://dailymed.nlm.nih.gov/dailymed/drugInfo.cfm?setid=bcbc5d92-e022-4a0d-ab4d-2b0d7aa68c58. Accessed April 2022.

Lithium

Screening laboratory tests	• Drug may be contraindicated in patients with Brugada syndrome (abnormal ECG and risk of sudden death). If the patient's history with respect to this syndrome is unclear, consult cardiology. Consider an alternative drug. • Check BUN, creatinine, and urinalysis. Dosage adjustment is required for those with mild to moderate renal impairment, and drug should be avoided for those with severe impairment. • TSH to establish baseline value. • Electrolyte panel to establish baseline values. Particularly important for sodium, potassium, and calcium. • ECG for patients older than 40 years and any patient with preexisting cardiac disease. Greater risk of lithium toxicity with significant cardiovascular disease. • Consider CBC to establish baseline values. • Pregnancy testing in patients of childbearing potential. Drug may cause fetal harm. • Metabolic syndrome screening: fasting glucose, lipid profile, weight and height, BMI calculation, waist circumference, blood pressure
Monitoring laboratory tests	• Lithium level within 1 week of initiation and after each change in dosage, then every 2–3 months for the first 6 months of treatment • BUN, creatinine, and urinalysis with each level check. Drug is associated with chronic tubulointerstitial nephropathy with proteinuria. Urinalysis helps evaluate tubular function. • TSH every 3 months for the first 6 months, then every 6 months • After 6 months on a stable dosage, check patient's drug level, BUN, creatinine, and urinalysis every 6–12 months. In older patients, any patient with serum levels above the recommended maintenance levels, and those with any evidence of worsening renal function, check every 3 months or more frequently. • Check serum calcium concentrations regularly. Long-term lithium treatment is associated with persistent hyperparathyroidism and hypercalcemia. • Metabolic syndrome monitoring: fasting glucose and blood pressure at 12 weeks, then yearly; fasting lipid profile at 12 weeks, then every 5 years; weight and BMI at 4 weeks, 8 weeks, and 12 weeks, then quarterly. Waist circumference yearly.

American Society of Health-System Pharmacists: AHFS Drug Information. Bethesda, MD, American Society of Health-System Pharmacists, 2016

U.S. Library of Medicine: Lithium carbonate capsule. DailyMed, March 31, 2020. Available at: https://dailymed.nlm.nih.gov/dailymed/drugInfo.cfm?setid=63b3790f-a9b5-47f4-bae1-ddf8b43c13c1. Accessed April 2022.

Lofexidine

Screening laboratory tests	• CMP to evaluate liver function, renal function, and electrolytes. Dosage adjustment is needed in patients with hepatic or renal impairment, and electrolyte abnormalities (low potassium or magnesium) increase the risk of QTc prolongation. • ECG to establish baseline QTc value and assess for arrhythmias or other abnormalities. Drug should be avoided if the QTc is prolonged at baseline or if marked bradycardia is present. • Pregnancy testing in patients of childbearing potential. Risk to fetus is unknown.
Monitoring laboratory tests	Monitor ECG for patients with baseline renal or hepatic impairment or electrolyte abnormalities or those who are coadministered methadone.

U.S. National Library of Medicine: Lucemyra: lofexidine hydrochloride tablet, film coated. DailyMed, March 7, 2020. Available at: https://dailymed.nlm.nih.gov/dailymed/drugInfo.cfm?setid=b748f308-ba71-4fd9-84ec-ec7e0f210885. Accessed April 2022.

Lumateperone

Screening laboratory tests	• LFTs (AST, ALT, total bilirubin) to determine general Child-Pugh classification (A—good hepatic function, B—moderately impaired hepatic function, and C—advanced hepatic dysfunction). Drug is not recommended for those with moderate to advanced hepatic dysfunction. • WBC count and differential. Preexisting leukopenia or neutropenia is a risk factor for a significant decline in WBC count or ANC values. If baseline values are low or the patient has a history of drug-induced leukopenia/neutropenia, obtain CBC with differential. • Fasting glucose, lipid profile, and weight for baseline values. • Pregnancy testing for patients of childbearing potential. Drug may cause extrapyramidal and/or withdrawal symptoms in neonates with third-trimester exposure.
Monitoring laboratory tests	• Obtain CBC with differential frequently during the first few months of therapy for patients with a low baseline WBC count or ANC or a history of drug-induced leukopenia/neutropenia. If ANC is <1,000/mm^3, discontinue drug and follow WBC count until recovery. • Periodic monitoring of metabolic parameters: fasting glucose, lipid profile, and weight. Drug is known to have a favorable metabolic profile compared to other antipsychotics, but labs are still recommended.

U.S. Food and Drug Administration: Caplyta (lumateperone) package insert. Available at: https://www.accessdata.fda.gov/drugsatfda_docs/label/2021/209500s005s006lbl.pdf. Accessed April 2022.

Lurasidone

Screening laboratory tests	• BUN, creatinine, and urinalysis. Dosage adjustment is needed for moderate to severe renal impairment. • LFTs (AST, ALT, total bilirubin). Dosage adjustment is needed for patients with moderate to severe hepatic impairment. • CBC with differential. Low initial values for WBC count or ANC or any history of leukopenia or neutropenia increases the risk of a more severe reduction in blood counts. • Pregnancy testing for patients of childbearing potential Lurasidone has a relatively lower risk of causing the metabolic syndrome. Even so, metabolic screening and monitoring are recommended. Metabolic syndrome screening includes the following: • Fasting glucose • Fasting lipid profile (triglycerides and high-density lipoprotein) • Waist circumference • Blood pressure • Weight, height, and BMI calculation
Monitoring laboratory tests	• CBC with differential, BUN, creatinine, urinalysis, and LFTs at least annually. Metabolic syndrome monitoring: • Fasting glucose at 12 weeks, then yearly • Lipid profile at 12 weeks, then at least every 5 years • Waist circumference yearly • Blood pressure at 12 weeks, then every 6 months • Weight and BMI at 4 weeks, 8 weeks, and 12 weeks, then quarterly

American Society of Health-System Pharmacists: AHFS Drug Information. Bethesda, MD, American Society of Health-System Pharmacists, 2016

U.S. National Library of Medicine: Lurasidone hydrochloride tablet, film coated. DailyMed, May 17, 2021. Available at: https://dailymed.nlm.nih.gov/dailymed/drugInfo.cfm?setid=1cc441b3-0a23-4c68-a90e-436030b7daf2. Accessed April 2022.

Memantine

Screening laboratory tests	• BUN, creatinine, and urinalysis. Dosage adjustment is needed for patients with severe renal impairment. • Consider LFTs (AST, ALT, total bilirubin). Drug should be administered with caution in patients with severe hepatic impairment.
Monitoring laboratory tests	Monitoring labs are not required.

American Society of Health-System Pharmacists: AHFS Drug Information. Bethesda, MD, American Society of Health-System Pharmacists, 2016

U.S. National Library of Medicine: Memantine hydrochloride capsule, extended release. DailyMed, February 11, 2022. Available at: https://dailymed.nlm.nih.gov/dailymed/drugInfo.cfm?setid=f2b7538d-8ca1-4ac7-a172-d268e2fa9a52. Accessed April 2022.

Methylphenidate

Screening laboratory tests	• ECG and echocardiogram in patients with physical findings suggestive of cardiac disease or a family history of sudden death or ventricular arrhythmia. • Consider an EEG in patients with a history suggestive of seizure disorder. • Pregnancy testing in patients of childbearing potential
Monitoring laboratory tests	• Routine laboratory monitoring is not required. • Prompt cardiac evaluation with ECG and echocardiogram if syncope, exertional chest pain, or other cardiac symptoms develop • EEG if signs/symptoms of seizure develop

American Society of Health-System Pharmacists: AHFS Drug Information. Bethesda, MD, American Society of Health-System Pharmacists, 2016

U.S. National Library of Medicine: Methylphenidate capsule, extended release. DailyMed, June 16. 2021. Available at: https://dailymed.nlm.nih.gov/dailymed/drugInfo.cfm?setid=1f8983ce-71b8-4c62-830d-e4692ddededa. Accessed April 2022.

Milnacipran

Screening laboratory tests	• BUN, creatinine, and urinalysis. Drug should be used with caution in patients with moderate to severe renal impairment. Dosage adjustment is required in severe renal impairment, and drug is not recommended in end-stage renal disease. • Consider LFTs (AST, ALT, total bilirubin). Although dosage adjustment is not required for hepatic impairment, drug should not be used for patients with chronic liver disease. Mild elevations in ALT and AST have been seen with treatment. • Serum sodium for baseline value. Hyponatremia has been reported, in many cases as a result of SIAD. • Consider an EEG in patients with a history suggestive of seizure disorder. • Pregnancy testing in patients of childbearing potential.
Monitoring laboratory tests	Although routine laboratory testing is not required, consider periodic checks of BUN, creatinine, urinalysis, LFTs, and serum sodium.

American Society of Health-System Pharmacists: AHFS Drug Information. Bethesda, MD, American Society of Health-System Pharmacists, 2016

U.S. National Library of Medicine: Milnacipran HCL tablet. DailyMed, April 12, 2022. Available at: https://dailymed.nlm.nih.gov/dailymed/drugInfo.cfm?setid=eaa14195-1b9c-423c-9412-d2fe0857e39d. Accessed April 2022.

Mitazapine

Screening laboratory tests	• ECG to establish baseline QTc. If QTc is >500 msec, consider risks/benefits. Plan for close monitoring of ECG. • BUN, creatinine, and urinalysis. Clearance of mirtazapine is significantly reduced in patients with moderate to severe renal impairment. • Consider LFTs (AST, ALT, total bilirubin). Clearance of drug may be reduced in patients with hepatic impairment. • Consider WBC count with differential. Neutropenia and agranulocytosis are very rare but have been reported. • Pregnancy testing for patients of childbearing potential Metabolic syndrome screening: • Fasting glucose • Fasting lipid profile • Waist circumference • Blood pressure • Weight, height, and BMI calculation
Monitoring laboratory tests	• Regular ECG to check QTc. If the QTc is >500 msec or QTc change is >20 msec, consult cardiology and consider change of drug. • Periodic check of BUN, creatinine, urinalysis, and CBC with differential. Leukopenia with clinical evidence of infection should prompt evaluation and monitoring for agranulocytosis. • Consider LFTs. Transaminase elevations have been noted in patients treated with this drug. Metabolic syndrome monitoring: • Fasting glucose at 12 weeks, then yearly • Lipid profile at 12 weeks, then at least every 5 years • Waist circumference yearly • Blood pressure at 12 weeks, then every 6 months • Periodic check of weight and BMI calculation

American Society of Health-System Pharmacists: AHFS Drug Information. Bethesda, MD, American Society of Health-System Pharmacists, 2016

U.S. National Library of Medicine: Mirtazapine tablet, film coated. DailyMed, March 31, 2022. Available at: https://dailymed.nlm.nih.gov/dailymed/drugInfo.cfm?setid=9675333e-3064-c8cb-a4b4-6c74d9a82f17. Accessed April 2022.

Monoamine oxidase inhibitors*

Screening laboratory tests	• The first generation of non-selective MAOIs is characterized by very significant drug interactions and food prohibitions. Transdermal selegiline—a selective MAO-B inhibitor—has similar interactions and prohibitions for all but the lowest dose. • BUN, creatinine, and eGFR for non-selective MAOI use. These drugs should be used with caution in patients with abnormal kidney function and should not be used for patients with severe renal impairment. • Liver function testing (AST, ALT, total bilirubin) for non-selective MAOI use. These drugs should not be used for patients with abnormal liver function tests or history of liver disease. • Transdermal selegiline has not been studied in patients with severe liver dysfunction. • Blood pressure for baseline values for all MAOIs. These drugs should not be used for patients with preexisting hypertension. Hypertensive crises seen with MAOIs have sometimes been fatal. In addition, postural hypotension mostly affects patients with preexisting hypertension. • Consider an EEG for patients with uncertain seizure control who are considering treatment with isocarboxazid. This drug is known to lower the seizure threshold. • Pregnancy testing for patients of childbearing potential. These drugs may cause fetal harm.
Monitoring laboratory tests	• Periodic monitoring of kidney function: BUN, creatinine, and eGFR • Periodic monitoring of liver function: AST, ALT, and total bilirubin. MAOI should be discontinued at the first sign of hepatic dysfunction or jaundice. • Frequent monitoring of blood pressure and pulse • Periodic monitoring of weight with phenelzine use • Frequent check of blood glucose in patients also treated with blood glucose–lowering drugs. MAOIs can contribute to hypoglycemic episodes. Dosage reduction of the MAOI may be needed. • If MAOI toxicity is suspected, electrolytes and lactic acid should be checked.

*Includes isocarboxazid, phenelzine, tranylcypromine, selegiline transdermal.

American Society of Health-System Pharmacists: AHFS Drug Information. Bethesda, MD, American Society of Health-System Pharmacists, 2016

U.S. National Library of Medicine: DailyMed. Available at: https://dailymed.nlm.nih.gov/dailymed. Accessed April 2022.

Naltrexone

Screening laboratory tests	• Contraindicated in any patient who has failed a naloxone challenge test or had a positive urine screen for opioids.
	• Hepatitis screening. Drug is contraindicated in any patient with acute hepatitis.
	• LFTs (AST, ALT, total bilirubin, albumin, INR). Drug is contraindicated in patients with liver failure.
	• BUN, creatinine, and eGFR. Caution is advised in administering drug to patients with renal impairment because the parent drug and its primary metabolite are excreted mostly in urine.
	• Pregnancy testing for patients of childbearing potential. Drug may cause fetal harm.
Monitoring laboratory tests	No specific recommendations for laboratory monitoring, but consider periodic checks of BUN, creatinine, and eGFR, as well as LFTs.

American Society of Health-System Pharmacists: AHFS Drug Information. Bethesda, MD, American Society of Health-System Pharmacists, 2016

U.S. National Library of Medicine: Naltrexone hydrochloride tablet, film coated. DailyMed, February 8, 2017. Available at: https://dailymed.nlm.nih.gov/dailymed/drugInfo.cfm?setid=49aa3d6d-2270-4615-aafa-b440859ab870. Accessed April 2022.

Nefazodone

Screening laboratory tests	• Treatment is associated with liver abnormalities ranging from asymptomatic reversible elevation of liver transaminases to liver failure resulting in transplant and/or death. Time to liver injury for most serious cases ranges from 2 weeks to 6 months on this drug. There is no way to predict who will develop liver failure. Drug is contraindicated in patients with active liver disease and in those previously withdrawn from nefazodone because of evidence of liver injury. • LFTs (AST, ALT, total bilirubin, albumin, INR) to exclude active liver disease and establish baseline values. Drug should be avoided in patients with baseline transaminase elevation. Drug is associated with weight gain and the metabolic syndrome. Screening for the metabolic syndrome includes the following tests: • Fasting glucose • Fasting lipid profile • Weight, height, and BMI calculation • Waist circumference • Blood pressure
Monitoring laboratory tests	• LFTs at least every 3 months. If serum ALT or AST is ≥3 times the upper limit of normal, drug should be discontinued, and the patient should not be rechallenged. Metabolic syndrome monitoring: • Weight and BMI at 4 weeks, 8 weeks, and 12 weeks, then quarterly • Waist circumference yearly • Blood pressure at 12 weeks, then every 6 months • Fasting glucose at 12 weeks, then yearly • Fasting lipid profile at 12 weeks, then every 5 years

American Society of Health-System Pharmacists: AHFS Drug Information. Bethesda, MD, American Society of Health-System Pharmacists, 2016

U.S. National Library of Medicine: Nefazodone hydrochloride tablet. DailyMed, December 24, 2008. Available at: https://dailymed.nlm.nih.gov/dailymed/drugInfo.cfm?setid=b1d149db-ad43-4f3f-aef1-fb0395ba4191. Accessed April 2022.

Nonbenzodiazepine hypnotics*

Screening laboratory tests	• Liver function testing (AST, ALT, total bilirubin). Dosage adjustment is required. • Caution is advised when these drugs are administered to patients with compromised respiratory function. • Pregnancy testing in patients of childbearing potential. May cause fetal harm.
Monitoring laboratory tests	Laboratory monitoring is not required.

*Includes eszopiclone, zaleplon, and zolpidem.

American Society of Health-System Pharmacists: AHFS Drug Information. Bethesda, MD, American Society of Health-System Pharmacists, 2016

U.S. National Library of Medicine: DailyMed. Available at: https://dailymed.nlm.nih.gov/dailymed/index.cfm. Accessed April 2022.

Olanzapine

Screening laboratory tests	• CBC with differential to establish baseline values. Patients with a history of clinically significant leukopenia or neutropenia are at greater risk of a more severe reduction in blood counts. • Consider checking baseline prolactin level. • Pregnancy testing for patients of childbearing potential. Metabolic syndrome screening: • Fasting glucose • Lipid profile • Weight, height, and BMI calculation • Waist circumference • Blood pressure
Monitoring laboratory tests	• CBC with differential should be checked frequently during the first few months of treatment. • Prolactin level at 3 months on a stable drug dosage if signs/symptoms of prolactin elevation are seen. Repeat prolactin level after any change in dosage if signs/symptoms of prolactin elevation are seen. • BUN, creatinine, urinalysis, and LFTs (AST, ALT, total bilirubin) at least annually. Metabolic syndrome monitoring: • Weight and BMI at 4 weeks, 8 weeks, and 12 weeks, then quarterly • Waist circumference yearly • Blood pressure at 12 weeks, then every 6 months • Fasting glucose at 12 weeks, then yearly • Fasting lipid profile at 12 weeks, then every 5 years

American Society of Health-System Pharmacists: AHFS Drug Information. Bethesda, MD, American Society of Health-System Pharmacists, 2016

U.S. National Library of Medicine: Olanzapine tablet. DailyMed, October 23, 2015. Available at: https://dailymed.nlm.nih.gov/dailymed/drugInfo.cfm?setid=e8626e68-088d-47ff-bf06-489a778815aa. Accessed April 2022.

Olanzapine-samidorphan

Screening laboratory tests	• CBC with differential to establish baseline values. Patients with a history of clinically significant leukopenia or neutropenia are at greater risk of a more severe reduction in blood counts. • Consider checking baseline prolactin level. • Pregnancy testing for patients of childbearing potential Metabolic syndrome screening is recommended despite the inclusion of samidorphan. Tests include: • Fasting glucose • Lipid profile • Weight, height, and BMI calculation • Waist circumference • Blood pressure
Monitoring laboratory tests	• CBC with differential should be checked frequently during the first few months of treatment. • Prolactin level at 3 months on stable drug dosage if signs/symptoms of prolactin elevation are seen. Repeat prolactin level after any change in dosage if signs/symptoms of prolactin elevation are seen. • BUN, creatinine, urinalysis, and LFTs (AST, ALT, total bilirubin) at least annually Metabolic syndrome monitoring: • Weight and BMI at 4 weeks, 8 weeks, and 12 weeks, then quarterly • Waist circumference yearly • Blood pressure at 12 weeks, then every 6 months • Fasting glucose at 12 weeks, then yearly • Lipid profile at 12 weeks, then every 5 years

U.S. National Library of Medicine: Lybalvi: olanzapine and samidorphan L-malate tablet, film coated. DailyMed, February 24, 2022. Available at: https://dailymed.nlm.nih.gov/dailymed/drugInfo.cfm?setid=32ffddd1-4e2b-45d9-9b36-bb730167ec80. Accessed April 2022.

Opioids*

Screening laboratory tests	• The greatest risk in using opioid drugs is that of respiratory depression. Extreme caution should be used when initiating opioids in patients with pulmonary disease, right heart failure, hypoxia, hypercapnia, or preexisting respiratory depression. Patients must be monitored closely for respiratory depression, especially within the first 24–72 hours of initiating therapy and after dosage increases. • Consider urine drug screen before or at any time during treatment if multidrug use or diversion is suspected. • BUN, creatinine, and eGFR. Dosage adjustments may be required for patients with renal impairment. • Liver function testing (AST, ALT, total bilirubin). Dosage adjustment may be required for patients with hepatic impairment. • Consider an ECG to establish baseline QTc. Opioids such as oxycodone and hydrocodone are known to prolong the QT interval. • Consider an EEG for patients with unclear seizure control. Hydrocodone is associated with increased seizure frequency. • Consider CYP450 genotyping if codeine use is planned. This drug should be avoided in patients designated ultrarapid metabolizers at CYP2D6 because of toxicity and in patients designated poor or intermediate metabolizers because of insufficient pain relief. • Pregnancy testing in patients of childbearing age. May cause fetal and neonatal harm.
Monitoring laboratory tests	• Consider urine drug screen at any time during treatment if multidrug use or diversion is suspected. • Adrenal insufficiency has been reported with opioid use, more often following more than 1 month of treatment. Presentation may include nonspecific symptoms and signs including nausea, vomiting, anorexia, fatigue, weakness, dizziness, and low blood pressure. If adrenal insufficiency is suspected, confirm the diagnosis with laboratory testing as soon as possible. (See the entry on **Adrenal Insufficiency** in the *Diseases and Conditions* chapter.) If adrenal insufficiency is diagnosed, the patient should be treated with physiological replacement doses of corticosteroids and weaned off the opioid to allow adrenal function to recover.

*Includes codeine, hydrocodone, hydromorphone, morphine, oxycodone.

American Society of Health-System Pharmacists: AHFS Drug Information. Bethesda, MD, American Society of Health-System Pharmacists, 2016

U.S. National Library of Medicine: DailyMed. Available at: https://dailymed.nlm.nih.gov/dailymed. Accessed April 2022.

Oxcarbazepine

Screening laboratory tests	• BUN, creatinine, and eGFR
	• Serum sodium level
	• Pregnancy testing in patients of childbearing potential. Drug may cause fetal harm.
Monitoring laboratory tests	• Regularly scheduled checks of serum sodium level. Prompt check of serum sodium level if signs/symptoms of hyponatremia or SIAD are present.
	• Monitor clinically for evidence of DRESS. Syndrome typically presents with fever, rash, lymphadenopathy, and/or facial swelling in association with other organ system involvement, including hepatitis, nephritis, hematological abnormalities, myocarditis, or myositis. Eosinophilia is often present. Syndrome resembles an acute viral infection and requires immediate intervention and drug discontinuation.
	• Reductions in thyroxine (T4) are associated with the use of oxcarbazepine, without concomitant changes in triiodothyronine (T3) or TSH; thyroid monitoring is not required.

American Society of Health-System Pharmacists: AHFS Drug Information. Bethesda, MD, American Society of Health-System Pharmacists, 2016

U.S. National Library of Medicine: Oxcarbazepine tablet, film coated. DailyMed, November 12, 2020. Available at: https://dailymed.nlm.nih.gov/dailymed/drugInfo.cfm?setid=682a1210-b26e-426e-8ffe-d25d91bdd608. Accessed April 2022.

Paliperidone

Screening laboratory tests	• BUN, creatinine, and urinalysis. Dosage adjustment is required for impaired renal function. • ECG to exclude bradycardia and baseline QTc prolongation. Drug should be avoided in patients with congenital long QTc syndrome and those with a history of cardiac arrhythmias. • Electrolytes (potassium and magnesium) to determine baseline values. Low values increase the risk of malignant heart rhythms and sudden death in patients with QTc prolongation. • CBC with differential to establish baseline values. Patients with a history of clinically significant leukopenia or neutropenia or drug-induced leukopenia/neutropenia are at greater risk of a more severe reduction in blood counts. • Prolactin level to establish baseline value. Paliperidone has a prolactin-elevating effect like that seen with risperidone. • Pregnancy testing for patients of childbearing potential. Drug may cause fetal harm. Metabolic syndrome screening: • Fasting glucose • Lipid profile • Weight, height, and BMI calculation • Waist circumference • Blood pressure
Monitoring laboratory tests	• CBC with differential should be checked frequently during the first few months of treatment. • Prolactin level at 3 months on a stable drug dosage if signs/symptoms of prolactin elevation are seen. Repeat prolactin level after any change in dosage if signs/symptoms of prolactin elevation are seen. • BUN, creatinine, urinalysis, and LFTs (AST, ALT, total bilirubin) at least annually • ECG at least annually Metabolic syndrome monitoring: • Weight and BMI at 4 weeks, 8 weeks, and 12 weeks, then quarterly • Waist circumference yearly • Blood pressure at 12 weeks, then every 6 months • Fasting glucose at 12 weeks, then yearly • Lipid profile at 12 weeks, then every 5 years

U.S. National Library of Medicine: Paliperidone tablet, extended release. DailyMed, March 9, 2021. Available at: https://dailymed.nlm.nih.gov/dailymed/drugInfo.cfm?setid=7b269778-803b-4ce2-a8c0-636fb131d16a. Accessed April 2022.

Paroxetine

Screening laboratory tests	• Fasting glucose, lipid profile, and weight for baseline values. Drug is associated with more metabolic abnormalities than other SSRIs.
	• Serum sodium to establish baseline value. Drug is associated with hyponatremia, in many cases as a result of SIAD.
	• Consider BUN, creatinine, eGFR. Dosing is limited in patients with severe renal impairment.
	• Consider LFTs (AST, ALT, total bilirubin). Dosing is limited in patients with severe hepatic impairment.
	• Consider an EEG in patients with uncertain seizure control. Drug is associated with seizures in susceptible individuals.
	• Pregnancy testing for patients of childbearing potential. Drug may cause fetal and neonatal harm.
Monitoring laboratory tests	• Periodic monitoring of metabolic parameters: fasting glucose, lipid profile, and weight
	• Periodic check of serum sodium. In patients with symptomatic hyponatremia, drug should be discontinued and appropriate medical intervention instituted.

American Society of Health-System Pharmacists: AHFS Drug Information. Bethesda, MD, American Society of Health-System Pharmacists, 2016

U.S. National Library of Medicine: Paroxetine: paroxetine hydrochloride tablet, film coated. DailyMed, November 30, 2021. Available at: https://dailymed.nlm.nih.gov/dailymed/drugInfo.cfm?setid=1383d713-79b9-45bd-bd06-65707f28bc99. Accessed April 2022.

Pimavanserin

Screening laboratory tests	• ECG to establish baseline QTc and exclude bradycardia and any cardiac arrhythmias.
	• Consider electrolytes (potassium and magnesium). Low levels increase the risk of *torsades de pointes* and/or sudden death in the presence of QTc prolongation.
Monitoring laboratory tests	ECG annually or more often in presence of QTc prolongation or cardiac symptoms

U.S. National Library of Medicine: Nuplazid: pimavanserin tartrate capsule. DailyMed, February 8, 2022. Available at: https://dailymed.nlm.nih.gov/dailymed/drugInfo.cfm?setid=1e6bea44-57d6-4bac-9328-46e1ee59f83b. Accessed April 2022.

Pitolisant

Screening laboratory tests	• BUN, creatinine, and urinalysis. Dosage adjustment is required in moderate to severe renal impairment.
	• LFTs (AST, ALT, total bilirubin). Dosage adjustment is required in moderate hepatic impairment. Drug is contraindicated in patients with severe hepatic impairment.
	• ECG to establish baseline QTc. Drug prolongs the QT interval, so its use should be avoided in patients with a history of cardiac arrhythmias, symptomatic bradycardia, hypokalemia, hypomagnesemia, or congenital prolongation of the QT interval. This risk may be increased by renal or hepatic impairment.
	• Consider electrolyte testing (potassium and magnesium).
	• Consider CYP2D6 genotyping. Maximum dosage restricted for poor metabolizers.
	• Need for pregnancy testing in patients of childbearing potential has not been established.
Monitoring laboratory tests	ECG at least yearly. If QTc is persistently >500 msec or QTc increases >20 msec, intervention needed.

U.S. National Library of Medicine: Wakix: pitolisant hydrochloride tablet, film coated. DailyMed, March 12, 2021. Available at: https://dailymed.nlm.nih.gov/dailymed/drugInfo.cfm?setid=8daa5562-824e-476c-9652-26ceef3d4b0e. Accessed April 2022.

Quetiapine

Screening laboratory tests	• LFTs (AST, ALT, total bilirubin). Dosage limitations are required in hepatic impairment. • CBC with differential to establish baseline values. Events of leukopenia/neutropenia and agranulocytosis have been reported. • TSH and free T4 (FT4) levels. Drug is associated with a dosage-related decrease in thyroid hormone levels. • Consider ECG to establish baseline QTc. Drug should be avoided in patients with preexisting QT prolongation, a history of bradycardia or cardiac rhythm disturbances, hypokalemia, hypomagnesemia, or concomitant use of other QT-prolonging drugs. • Consider checking potassium and magnesium levels. • Consider serum prolactin level. Drug is associated with hyperprolactinemia in some patients. • Consider an EEG in patients with uncertain seizure control. Metabolic syndrome screening: • Fasting glucose • Fasting lipid profile • Weight, height, and BMI calculation • Waist circumference • Blood pressure
Monitoring laboratory tests	• Patients with preexisting leukopenia or a history of drug-induced leukopenia/neutropenia should have a CBC with differential performed frequently during the first few months of therapy. Drug should be stopped at the first sign of further decline in WBC count in the absence of other causative factors. Drug should also be stopped in patients with severe neutropenia (ANC <1,000/mm^3), and these patients should have CBC followed until recovery. • TSH and FT4 should be checked as clinically indicated. • Prolactin should be checked as clinically indicated. • Periodic check of ECG and potassium and magnesium levels Metabolic syndrome monitoring: • Fasting glucose at 12 weeks, then yearly • Lipid profile at 12 weeks, then at least every 5 years • Waist circumference yearly • Blood pressure at 12 weeks, then every 6 months • Weight and BMI at 4 weeks, 8 weeks, and 12 weeks, then quarterly

American Society of Health-System Pharmacists: AHFS Drug Information. Bethesda, MD, American Society of Health-System Pharmacists, 2016

U.S. National Library of Medicine: Quetiapine fumarate: quetiapine tablet. DailyMed, April 20, 2022. Available at: https://dailymed.nlm.nih.gov/dailymed/drugInfo.cfm?setid=07e4f3f4-42cb-4b22-bf8d-8c3279d26e97. Accessed April 2022.

Ramelteon

Screening laboratory tests	• Consider LFTs (AST, ALT, total bilirubin). Drug should be used with caution in those with moderate hepatic impairment and is not recommended for those with severe impairment. • Consider prolactin level to establish baseline. Drug is associated with increased prolactin levels. • Consider PSG for patients with suspected obstructive sleep apnea (OSA). Drug is not recommended for patients with severe OSA. • Pregnancy testing for patients of childbearing potential. Drug may cause fetal harm.
Monitoring laboratory tests	• No standard monitoring is required. • For patients presenting with unexplained amenorrhea, galactorrhea, decreased libido, or problems with fertility, assessment of prolactin and testosterone levels should be considered as appropriate.

American Society of Health-System Pharmacists: AHFS Drug Information. Bethesda, MD, American Society of Health-System Pharmacists, 2016

U.S. National Library of Medicine: Ramelteon tablet. DailyMed, March 28, 2022. Available at: https://dailymed.nlm.nih.gov/dailymed/drugInfo.cfm?setid=a89dae05-6c39-4072-b8ee-c4c35b46f7d4. Accessed April 2022.

Risperidone

Screening laboratory tests	• BUN, creatinine, and eGFR. Dosage limitations are required for patients with severely impaired renal function. • LFTs (AST, ALT, total bilirubin). Dosage limitations are required for patients with severe hepatic dysfunction. • Prolactin level to establish baseline value. Drug is associated with higher levels of prolactin elevation than other drugs in its class. • Consider CBC with differential. Drug is associated with neutropenia and agranulocytosis, although less often than other drugs in its class. Preexisting low WBC count or a history of drug-induced leukopenia/neutropenia increases this risk. • Weight and BMI calculation to establish baselines. Drug is associated with weight gain. • Consider an EEG in patients with unclear seizure control. Drug is associated with development of seizures. • Pregnancy testing in patients of childbearing potential
Monitoring laboratory tests	• Weight and BMI calculation at 4 weeks, 8 weeks, and 12 weeks, then quarterly • Periodic CBC with differential. If severe neutropenia develops (ANC <1,000/mm^3), drug should be discontinued and WBC/ANC followed until recovery.

American Society of Health-System Pharmacists: AHFS Drug Information. Bethesda, MD, American Society of Health-System Pharmacists, 2016

U.S. National Library of Medicine: Risperidone: risperidone tablet, coated. DailyMed, May 31, 2010. Available at: https://dailymed.nlm.nih.gov/dailymed/drugInfo.cfm?setid=c0c3eeb6-8a75-0b20-2008-396e63cddcdb. Accessed April 2022.

Rivastigmine

Screening laboratory tests	No requirements regarding laboratory screening. The following tests should be considered:
	• ECG to exclude supraventricular conduction abnormalities. Drug may have vagotonic effects on the heart, and this could be particularly problematic for those with sick sinus syndrome or related conduction abnormalities.
	• BUN, creatinine, and urinalysis. Patients with moderate to severe renal impairment may have difficulty tolerating anything but low dosages.
	• LFTs (AST, ALT, and total bilirubin). Patients with mild to moderate hepatic impairment may have difficulty tolerating anything but low dosages. Drug has not been studied in patients with severe hepatic impairment.
Monitoring laboratory tests	No recommendations regarding laboratory monitoring.

American Society of Health-System Pharmacists: AHFS Drug Information. Bethesda, MD, American Society of Health-System Pharmacists, 2016

U.S. National Library of Medicine: Rivastigmine tartrate capsule. DailyMed, February 19, 2018. Available at: https://dailymed.nlm.nih.gov/dailymed/drugInfo.cfm?setid=3d257f22-b504-4707-9b29-5ce9032667ca. Accessed April 2022.

Serdexmethylphenidate/Dexmethylphenidate

Screening laboratory tests	No requirements regarding laboratory testing. The following tests should be considered:
	• Baseline blood pressure and heart rate
	• ECG to exclude baseline abnormalities. Drug must be avoided in patients with known structural cardiac abnormalities, cardiomyopathy, serious heart rhythm abnormalities, coronary artery disease, and other serious heart problems.
	• TSH to exclude hyperthyroidism. Drug must be used with caution in hyperthyroid patients.
	• Pregnancy testing in patients of childbearing age
Monitoring laboratory tests	• Monitor all patients for hypertension and tachycardia.
	• Further cardiac evaluation indicated for patients who develop exertional chest pain, unexplained syncope, or arrhythmias during treatment.

U.S. National Library of Medicine: Azstarys: serdexmethylphenidate and dexmethylphenidate capsule. DailyMed, December 31, 2021. Available at: https://dailymed.nlm.nih.gov/dailymed/drugInfo.cfm?setid=00b5e716-5564-4bbd-acaf-df2bc45a5663. Accessed April 2022.

Sertraline

Screening laboratory tests	• Serum sodium to establish baseline value. Drug is associated with hyponatremia, in many cases as a result of SIAD.
	• Consider an EEG in patients with uncertain seizure control. Drug is associated with seizures in susceptible individuals.
	• Pregnancy testing for patients of childbearing potential. Drug may cause fetal and neonatal harm.
Monitoring laboratory tests	Check serum sodium if any clinical evidence of hyponatremia is found. In patients with symptomatic hyponatremia, drug should be discontinued and appropriate medical intervention instituted.

American Society of Health-System Pharmacists: AHFS Drug Information. Bethesda, MD, American Society of Health-System Pharmacists, 2016

U.S. National Library of Medicine: Sertraline hydrochloride: sertraline hydrochloride tablet. DailyMed, May 16, 2008. Available at: https://dailymed.nlm.nih.gov/dailymed/drugInfo.cfm?setid=8c8bcba9-eaeb-aa44-f9ea-b580de55a439. Accessed April 2022.

Sildenafil

Screening laboratory tests	• No recommendations regarding laboratory screening. No dosage adjustment is required for any degree of renal impairment. No dosage adjustment is needed for mild to moderate hepatic impairment. Drug has not been studied in severe hepatic impairment.
	• Because drug is a potent vasodilator, it should be used with caution in patients with left ventricular outflow obstruction (e.g., aortic stenosis) and in those with impaired autonomic control of blood pressure. In addition, data are inadequate regarding the safety of this drug in patients who have experienced an MI, stroke, or life-threatening arrhythmia within the prior 6 months; in those with resting hypotension (blood pressure [BP] <90/50) or hypertension (BP >170/110); or in patients with cardiac failure or coronary artery disease causing unstable angina.
Monitoring laboratory tests	No recommendations regarding laboratory monitoring.

American Society of Health-System Pharmacists: AHFS Drug Information. Bethesda, MD, American Society of Health-System Pharmacists, 2016

U.S. National Library of Medicine: Sildenafil citrate: sildenafil tablet, film coated. DailyMed, April 14, 2021. Available at: https://dailymed.nlm.nih.gov/dailymed/drugInfo.cfm?setid=ce683bbc-a1d2-4f23-b3d1-d9333d91dc55. Accessed April 2022.

Suvorexant

Screening laboratory tests	• Drug is contraindicated in patients with narcolepsy. If diagnosis is uncertain, a multiple sleep latency test could be performed.
	• Consider LFTs (AST, ALT, total bilirubin). Drug is not recommended in severe hepatic impairment.
	• Drug has not been studied in patients with severe obstructive sleep apnea or severe chronic obstructive pulmonary disease.
	• Exposure to suvorexant is increased in females and in patients with a BMI in the obese range.
	• Pregnancy testing for patients of childbearing potential. Drug may cause fetal harm.
Monitoring laboratory tests	Laboratory monitoring is not required.

American Society of Health-System Pharmacists: AHFS Drug Information. Bethesda, MD, American Society of Health-System Pharmacists, 2016

U.S. National Library of Medicine: Belsomra: suvorexant tablet, film coated. DailyMed, April 30, 2021. Available at: https://dailymed.nlm.nih.gov/dailymed/drugInfo.cfm?setid=e5b72731-1acb-45b7-9c13-290ad12d3951. Accessed April 2022.

Tasimelteon

Screening laboratory tests	• Consider LFTs (AST, ALT, total bilirubin). Drug is known to cause an elevation in serum transaminase levels (especially ALT) but not clinically apparent liver injury. Drug is not recommended in patients with severe hepatic impairment.
	• Pregnancy testing in patients of childbearing potential. Drug may cause fetal harm.
Monitoring laboratory tests	Laboratory monitoring not required.

American Society of Health-System Pharmacists: AHFS Drug Information. Bethesda, MD, American Society of Health-System Pharmacists, 2016

U.S. National Library of Medicine: Hetlioz: tasimelteon capsule. DailyMed, December 10, 2020. Available at: https://dailymed.nlm.nih.gov/dailymed/drugInfo.cfm?setid=ca4a9b63-708e-49e9-8f9b-010625443b90. Accessed April 2022.

Topiramate

Screening laboratory tests	• BUN, creatinine, and eGFR. Dosage adjustment is required in renal impairment.
	• Electrolyte panel or metabolic panel to check bicarbonate level. Topiramate causes a hyperchloremic, non-anion gap metabolic acidosis (decreased serum bicarbonate level in the absence of chronic respiratory alkalosis) due to renal carbonate loss from carbonic anhydrase inhibition.
	• Pregnancy testing in patients of childbearing potential. Drug is toxic to fetus.
Monitoring laboratory tests	• BUN, creatinine, and eGFR periodically during treatment
	• Electrolyte panel or metabolic panel to check bicarbonate level periodically during treatment
	• Ammonia level in patients coadministered valproate who develop encephalopathy, characterized by acute alterations in level of consciousness and/or cognitive function with lethargy and/or vomiting. In most cases, encephalopathy abates with discontinuation of treatment.

American Society of Health-System Pharmacists: AHFS Drug Information. Bethesda, MD, American Society of Health-System Pharmacists, 2016

U.S. Food and Drug Administration: Topamax (topiramate) package insert. Available at: https://www.accessdata.fda.gov/drugsatfda_docs/label/2017/020505s057_020844s048lbl.pdf. Accessed April 2022.

Tramadol

Screening laboratory tests	• BUN, creatinine, and cGFR. Dosage adjustment may be required in patients with renal impairment.
	• LFTs (AST, ALT, total bilirubin). Dosage reduction is recommended for patients with advanced liver disease.
	• An EEG should be considered in patients with a history suggestive of seizure disorder.
	• Pregnancy testing in patients of childbearing potential
Monitoring laboratory tests	No routine monitoring recommended by manufacturer.

American Society of Health-System Pharmacists: AHFS Drug Information. Bethesda, MD, American Society of Health-System Pharmacists, 2016

U.S. National Library of Medicine: Tramadol HCL: tramadol hydrochloride tablet. DailyMed, March 30, 2007. Available at: https://dailymed.nlm.nih.gov/dailymed/drugInfo.cfm?setid=ae7c54b1-b440-4cca-97e8-e5b825413d32. Accessed April 2022.

Trazodone

Screening laboratory tests	• BUN, creatinine, and eGFR. Drug should be used with caution in patients with renal impairment.
	• LFTs (AST, ALT, total bilirubin). Drug undergoes significant hepatic metabolism and has active metabolite *m*-chlorophenylpiperazine (m-CPP). It should be used with caution in patients with hepatic impairment.
	• Serum sodium level. Drug is known to cause hyponatremia, in many cases due to SIAD.
	• Serum potassium and magnesium levels. Hypokalemia and hypomagnesemia increase the risk of malignant cardiac rhythms.
	• Consider an ECG for patients with preexisting cardiac disease because drug may be arrhythmogenic. Trazodone should be avoided in patients with a history of cardiac arrhythmias or other factors that increase the risk of *torsades de pointes* and/or sudden death, including symptomatic bradycardia, hypokalemia or hypomagnesemia, and presence of congenital prolongation of the QT interval. It is not recommended for use during the initial recovery phase of MI. Drug prolongs the QTc interval, so other QTc-prolonging drugs should be avoided.
	• Pregnancy testing for patients of childbearing potential. Drug may cause fetal harm.
Monitoring laboratory tests	• ECG if the patient develops palpitations or other cardiac signs/symptoms.
	• Periodic check of serum sodium. If the patient develops symptomatic hyponatremia, trazodone should be stopped, and the patient should be treated urgently.
	• Periodic check of renal tests and LFTs, potassium, and magnesium

American Society of Health-System Pharmacists: AHFS Drug Information. Bethesda, MD, American Society of Health-System Pharmacists, 2016

U.S. National Library of Medicine: Trazodone hydrochloride tablet. DailyMed, December 23, 2021. Available at: https://dailymed.nlm.nih.gov/dailymed/drugInfo.cfm?setid=ed3039d8-3d27-4b71-a4b0-812943c9457f. Accessed April 2022.

Tricyclic antidepressants*

Screening laboratory tests	• Nortriptyline is contraindicated in patients with Brugada syndrome (syncope, abnormal ECG, and risk of sudden death). If a patient's history with respect to this syndrome is unclear, consult Cardiology and consider an alternative drug. It is not known whether this might be a class effect with TCAs.
	• ECG to establish baseline QTc and evaluate for arrhythmias, conduction defects, and evidence of cardiovascular disease. Caution is advised in treating patients with cardiovascular disease with TCAs; gradual dosage titration is recommended.
	• Liver function testing (AST, ALT, total bilirubin). Caution is advised in treating patients with liver impairment.
	• BUN, creatinine, and eGFR. Caution is advised in treating patients with renal impairment.
	• CBC with differential and platelets. TCAs are associated with a variety of hematological abnormalities, including agranulocytosis and thrombocytopenia.
	• Serum sodium to determine baseline value. TCA use is associated with hyponatremia and SIAD.
	• Consider checking TSH before initiating clomipramine. Thyroid dysfunction increases the risk of cardiac toxicity, including arrhythmias.
	• EEG before initiating clomipramine (and possibly other TCAs) because this drug significantly lowers the seizure threshold. Seizures precede cardiac dysrhythmias and death in some patients.
	• Consider CYP2D6 genotyping before initiating amitriptyline. Poor metabolizers have higher-than-expected plasma concentrations of this drug.
	• Pregnancy testing in patients of childbearing potential. TCAs may cause fetal and neonatal harm.
Monitoring laboratory tests	• Periodic ECG to determine QTc. If the QTc is >500 msec or if the QTc increases >20 msec, consult Cardiology and consider discontinuing drug.
	• Periodic check of BUN, creatinine, eGFR, and LFTs (AST, ALT, total bilirubin)
	• Periodic check of CBC with differential and platelets. In addition to routine testing, these labs should be performed in any patient who develops fever and sore throat during treatment. The drug should be stopped if there is evidence of neutropenia.
	• Check serum sodium if the patient develops symptoms of SIAD or hyponatremia, including headache, difficulty concentrating, memory impairment, confusion, weakness, and unsteadiness, which may lead to falls. More severe and/or acute cases can be associated with hallucinations, syncope, seizures, coma, respiratory arrest, and death.
	• Regular blood pressure checks
	• TCA drug level as clinically indicated to exclude toxicity or non-absorption/noncompliance
	• Serum prolactin level for patients with any evidence of hyperprolactinemia

Tricyclic antidepressants* *(continued)*

Monitoring laboratory tests *(continued)*	• Rare cases of DRESS syndrome have been reported with the use of clomipramine. DRESS syndrome typically presents with fever, rash, lymphadenopathy, and/or facial swelling in association with other organ system involvement, including hepatitis, nephritis, hematological abnormalities, myocarditis, or myositis. Eosinophilia is often present. The syndrome resembles an acute viral infection and requires urgent intervention and drug discontinuation.

*Includes amitriptyline, clomipramine, desipramine, doxepin, imipramine, and nortriptyline.

American Society of Health-System Pharmacists: AHFS Drug Information. Bethesda, MD, American Society of Health-System Pharmacists, 2016

U.S. National Library of Medicine: DailyMed. Available at: https://dailymed.nlm.nih.gov/dailymed. Accessed April 2022.

Valproate/Divalproex

Screening laboratory tests	• CBC with platelets. Drug causes thrombocytopenia with high-dosage therapy as well as leukopenia and other hematological abnormalities. • Coagulation testing (PT/INR, activated partial thromboplastin time [aPTT], thrombin time). Drug is associated with abnormal bleeding events. • LFTs (AST, ALT, total bilirubin) • TSH • Pregnancy testing in patients of childbearing potential. Drug may cause fetal harm.
Monitoring laboratory tests	• CBC with platelets every week during initial drug titration • After dosage stabilized, CBC with platelets and coagulation studies (PT/INR, aPTT, thrombin time) is performed quarterly. • LFTs every week during initial drug titration. • After dosage stabilized, LFTs at frequent intervals during the first 6 months of treatment • LFTs, serum ammonia, TSH, amylase, and lipase every 6 months thereafter • Valproate levels as needed to check noncompliance or toxicity due to interacting drugs or changes in clearance • Check valproate level in patients who have medication residue in stool. • Drug is associated with DRESS syndrome. If patient develops symptoms suggestive of this syndrome, immediate evaluation is indicated. Valproate should be discontinued.

American Society of Health-System Pharmacists: AHFS Drug Information. Bethesda, MD, American Society of Health-System Pharmacists, 2016

U.S. National Library of Medicine: Depakote: divalproex sodium tablet, delayed release. DailyMed, October 1, 2021. Available at: https://dailymed.nlm.nih.gov/dailymed/drugInfo.cfm?setid=f911748c-fb3a-fe1a-ab2a-4b40455e05ef. Accessed April 2022.

Vardenafil

Screening laboratory tests	• No specific requirements for laboratory screening. No dosage adjustment is required for mild, moderate, or severe renal impairment, but drug should not be used in patients who are on renal dialysis. • Consider LFTs (AST, ALT, total bilirubin). Dosage adjustment needed for patients with moderate hepatic impairment. Drug should not be used in patients with severe hepatic impairment. • Consider an ECG to obtain baseline QTc value. Patients with congenital long QT syndrome and those taking certain antiarrhythmics should avoid this drug. • Drug should be used with caution in patients with ventricular outflow obstruction (e.g., aortic stenosis) because of vasodilating effects. Drug is not recommended for patients with unstable angina, hypotension (resting systolic blood pressure <90 mmHg), uncontrolled hypertension (>170/110 mmHg), severe cardiac failure, or a recent history of stroke, life-threatening arrhythmia, or MI (within the past 6 months).
Monitoring laboratory tests	No specific requirements for laboratory monitoring.

American Society of Health-System Pharmacists: AHFS Drug Information. Bethesda, MD, American Society of Health-System Pharmacists, 2016

U.S. National Library of Medicine: Vardenafil hydrochloride tablet, film coated. DailyMed, October 18, 2021. Available at: https://dailymed.nlm.nih.gov/dailymed/drugInfo.cfm?setid=d2dce236-257e-44b6-93a9-9f0280257c6a. Accessed April 2022.

Varenicline

Screening laboratory tests	• No specific requirements for laboratory screening. No dosage adjustment is needed for patients with mild to moderate renal impairment. Dosage adjustment is needed for patients with severe renal impairment as well as for patients who are on hemodialysis. No dosage adjustment is needed for patients with hepatic impairment. • Consider an EEG for patients with a history of seizure with unclear seizure stabilization. Drug is associated with new or worsening seizures. • Pregnancy testing in patients of childbearing potential. Drug is not recommended in pregnancy.
Monitoring laboratory tests	No specific requirements for laboratory monitoring.

American Society of Health-System Pharmacists: AHFS Drug Information. Bethesda, MD, American Society of Health-System Pharmacists, 2016

U.S. National Library of Medicine: Varenicline: varenicline tartrate tablet, film coated. DailyMed, January 21, 2022. Available at: https://dailymed.nlm.nih.gov/dailymed/drugInfo.cfm?setid=f0ff4f27-5185-4881-a749-c6b7a0ca5696. Accessed April 2022.

Venlafaxine

Screening laboratory tests	• BUN, creatinine, and eGFR. Dosage reduction is needed for any degree of renal impairment.
	• LFTs (AST, ALT, total bilirubin). Dosage reduction is needed for any degree of hepatic impairment.
	• Consider serum sodium to establish baseline value. Drug is associated with hyponatremia, in many cases as a result of SIAD.
	• Blood pressure. Hypertension should be controlled before treatment is initiated.
	• Consider lipid panel to establish baseline values. Drug is associated with small increases in cholesterol and triglyceride levels.
	• Consider EEG in patients with uncertain seizure control. Drug is associated with seizures in susceptible individuals.
	• Consider ECG in patients at risk for QTc prolongation because of coadministered drugs or other factors. QTc prolongation has been reported with venlafaxine, although rarely.
	• Pregnancy testing for patients of childbearing potential. Drug may cause fetal harm.
Monitoring laboratory tests	• Periodic check of sodium, BUN, creatinine, GFR, LFTs, and lipid panel may show changes due to the long-term use of this drug.
	• Blood pressure should be monitored regularly.

American Society of Health-System Pharmacists: AHFS Drug Information. Bethesda, MD, American Society of Health-System Pharmacists, 2016

U.S. National Library of Medicine: Venlafaxine hydrochloride capsule, extended release. DailyMed, March 3, 2022. Available at: https://dailymed.nlm.nih.gov/dailymed/drugInfo.cfm?setid=6c7c6190-b35f-4228-ba3d-2cb3149c81b3. Accessed April 2022.

Vilazodone

Screening laboratory tests	Screening laboratory tests are not required, but pregnancy testing for patients of childbearing potential should be considered.
Monitoring laboratory tests	Monitoring laboratory tests are not required.

American Society of Health-System Pharmacists: AHFS Drug Information. Bethesda, MD, American Society of Health-System Pharmacists, 2016

U.S. National Library of Medicine: Viibryd: vilazodone hydrochloride tablet. DailyMed, March 24, 2021. Available at: https://dailymed.nlm.nih.gov/dailymed/drugInfo.cfm?setid=f917f30d-f2a7-43eb-836f-53eaa2a31cb0. Accessed April 2022.

Vortioxetine

Screening laboratory tests	• Consider CYP2D6 genotyping. Dosing is limited in patients who are poor metabolizers of CYP2D6. • Pregnancy testing in patients of childbearing potential. Drug may cause fetal harm.
Monitoring laboratory tests	Monitoring laboratory tests are not required.

American Society of Health-System Pharmacists: AHFS Drug Information. Bethesda, MD, American Society of Health-System Pharmacists, 2016

U.S. National Library of Medicine: Trintellix: vortioxetine tablet, film coated. DailyMed, September 27, 2021. Available at: https://dailymed.nlm.nih.gov/dailymed/drugInfo.cfm?setid=1a5b68e2-14d0-419d-9ec6-1ca97145e838. Accessed April 2022.

Ziprasidone

Screening laboratory tests	• ECG before treatment is initiated to determine baseline QTc measurement and evaluate for other abnormalities. Drug should be avoided in patients with a known history of QT prolongation, recent MI, or uncompensated heart failure and those with any history of cardiac arrhythmia. • Serum potassium and magnesium levels. Low levels increase the risk of malignant cardiac rhythms. • Consider LFTs (AST, ALT, total bilirubin, albumin, PT/INR). Liver dysfunction (Child-Pugh Class A/B) increases drug exposure and prolongs the half-life of ziprasidone. • Consider CBC with differential. This class of drugs carries a risk of neutropenia and agranulocytosis. • Consider an EEG. Drug is associated with seizures in susceptible patients. • Consider prolactin level to establish baseline value. Drug is associated with prolactin elevation. • Pregnancy testing in patients of childbearing potential
Monitoring laboratory tests	• ECG every 6 months, or more often as clinically indicated. Drug should be discontinued if QTc is >500 msec or change in QTc is >20 msec. • Clinical and laboratory monitoring for DRESS syndrome. DRESS typically presents with fever, rash, lymphadenopathy, and/or facial swelling in association with other organ system involvement, including hepatitis, nephritis, hematological abnormalities, myocarditis, or myositis. Eosinophilia is often present. DRESS resembles acute viral infection and requires urgent intervention and drug discontinuation.

American Society of Health-System Pharmacists: AHFS Drug Information. Bethesda, MD, American Society of Health-System Pharmacists, 2016

U.S. National Library of Medicine: Ziprasidone capsule. DailyMed, December 16, 2020. Available at: https://dailymed.nlm.nih.gov/dailymed/drugInfo.cfm?setid=8f78b278-a0b3-47ce-bbad-5dad7012896a. Accessed April 2022.

APPENDIX A

Therapeutic and Toxic Drug Levels at a Glance

Drug	Therapeutic level, *ng/mL*	Toxic level, *ng/mL*
Alprazolam		
1–4 mg/day	10–40	>100
6–9 mg/day	50–100	
Amitriptyline+nortriptyline	95–250	>500
Amoxapine	200–400	—
Aripiprazole+dehydroaripiprazole	100–350	≥1,000
Asenapine	1–5	≥10
Brexpiprazole	40–140	≥280
Buprenorphine	1 ng/mL cutoff*	—
Bupropion	10–100	≥400
Hydroxybupropion	850–1,500	≥2,000
Carbamazepine, total	4,000–12,000	>15,000
Carbamazepine, free	1,000–3,000	>3,800
Carbamazepine, % free (calculated)	8%–35%	—
Cariprazine	5–15	≥40
Citalopram	50–110	—
Chlordiazepoxide	500–3,000	>5,000
Nordiazepam	100–1,500	>2,500
Chlorpromazine	30–300	≥600
Clomipramine	230–450	>900
Clonazepam	20–70	>80
Clozapine	350–600	≥1,000
Desipramine	100–300	>500
Desvenlafaxine	100–400	—
Diazepam	200–1,000	—
Nordiazepam	100–1,500	>2,500
Doxepin+nordoxepin	100–300	>300
Duloxetine	30–120	—
Escitalopram	15–80	—
Fluoxetine+norfluoxetine	120–500	—
Fluphenazine	1–10	≥15
Fluvoxamine	60–230	—
Gabapentin	2,000–20,000	—
Haloperidol	1–10	≥15
Iloperidone	5–10	≥20
Imipramine+desipramine	175–300	>500
Lamotrigine	3,000–15,000	≥20,000
Levetiracetam	10,000–40,000	—
Levomilnacipran	80–120	—
Lithium		
Adults	0.6–1.0 mEq/L	≥1.5 mEq/L
Elderly patients	0.4–0.8 mEq/L	—

Drug	Therapeutic level, *ng/mL*	Toxic level, *ng/mL*
Lorazepam 1–10 mg/day	50–240	>300
Lurasidone	14–40	≥120
Milnacipran	50–110	—
Mirtazapine	30–80	—
Nortriptyline	50–150	>500
Olanzapine	20–80	≥100
Oxazepam	200–500	>2,000
Oxcarbazepine (monohydroxy-carbazepine)	3,000–35,000	>40,000
Paliperidone	20–60	>120
Paroxetine	20–65	—
Perphenazine	0.6–2.4	≥5
Phenytoin, total	10,000–20,000	>30,000
Phenytoin, free	1,000–2,500	>2,500
Phenytoin, % free (calculated)	8%–14%	—
Quetiapine	100–500	≥1,000
Risperidone	20–60	Risperidone+
9-hydroxyrisperidone	20–60	9-hydroxyrisperidone >120
Sertraline	10–150	>300
Topiramate	5,000–20,000	—
Trazodone	500–2,500	≥4,000
Valproate, total	50,000–125,000	>150,000
Valproate, free	6,000–22,000	>30,000
Valproate, % free (calculated)	5%–18%	—
Venlafaxine+o-desmethylvenlafaxine	195–400	≥800
Vortioxetine	10–40	—
Ziprasidone	50–130	≥400

*Therapeutic levels are trough levels, and toxic levels are random. The buprenorphine level noted is a cut-off, meaning that the concentration of the drug must be at or above that level to be reported as positive.

References

ARUP Laboratories: Laboratory Test Directory. Salt Lake City, UT, ARUP Laboratories, 2022. Available at: https://www.aruplab.com/testing. Accessed April 2022.

Eap CB, Gründer G, Baumann P, et al: Tools for optimising pharmacotherapy in psychiatry (therapeutic drug monitoring, molecular brain imaging and pharmacogenetic tests): focus on antidepressants. World J Biol Psychiatry 22(8):561–628, 2021

Schoretsanitis G, Kane JM, Correll CU, et al: Blood levels to optimize antipsychotic treatment in clinical practice: a joint consensus statement of the American Society of Clinical Psychopharmacology and the Therapeutic Drug Monitoring Task Force of the Arbeitsgemeinschaft für Neuropsychopharmakologie und Pharmakopsychiatrie. J Clin Psychiatry 81(3):19cs13169, 2020

Vogel F, Gansmüller R, Leiblein T, et al: The use of ziprasidone in clinical practice: analysis of pharmacokinetic and pharmacodynamic aspects from data of a drug monitoring survey. Eur Psychiatry 24(3):143–148, 2009

APPENDIX B

Additional Information on Neuroimaging

Neuroimaging signal appearance: MRI and CT

Tissue	MRI T1	MRI T2	CT
Dense bone	Dark	Dark	Bright
Air	Dark	Dark	Dark
Fat	Bright	Bright	Dark
Water	Dark	Bright	Dark
Brain gray matter	Gray	Intermediate	Intermediate
Brain white matter	White	Intermediate	Intermediate
Infarct	Dark	Bright	Dark
Blood	Bright[a]	Bright[a]	Bright
Tumor	Dark	Bright	Dark[b]
Multiple sclerosis plaque	Dark	Bright	Dark[c]
Edema	Dark	Bright	Dark
Inflammation	Dark	Bright	Dark
Infection	Dark	Bright	Dark
Calcification	Dark	Dark	Bright
Protein-rich fluid	Bright	Dark	—

[a]Unless fresh or old.
[b]Unless calcified.
[c]Often isodense.

Approach to reading a head CT scan

1. Identification: Check the patient's name, date of birth, and date of exam.
2. Orientation: Orient yourself to right/left sides and anterior/posterior aspects of the brain.
3. Locate the scale marker for measurement.
4. Note plane of exam: axial (usual), coronal, or sagittal (less common).
5. Note windows: brain, bone, or subdural.
6. Note slice thickness: written on the scan.
7. Note whether contrast material was given.
8. Look for midline shift:
    a. Draw an imaginary line between the midline inner table protuberances (frontal and occipital).
    b. Determine which midline structure is most displaced.
    c. Use the scale marker to measure the distance between the midline and the displaced structure.
    d. Note the direction of shift (right/left).
    e. Look for mass effect on one side or atrophy on the other side to explain displacement.
    f. Quantify displacement (in millimeters or centimeters, using scale marker).
9. Examine the ventricles: Look for abnormal size, shape, density (bright/dark), asymmetry.
10. Examine the cisterns: Look for abnormal size, shape, density (bright/dark), asymmetry.
11. Examine the sulci: Look for widening of sulci in atrophy, effacement with mass lesions, changes in density.
12. Examine the brain from superficial to deep, looking for abnormalities in size, shape, symmetry, density, displacement, gray-white matter differentiation, integrity, and presence of lesions.
    a. Lobes, gyri, corona radiata
    b. Basal structures (basal ganglia, internal capsule, thalamus, corpus callosum)
    c. Cerebellum and brainstem

APPENDIX C
Additional Cardiac-Related Information

Ten rules for a normal electrocardiogram

1. The PR interval should be 120–200 ms (three to five small squares).
2. The QRS complex should not be wider than 110 ms (fewer than three small squares).
3. The QRS complex should be mostly upright in leads I and II.
4. The QRS and T waves should have the same general polarity (up or down) in limb leads.
5. All waves in aVR are downgoing (negative).
6. The R wave should grow across precordial leads (V_1 to V_6), at least to V_4.
7. The ST segment should start at baseline (be isoelectric) in all leads except V_1 and V_2, where it may start above the baseline.
8. P waves should be upright in leads I, II, and V_2 to V_6.
9. Q waves should be absent, except for small Q waves of <0.04 seconds in I, II, and V_2 to V_6.
10. The T wave must be upright in I, II, and V_2 to V_6.

Source.   Douglas Chamberlain, M.D., F.R.C.P., Brighton and Sussex Medical School, University of Brighton, United Kingdom. Used with permission.

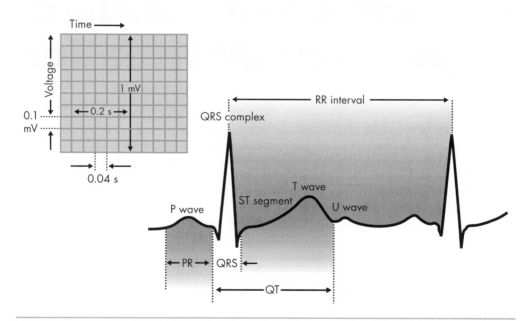

Figure C–1.   Waves and intervals on the electrocardiogram. Note that QT is corrected as follows: QTc=QT×(120+heart rate)/180.

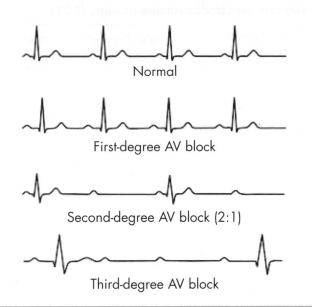

Normal

First-degree AV block

Second-degree AV block (2:1)

Third-degree AV block

FIGURE C–2. Heart blocks on the electrocardiogram.
AV=atrioventricular.

Cardiovascular risk assessment

The American College of Cardiology has developed a new tool for calculating a patient's 10-year atherosclerotic cardiovascular disease (ASCVD) risk—the ASCVD Risk Estimator Plus—for use with patients without existing ASCVD (primary prevention). The estimator requires the following input data: age, sex, race, systolic blood pressure, diastolic blood pressure, total cholesterol, high-density lipoprotein cholesterol, low-density lipoprotein cholesterol, diabetes history, smoking history, antihypertensive use, statin use, and aspirin use. The tool is available at https://tools.acc.org/ASCVD-Risk-Estimator-Plus/?_ga=2.97656095.1633232292. 1650655285%E2%80%93921864359.1650655285#!/calculate/estimate.

Medical evaluation for electroconvulsive therapy (ECT)

The 2001 Consensus Statement from the American Psychiatric Association listed no absolute contraindications to ECT. Several preexisting medical conditions can elevate the risk associated with ECT, however, such that a pre-procedure evaluation is performed. In general, ECT is considered a low-risk procedure.

Physiological changes during ECT include the following:

- Initially, stimulation of the vagus nerve causes bradycardia and, in some patients, asystole for up to 5 seconds.

- With the onset of seizure activity, sympathetic tone increases, and tachycardia and hypertension occur. At this time, the patient may be at risk of cardiac dysrhythmia, ischemia, or hypertensive crisis.

- There is an expected increase of 25 mmHg in systolic and diastolic blood pressures during ECT.

- Also, with onset of seizure activity, blood flow to the brain and brain metabolism increase dramatically. Increased blood flow causes increased intracranial pressure.

- Anesthesia used with ECT depresses the respiratory drive.

Risks of ECT include the following:

- Cardiac dysrhythmia—ventricular ectopy, most likely to occur in those with previous dysrhythmia.

- Cardiac ischemia—most likely to occur in those with coronary artery disease (CAD). In general, the risk factors for complications with ECT include not only CAD but also cerebrovascular disease, diabetes, kidney disease (creatinine >2 mg/dL), and congestive heart failure. Hypertension (≥140/90) is controlled before ECT commences.

- Increased intracranial pressure—may be problematic in patients with preexisting hydrocephalus, tumor, or aneurysm. Caution is advised in treating these patients.

- Prolonged seizure in patients taking medication that lowers the seizure threshold and in those with electrolyte derangements.

- Bronchospasm in those with chronic obstructive pulmonary disease or asthma. Caution is advised in treating these patients.

- Apnea in patients unable to metabolize succinylcholine.

Laboratory workup in preparation for ECT includes the following:

- ECG in patients older than 50 years, those with a previous abnormal ECG, and those with known cardiac disease or with symptoms suggestive of cardiac disease.

- Neuroimaging to rule out increased intracranial pressure in patients with abnormal neurological exams or known intracranial masses.

- Electrolytes, BUN, and creatinine in patients taking diuretics or antihypertensives and those with malnutrition, congestive heart failure, diabetes, or known renal disease.

- Pregnancy test for patients of childbearing age.

- Echocardiogram for patients with aortic stenosis, if not done within the past year or if symptoms have changed. Reconsider ECT if aortic stenosis is moderate or severe. Consult with cardiology.

- Pacemaker testing before and after ECT. Magnet should be placed at the patient's bedside for use in the event of bradycardia from pacemaker inhibition.

Medical evaluation for electroconvulsive therapy (ECT) *(continued)*

- Continuous ECG monitoring during ECT for patients with implantable cardioverter-defibrillator devices. Detection mode is turned OFF during ECT. Proper patient grounding is essential. An external defibrillator should be placed at the patient's bedside.

- Elevation of INR should be maintained for patients on chronic anticoagulation, up to 3.5 unless the patient is at risk of intracranial hemorrhage (e.g., from tumor or aneurysm).

- Blood glucose should be checked before and after ECT for patients with diabetes.

- For pregnant patients, before and after ECT, noninvasive fetal monitoring should be done after 14 weeks and a nonstress test with a tocometer should be done after 24 weeks.

American Psychiatric Association: The Practice of Electroconvulsive Therapy: Recommendations for Treatment, Training, and Privileging, 2nd Edition. A Task Force Report of the American Psychiatric Association. Washington, DC, American Psychiatric Association, 2001

Tess AV, Smetana GW: Medical evaluation of patients undergoing electroconvulsive therapy. N Engl J Med 360:1437–1444, 2009

APPENDIX D
The Bilirubin Cycle

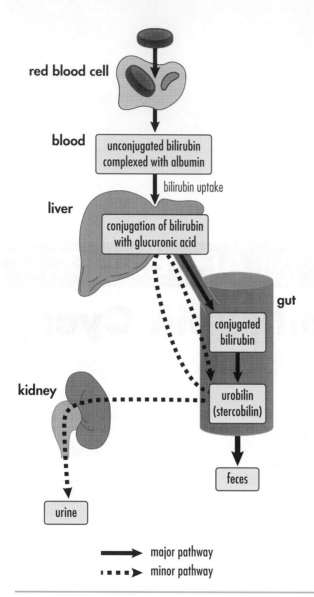

Bilirubin is derived mainly from red blood cell (hemoglobin) breakdown. This is unconjugated bilirubin. It travels with albumin to the liver.

In the liver, bilirubin is conjugated with glucuronic acid, making it water-soluble. It can then be excreted in feces and urine.

Prehepatic disease such as hemolytic anemia causes increased unconjugated bilirubin.

Posthepatic disease such as bile duct obstruction causes increased conjugated bilirubin.

Liver disease such as hepatitis causes increased conjugated and unconjugated bilirubin.

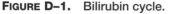

FIGURE D–1. Bilirubin cycle.

Red blood cell breakdown gives rise to bilirubin in the circulation, which binds to albumin and travels to the liver. There, bilirubin is conjugated with glucuronic acid and secreted into bile and then to the GI tract. In the gut, the glucuronic acid is removed, and the bilirubin is converted to urobilinogen and then to the brown-colored stercobilin.

APPENDIX E

The Syndrome of Inappropriate Antidiuresis

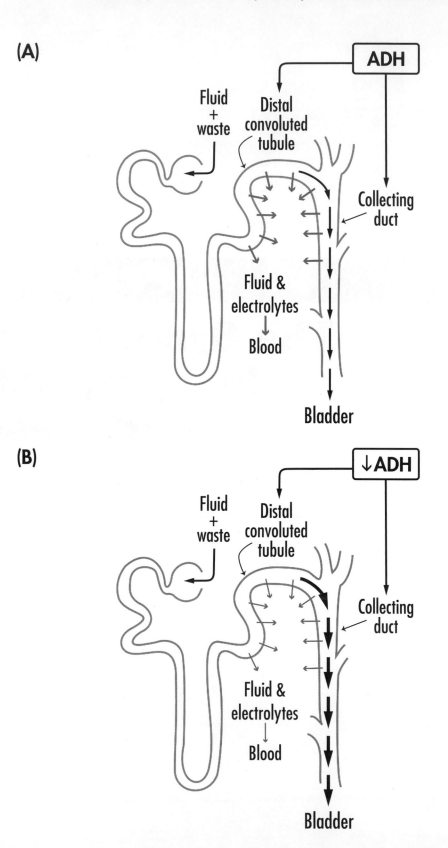

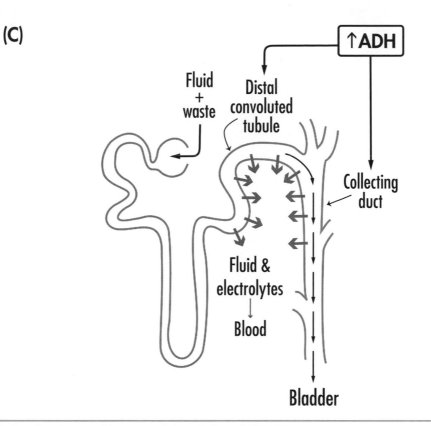

FIGURE E–1. Syndrome of inappropriate antidiuresis (SIAD).

(A) Antidiuretic hormone (ADH) acts on the nephron, which controls water excretion. **(B)** When serum ADH level is decreased, the nephron excretes water. **(C)** When the serum ADH level is increased, the nephron retains water. Serum becomes dilute, while urine becomes concentrated. At the same time, serum sodium decreases and urine sodium increases. Under normal conditions, a drop in serum osmolality signals osmoreceptors in the hypothalamus to reduce ADH secretion. In certain conditions and with certain drugs, however, ADH continues to be secreted when serum osmolality is low. This is SIAD, in which serum osmolality is low, urine osmolality is high, serum sodium is low, and urine sodium is high.

References

Laboratory Tests Section

Abi-Saleh B, Iskandar SB, Elgharib N, et al: C-reactive protein: the harbinger of cardiovascular diseases. South Med J 101(5):525–533, 2008

Adrogue HJ, Madias NE: Hyponatremia. N Engl J Med 342(21):1581–1589, 2000

Agarwal N, Port JD, Bazzocchi M, et al: Update on the use of MR for assessment and diagnosis of psychiatric diseases. Radiology 255(1):23–41, 2010

Agrawal S, Dhiman RK, Limdi JK: Evaluation of abnormal liver function tests. Postgrad Med J 92(1086):223–34, 2016

Ahmadi L, Goldman MB: Primary polydipsia: update. Best Pract Res Clin Endocrinol Metab 34(5):101469, 2020

Akhavizadegan H, Hosamirudsari H, Alizadeh M, et al: Can laboratory tests at the time of admission guide us to the prognosis of patients with COVID-19? J Prev Med Hyg 62(2):E321–E325, 2021

Ali SN, Bazzano LA. Hyponatremia in association with second-generation antipsychotics: a systematic review of case reports. Ochsner J 18(3):230–235, 2018

Aljomah AS, Hammami MM: Superfluous amylase/lipase testing at a tertiary care hospital: a retrospective study. Ann Saudi Med 39(5):354–358, 2019

Allen JA, Peterson A, Sufit R, et al: Post-epidemic eosinophilia-myalgia syndrome associated with L-tryptophan. Arthritis Rheum 63(11):3633–3639, 2011

Allen JP, Sillanaukee P, Strid N, et al: Biomarkers of heavy drinking, in Assessing Alcohol Problems: A Guide for Clinicians and Researchers. Bethesda, MD, National Institute on Alcohol Abuse and Alcoholism, 2004. Available at: https://pubs.niaaa.nih.gov/publications/assessingalcohol/allen.pdf. Accessed July 28, 2022.

Almeida PH, Matielo CEL, Curvelo LA, et al: Update on the management and treatment of viral hepatitis. World J Gastroenterol 27(23):3249–3261, 2021

Amen DG, Trujillo M, Newberg A, et al: Brain SPECT imaging in complex psychiatric cases: an evidence-based, underutilized tool. Open Neuroimag J 5:40–48, 2011

American Cancer Society: American Cancer Society recommendations for the early detection of breast cancer, in Breast Cancer Early Detection and Diagnosis. Kennesaw, GA, American Cancer Society, 2022. Available at: https://www.cancer.org/cancer/breast-cancer/screening-tests-and-early-detection/american-cancer-society-recommendations-for-the-early-detection-of-breast-cancer.html. Accessed July 22, 2022.

American College of Radiology Committee on Appropriateness Criteria: American College of Radiology Appropriateness Criteria for Acute Mental Status Change, Delirium, and New Onset Psychosis. Reston, VA, American College of Radiology, 2018. Available at: https://acsearch.acr.org/docs/3102409/Narrative. Accessed July 28, 2022.

American College of Radiology Committee on Appropriateness Criteria: American College of Radiology Appropriateness Criteria for Cerebrovascular Disease. Reston, VA, American College of Radiology, 2016. Available at: https://acsearch.acr.org/docs/69478/Narrative. Accessed July 22, 2022.

American Society of Health-System Pharmacists: AHFS Drug Information. Bethesda, MD, American Society of Health-System Pharmacists, 2016

Anam AK, Insogna K: Update on osteoporosis screening and management. Med Clin North Am 105(6):1117–1134, 2021

Andrade L, Paiva T: Ambulatory versus laboratory polysomnography in obstructive sleep apnea: comparative assessment of quality, clinical efficacy, treatment compliance, and quality of life. J Clin Sleep Med 14(8):1323–1331, 2018

Andrès E, Loukili NH, Noel E, et al: Vitamin B12 (cobalamin) deficiency in elderly patients. CMAJ 171(3):251–259, 2004

Angelini C, Marozzo R, Pegoraro V, et al: Diagnostic challenges in metabolic myopathies. Expert Rev Neurother 20(12):1287–1298, 2020

Anglin RE, Samaan Z, Walter SD, et al: Vitamin D deficiency and depression in adults: systematic review and meta-analysis. Br J Psychiatry 202:100–107, 2013

Anniss AM, Young A, O'Driscoll DM: Importance of urinary drug screening in the multiple sleep latency test and maintenance of wakefulness test. J Clin Sleep Med 12(12):1633–1640, 2016

Annweiler C, Dursun E, Féron F, et al: "Vitamin D and cognition in older adults": updated international recommendations. J Intern Med 277(1):45–57, 2015

Arboleda-Velasquez JF, Lopera F, O'Hare M, et al: Resistance to autosomal dominant Alzheimer's disease in an APOE3 Christchurch homozygote: a case report. Nat Med 25(11):1680–1683, 2019

Arnett DK, Blumenthal RS, Albert MA, et al: 2019 ACC/AHA guideline on the primary prevention of cardiovascular disease: a report of the American College of Cardiology/American Heart Association Task Force on Clinical Practice Guidelines. Circulation 140(11):e596–e646, 2019

ARUP Laboratories: Drug plasma half-life and urine detection window, in Laboratory Test Directory. Salt Lake City, UT, ARUP Laboratories, 2021. Available at: https://www.aruplab.com/files/resources/pain-management/DrugAnalytesPlasmaUrine.pdf. Accessed July 22, 2022.

ARUP Laboratories: Laboratory Test Directory. Salt Lake City, UT, ARUP Laboratories, 2022. Available at: https://www.aruplab.com. Accessed July 22, 2022.

Atallah-Yunes SA, Ready A, Newburger PE: Benign ethnic neutropenia. Blood Rev 37:100586, 2019

Atar D, Jukema JW, Molemans B, et al: New cardiovascular prevention guidelines: How to optimally manage dyslipidaemia and cardiovascular risk in 2021 in patients needing secondary prevention? Atherosclerosis 319:51–61, 2021

Ates Bulut E, Soysal P, Aydin AE, et al: Vitamin B12 deficiency might be related to sarcopenia in older adults. Exp Gerontol 95:136–140, 2017

Auerbach M, Adamson JW: How we diagnose and treat iron deficiency anemia. Am J Hematol 91(1):31–38, 2016

Azar RR, Sarkis A, Giannitsis E: A practical approach for the use of high-sensitivity cardiac troponin assays in the evaluation of patients with chest pain. Am J Cardiol 139:1–7, 2021

Barbesino G: Thyroid function changes in the elderly and their relationship to cardiovascular health: a mini-review. Gerontology 65(1):1–8, 2019

Barceloux DG, Krenzelok EP, Olson K, et al: American Academy of Clinical Toxicology practice guidelines on the treatment of ethylene glycol poisoning. Ad Hoc Committee. J Toxicol Clin Toxicol 37(5):537–560, 1999

Barlass U, Wiliams B, Dhana K, et al: Marked elevation of lipase in COVID-19 disease: a cohort study. Clin Transl Gastroenterol 11(7):e00215, 2020

Barocas DA, Boorjian SA, Alvarez RD, et al: Microhematuria: AUA/SUFU guideline. J Urol 204:778, 2020

Barrons RW, Nguyen LT: Succinylcholine-induced rhabdomyolysis in adults: case report and review of the literature. J Pharm Pract 33(1):102–107, 2020

Barstow C, Braun M: Electrolytes: calcium disorders. FP Essent 459:29–34, 2017

Bart G, Piccolo P, Zhang L, et al: Markers for hepatitis A, B and C in methadone-maintained patients: an unexpectedly high co-infection with silent hepatitis B. Addiction 103(4):681–686, 2008

Becker GJ, Garigali G, Fogazzi GB: Advances in urine microscopy. Am J Kidney Dis 67(6):954–964, 2016

Belteczki Z, Ujvari J, Dome P: Clozapine withdrawal-induced malignant catatonia or neuroleptic malignant syndrome: a case report and a brief review of the literature. Clin Neuropharmacol 44(4):148–153, 2021

Ben-Yehuda O: High-sensitivity C-reactive protein in every chart? The use of biomarkers in individual patients. J Am Coll Cardiol 49(21):2139–2141, 2007

Bender A, Hagan KE, Kingston N: The association of folate and depression: a meta-analysis. J Psychiatr Res 95:9–18, 2017

Bennys K, Portet F, Touchon J, et al: Diagnostic value of event-related evoked potentials N200 and P300 subcomponents in early diagnosis of Alzheimer's disease and mild cognitive impairment. J Clin Neurophysiol 24(5):405–412, 2007

Benoit SW, Ciccia EA, Devarajan P: Cystatin C as a biomarker of chronic kidney disease: latest developments. Expert Rev Mol Diagn 20(10):1019–1026, 2020

Benseler SM, Silverman ED: Neuropsychiatric involvement in pediatric systemic lupus erythematosus. Lupus 16(8):564–571, 2007

Benvenga S: L-T4 Therapy in the presence of pharmacological interferents. Front Endocrinol (Lausanne) 11:607446, 2020

Bertolini A, van de Peppel IP, Bodewes FAJA, et al: Abnormal liver function tests in patients with COVID-19: relevance and potential pathogenesis. Hepatology 72(5):1864–1872, 2020

Bielecka-Dabrowa A, Cichocka-Radwan A, Lewek J, et al: Cardiac manifestations of COVID-19. Rev Cardiovasc Med 22(2):365–371, 2021

Blanco Vela CI, Bosques Padilla FJ: Determination of ammonia concentrations in cirrhosis patients-still confusing after all these years? Ann Hepatol 10 (Suppl 2):S60–S65, 2011

Blennow K, Zetterberg H: Biomarkers for Alzheimer's disease: current status and prospects for the future. J Intern Med 284(6):643–663, 2018

Bobbitt WH, Williams RM, Freed CR: Severe ethylene glycol intoxication with multisystem failure. West J Med 144(2):225–228, 1986

Boldt J: Use of albumin: an update. Br J Anaesth 104(3):276–284, 2010

Borges L, Pithon-Curi TC, Curi R, et al: COVID-19 and neutrophils: the relationship between hyperinflammation and neutrophil extracellular traps. Mediators Inflamm 2020:8829674, 2020

Borghi C, Agabiti-Rosei E, Johnson RJ, et al: Hyperuricaemia and gout in cardiovascular, metabolic and kidney disease. Eur J Intern Med 80:1–11, 2020

Bortolotti F, Sorio D, Bertaso A, et al: Analytical and diagnostic aspects of carbohydrate deficient transferrin (CDT): a critical review over years 2007–2017. J Pharm Biomed Anal 147:2–12, 2018

Boulos MI, Jairam T, Kendzerska T, et al: Normal polysomnography parameters in healthy adults: a systematic review and meta-analysis. Lancet Respir Med 7(6):533–543, 2019

Bowen BC, Quencer RM, Margosian P, et al: MR angiography of occlusive disease of the arteries in the head and neck: current concepts. AJR Am J Roentgenol 162(1):9–18, 1994

Bowen R, Benavides R, Colón-Franco JM, et al: Best practices in mitigating the risk of biotin interference with laboratory testing. Clin Biochem 74:1–11, 2019

Boxhoorn L, Voermans RP, Bouwense SA, et al: Acute pancreatitis. Lancet 396(10252):726–734, 2020

Bradley P, Shiekh M, Mehra V, et al: Improved efficacy with targeted pharmacogenetic-guided treatment of patients with depression and anxiety: a randomized clinical trial demonstrating clinical utility. J Psychiatr Res 96:100–107, 2018

Bradley R, Fitzpatrick AL, Jenny NS, et al: Associations between total serum GGT activity and metabolic risk: MESA. Biomark Med 7(5):709–721, 2013

Brahmi N, Kouraichi N, Abderrazek H, et al: Clinical experience with carbamazepine overdose: relationship between serum concentration and neurological severity. J Clin Psychopharmacol 28(2):241–243, 2008

Brant-Zawadzki M, Heiserman JE: The roles of MR angiography, CT angiography, and sonography in vascular imaging of the head and neck. AJNR Am J Neuroradiol 18(10):1820–1825, 1997

Bray C, Bell LN, Liang H, et al: Erythrocyte sedimentation rate and C-reactive protein measurements and their relevance in clinical medicine. WMJ 115(6):317–321, 2016

Brent J: Current management of ethylene glycol poisoning. Drugs 61(7):979–988, 2001

Brewer CP, Dawson B, Wallman KE, et al: Effect of sodium phosphate supplementation on repeated high-intensity cycling efforts. J Sports Sci 33(11):1109–111, 2015

Brosnan EM, Anders CK: Understanding patterns of brain metastasis in breast cancer and designing rational therapeutic strategies. Ann Transl Med 6(9):163, 2018

Brown JS: Environmental and Chemical Toxins and Psychiatric Illness. Washington, DC, American Psychiatric Publishing, 2002

Brun JF, Varlet-Marie E, Richou M, et al: Seeking the optimal hematocrit: may hemorheological modelling provide a solution? Clin Hemorheol Microcirc 69(4):493–501, 2018

Brunzell JD: Clinical practice. Hypertriglyceridemia. N Engl J Med 357(10):1009–1017, 2007

Cabral BMI, Edding SN, Portocarrero JP, et al: Rhabdomyolysis. Dis Mon 66(8):101015, 2020

Cai Z, Li S, Matuskey D, et al: PET imaging of synaptic density: a new tool for investigation of neuropsychiatric diseases. Neurosci Lett 691:44–50, 2019

Cappell MS: Acute pancreatitis: etiology, clinical presentation, diagnosis, and therapy. Med Clin North Am 92(4):889–923, ix–x, 2008

Carranza C, Pedraza-Sanchez S, de Oyarzabal-Mendez E, et al: Diagnosis for latent tuberculosis infection: new alternatives. Front Immunol 11:2006, 2020

Carrick AI, Costner HB: Rapid fire: hypercalcemia. Emerg Med Clin North Am 36(3):549–555, 2018

Carson AP, Fox CS, McGuire DK, et al: Low hemoglobin A1c and risk of all-cause mortality among US adults without diabetes. Circ Cardiovasc Qual Outcomes 3(6):661–667, 2010

Castaneda D, Gonzalez AJ, Alomari M, et al: From hepatitis A to E: a critical review of viral hepatitis. World J Gastroenterol 27(16):1691–1715, 2021

Castanheira FVS, Kubes P: Neutrophils and NETs in modulating acute and chronic inflammation. Blood 133(20):2178–2185, 2019

Caton MT Jr, Wiggins WF, Nunez D: Three-dimensional cinematic rendering to optimize visualization of cerebrovascular anatomy and disease in CT angiography. J Neuroimaging 30(3):286–296, 2020

Caye A, Pilz LK, Maia AL, et al: The impact of selective serotonin reuptake inhibitors on the thyroid function among patients with major depressive disorder: a systematic review and meta-analysis. Eur Neuropsychopharmacol 33:139–145, 2020

Centers for Disease Control and Prevention: Types of HIV tests, in HIV: Testing. Atlanta, GA, Centers for Disease Control and Prevention, June 22, 2022. Available at: https://www.cdc.gov/hiv/basics/hiv-testing/test-types.html. Accessed July 21, 2022.

Chaconas G, Castellanos M, Verhey TB: Changing of the guard: how the Lyme disease spirochete subverts the host immune response. J Biol Chem 295(2):301–313, 2020

Chaulin A: Clinical and diagnostic value of highly sensitive cardiac troponins in arterial hypertension. Vasc Health Risk Manag 7:431–443, 2021

Chemali KR, Tsao B: Electrodiagnostic testing of nerves and muscles: when, why, and how to order. Cleve Clin J Med 72(1):37–48, 2005

Chen M, Zhou W, Xu W: Thyroid function analysis in 50 patients with COVID-19: a retrospective study. Thyroid 31(1):8–11, 2021

Chen S, Honda T, Ohara T, et al: Serum homocysteine and risk of dementia in Japan. J Neurol Neurosurg Psychiatry 91(5):540–546, 2020

Chen S, Li J, Liu Z, et al: Comparing the value of cystatin C and serum creatinine for evaluating the renal function and predicting the prognosis of COVID-19 patients. Front Pharmacol 12:587816, 2021

Chernecky CC, Berger BJ: Laboratory Tests and Diagnostic Procedures, 5th Edition. St. Louis, MO, WB Saunders, 2008

Chrostek L, Cylwik B, Szmitkowski M, et al: The diagnostic accuracy of carbohydrate-deficient transferrin, sialic acid and commonly used markers of alcohol abuse during abstinence. Clin Chim Acta 364(1–2):167–171, 2006

Chrysant SG: The current debate over treatment of subclinical hypothyroidism to prevent cardiovascular complications. Int J Clin Pract 74(7):e13499, 2020

Chu CM, Lowder JL: Diagnosis and treatment of urinary tract infections across age groups. Am J Obstet Gynecol 219(1):40–51, 2018

Clark SR, Warren NS, Kim G, et al: Elevated clozapine levels associated with infection: a systematic review. Schizophr Res 192:50–56, 2018

Clyne B, Jerrard DA: Syphilis testing. J Emerg Med 18:361–367, 2000

Cohen BM, Sommer BR, Vuckovic A: Antidepressant-resistant depression in patients with comorbid subclinical hypothyroidism or high-normal TSH levels. Am J Psychiatry 175(7):598–604, 2018

Cohen SM: Crystalluria and chronic kidney disease. Toxicol Pathol 46(8):949–955, 2018

Cohn RM, Roth KS: Hyperammonemia, bane of the brain. Clin Pediatr (Phila) 43:683–689, 2004

Collins JF, Lieberman DA, Durbin TE, et al: Accuracy of screening for fecal occult blood on a single stool sample obtained by digital rectal examination: a comparison with recommended sampling practice. Ann Intern Med 142(2):81–85, 2005

Cortese F, Scicchitano P, Cortese AM, et al: Uric acid in metabolic and cerebrovascular disorders: a review. Curr Vasc Pharmacol 18(6):610–618, 2020

Corti A, Belcastro E, Dominici S, et al: The dark side of gamma-glutamyltransferase (GGT): pathogenic effects of an "antioxidant" enzyme. Free Radic Biol Med 160:807–819, 2020

Coughlin JM, Horti AG, Pomper MG: Opportunities in precision psychiatry using PET neuroimaging in psychosis. Neurobiol Dis 131:104428, 2019

Coughlin JM, Yang T, Rebman AW, et al: Imaging glial activation in patients with post-treatment Lyme disease symptoms: a pilot study using [11C]DPA-713 PET. J Neuroinflammation 15(1):346, 2018

Cure JK: Imaging of vascular lesions of the head and neck. Facial Plast Surg Clin North Am 9(4):525–549, 2001

Currie S, Hadjivassiliou M, Craven IJ, et al: Magnetic resonance spectroscopy of the brain. Postgrad Med J 89(1048):94–106, 2013

Czarnywojtek A, Zgorzalewicz-Stachowiak M, Czarnocka B, et al: Effect of lithium carbonate on the function of the thyroid gland: mechanism of action and clinical implications. J Physiol Pharmacol 71(2):10.26402/jpp.2020.2.03, 2020

Dadiomov D: Laboratory testing for substance use disorders, in Absolute Addiction Psychiatry Review. Edited by Marienfeld C. Cham, Switzerland, Springer, 2020, pp 17–30

Därr R, Kuhn M, Bode C, et al: Accuracy of recommended sampling and assay methods for the determination of plasma-free and urinary fractionated metanephrines in the diagnosis of pheochromocytoma and paraganglioma: a systematic review. Endocrine 56(3):495–503, 2017

Dasgupta A, Bernard DW: Herbal remedies: effects on clinical laboratory tests. Arch Pathol Lab Med 130(4):521–528, 2006

Daube JR: Clinical Neurophysiology. Philadelphia, PA, FA Davis, 1996

Davis J, Desmond M, Berk M: Lithium and nephrotoxicity: a literature review of approaches to clinical management and risk stratification. BMC Nephrol 19(1):305, 2018

de Leon J, Armstrong S, Cozza K: Clinical guidelines for psychiatrists for the use of pharmacogenetic testing for CYP450 2D6 and CYP450 2C19. Psychosomatics 47(1):75–85, 2006 de Leon J, Ruan CJ, Schoretsanitis G, et al: A rational use of clozapine based on adverse drug reactions, pharmacokinetics, and clinical pharmacopsychology. Psychother Psychosom 89(4):200–214, 2020

de Leon J, Schoretsanitis G, Kane JM, et al: Using therapeutic drug monitoring to personalize clozapine dosing in Asians. Asia Pac Psychiatry 12(2):e12384, 2020

de Leon MJ, DeSanti S, Zinkowski R, et al: MRI and CSF studies in the early diagnosis of Alzheimer's disease. J Intern Med 256(3):205–223, 2004

De Luca A, Morella A, Consoli F, et al: A novel triplet-primed PCR assay to detect the full range of trinucleotide CAG repeats in the Huntingtin gene (HTT). Int J Mol Sci 22(4):1689, 2021

Deal CL, Tony M, Höybye C, et al: Growth Hormone Research Society workshop summary: consensus guidelines for recombinant human growth hormone therapy in Prader-Willi syndrome. J Clin Endocrinol Metab 98(6):E1072–E1087, 2013

Dean RA, Shaw LM: Use of cerebrospinal fluid biomarkers for diagnosis of incipient Alzheimer disease in patients with mild cognitive impairment. Clin Chem 56(1):7–9, 2009

Del Nonno F, Nardacci R, Colombo D, et al: Hepatic failure in COVID-19: is iron overload the dangerous trigger? Cells 10(5):1103, 2021

Delanaye P, Cavalier E, Pottel H: Serum creatinine: not so simple! Nephron 136(4):302–308, 2017

Devillé WL, Yzermans JC, van Duijn NP, et al: The urine dipstick test useful to rule out infections: a meta-analysis of the accuracy. BMC Urol 4:4, 2004

Devreese KMJ: COVID-19-related laboratory coagulation findings. Int J Lab Hematol 43(Suppl 1):36–42, 2021

Dewan R, Chia R, Ding J, et al: Pathogenic Huntingtin repeat expansions in patients with frontotemporal dementia and amyotrophic lateral sclerosis. Neuron 109(3):448–460, 2021

Doran B, Guo Y, Xu J, et al: Prognostic value of fasting versus nonfasting low-density lipoprotein cholesterol levels on long-term mortality: insight from the National Health and Nutrition Examination Survey III (NHANES-III). Circulation 130(7):546–553, 2014

Dorin RI, Qualls CR, Crapo LM: Diagnosis of adrenal insufficiency. Ann Intern Med 139(3):194–204, 2003

Dørup I: Magnesium and potassium deficiency: its diagnosis, occurrence and treatment in diuretic therapy and its consequences for growth, protein synthesis and growth factors. Acta Physiol Scand Suppl 618:1–55, 1994

Dos Santos DT, Imthon AK, Strelow MZ, et al: Parkinsonism-hyperpyrexia syndrome after amantadine withdrawal: case report and review of the literature. Neurologist 26(4):149–152, 2021

Dubin D: Rapid Interpretation of EKGs, 3rd Edition. Tampa, FL, Cover Publishing, 1984

Dumes AA: Lyme disease and the epistemic tensions of "medically unexplained illnesses." Med Anthropol 39(6):441–456, 2020

Dworakowska D, Morley S, Mulholland N, et al: COVID-19-related thyroiditis: a novel disease entity? Clin Endocrinol (Oxf) 95(3):369–377, 2021

Eap CB, Gründer G, Baumann P, et al: Tools for optimising pharmacotherapy in psychiatry (therapeutic drug monitoring, molecular brain imaging and pharmacogenetic tests): focus on antidepressants. World J Biol Psychiatry 22(8):561–628, 2021

Eyrich NW, Morgan TM, Tosoian JJ: Biomarkers for detection of clinically significant prostate cancer: contemporary clinical data and future directions. Transl Androl Urol 10(7):3091–3103, 2021

Faria AC, Carmo H, Carvalho F, et al: Drinking to death: hyponatraemia induced by synthetic phenethylamines. Drug Alcohol Depend 212:108045, 2020

Farrugia FA, Martikos G, Tzanetis P, et al: Pheochromocytoma, diagnosis and treatment: review of the literature. Endocr Regul 51(3):168–181, 2017

Fauci AS, Braunwald E, Kasper DL, et al (eds): Harrison's Principles of Internal Medicine, 17th Edition. New York, McGraw-Hill, 2008

Favaloro EJ, Henry BM, Lippi G: COVID-19 and antiphospholipid antibodies: time for a reality check? Semin Thromb Hemost 48(1):72–92, 2021

Favresse J, Burlacu MC, Maiter D, et al: Interferences with thyroid function immunoassays: clinical implications and detection algorithm. Endocr Rev 39(5):830–850, 2018

Ferguson TW, Komenda P, Tangri N: Cystatin C as a biomarker for estimating glomerular filtration rate. Curr Opin Nephrol Hypertens 24(3):295–300, 2015

Fernandes ML, Oliveira WM, Santos MV, et al: Sedation for electroencephalography with dexmedetomidine or chloral hydrate: a comparative study on the qualitative and quantitative electroencephalogram pattern. J Neurosurg Anesthesiol 27(1):21–25, 2015

Ferrell PB Jr, McLeod HL: Carbamazepine, HLA-B*1502 and risk of Stevens-Johnson syndrome and toxic epidermal necrolysis: US FDA recommendations. Pharmacogenomics 9(10):1543–1546, 2008

Filippatos TD, Makri A, Elisaf MS, et al: Hyponatremia in the elderly: challenges and solutions. Clin Interv Aging 12:1957–1965, 2017

Fischbach FT, Fischbach MA: A Manual of Laboratory and Diagnostic Tests, 10th Edition. Philadelphia, PA, Wolters Kluwer Health/Lippincott Williams & Wilkins, 2018

Fleming J, Chetty M: Therapeutic monitoring of valproate in psychiatry: how far have we progressed? Clin Neuropharmacol 29(6):350–360, 2006

Flockhart DA: Drug interactions and the cytochrome P450 system: the role of cytochrome P450 2C19. Clin Pharmacokinet 29(suppl):45–52, 1995

Fogazzi GB, Delanghe J: Microscopic examination of urine sediment: phase contrast versus bright field. Clin Chim Acta 487:168–173, 2018

Fond G, Garosi A, Faugere M, et al: Peripheral inflammation is associated with brain SPECT perfusion changes in schizophrenia. Eur J Nucl Med Mol Imaging 49(3):905–912, 2021

Fontana RJ, Engle RE, Gottfried M, et al: Role of hepatitis E virus infection in North American patients with severe acute liver injury. Clin Transl Gastroenterol 11(11):e00273, 2020

Forlenza OV, De-Paula VJ, Diniz BS: Neuroprotective effects of lithium: implications for the treatment of Alzheimer's disease and related neurodegenerative disorders. ACS Chem Neurosci 5(6):443–450, 2014

Foulser P, Abbasi Y, Mathilakath A, et al: Do not treat the numbers: lithium toxicity. BMJ Case Rep 2017:bcr2017220079, 2017

Frame IJ, Joshi PH, Mwangi C, et al: Susceptibility of cardiac troponin assays to biotin interference. Am J Clin Pathol 151(5):486–493, 2019

Fuhrman MP, Charney P, Mueller CM: Hepatic proteins and nutrition assessment. J Am Diet Assoc 104(8):1258–1264, 2004

Fujii H, Doi H, Ko T, et al: Frequently abnormal serum gamma-glutamyl transferase activity is associated with future development of fatty liver: a retrospective cohort study. BMC Gastroenterol 20(1):217, 2020

Galanter M, Kleber HD (eds): The American Psychiatric Publishing Textbook of Substance Abuse Treatment, 4th Edition. Washington, DC, American Psychiatric Publishing, 2008

Gallucci-Neto J, Brunoni AR, Ono CR, et al: Ictal SPECT in psychogenic nonepileptic and epileptic seizures. J Acad Consult Liaison Psychiatry 62(1):29–37, 2021

Garcia C, Biller BM, Klibanski A: The role of the clinical laboratory in the diagnosis of Cushing syndrome. Am J Clin Pathol 120(suppl):S38–S45, 2003

Garcia D, Erkan D: Diagnosis and management of the antiphospholipid syndrome. N Engl J Med 378(21):2010–2021, 2018

Garcia-Carbonero R, Matute Teresa F, Mercader-Cidoncha E, et al: Multidisciplinary practice guidelines for the diagnosis, genetic counseling and treatment of pheochromocytomas and paragangliomas. Clin Transl Oncol 23(10):1995–2019, 2021

George JA, Khoza S: SARS-CoV-2 infection and the kidneys: an evolving picture. Adv Exp Med Biol 1327:107–118, 2021

Germon K: Fluid and electrolyte problems associated with diabetes insipidus and syndrome of inappropriate antidiuretic hormone. Nurs Clin North Am 22(4):785–796, 1987

Gezer S: Antiphospholipid syndrome. Dis Mon 49(12):696–741, 2003

Gharzeddine K, Hatzoglou V, Holodny AI, et al: MR perfusion and MR spectroscopy of brain neoplasms. Radiol Clin North Am 57(6):1177–1188, 2019

Ghio L, Fornaro G, Rossi P: Risperidone-induced hyperamylasemia, hyperlipasemia, and neuroleptic malignant syndrome: a case report. J Clin Psychopharmacol 29(4):391–392, 2009

Ghishan FK, Kiela PR: Vitamins and minerals in inflammatory bowel disease. Gastroenterol Clin North Am 46(4):797–808, 2017

Giakoumatos CI, Nanda P, Mathew IT, et al: Effects of lithium on cortical thickness and hippocampal subfield volumes in psychotic bipolar disorder. J Psychiatr Res 61:180–187, 2015

Giannakopoulos B, Passam F, Ioannou Y, et al: How we diagnose the antiphospholipid syndrome. Blood 113(5):985–994, 2009

Gianni AD, De Donatis D, Valente S, et al: Eating disorders: do PET and SPECT have a role? A systematic review of the literature. Psychiatry Res Neuroimaging 300:111065, 2020

Giannini EG, Testa R, Savarino V: Liver enzyme alteration: a guide for clinicians. CMAJ 172(3):367–379, 2005

Giboney PT: Mildly elevated liver transaminase levels in the asymptomatic patient. Am Fam Physician 71(6):1105–1110, 2005

Giesen LG, Cousins G, Dimitrov BD, et al: Predicting acute uncomplicated urinary tract infection in women: a systematic review of the diagnostic accuracy of symptoms and signs. BMC Fam Pract 11:78, 2010

Ginsberg C, Houben AJHM, Malhotra R, et al: Serum phosphate and microvascular function in a population-based cohort. Clin J Am Soc Nephrol 14(11):1626–1633, 2019

Gong R, Wang P, Dworkin L: What we need to know about the effect of lithium on the kidney. Am J Physiol Renal Physiol 311(6):F1168–F1171, 2016

Goodwill AM, Szoeke C: A systematic review and meta-analysis of the effect of low vitamin D on cognition. J Am Geriatr Soc 65(10):2161–2168, 2017

Gopal DV, Rosen HR: Abnormal findings on liver function tests: interpreting results to narrow the diagnosis and establish a prognosis. Postgrad Med 107(2):100–102, 105–109, 113–114, 2000

Grigsby J, Brega AG, Bennett RE, et al: Clinically significant psychiatric symptoms among male carriers of the fragile X premutation, with and without FXTAS, and the mediating influence of executive functioning. Clin Neuropsychol 30(6):944–959, 2016

Guilliams M, Mildner A, Yona S: Developmental and functional heterogeneity of monocytes. Immunity 49(4):595–613, 2018

Gulani V, Calamante F, Shellock FG, et al: International Society for Magnetic Resonance in Medicine. Gadolinium deposition in the brain: summary of evidence and recommendations. Lancet Neurol 16(7):564–570, 2017

Guo W, Zhou Q, Jia Y, et al: Increased levels of glycated hemoglobin A1c and iron deficiency anemia: a review. Med Sci Monit 25:8371–8378, 2019

Gupta RK, Jobanputra KJ, Yadav A: MR spectroscopy in brain infections. Neuroimaging Clin N Am 23(3):475–498, 2013

Hagerman RJ, Hagerman P: Fragile X-associated tremor/ataxia syndrome: features, mechanisms and management. Nat Rev Neurol 12(7):403–412, 2016

Hales RE, Yudofsky SC, Gabbard GO (eds): The American Psychiatric Publishing Textbook of Psychiatry. Washington, DC, American Psychiatric Publishing, 2008

Hall DA, Berry-Kravis E: Fragile X syndrome and fragile X-associated tremor ataxia syndrome. Handb Clin Neurol 147:377–391, 2018

Hall SA, Esche GR, Araujo AB, et al: Correlates of low testosterone and symptomatic androgen deficiency in a population-based sample. J Clin Endocrinol Metab 93(10):3870–3877, 2008

Hameed AM, Lam VW, Pleass HC: Significant elevations of serum lipase not caused by pancreatitis: a systematic review. HPB (Oxford) 17(2):99–112, 2015

Hanly JG, Urowitz MB, Siannis F, et al: Autoantibodies and neuropsychiatric events at the time of systemic lupus erythematosus diagnosis: results from an international inception cohort study. Arthritis Rheum 58(3):843–853, 2008

Hansson O, Lehmann S, Otto M, et al: Advantages and disadvantages of the use of the CSF amyloid β (Aβ) 42/40 ratio in the diagnosis of Alzheimer's disease. Alzheimers Res Ther 11(1):34, 2019

Harris RH, Sasson G, Mehler PS: Elevation of liver function tests in severe anorexia nervosa. Int J Eat Disord 46(4):369–374, 2013

Harvard Health Publishing: Testosterone: what it does and doesn't do. Harvard Medical School Blog, August 29, 2019. Available at: https://www.health.harvard.edu/medications/testosterone--what-it-does-and-doesnt-do. Accessed July 22, 2022.

Hasan MN, Fraiwan A, An R, et al: Paper-based microchip electrophoresis for point-of-care hemoglobin testing. Analyst 145(7):2525–2542, 2020

Haverfield EV, Esplin ED, Aguilar SJ, et al: Physician-directed genetic screening to evaluate personal risk for medically actionable disorders: a large multi-center cohort study. BMC Med 19(1):199, 2021

Haynes J, Haynes R: Proteinuria. BMJ 332(7536):284, 2006

Hellwig S, Domschke K: Update on PET imaging biomarkers in the diagnosis of neuropsychiatric disorders. Curr Opin Neurol 32(4):539–547, 2019

Henderson TA, Cohen P, van Lierop M, et al: A reckoning to keep doing what we are already doing with PET and SPECT functional neuroimaging. Am J Psychiatry 177(7):637–638, 2020

Hiemke C, Bergemann N, Clement HW, et al: Consensus guidelines for therapeutic drug monitoring in neuropsychopharmacology: update 2017. Pharmacopsychiatry 51(1–02):9–62, 2018

Hill MH, Flatley JE, Barker ME, et al: A vitamin B-12 supplement of 500 μg/d for eight weeks does not normalize urinary methylmalonic acid or other biomarkers of vitamin B-12 status in elderly people with moderately poor vitamin B-12 status. J Nutr 143(2):142–147, 2013

Hinds K, Sutcliffe K: Heterodox and orthodox discourses in the case of Lyme disease: a synthesis of arguments. Qual Health Res 29(11):1661–1673, 2019

HIV.gov: U.S. statistics, in HIV Basics, Overview: Data and Trends. Washington, DC, U.S. Department of Health and Human Services, 2022. Available at: https://www.hiv.gov/hiv-basics/overview/data-and-trends/statistics. Accessed July 21, 2022.

HIVinfo: HIV overview: HIV testing, in Understanding HIV: Facts Sheets. Bethesda, MD, National Institutes of Health, 2021. Available at: https://hivinfo.nih.gov/understanding-hiv/fact-sheets/hiv-testing. Accessed July 21, 2022.

Holt RE: The role of computed tomography of the brain in psychiatry. Psychiatr Med 1(3):275–285, 1983

Hong SH, Lee JS, Kim JA, et al: Gamma-glutamyl transferase variability and the risk of hospitalisation for heart failure. Heart 106(14):1080–1086, 2020

Hong Y, Seese L, Hickey G, et al: Preoperative prealbumin does not impact outcomes after left ventricular assist device implantation. J Card Surg 35(5):1029–1036, 2020

Hopyan J, Ciarallo A, Dowlatshahi D, et al: Certainty of stroke diagnosis: incremental benefit with CT perfusion over noncontrast CT and CT angiography. Radiology 255(1):142–153, 2010

Hsieh YP, Chang CC, Kor CT, et al: Mean corpuscular volume and mortality in patients with CKD. Clin J Am Soc Nephrol 12(2):237–244, 2017

Hussain HM, Zakaria M: Drug-induced lupus secondary to sertraline. Aust N Z J Psychiatry 42(12):1074–1075, 2008

Imperiale TF, Ransohoff DF, Itzkowitz SH, et al: Fecal DNA versus fecal occult blood for colorectal-cancer screening in an average-risk population. N Engl J Med 351(26):2704–2714, 2004

Irani DN: Cerebrospinal Fluid in Clinical Practice. Philadelphia, PA, Saunders Elsevier, 2009

Ismail OZ, Bhayana V: Lipase or amylase for the diagnosis of acute pancreatitis? Clin Biochem 50(18):1275–1280, 2017

Iyer KS, Dayal S: Modulators of platelet function in aging. Platelets 31(4):474–482, 2020

Jack CR Jr, Bennett DA, Blennow K, et al: NIA-AA research framework: toward a biological definition of Alzheimer's disease. Alzheimers Dement 14(4):535–562, 2018

Jacobi A, Chung M, Bernheim A, et al: Portable chest X-ray in coronavirus disease-19 (COVID-19): a pictorial review. Clin Imaging 64:35–42, 2020

Jacobson S, Jerrier H: EEG in delirium. Semin Clin Neuropsychiatry 5(2):86–92, 2000

Jacobson SA, Pies RW, Katz IR: Clinical Manual of Geriatric Psychopharmacology. Washington, DC, American Psychiatric Publishing, 2007

Jain P, Chaney AM, Carlson ML, et al: Neuroinflammation PET imaging: current opinion and future directions. J Nucl Med 61(8):1107–1112, 2020

Jaipersad AS, Lip GY, Silverman S, et al: The role of monocytes in angiogenesis and atherosclerosis. J Am Coll Cardiol 63(1):1–11, 2014

Jessel CD, Mostafa S, Potiriadis M, et al: Use of antidepressants with pharmacogenetic prescribing guidelines in a 10-year depression cohort of adult primary care patients. Pharmacogenet Genomics 30(7):145–152, 2020

Jha AK, Kumar G, Dayal VM, et al: Neurological manifestations of hepatitis E virus infection: an overview. World J Gastroenterol 27(18):2090–2104, 2021

Jiang B, Yao G, Yao C, et al: The effect of folate and VitB12 in the treatment of MCI patients with hyperhomocysteinemia. J Clin Neurosci 81:65–69, 2020

John TM, Taege AJ: Appropriate laboratory testing in Lyme disease. Cleve Clin J Med 86(11):751–759, 2019

Johnson EB, Ziegler G, Penny W, et al: Dynamics of cortical degeneration over a decade in Huntington's disease. Biol Psychiatry 89(8):807–816, 2021

Johnston DE: Special considerations in interpreting liver function tests. Am Fam Physician 59(8):2223–2230, 1999

Kachian ZR, Cohen-Zimerman S, Bega D, et al: Suicidal ideation and behavior in Huntington's disease: systematic review and recommendations. J Affect Disord 250:319–329, 2019

Kanbay M, Yilmaz S, Dincer N, et al: Antidiuretic hormone and serum osmolarity physiology and related outcomes: what is old, what is new, and what is unknown? J Clin Endocrinol Metab 104(11):5406–5420, 2019

Kang M, Galuska MA, Ghassemzadeh S: Benzodiazepine toxicity, in StatPearls. Treasure Island, FL, StatPearls Publishing, 2021. Available at: https://www.statpearls.com/ArticleLibrary/viewarticle/30312. Accessed September 1, 2021.

Kapur VK, Auckley DH, Chowdhuri S, et al: Clinical practice guideline for diagnostic testing for adult obstructive sleep apnea: an American Academy of Sleep Medicine clinical practice guideline. J Clin Sleep Med 13(3):479–504, 2017

Karaca Z, Grossman A, Kelestimur F: Investigation of the Hypothalamo-pituitary-adrenal (HPA) axis: a contemporary synthesis. Rev Endocr Metab Disord 22(2):179–204, 2021

Karazniewicz-Łada M, Główka AK, Mikulska AA, et al: Pharmacokinetic drug-drug interactions among antiepileptic drugs, including CBD, drugs used to treat COVID-19 and nutrients. Int J Mol Sci 22(17):9582, 2021

Katz KD, Brooks DE: Organophosphate toxicity clinical presentation. Medscape, December 30, 2020. Available at: https://emedicine.medscape.com/article/167726-clinical. Accessed June 1, 2021.

Katz U, Zandman-Goddard G: Drug-induced lupus: an update. Autoimmun Rev 10(1):46–50, 2010

Kaul S, Gupta M, Bandyopadhyay D, et al: Gout pharmacotherapy in cardiovascular diseases: a review of utility and outcomes. Am J Cardiovasc Drugs 21(5):499–512, 2021

Khare S, Anjum F: Adrenocorticotropic hormone test, StatPearls. Treasure Island, FL, StatPearls Publishing, 2021. Available at: https://www.statpearls.com/ArticleLibrary/viewarticle/20072. Accessed July 28, 2022.

Kho J, Mandal AKJ, Geraldes R, et al: COVID-19 encephalitis and Wernicke's encephalopathy. J Med Virol 93(9):5248–5251, 2021

Khosravi M, Sotoudeh G, Amini M, et al: The relationship between dietary patterns and depression mediated by serum levels of Folate and vitamin B12. BMC Psychiatry 20(1):63, 2020

Killip S, Bennett JM, Chambers MD: Iron deficiency anemia. Am Fam Physician 75(5):671–678, 2007

Kim EJ, Wierzbicki AS: Investigating raised creatine kinase. BMJ 373:n1486, 2021

Kim JJ, Kim YS, Kumar V: Heavy metal toxicity: an update of chelating therapeutic strategies. J Trace Elem Med Biol 54:226–231, 2019

Kim JM, Stewart R, Kim SW, et al: Predictive value of folate, vitamin B12 and homocysteine levels in late-life depression. Br J Psychiatry 192(4):268–274, 2008

Klein DA, Paradise SL, Goodwin ET: Caring for transgender and gender-diverse persons: what clinicians should know. Am Fam Physician 98(11):645–653, 2018

Kluge M, Himmerich H, Wehmeier PM, et al: Sleep propensity at daytime as assessed by Multiple Sleep Latency Tests (MSLT) in patients with schizophrenia increases with clozapine and olanzapine. Schizophr Res 135(1–3):123–127, 2012

Koenig G, Seneff S: Gamma-glutamyltransferase: a predictive biomarker of cellular antioxidant inadequacy and disease risk. Dis Markers 2015:818570, 2015

Kolla BP, Jahani Kondori M, Silber MH, et al: Advance taper of antidepressants prior to multiple sleep latency testing increases the number of sleep-onset rapid eye movement periods and reduces mean sleep latency. J Clin Sleep Med 16(11):1921–1927, 2020

Kounin G, Bashir Q: Mechanism and role of antidiuretic hormone. Surg Neurol 53(5):508–510, 2000

Kubo M: Mast cells and basophils in allergic inflammation. Curr Opin Immunol 54:74–79, 2018

Kuloglu M, Atmaca M, Ustundag B, et al: Serum iron levels in schizophrenic patients with or without akathisia. Eur Neuropsychopharmacol 13(2):67–71, 2003

Kundra A, Jain A, Banga A, et al: Evaluation of plasma ammonia levels in patients with acute liver failure and chronic liver disease and its correlation with the severity of hepatic encephalopathy and clinical features of raised intracranial tension. Clin Biochem 38(8):696–699, 2005

Landel V, Annweiler C, Millet P, et al: Vitamin D, cognition and Alzheimer's disease: the therapeutic benefit is in the D-tails. J Alzheimers Dis 53(2):419–444, 2016

Lane NE: Epidemiology, etiology, and diagnosis of osteoporosis. Am J Obstet Gynecol 194(2 Suppl):S3–S11, 2006

Langan RC, Goodbred AJ: Vitamin B12 deficiency: recognition and management. Am Fam Physician 96(6):384–389, 2017

Lange S, Medrzycka-Dabrowska W, Friganovic A, et al: Delirium in critical illness patients and the potential role of thiamine therapy in prevention and treatment: findings from a scoping review with implications for evidence-based practice. Int J Environ Res Public Health 18(16):8809, 2021

Lantos PM, Rumbaugh J, Bockenstedt LK, et al: Clinical practice guidelines by the Infectious Diseases Society of America (IDSA), American Academy of Neurology (AAN), and American College of Rheumatology (ACR): 2020 guidelines for the prevention, diagnosis, and treatment of Lyme disease. Arthritis Care Res (Hoboken) 73(1):1–9, 2021

Lantos PM: Chronic Lyme disease. Infect Dis Clin North Am 29(2):325–340, 2015

Laoutidis ZG, Kioulos KT: Antipsychotic-induced elevation of creatine kinase: a systematic review of the literature and recommendations for the clinical practice. Psychopharmacology (Berl) 231(22):4255–4270, 2014

Le Bihan D: Diffusion MRI: what water tells us about the brain. EMBO Mol Med 6(5):569–573, 2014

Le Bihan D, Johansen-Berg H: Diffusion MRI at 25: exploring brain tissue structure and function. Neuroimage 61(2):324–341, 2012

Le-Niculescu H, Roseberry K, Gill SS, et al: Precision medicine for mood disorders: objective assessment, risk prediction, pharmacogenomics, and repurposed drugs. Mol Psychiatry 26(7):2776–2804, 2021

Leavitt BR, Kordasiewicz HB, Schobel SA: Huntingtin-Lowering therapies for Huntington disease: a review of the evidence of potential benefits and risks. JAMA Neurol 77(6):764–772, 2020

Lee Y, Siddiqui WJ: Cholesterol levels, in StatPearls. Treasure Island, FL, StatPearls Publishing, July 26, 2021. Available at: https://www.statpearls.com/ArticleLibrary/viewarticle/19466. Accessed September 1, 2021.

Lee YB, Han K, Park S, et al: Gamma-glutamyl transferase variability and risk of dementia: a nationwide study. Int J Geriatr Psychiatry 35(10):1105–1114, 2020

Lerner V, Kanevsky M, Dwolatzky T, et al: Vitamin B12 and folate serum levels in newly admitted psychiatric patients. Clin Nutr 25(1):60–67, 2006

Lessey G, Stavropoulos K, Papademetriou V: Mild to moderate chronic kidney disease and cardiovascular events in patients with type 2 diabetes mellitus. Vasc Health Risk Manag 15:365–373, 2019

Leuzy A, Chiotis K, Lemoine L, et al: Tau PET imaging in neurodegenerative tauopathies—still a challenge. Mol Psychiatry 24(8):1112–1134, 2019

Levey AS, Inker LA, Aziz O, et al: CKD-EPI equations for glomerular filtration rate (GFR), in MDCalc.com, 2022. Available at: https://www.mdcalc.com/ckd-epi-equations-glomerular-filtration-rate-gfr. Accessed July 22, 2022.

Levitt DG, Levitt MD: Human serum albumin homeostasis: a new look at the roles of synthesis, catabolism, renal and gastrointestinal excretion, and the clinical value of serum albumin measurements. Int J Gen Med 9:229–255, 2016

Li J, Hovey KM, Andrews CA, et al: Association of dietary magnesium intake with fatal coronary heart disease and sudden cardiac death. J Womens Health (Larchmt) 29(1):7–12, 2020

Li S, Guo Y, Men J, et al: The preventive efficacy of vitamin B supplements on the cognitive decline of elderly adults: a systematic review and meta-analysis. BMC Geriatr 21(1):367, 2021

Lien YH, Shapiro JI: Hyponatremia: clinical diagnosis and management. Am J Med 120(8):653–658, 2007

Lim EW, Aarsland D, Ffytche D, et al: Amyloid-β and Parkinson's disease. J Neurol 266(11):2605–2619, 2019

Lin MS, Shih SR, Li HY, et al: Serum C-reactive protein levels correlates better to metabolic syndrome defined by International Diabetes Federation than by NCEP ATP III in men. Diabetes Res Clin Pract 77(2):286–292, 2007

Ling M, Murali M: Antinuclear antibody tests. Clin Lab Med 39(4):513–524, 2019

Liu BA, Mittmann N, Knowles SR, et al: Hyponatremia and the syndrome of inappropriate secretion of antidiuretic hormone associated with the use of selective serotonin reuptake inhibitors: a review of spontaneous reports. CMAJ 155(5):519–527, 1996

Liu YS, Lin KY, Masur J, et al: Outcomes after recurrent intentional methanol exposures not treated with alcohol dehydrogenase inhibitors or hemodialysis. J Emerg Med 58(6):910–916, 2020

Lo Gullo A, Rifici C, Caliri S, et al: Refeeding syndrome in a woman with pancreatitis: a case report. J Int Med Res 49(2):300060520986675, 2021

Løberg M, Lousdal ML, Bretthauer M, et al: Benefits and harms of mammography screening. Breast Cancer Res 17(1):63, 2015

Lohr JW: Hyperuricemia. Medscape, July 1, 2022. Available at: https://emedicine.medscape.com/article/241767-overview. Accessed July 22, 2022.

Luddington NS, Mandadapu A, Husk M, et al: Clinical implications of genetic variation in the serotonin transporter promoter region: a review. Prim Care Companion J Clin Psychiatry 11(3):93–102, 2009

Luo J, Wang LP, Hu HF, et al: Cystatin C and cardiovascular or all-cause mortality risk in the general population: a meta-analysis. Clin Chim Acta 450:39–45, 2015

Mair J, Lindahl B, Müller C, et al: What to do when you question cardiac troponin values. Eur Heart J Acute Cardiovasc Care 7(6):577–586, 2018

Malabanan AO, Meikle AW, Swenson L: Endocrine Disorders: Choose the Right Tests. The Primary Care Guide to Diagnostic Testing. Columbus, OH, Anadem Publishing, 2004

Malcangio M: Role of the immune system in neuropathic pain. Scand J Pain 20(1):33–37, 2019

Maloberti A, Giannattasio C, Bombelli M, et al: Hyperuricemia and risk of cardiovascular outcomes: the experience of the URRAH (Uric Acid Right for Heart Health) Project. High Blood Press Cardiovasc Prev 27(2):121–128, 2020

Mank V, Brown K: Leukocytosis, in StatPearls. Treasure Island, FL, StatPearls Publishing, September 19, 2021. Available at: https://www.statpearls.com/ArticleLibrary/viewarticle/24216. Accessed July 28, 2022.

Marques AR: Laboratory diagnosis of Lyme disease: advances and challenges. Infect Dis Clin North Am 29(2):295–307, 2015

Márquez DF, Ruiz-Hurtado G, Segura J, et al: Microalbuminuria and cardiorenal risk: old and new evidence in different populations. F1000Res 8:F1000, 2019

Marwick KF, Taylor M, Walker SW: Antipsychotics and abnormal liver function tests: systematic review. Clin Neuropharmacol 35(5):244–253, 2012

Masajtis-Zagajewska A, Nowicki M: New markers of urinary tract infection. Clin Chim Acta 471:286–291, 2017

Matull WR, Pereira SP, O'Donohue JW: Biochemical markers of acute pancreatitis. J Clin Pathol 59(4):340–344, 2006

Mayo Clinic Laboratories: Test Catalog. Rochester, MN, Mayo Clinic, 2022. Available at: https://www.mayocliniclabs.com/test-catalog. Accessed July 28, 2022.

McAllister B, Gusella JF, Landwehrmeyer GB, et al: Timing and impact of psychiatric, cognitive, and motor abnormalities in Huntington disease. Neurology 96(19):e2395–e2406, 2021

McConnell LM, Sanders GD, Owens DK: Evaluation of genetic tests: APOE genotyping for the diagnosis of Alzheimer disease. Genet Test 3(1):47–53, 1999

McPherson RA, Pincus MR: Henry's Clinical Diagnosis and Management by Laboratory Methods, 24th Edition. Philadelphia, PA, Elsevier, 2022

Mead P, Petersen J, Hinckley A: Updated CDC recommendation for serologic diagnosis of Lyme disease. MMWR Morb Mortal Wkly Rep 68(32):703, 2019

Mehrpour O, Sadeghi M: Toll of acute methanol poisoning for preventing COVID-19. Arch Toxicol 94(6):2259–2260, 2020

Mehta N, Vannozzi R: Lithium-induced electrocardiographic changes: a complete review. Clin Cardiol 40(12):1363–1367, 2017

Melmed S: Pathogenesis and diagnosis of growth hormone deficiency in adults. N Engl J Med 380(26):2551–2562, 2019

Meltzer HY, Cola PA, Parsa M: Marked elevations of serum creatine kinase activity associated with antipsychotic drug treatment. Neuropsychopharmacology 15(4):395–405, 1996

Meyer JH, Cervenka S, Kim, et al: Neuroinflammation in psychiatric disorders: PET imaging and promising new targets. Lancet Psychiatry 7(12):1064–1074, 2020

Mielech A, Puscion-Jakubik A, Markiewicz-Zukowska R, et al: Vitamins in Alzheimer's disease: review of the latest reports. Nutrients 12(11):3458, 2020

Minovic I, Kieneker LM, Gansevoort RT, et al: Vitamin B6, inflammation, and cardiovascular outcome in a population-based cohort: the Prevention of Renal and Vascular End-Stage Disease (PREVEND) study. Nutrients 12(9):2711, 2020

Mitchell AJ: CSF phosphorylated tau in the diagnosis and prognosis of mild cognitive impairment and Alzheimer's disease: a meta-analysis of 51 studies. J Neurol Neurosurg Psychiatry 80(9):966–975, 2009

Mitelman SA: Transdiagnostic neuroimaging in psychiatry: a review. Psychiatry Res 277:23–38, 2019

Miyagawa T, Przybelski SA, Maltais D, et al: The value of multimodal imaging with 123I-FP-CIT SPECT in differential diagnosis of dementia with Lewy bodies and Alzheimer's disease dementia. Neurobiol Aging 99:11–18, 2021

Moeller KE, Lee KC, Kissack JC: Urine drug screening: practical guide for clinicians. Mayo Clin Proc 83(1):66–76, 2008

Moore A, Nelson C, Molins C, et al: Current guidelines, common clinical pitfalls, and future directions for laboratory diagnosis of Lyme disease, United States. Emerg Infect Dis 22(7):1169–1177, 2016

Morris DW, Trivedi MH, Rush AJ: Folate and unipolar depression. J Altern Complement Med 14(3):277–285, 2008

Morris G, Fernandes BS, Puri BK, et al: Leaky brain in neurological and psychiatric disorders: drivers and consequences. Aust N Z J Psychiatry 52(10):924–948, 2018

Mounsey AL, Zeitler MR: Cerebrospinal fluid biomarkers for detection of Alzheimer disease in patients with mild cognitive impairment. Am Fam Physician 97(11):714–715, 2018

Mueller C, McDonald K, de Boer RA, et al: Heart Failure Association of the European Society of Cardiology practical guidance on the use of natriuretic peptide concentrations. Eur J Heart Fail 21(6):715–731, 2019

Mulhall JP, Trost LW, Brannigan RE, et al: Evaluation and management of testosterone deficiency: AUA guideline. J Urol 200(2):423–432, 2018

NACB LMPG Committee Members, Myers GL, Christenson RH, et al: National Academy of Clinical Biochemistry Laboratory Medicine Practice guidelines: emerging biomarkers for primary prevention of cardiovascular disease. Clin Chem 55(2):378–384, 2009

Nader DN: Neutrophilia. Medscape, October 3, 2019. Available at: https://emedicine.medscape.com/article/208576-overview. Accessed July 22, 2022.

Narayan AK, Lee CI, Lehman CD: Screening for breast cancer. Med Clin North Am 104(6):1007–1021, 2020

Nathan DM, Griffin A, Perez FM, et al: Accuracy of a point-of-care hemoglobin A1c assay. J Diabetes Sci Technol 13(6):1149–1153, 2019

National Institute on Alcohol Abuse and Alcoholism: Biomarkers of heavy drinking, in Assessing Alcohol Problems: A Guide for Clinicians and Researchers. Edited by Allen JP, Wilson VB. Available at: https://pubs.niaaa.nih.gov/publications/assessingalcohol/allen.pdf. Accessed June 2021.

National Institutes of Health: Vitamin B6: fact sheet for health professionals, in Health Information: Dietary Supplement Fact Sheets. Bethesda, MD, National Institutes of Health, June 2, 2022. Available at: https://ods.od.nih.gov/factsheets/VitaminB6-HealthProfessional. Accessed July 28, 2022.

Nelson SM, Sarabia SR, Christilaw E, et al: Phosphate-containing prescription medications contribute to the daily phosphate intake in a third of hemodialysis patients. J Ren Nutr 27(2):91–96, 2017

Niemelä O: Biomarker-based approaches for assessing alcohol use disorders. Int J Environ Res Public Health 13(2):166, 2016

Nigrovic LE, Lewander DP, Balamuth F, et al: The Lyme Disease Polymerase Chain Reaction Test has low sensitivity. Vector Borne Zoonotic Dis 20(4):310–313, 2020

Nijdam MJ, van Amsterdam JGC, Gersons BPR, Olff M: Dexamethasone-suppressed cortisol awakening response predicts treatment outcome in posttraumatic stress disorder. J Affect Disord 184:205–208, 2015

Nolen WA, Licht RW, Young AH, et al: What is the optimal serum level for lithium in the maintenance treatment of bipolar disorder? A systematic review and recommendations from the ISBD/IGSLI Task Force on treatment with lithium. Bipolar Disord 21(5):394–409, 2019

O'Connor EE, Zeffiro TA: Why is clinical fMRI in a resting state? Front Neurol 10:420, 2019

Odai T, Terauchi M, Suzuki R, et al: Depressive symptoms in middle-aged and elderly women are associated with a low intake of vitamin B6: a cross-sectional study. Nutrients 12(11):3437, 2020

Oh RC, Trivette ET, Westerfield KL: Management of hypertriglyceridemia: common questions and answers. Am Fam Physician 102(6):347–354, 2020

OneCare Media: Testing.com: Your Trusted Guide. Understand Your Tests, Empower Your Health. Seattle, WA, OneCare Media, 2022. Available at: https://www.testing.com. Accessed July 20, 2022.

Oudman E, Wijnia JW, Oey MJ, et al: Preventing Wernicke's encephalopathy in anorexia nervosa: a systematic review. Psychiatry Clin Neurosci 72(10):774–779, 2018

Oz G, Alger JR, Barker PB, et al: Clinical proton MR spectroscopy in central nervous system disorders. Radiology 270(3):658–679, 2014

Oz MD, Baskak B, Uckun Z, et al: Association between serotonin 2A receptor (HTR2A), serotonin transporter (SLC6A4) and brain-derived neurotrophic factor (BDNF) gene polymorphisms and citalopram/sertraline induced sexual dysfunction in MDD patients. Pharmacogenomics J 20(3):443–450, 2020

Pagani M, Carletto S, Ostacoli L: PET and SPECT in psychiatry: the past and the future. Eur J Nucl Med Mol Imaging 46(10):1985–1987, 2019

Palladino M: Complete blood count alterations in COVID-19 patients: a narrative review. Biochem Med (Zagreb) 31(3):030501, 2021

Park YM: Serum prolactin levels in patients with major depressive disorder receiving selective serotonin-reuptake inhibitor monotherapy for 3 months: a prospective study. Psychiatry Investig 14(3):368–371, 2017

Pasala S, Carmody JB: How to use…serum creatinine, cystatin C and GFR. Arch Dis Child Educ Pract Ed 102(1):37–43, 2017

Patel AA, Budoff MJ: Screening for heart disease: C-reactive protein versus coronary artery calcium. Expert Rev Cardiovasc Ther 8(1):125–131, 2010

Patel MR, Edelman RR: MR angiography of the head and neck. Top Magn Reson Imaging 8(6):345–365, 1996

Peacock M: Calcium metabolism in health and disease. Clin J Am Soc Nephrol 5(Suppl):S23–S30, 2010

Pearlson GD, Veroff AE, McHugh PR: The use of computed tomography in psychiatry: recent applications to schizophrenia, manic-depressive illness and dementia syndromes. Johns Hopkins Med J 149(5):194–202, 1981

Peaston RT, Graham KS, Chambers E, et al: Performance of plasma free metanephrines measured by liquid chromatography-tandem mass spectrometry in the diagnosis of pheochromocytoma. Clin Chim Acta 411(7–8):546–552, 2010

Peeri NC, Egan KM, Chai W, Tao MH: Association of magnesium intake and vitamin D status with cognitive function in older adults: an analysis of US National Health and Nutrition Examination Survey (NHANES) 2011 to 2014. Eur J Nutr 60(1):465–474, 2021

Peitl V, Badžim VA, Šiško Markoš I, et al: Improvements of frontotemporal cerebral blood flow and cognitive functioning in patients with first episode of schizophrenia treated with long-acting aripiprazole. J Clin Psychopharmacol 41(6):638–643, 2021

Pepe J, Colangelo L, Biamonte F, et al: Diagnosis and management of hypocalcemia. Endocrine 69(3):485–495, 2020

Petersen RC, Waring SC, Smith GE, et al: Predictive value of APOE genotyping in incipient Alzheimer's disease. Ann N Y Acad Sci 802:58–69, 1996

Peterson CT, Rodionov DA, Osterman AL, et al: B vitamins and their role in immune regulation and cancer. Nutrients 12(11):3380, 2020

Petit P, Lonjon R, Cociglio M, et al: Carbamazepine and its 10,11-epoxide metabolite in acute mania: clinical and pharmacokinetic correlates. Eur J Clin Pharmacol 41(6):541–546, 1991

Piano S, Dalbeni A, Vettore E, et al: Abnormal liver function tests predict transfer to intensive care unit and death in COVID-19. Liver Int 40(10):2394–2406, 2020

Piera-Velazquez S, Wermuth PJ, Gomez-Reino JJ, et al: Chemical exposure-induced systemic fibrosing disorders: novel insights into systemic sclerosis etiology and pathogenesis. Semin Arthritis Rheum 50(6):1226–1237, 2020

Pietrangelo A: Hereditary hemochromatosis: pathogenesis, diagnosis, and treatment. Gastroenterology 139(2):393–408, 408.e1–408.e2, 2010

Pisetsky DS. Antinuclear antibody testing: misunderstood or misbegotten? Nat Rev Rheumatol 13(8):495–502, 2017

Plante DT: Sleep propensity in psychiatric hypersomnolence: a systematic review and meta-analysis of multiple sleep latency test findings. Sleep Med Rev 31:48–57, 2017

Plenge P, Yang D, Salomon K, et al: The antidepressant drug vilazodone is an allosteric inhibitor of the serotonin transporter. Nat Commun 12(1):5063, 2021

Polat DS, Evans WP, Dogan BE: Contrast-enhanced digital mammography: technique, clinical applications, and pitfalls. AJR Am J Roentgenol 215(5):1267–1278, 2020

Polegato BF, Pereira AG, Azevedo PS, et al: Role of thiamin in health and disease. Nutr Clin Pract 34(4):558–564, 2019

Polkinghorne KR: Detection and measurement of urinary protein. Curr Opin Nephrol Hypertens 15(6):625–630, 2006

Praetorius Björk M, Johansson B: Gamma-glutamyltransferase (GGT) as a biomarker of cognitive decline at the end of life: contrasting age and time to death trajectories. Int Psychogeriatr 30(7):981–990, 2018

Price RW, Epstein LG, Becker JT, et al: Biomarkers of HIV-1 CNS infection and injury. Neurology 69(19):1781–1788, 2007

Prinz M, Priller J: The role of peripheral immune cells in the CNS in steady state and disease. Nat Neurosci 20(2):136–144, 2017

Qaseem A, Horwitch CA, Vijan S, et al: Testosterone treatment in adult men with age-related low testosterone: a clinical guideline from the American College of Physicians. Ann Intern Med 172(2):126–133, 2020

Rack M, Davis J, Roffwarg HP, et al: The multiple sleep latency test in the diagnosis of narcolepsy. Am J Psychiatry 162(11):2198–2199, 2005

Radin MS: Pitfalls in hemoglobin A1c measurement: when results may be misleading. J Gen Intern Med 29(2):388–394, 2014

Rajizadeh A, Mozaffari-Khosravi H, Yassini-Ardakani M, et al: Effect of magnesium supplementation on depression status in depressed patients with magnesium deficiency: a randomized, double-blind, placebo-controlled trial. Nutrition 35:56–60, 2017

Raman M, Middleton RJ, Kalra PA, et al: Estimating renal function in old people: an in-depth review. Int Urol Nephrol 49(11):1979–1988, 2017

Rebeck GW: The role of APOE on lipid homeostasis and inflammation in normal brains. J Lipid Res 58(8):1493–1499, 2017

Reddy P, Edwards LR: Magnesium supplementation in vitamin D deficiency. Am J Ther 26(1):e124–e132, 2019

Reed RC, Dutta S: Does it really matter when a blood sample for valproic acid concentration is taken following once-daily administration of divalproex-ER? Ther Drug Monit 28(3):413–418, 2006

Reiber H, Peter JB: Cerebrospinal fluid analysis: disease-related data patterns and evaluation programs. J Neurol Sci 184(2):101–122, 2001

Reisfield GM, Bertholf RL: "Practical guide" to urine drug screening clarified. Mayo Clin Proc 83(7):848–849, 2008

Remacha AF, Sardà MP, Canals C, et al: Role of serum holotranscobalamin (holoTC) in the diagnosis of patients with low serum cobalamin: comparison with methylmalonic acid and homocysteine. Ann Hematol 93(4):565–569, 2014

Reust CE, Hall L: Clinical inquiries: what is the differential diagnosis of an elevated alkaline phosphatase (AP) level in an otherwise asymptomatic patient? J Fam Pract 50(6):496–497, 2001

Reynolds RM, Padfield PL, Seckl JR: Disorders of sodium balance. BMJ 332(7543):702–705, 2006

Richa V, Rahul G, Sarika A: Macroprolactin; a frequent cause of misdiagnosed hyperprolactinemia in clinical practice. J Reprod Infertil 11(3):161–167, 2010

Richieri R, Boyer L, Faget-Agius C, et al: Determinants of brain SPECT perfusion and connectivity in treatment-resistant depression. Psychiatry Res 231(2):134–140, 2015

Rimer JD, Kolbach-Mandel AM, Ward MD, et al: The role of macromolecules in the formation of kidney stones. Urolithiasis 5(1):57–74, 2017

Rinck D, Frieling H, Freitag A, et al: Combinations of carbohydrate-deficient transferrin, mean corpuscular erythrocyte volume, gamma-glutamyltransferase, homocysteine and folate increase the significance of biological markers in alcohol dependent patients. Drug Alcohol Depend 89(1):60–65, 2007

Ritter JP, Ghirimoldi FM, Manuel LSM, et al: Cost of unnecessary amylase and lipase testing at multiple academic health systems. Am J Clin Pathol 153(3):346–352, 2020

Roberts CG, Ladenson PW: Hypothyroidism. Lancet 363(9411):793–803, 2004

Robertson GL: Antidiuretic hormone: normal and disordered function. Endocrinol Metab Clin North Am 30(3):671–694, vii, 2001

Robinson AG: Disorders of antidiuretic hormone secretion. Clin Endocrinol Metab 14(1):55–88, 1985

Romoli M, Perucca E, Sen A: Pyridoxine supplementation for levetiracetam-related neuropsychiatric adverse events: a systematic review. Epilepsy Behav 103(Pt A):106861, 2020

Rompianesi G, Hann A, Komolafe O, et al: Serum amylase and lipase and urinary trypsinogen and amylase for diagnosis of acute pancreatitis. Cochrane Database Syst Rev 4(4):CD012010, 2017

Roomruangwong C, Kanchanatawan B, Sirivichayakul S, et al: Antenatal depression and hematocrit levels as predictors of postpartum depression and anxiety symptoms. Psychiatry Res 238:211–217, 2016

Rose VL: American College of Cardiology and American Heart Association address the use of echocardiography. Am Fam Physician 56(5):1489–1490, 1997

Rouse JK, Shirley SR, Holley AB, et al: Split-night polysomnography overestimates apnea-hypopnea index in high-risk professions. Mil Med 184(5–6):e137–e140, 2019

Rundo JV, Downey R III: Polysomnography. Handb Clin Neurol 160:381–392, 2019

Sadock BJ, Sadock VA, Ruiz P (eds): Kaplan and Sadock's Comprehensive Textbook of Psychiatry. Philadelphia, PA, Lippincott Williams & Wilkins, 2009

Sailer C, Winzeler B, Christ-Crain M: Primary polydipsia in the medical and psychiatric patient: characteristics, complications and therapy. Swiss Med Wkly 147:w14514, 2017

Salcedo-Arellano MJ, Dufour B, McLennan Y, et al: Fragile X syndrome and associated disorders: clinical aspects and pathology. Neurobiol Dis 136:104740, 2020

Sammaritano LR: Antiphospholipid syndrome. Best Pract Res Clin Rheumatol 34(1):101463, 2020

Santos E, Emeka-Nwonovo C, Wang JY, et al: Developmental aspects of FXAND in a man with the FMR1 premutation. Mol Genet Genomic Med 8(2):e1050, 2020

Saud A, Naveen R, Aggarwal R, et al: COVID-19 and myositis: what we know so far. Curr Rheumatol Rep 23(8):63, 2021

Saxena A, Ng EYK, Lim ST: Imaging modalities to diagnose carotid artery stenosis: progress and prospect. Biomed Eng Online 18(1):66, 2019

Saxena K: Clinical features and management of poisoning due to potassium chloride. Med Toxicol Adverse Drug Exp 4(6):429–443, 1989

Schattner E: Correcting a decade of negative news about mammography. Clin Imaging 60(2):265–270, 2020

Scheitz JF, Stengl H, Nolte CH, et al: Neurological update: use of cardiac troponin in patients with stroke. J Neurol 268(6):2284–2292, 2021

Scherf-Clavel M, Wurst C, Nitschke F, et al: Extent of cortisol suppression at baseline predicts improvement in HPA axis function during antidepressant treatment. Psychoneuroendocrinology 114:104590, 2020

Schmitz B, Wang X, Barker PB, et al: Effects of aging on the human brain: a proton and phosphorus MR spectroscopy study at 3T. J Neuroimaging 28(4):416–421, 2018

Schoot TS, Molmans THJ, Grootens KP, et al: Systematic review and practical guideline for the prevention and management of the renal side effects of lithium therapy. Eur Neuropsychopharmacol 31:16–32, 2020

Schoretsanitis G, Kane JM, Correll CU, et al: Blood levels to optimize antipsychotic treatment in clinical practice: a joint consensus statement of the American Society of Clinical Psychopharmacology and the Therapeutic Drug Monitoring Task Force of the Arbeitsgemeinschaft für Neuropsychopharmakologie und Pharmakopsychiatrie. J Clin Psychiatry 81(3):19cs13169, 2020

Schorgg P, Bärnighausen T, Rohrmann S, et al: Vitamin B6 status among Vegetarians: findings from a population-based survey. Nutrients 13(5):1627, 2021

Schreiner AD, Rockey DC: Evaluation of abnormal liver tests in the adult asymptomatic patient. Current Opinion in Gastroenterology 34(4):272–279, 2018

Schriefer ME: Lyme disease diagnosis: serology. Clin Lab Med 35(4):797–814, 2015

Schutzer SE, Body BA, Boyle J, et al: Direct diagnostic tests for Lyme disease. Clin Infect Dis 68(6):1052–1057, 2019

Sciascia S, Costanzo P, Radin M, et al: Safety and tolerability of mRNA COVID-19 vaccines in people with antiphospholipid antibodies. Lancet Rheumatol 3(12):e832, 2021

Sebastiani P, Gurinovich A, Nygaard M, et al: APOE alleles and extreme human longevity. J Gerontol A Biol Sci Med Sci 74(1):44–51, 2019

Seehusen DA, Reeves MM, Fomin DA: Cerebrospinal fluid analysis. Am Fam Physician 68(6):1103–1108, 2003

Sefidbakht S, Lotfi M, Jalli R, et al: Methanol toxicity outbreak: when fear of COVID-19 goes viral. Emerg Med J 37(7):416, 2020

Selkoe DJ, Hardy J: The amyloid hypothesis of Alzheimer's disease at 25 years. EMBO Mol Med 8(6):595–608, 2016

658

Selvin E, Paynter NP, Erlinger TP: The effect of weight loss on C-reactive protein: a systematic review. Arch Intern Med 167(1):31–39, 2007

Seshadri S, Beiser A, Selhub J, et al: Plasma homocysteine as a risk factor for dementia and Alzheimer's disease. N Engl J Med 346(7):476–483, 2002

Shapiro ED. Clinical practice. Lyme disease. N Engl J Med 370(18):1724–1731, 2014

Sharma RA, Varga AW, Bubu OM, et al: Obstructive sleep apnea severity affects amyloid burden in cognitively normal elderly: a longitudinal study. Am J Respir Crit Care Med 197(7):933–943, 2018

Sharp VJ, Barnes KT, Erickson BA: Assessment of asymptomatic microscopic hematuria in adults. Am Fam Physician 88(11):747–754, 2013

Shaul ME, Fridlender ZG: Tumour-associated neutrophils in patients with cancer. Nat Rev Clin Oncol 16(10):601–620, 2019

Siebert DM, Rao AL: The use and abuse of human growth hormone in sports. Sports Health 10(5):419–426, 2018

Silvestre-Roig C, Braster Q, Ortega-Gomez A, et al: Neutrophils as regulators of cardiovascular inflammation. Nat Rev Cardiol 17(6):327–340, 2020

Simerville JA, Maxted WC, Pahira JJ: Urinalysis: a comprehensive review. Am Fam Physician 71:1153–1162, 2005

Sinha S, Kataria A, Kolla BP, et al: Wernicke encephalopathy: clinical pearls. Mayo Clin Proc 94(6):1065–1072, 2019

Siragy HM: Hyponatremia, fluid-electrolyte disorders, and the syndrome of inappropriate antidiuretic hormone secretion: diagnosis and treatment options. Endocr Pract 12(4):446–457, 2006

Skoberne A, Konieczny A, Schiffer: Glomerular epithelial cells in the urine: what has to be done to make them worthwhile? Am J Physiol Renal Physiol 296(2):F230–F241, 2009

Skov L, Holm KM, Johansen SS, et al: Postmortem brain and blood reference concentrations of alprazolam, bromazepam, chlordiazepoxide, diazepam, and their metabolites and a review of the literature. J Anal Toxicol 40(7):529–36, 2016

Slough C, Masters SC, Hurley RA, et al: Clinical positron emission tomography (PET) neuroimaging: advantages and limitations as a diagnostic tool. J Neuropsychiatry Clin Neurosci 28(2):A4–A71, 2016

Smith AD, Refsum H, Bottiglieri T, et al: Homocysteine and dementia: an international consensus statement. J Alzheimers Dis 62(2):561–570, 2018

Soh SB, Aw TC: Laboratory testing in thyroid conditions: pitfalls and clinical utility. Ann Lab Med 39(1):3–14, 2019

Spaulding SW, Lippes H: Hyperthyroidism: causes, clinical features, and diagnosis. Med Clin North Am 69(5):937–951, 1985

Stabler SP: Clinical practice: vitamin B12 deficiency. N Engl J Med 368(2):149–160, 2013

Sullivan SS, Kushida CA: Multiple sleep latency test and maintenance of wakefulness test. Chest 134(4):854–861, 2008

Sun J, Han W, Wu S, et al: Associations between hyperhomocysteinemia and the presence and severity of acute coronary syndrome in young adults ≤<t#>35 years of age. BMC Cardiovasc Disord 21(1):47, 2021

Svensson JE, Svanborg C, Plavén-Sigray P, et al: Serotonin transporter availability increases in patients recovering from a depressive episode. Transl Psychiatry 11(1):264, 2021

Syed Iqbal H, Balakrishnan P, Murugavel KG, et al: Performance characteristics of a new rapid immunochromatographic test for the detection of antibodies to human immunodeficiency virus (HIV) types 1 and 2. J Clin Lab Anal 22(3):178–185, 2008

Tarleton EK, Littenberg B: Magnesium intake and depression in adults. J Am Board Fam Med 28(2):249–256, 2015

Taylor MM, Hawkins K, Gonzalez A, et al: Use of the serologic testing algorithm for recent HIV seroconversion (STARHS) to identify recently acquired HIV infections in men with early syphilis in Los Angeles County. J Acquir Immune Defic Syndr 38(5):505–508, 2005

Territo M: Overview of leukopenias, in Merck Manual: Professional Version. Rahway, NJ, Marck Sharp & Dohme, August 2021. Available at: https://www.merckmanuals.com/professional/hematology-and-oncology/leukopenias/overview-of-leukopenias. Accessed July 28, 2022.

Theal RM, Scott K: Evaluating asymptomatic patients with abnormal liver function test results. Am Fam Physician 53(6):2111–2119, 1996

Thomas Z, Fraser GL: An update on the diagnosis of adrenal insufficiency and the use of corticotherapy in critical illness. Ann Pharmacother 41(9):1456–1465, 2007

Tojo K, Sugawara Y, Oi Y, et al: The U-shaped association of serum iron level with disease severity in adult hospitalized patients with COVID-19. Sci Rep 11(1):13431, 2021

Torpy DJ, Stratakis CA, Chrousos GP: Hyper- and hypoaldosteronism. Vitam Horm 57:177–216, 1999

Torre DL, Falorni A: Pharmacological causes of hyperprolactinemia. Ther Clin Risk Manag 3(5):929–951, 2007

Toyohara J: Importance of P-gp PET Imaging in Pharmacology. Curr Pharm Des 22(38):5830–5836, 2016

Truong T, Hetzel F, Stiff KM, et al: Case of hypoactive delirium precipitated by thiamine deficiency. BMJ Case Rep 14(3):e239886, 2021

UCSF Health: Prolactin blood test, in Conditions and Treatments: Medical Tests. San Francisco, CA, University of California San Francisco, 2022. Available at: https://www.ucsfhealth.org/medical-tests/prolactin-blood-test. Accessed July 28, 2022.

U.S. Food and Drug Administration: Table of pharmacogenetic associations, in Products and Medical Procedures: In Vitro Diagnostics: Precision Medicine. Washington, DC, U.S. Food and Drug Administration, May 24, 2022. Available at: https://www.fda.gov/medical-devices/precision-medicine/table-pharmacogenetic-associations#section1. Accessed July 28, 2022.

U.S. National Library of Medicine: Health topics, in MedlinePlus. Washington DC, U.S. Department of Health and Human Services, 2022. Available at: https://medlineplus.gov/health-topics.html. Accessed July 28, 2022.

U.S. National Library of Medicine: DailyMed. Bethesda, National Institutes of Health, 2022. Available at: https://dailymed.nlm.nih.gov/dailymed. Accessed July 28, 2022.

Vaidya A, Carey RM: Evolution of the primary aldosteronism syndrome: updating the approach. J Clin Endocrinol Metab 105(12):3771–3783, 2020

van der Plas E, Langbehn DR, Conrad AL, et al: Abnormal brain development in child and adolescent carriers of mutant huntingtin. Neurology 93(10):e1021–e1030, 2019

Van Poppel H, Roobol MJ, Chapple CR, et al: Prostate-specific antigen testing as part of a risk-adapted early detection strategy for prostate cancer: European Association of Urology position and recommendations for 2021. Eur Urol 80(6)703–711, 2021

Varricchi G, Raap U, Rivellese F, et al: Human mast cells and basophils-How are they similar how are they different? Immunol Rev 282(1):8–34, 2018

Vasudeva SS: Meningitis workup, in Drugs and Diseases: Infectious Disease. Medscape, July 11, 2022. Available at: https://emedicine.medscape.com/article/232915-workup. Accessed July 21, 2022.

Veasey SC, Rosen IM: Obstructive sleep apnea in adults. N Engl J Med 380(15):1442–1449, 2019

Veda P: Evaluation of macrocytosis in routine hemograms. Indian J Hematol Blood Transfus 29(1):26–30, 2013

Verrotti A, Coppola G, Parisi P, et al: Bone and calcium metabolism and antiepileptic drugs. Clin Neurol Neurosurg 112(1):1–10, 2010

Vinkers CH, Kuzminskaite E, Lamers F, et al: An integrated approach to understand biological stress system dysregulation across depressive and anxiety disorders. J Affect Disord 283:139–146, 2021

Vogel F, Gansmüller R, Leiblein T, et al: The use of ziprasidone in clinical practice: analysis of pharmacokinetic and pharmacodynamic aspects from data of a drug monitoring survey. Eur Psychiatry 24(3):143–148, 2009

Waddell LA, Greig J, Mascarenhas M, et al: The accuracy of diagnostic tests for Lyme disease in humans: a systematic review and meta-analysis of North American research. PLoS One 11(12):e0168613, 2016

Wald DS, Bestwick JP: Association between serum calcium, serum phosphate and aortic stenosis with implications for prevention. Eur J Prev Cardiol 25(5):551–556, 2018

Weir MR: Microalbuminuria and cardiovascular disease. Clin J Am Soc Nephrol 2(3):581–590, 2007

Wen J, Sawmiller D, Wheeldon B, et al: A review for lithium: pharmacokinetics, drug design, and toxicity. CNS Neurol Disord Drug Targets 18(10):769–778, 2019

White PC: Disorders of aldosterone biosynthesis and action. N Engl J Med 331:250–258, 1994

Williams JC Jr, Gambaro G, Rodgers A, et al: Urine and stone analysis for the investigation of the renal stone former: a consensus conference. Urolithiasis 49(1):1–16, 2021

Wolffenbuttel BHR, Wouters HJCM, de Jong WHA, et al: Association of vitamin B12, methylmalonic acid, and functional parameters. Neth J Med 78(1):10–24, 2020

Woreta TA, Alqahtani SA: Evaluation of abnormal liver tests. Med Clin North Am 98(1):1–16, 2014

Wright LA, Hirsch IB: Metrics beyond hemoglobin A1C in diabetes management: time in range, hypoglycemia, and other parameters. Diabetes Technol Ther 19(S2):S16–S26, 2017

Wu AHB: Tietz Clinical Guide to Laboratory Tests, 4th Edition. St. Louis, MO, WB Saunders, 2006

Xie C, Huang W, Young RL, et al: Role of bile acids in the regulation of food intake, and their dysregulation in metabolic disease. Nutrients 13(4):1104, 2021

Yamazaki Y, Zhao N, Caulfield TR, et al: Apolipoprotein E and Alzheimer disease: pathobiology and targeting strategies. Nat Rev Neurol 15(9):501–518, 2019

Yang Q, Lu Y, Deng Y, et al: Homocysteine level is positively and independently associated with serum creatinine and urea nitrogen levels in old male patients with hypertension. Sci Rep 10(1):18050, 2020

Yip L, Bixler D, Brooks DE, et al: Serious adverse health events, including death, associated with ingesting alcohol-based hand sanitizers containing methanol: Arizona and New Mexico, May–June 2020. MMWR Morb Mortal Wkly Rep 69(32):1070–1073, 2020

Ylli D, Wartofsky L, Burman KD: Evaluation and treatment of amiodarone-induced thyroid disorders. J Clin Endocrinol Metab 106(1):226–236, 2021

Young H: Guidelines for serological testing for syphilis. Sex Transm Infect 76(5):403–405, 2000

Zagzag J, Hu MI, Fisher SB, et al: Hypercalcemia and cancer: differential diagnosis and treatment. CA Cancer J Clin 68(5):377–386, 2018

Zakharov S, Pelclova D, Navratil T, et al: Fomepizole versus ethanol in the treatment of acute methanol poisoning: comparison of clinical effectiveness in a mass poisoning outbreak. Clin Toxicol (Phila) 53(8):797–806, 2015

Zarifi C, Vyas S: Spice-y kidney failure: a case report and systematic review of acute kidney injury attributable to the use of synthetic cannabis. Perm J 21:16–160, 2017

Zhang XH, Liang H: Systematic review with network meta-analysis: diagnostic values of ultrasonography, computed tomography, and magnetic resonance imaging in patients with ischemic stroke. Medicine (Baltimore) 98(30):e16360, 2019

Zhang Z, Pereira SL, Luo M, et al: Evaluation of blood biomarkers associated with risk of malnutrition in older adults: a systematic review and meta-analysis. Nutrients 9(8):829, 2017

Zhu A, Kaneshiro M, Kaunitz JD: Evaluation and treatment of iron deficiency anemia: a gastroenterological perspective. Dig Dis Sci 55(3):548–559, 2010

Zik C: Late life vitamin B12 deficiency. Clin Geriatr Med 35(3):319–325, 2019

Zu H, Wang H, Li C, et al: Preoperative prealbumin levels on admission as an independent predictive factor in patients with gastric cancer. Medicine (Baltimore) 99(11):e19196, 2020

Zuo Y, Yalavarthi S, Shi H, et al: Neutrophil extracellular traps in COVID-19. JCI Insight 5(11):e138999, 2020

Diseases and Conditions Section

Abboud H, Probasco JC, Irani S, et al: Autoimmune encephalitis: proposed best practice recommendations for diagnosis and acute management. J Neurol Neurosurg Psychiatry 92(7):757–768, 2021

Abdel-Naby S, Hassanein M: Neuropsychiatric manifestations of chronic manganese poisoning. J Neurol Neurosurg Psychiatry 28:282–288, 1965

Abrol E, Coutinho E, Chou M, et al: Psychosis in systemic lupus erythematosus (SLE): 40-year experience of a specialist centre. Rheumatology (Oxford) 60(12):5620–5629, 2021

Abussuud ZA, Geneta VP: Rheumatoid meningitis. World Neurosurg 137:98–101, 2020

Abutaleb A, Kottilil S: Hepatitis A: epidemiology, natural history, unusual clinical manifestations, and prevention. Gastroenterol Clin North Am 49(2):191–199, 2020

Adamou M, Jones SL, Wetherhill S: Predicting diagnostic outcome in adult autism spectrum disorder using the autism diagnostic observation schedule, second edition. BMC Psychiatry 21(1):24, 2021

Adra N, Goodheart AE, Rapalino O, et al: MRI shrimp sign in cerebellar progressive multifocal leukoencephalopathy: description and validation of a novel observation. AJNR Am J Neuroradiol 42(6):1073–1079, 2021

Adrogué HJ, Madias NE: Hypernatremia. N Engl J Med 342(20):1493–1499, 2000

Aghagoli G, Gallo Marin B, et al: Neurological involvement in COVID-19 and potential mechanisms: a review. Neurocrit Care 34(3):1062–1071, 2021

Ahmadi L, Goldman MB: Primary polydipsia: update. Best Pract Res Clin Endocrinol Metab 34(5):101469, 2020

Akiyama Y, Ishikane M, Ohmagari N: Epstein-Barr virus induced skin rash in infectious mononucleosis. IDCases 26:e01298, 2021

Aksamit AJ: Chronic meningitis. N Engl J Med 385(10):930–936, 2021

Alagesan M, Chidambaram Y: Pellagra. N Engl J Med 386(10):e24, 2022

Alexandri M, Reynolds BZ, Smith H, et al: Wernicke's encephalopathy and cranial nerve VII palsy in a 24-year-old patient with COVID-19. Int J Emerg Med 15(1):6, 2022

Alfano G, Ferrari A, Fontana F, et al: Hypokalemia in patients with COVID-19. Clin Exp Nephrol 25(4):401–409, 2021

Almeida MQ, Mendonca BB: Adrenal insufficiency and glucocorticoid use during the COVID-19 pandemic. Clinics (Sao Paulo) 75:e2022, 2020

Almeida PH, Matielo CEL, Curvelo LA, et al: Update on the management and treatment of viral hepatitis. World J Gastroenterol 27(23):3249–3261, 2021

Alsharif W, Qurashi A: Effectiveness of COVID-19 diagnosis and management tools: a review. Radiography (Lond) 27(2):682–687, 2021

Altuna-Azkargorta M, Mendioroz-Iriarte M: Blood biomarkers in Alzheimer's disease. Neurologia (Engl Ed) 36(9):704–710, 2021

Alves C, Franco RR: Prader-Willi syndrome: endocrine manifestations and management. Arch Endocrinol Metab 64(3):223–234, 2020

Alwani M, Yassin A, Talib R, et al: Cardiovascular disease, hypogonadism and erectile dysfunction: early detection, prevention and the positive effects of long-term testosterone treatment: prospective observational, real-life data. Vasc Health Risk Manag 17:497–508, 2021

American Diabetes Association: Classification and diagnosis of diabetes: standards of medical care in diabetes 2021. Diabetes Care 44(Suppl 1):S152S33, 2021

American Psychiatric Association: Diagnostic and Statistical Manual of Mental Disorders, 5th Edition, Text Revision. Washington, DC, American Psychiatric Association, 2022

Anamnart C, Tisavipat N, Owattanapanich W, et al: Newly diagnosed neuromyelitis optica spectrum disorders following vaccination: case report and systematic review. Mult Scler Relat Disord 58:103414, 2022

Anbarasan D, Kitchin M, Adler LA: Screening for adult ADHD. Curr Psychiatry Rep 22(12):72, 2020

Andalib S, Biller J, Di Napoli M, et al: Peripheral nervous system manifestations associated with COVID-19. Curr Neurol Neurosci Rep 21(3):9, 2021

Anderson JL, Morrow DA: Acute myocardial infarction. N Engl J Med 376(21):2053–2064, 2017

Anderson ND: State of the science on mild cognitive impairment (MCI). CNS Spectr 24(1):78–87, 2019

Anderson NE, Chung K, Willoughby E, et al: Neurological manifestations of phaeochromocytomas and secretory paragangliomas: a reappraisal. J Neurol Neurosurg Psychiatry 84(4):452–457, 2013

Andresen-Streichert H, Müller A, Glahn A, et al: Alcohol biomarkers in clinical and forensic contexts. Dtsch Arztebl Int 115(18):309–315, 2018

Andrews JP, Taylor J, Saunders D, et al: Peduncular psychosis. BMJ Case Rep 2016:bcr2016216165, 2016

Aneja J, Kuppili PP, Paul K, et al: Antiphospholipid syndrome presenting as treatment resistant bipolar disorder and thrombocytopenia in a young male. J Neuroimmunol 343:577238, 2020

Anglin RE, Rosebush PI, Mazurek MF: The neuropsychiatric profile of Addison's disease: revisiting a forgotten phenomenon. J Neuropsychiatry Clin Neurosci 18(4):450–459, 2006

Antonarakis SE, Skotko BG, Rafii MS, et al: Down syndrome. Nat Rev Dis Primers 6(1):9, 2020

Antshel KM, Fremont W, Roizen NJ, et al: ADHD, major depressive disorder, and simple phobias are prevalent psychiatric conditions in youth with velocardiofacial syndrome. J Am Acad Child Adolesc Psychiatry 45(5):596–603, 2006

Aomura D, Kurasawa Y, Harada M, et al: Brain MRI detection of early Wernicke's encephalopathy in a hemodialysis patient. Clin Case Rep 10(3):e05539, 2022

Appleby N, Angelov D: Clinical and laboratory assessment of a patient with thrombocytosis. Br J Hosp Med (Lond) 78(10):558–564, 2017

Arca KN, Halker Singh RB: Dehydration and headache. Curr Pain Headache Rep 25(8):56, 2021

Arca KN, Halker Singh RB: The hypertensive headache: a review. Curr Pain Headache Rep 23(5):30, 2019

Aringer M, Costenbader K, Daikh D, et al: 2019 European League Against Rheumatism/American College of Rheumatology classification criteria for systemic lupus erythematosus. Arthritis Rheumatol 71(9):1400–1412, 2019

Aringer M: Inflammatory markers in systemic lupus erythematosus. J Autoimmun 110:102374, 2020

Armstrong MJ, Okun MS: Diagnosis and treatment of Parkinson disease: a review. JAMA 323(6):548–560, 2020

Arora N, Wasti K, Suri V, et al: "Face of a giant panda" and "beating wings" in a young male. Cureus 14(2):e22429, 2022

Arumugam A, Raja K, Venugopalan M, et al: Down syndrome: a narrative review with a focus on anatomical features. Clin Anat 29(5):568–577, 2016

ARUP Laboratories: ARUP Consult: The Physician's Guide to Laboratory Test Selection and Interpretation. Salt Lake City, UT, ARUP Laboratories, 2022. Available at: https://www.arupconsult.com. Accessed July 20, 2022.

ARUP Laboratories: Laboratory Test Directory. Salt Lake City, UT, ARUP Laboratories, 2022. Available at: https://www.aruplab.com. Accessed July 20, 2022.

Arvanitakis Z, Shah RC, Bennett DA: Diagnosis and management of dementia: review. JAMA 322(16):1589–1599, 2019

Arvikar SL, Steere AC: Diagnosis and treatment of Lyme arthritis. Infect Dis Clin North Am 29(2):269–280, 2015

Atarashi R, Sano K, Satoh K, et al: Real-time quaking-induced conversion: a highly sensitive assay for prion detection. Prion 5(3):150–153, 2011

Atri A: The Alzheimer's disease clinical spectrum: diagnosis and management. Med Clin North Am 103(2):263–293, 2019

Avari JN, Young RC: A patient with bipolar disorder and antiphospholipid syndrome. J Geriatr Psychiatry Neurol 25(1):26–28, 2012

Axisa PP, Hafler DA: Multiple sclerosis: genetics, biomarkers, treatments. Curr Opin Neurol 29(3):345–353, 2016

Babaei A, Szabo A, Shad S, et al: Chronic daily opioid exposure is associated with dysphagia, esophageal outflow obstruction, and disordered peristalsis. Neurogastroenterol Motil 31(7):e13601, 2019

Bagash H, Marwat A, Marwat A, et al: A case of chronic Wernicke encephalopathy (WE): an underdiagnosed phenomena. Cureus 13(10):e19100, 2021

BaHammam AS, Alnakshabandi K, Pandi-Perumal SR: Neuropsychiatric correlates of narcolepsy. Curr Psychiatry Rep 22(8):36, 2020

Baig AM: Deleterious outcomes in long-hauler COVID-19: the effects of SARS-CoV-2 on the CNS in chronic COVID syndrome. ACS Chem Neurosci 11(24):4017–4020, 2020

Baig FA, Khan S, Rizwan A: Frequency of vitamin B12 deficiency in type 2 diabetic patients taking metformin. Cureus 14(3):e22924, 2022

Baj J, Flieger W, Flieger M, et al: Autism spectrum disorder: trace elements imbalances and the pathogenesis and severity of autistic symptoms. Neurosci Biobehav Rev 129:117–132, 2021

Bakchoul T, Marini I: Drug-associated thrombocytopenia. Hematology Am Soc Hematol Educ Program 2018(1):576–583, 2018

Balani SG, Umarji GM, Bellare RA, et al: Chronic manganese poisoning. J Postgrad Med 13:116–121, 1967

Ballantyne F III, Vander Ark C: The difficult diagnosis of hypokalemia. Am Fam Physician 33:256–258, 1986

Ballard C, Mobley W, Hardy J, et al: Dementia in Down's syndrome. Lancet Neurol 15(6):622–636, 2016

Banaschewski T, Becker K, Döpfner M, et al: Attention-deficit/hyperactivity disorder. Dtsch Arztebl Int 114(9):149–159, 2017

Bancos I, Hahner S, Tomlinson J, et al: Diagnosis and management of adrenal insufficiency. Lancet Diabetes Endocrinol 3(3):216–226, 2015

Bandmann O, Weiss KH, Kaler SG: Wilson's disease and other neurological copper disorders. Lancet Neurol 14(1):103–113, 2015

Bang J, Spina S, Miller BL: Frontotemporal dementia. Lancet 386(10004):1672–1682, 2015

Barbesino G: Thyroid function changes in the elderly and their relationship to cardiovascular health: a mini-review. Gerontology 65(1):1–8, 2019

Barbhaiya M, Costenbader KH: Environmental exposures and the development of systemic lupus erythematosus. Curr Opin Rheumatol 28(5):497–505, 2016

Barbot M, Zilio M, Scaroni C: Cushing's syndrome: overview of clinical presentation, diagnostic tools and complications. Best Pract Res Clin Endocrinol Metab 34(2):101380, 2020

Baroni L, Bonetto C, Rizzo G, et al: Association between cognitive impairment and vitamin B12, folate, and homocysteine status in elderly adults: a retrospective study. J Alzheimers Dis 70(2):443–453, 2019

Barra A, Camardese G, Tonioni F, et al: Plasma magnesium level and psychomotor retardation in major depressed patients. Magnes Res 20(4):245–249, 2007

Barrell K, Smith AG: Peripheral neuropathy. Med Clin North Am 103(2):383–397, 2019

Bart G, Piccolo P, Zhang L, et al: Markers for hepatitis A, B, and C in methadone maintained patients: an unexpectedly high co-infection with silent hepatitis B. Addiction 103:681–686, 2008

Bartsch T, Rempe T, Leypoldt F, et al: The spectrum of progressive multifocal leukoencephalopathy: a practical approach. Eur J Neurol 26(4):566-e41, 2019

Barzegar M, Mirmosayyeb O, Ebrahimi N, et al: COVID-19 susceptibility and outcomes among patients with neuromyelitis optica spectrum disorder (NMOSD): a systematic review and meta-analysis. Mult Scler Relat Disord 57:103359, 2022

Bassetti CLA, Adamantidis A, Burdakov D, et al: Narcolepsy: clinical spectrum, aetiopathophysiology, diagnosis and treatment. Nat Rev Neurol 15(9):519–539, 2019

Battaglia F, Quartarone A, Bagnato S, et al: Brain dysfunction in uremia: a question of cortical hyperexcitability? Clin Neurophysiol 116:1507–1514, 2005

Bauduin SEEC, van der Wee NJA, van der Werff SJA: Structural brain abnormalities in Cushing's syndrome. Curr Opin Endocrinol Diabetes Obes 25(4):285–289, 2018

Bearelly P, Oates R: Recent advances in managing and understanding Klinefelter syndrome. F1000Res 8:F1000, 2019

Beckert BW, Concannon MJ, Henry SL, et al: The effect of herbal medicines on platelet function: an in vivo experiment and review of the literature. Plast Reconstr Surg 120:2044–2050, 2007

Beerepoot S, Nierkens S, Boelens JJ, et al: Peripheral neuropathy in metachromatic leukodystrophy: current status and future perspective. Orphanet J Rare Dis 14(1):240, 2019

Bellis SA, Kuhn I, Adams S, et al: The consequences of hyperphagia in people with Prader-Willi syndrome: a systematic review of studies of morbidity and mortality. Eur J Med Genet 65(1):104379, 2022

Ben Ammar H, Hakiri A, Khelifa E, et al: Metachromatic leukodystrophy presenting as a bipolar disorder: A case report. Encephale 48(1):108–109, 2022

Ben Salem C, Badreddine A, Fathallah N, et al: Drug-induced hyperkalemia. Drug Saf 37(9):677–692, 2014

Benítez-Mejía JF, Morales-Cuellar J, Restrepo-López JS, et al: Psycogenic polydipsia and severe hyponatremia in bipolar affective disorder. Actas Esp Psiquiatr 49(6):288–290, 2021

Bennett B, Mansingh A, Fenton C, et al: Graves' disease presenting with hypomania and paranoia to the acute psychiatry service. BMJ Case Rep 14(2):e236089, 2021

Bent S, Nallamothu BK, Simel DL, et al: Does this woman have an acute uncomplicated urinary tract infection? JAMA 287:2701–2710, 2002

Benton D: Hypoglycemia and aggression: a review. Int J Neurosci 41:163–168, 1988

Bentz M, Westwood H, Jepsen JRM, et al: The autism diagnostic observation schedule: patterns in individuals with anorexia nervosa. Eur Eat Disord Rev 28(5):571–579, 2020

Benzoni C, Moscatelli M, Fenu S, et al: Metachromatic leukodystrophy with late adult-onset: diagnostic clues and differences from other genetic leukoencephalopathies with dementia [published correction appears in J Neurol. J Neurol 268(5):1972–1976, 2021

Beretta S, Stabile A, Balducci C, et al: COVID-19-associated immune-mediated encephalitis mimicking acute-onset Creutzfeldt-Jakob disease. Ann Clin Transl Neurol 8(12):2314–2318, 2021

Berger JR, Aksamit AJ, Clifford DB, et al: PML diagnostic criteria: consensus statement from the AAN Neuroinfectious Disease section. Neurology 80(15):1430–1438, 2013

Bergink V, Rasgon N, Wisner KL: Postpartum psychosis: madness, mania, and melancholia in motherhood. Am J Psychiatry 173(12):1179–1188, 2016

Bergstrom J: Toxicity of uremia: physiopathology and clinical signs. Contrib Nephrol 71:1–9, 1989

Berkins S, Schiöth HB, Rukh G: Depression and vegetarians: association between dietary vitamin B6, B12, and folate intake and global and subcortical brain volumes. Nutrients 13(6):1790, 2021

Berlinska A, Swiatkowska-Stodulska R, Sworczak K: Old problem, new concerns: hypercortisolemia in the time of COVID-19. Front Endocrinol (Lausanne) 12:711612, 2021

Beyer G, Habtezion A, Werner J, et al: Chronic pancreatitis. Lancet 396(10249):499–512, 2020

Bhatt K, Yoo J, Bridges A: Ketamine-induced manic episode. Prim Care Companion CNS Disord 23(3):20l02811, 2021

Bieniek KF, Cairns NJ, Crary JF, et al: The second NINDS/NIBIB consensus meeting to define neuropathological criteria for the diagnosis of chronic traumatic encephalopathy. J Neuropathol Exp Neurol 80(3):210–219, 2021

Bilezikian JP, Bandeira L, Khan A, et al: Hyperparathyroidism. Lancet 391(10116):168–178, 2018

Bilezikian JP: Hypoparathyroidism. J Clin Endocrinol Metab 105(6):1722–1736, 2020

Bird RP: The emerging role of vitamin B6 in inflammation and carcinogenesis. Adv Food Nutr Res 83:151–194, 2018

Bissell DM, Anderson KE, Bonkovsky HL: Porphyria. N Engl J Med 377(9):862–872, 2017

Black DM, Rosen CJ: Clinical Practice. Postmenopausal osteoporosis. N Engl J Med 374(3):254–262, 2016

Bloem BR, Okun MS, Klein C: Parkinson's disease. Lancet 397(10291):2284–2303, 2021

Bokhari SR, Siriki R, Teran FJ, et al: Fatal hypermagnesemia due to laxative use. Am J Med Sci 355(4):390–395, 2018

Bommersbach TJ, Lapid MI, Leung JG, et al: Management of psychotropic drug-induced DRESS syndrome: a systematic review. Mayo Clin Proc 91(6):787–801, 2016

Bonomi M, Rochira V, Pasquali D, et al: Klinefelter syndrome (KS): genetics, clinical phenotype and hypogonadism. J Endocrinol Invest 40(2):123–134, 2017

Boog GHP, Lopes JVZ, Mahler JV, et al: Diagnostic tools for neurosyphilis: a systematic review. BMC Infect Dis 21(1):568, 2021

Bosman W, Hoenderop JGJ, de Baaij JHF: Genetic and drug-induced hypomagnesemia: different cause, same mechanism. Proc Nutr Soc 80(3):327–338, 2021

Brackenridge CJ, Jones IH: Relation of hypermagnesaemia to activity and neuroleptic drug therapy in schizophrenic states. J Neurol Neurosurg Psychiatry 34(2):195–199, 1971

Bradshaw MJ, Pawate S, Koth LL, et al: Neurosarcoidosis: pathophysiology, diagnosis, and treatment. Neurol Neuroimmunol Neuroinflamm 8(6):e1084, 2021

Brar K, Kaushik SS, Lippmann S: Catatonia update. Prim Care Companion CNS Disord 19(5):16br02023, 2017

Braun MM, Barstow CH, Pyzocha NJ: Diagnosis and management of sodium disorders: hyponatremia and hypernatremia. Am Fam Physician 91(5):299–307, 2015

Breton A, Casey D, Arnaoutoglou NA: Cognitive tests for the detection of mild cognitive impairment (MCI), the prodromal stage of dementia: meta-analysis of diagnostic accuracy studies. Int J Geriatr Psychiatry 34(2):233–242, 2019

Brissot P, Pietrangelo A, Adams PC: Haemochromatosis. Nat Rev Dis Primers 4:18016, 2018

Brodie D, Schluger NW: The diagnosis of tuberculosis. Clin Chest Med 26(2):247–271, 2005

Brook I: Microbiology and treatment of brain abscess. J Clin Neurosci 38:8–12, 2017

Brouwer MC, van de Beek D: Epidemiology, diagnosis, and treatment of brain abscesses. Curr Opin Infect Dis 30(1):129–134, 2017

Brust JC: A 74-year-old man with memory loss and neuropathy who enjoys alcoholic beverages. JAMA 299(9):1046–1054, 2008

Budhram A, Leung A, Nicolle MW, et al: Diagnosing autoimmune limbic encephalitis. CMAJ 191(19):E529–E534, 2019

Buffington MA, Abreo K: Hyponatremia: a review. J Intensive Care Med 31(4):223–236, 2016

Bull MJ: Down syndrome. N Engl J Med 382(24):2344–2352, 2020

Bunevicius R, Prange AJ Jr: Psychiatric manifestations of Graves' hyperthyroidism: pathophysiology and treatment options. CNS Drugs 20(11):897–909, 2006

Burman D: Sleep disorders: insomnia. FP Essent 460:22–28, 2017

Busch JR, Löchte L, Lindh AS, et al: Lethal small bowel obstruction due to pica. J Forensic Sci 67(1):374–376, 2022

Bush G, Fink M, Petrides G, et al: Catatonia. I. Rating scale and standardized examination. Acta Psychiatr Scand 93(2):129–136, 1996

Butler MG, Miller JL, Forster JL: Prader-Willi syndrome: clinical genetics, diagnosis and treatment approaches: an update. Curr Pediatr Rev 15(4):207–244, 2019

Buysse DJ: Insomnia. JAMA 309(7):706–716, 2013

Cai W, Mueller C, Li Y-J, et al: Post stroke depression and risk of stroke recurrence and mortality: a systematic review and meta-analysis. Ageing Res Rev 50:102–109, 2019

Cai X, Ebell MH, Haines L: Accuracy of signs, symptoms, and hematologic parameters for the diagnosis of infectious mononucleosis: a systematic review and meta-analysis. J Am Board Fam Med 34(6):1141–1156, 2021

Cain KP, McCarthy KD, Heilig CM, et al: An algorithm for tuberculosis screening and diagnosis in people with HIV. N Engl J Med 362(8):707–716, 2010

Calissendorff J, Falhammar H: To treat or not to treat subclinical hypothyroidism: what is the evidence? Medicina (Kaunas) 56(1):40, 2020

Calpena Martínez S, Arapiles Muñoz A: The value of the classic signs: hypocalcemia. Med Clin (Barc) 157(11):554, 2021

Camacho PM, Petak SM, Binkley N, et al: American Association of Clinical Endocrinologists/ American College of Endocrinology clinical practice guidelines for the diagnosis and treatment of postmenopausal osteoporosis: 2020 update. Endocr Pract 26(Suppl 1):1–46, 2020

Campbell NL, Unverzagt F, LaMantia MA, et al: Risk factors for the progression of mild cognitive impairment to dementia. Clin Geriatr Med 29(4):873–893, 2013

Cantiera M, Tattevin P, Sonneville R: Brain abscess in immunocompetent adult patients. Rev Neurol (Paris) 175(7–8):469–474, 2019

Cao B, Wang DF, Xu MY, et al: Lower folate levels in schizophrenia: a meta-analysis. Psychiatry Res 245:1–7, 2016

Cao S, Wang X, Cestodio K: Pellagra: an almost-forgotten differential diagnosis of chronic diarrhea: more prevalent than we think. Nutr Clin Pract 35(5):860–863, 2020

Cardones AR: Drug reaction with eosinophilia and systemic symptoms (DRESS) syndrome. Clin Dermatol 38(6):702–711, 2020

Cariccio VL, Samà A, Bramanti P, et al: Mercury involvement in neuronal damage and in neurodegenerative diseases. Biol Trace Elem Res 187(2):341–356, 2019

Carod-Artal FJ: Post-COVID-19 syndrome: epidemiology, diagnostic criteria and pathogenic mechanisms involved. Rev Neurol 72(11):384–396, 2021

Carranza C, Pedraza-Sanchez S, de Oyarzabal-Mendez E, et al: Diagnosis for latent tuberculosis infection: new alternatives. Front Immunol 11:2006, 2020

Carrasquillo JA, Chen CC, Jha A, et al: Imaging of pheochromocytoma and paraganglioma. J Nucl Med 62(8):1033–1042, 2021

Carroll VK, Rado JT: Is a medical illness causing your patient's depression? Endocrine, neurologic, infectious, or malignant processes could cause mood symptoms. Current Psychiatry 8(8):43, 2009

Castaneda D, Gonzalez AJ, Alomari M, et al: From hepatitis A to E: a critical review of viral hepatitis. World J Gastroenterol 27(16):1691–1715, 2021

Castelli G, Desai KM, Cantone RE: Peripheral neuropathy: evaluation and differential diagnosis. Am Fam Physician 102(12):732–739, 2020

Centers for Disease Control and Prevention: CDC's diagnostic criteria for Creutzfeldt-Jakob disease (CJD), in Creutzfeldt-Jakob Disease, Classic (CJD): Diagnostic Criteria. Atlanta, GA, Centers for Disease Control and Prevention, 2018. Available at: https://www.cdc.gov/prions/cjd/diagnostic-criteria.html. Accessed January 2, 2022.

Centers for Disease Control and Prevention: Testing recommendations for hepatitis C virus infection, in Viral Hepatitis. Atlanta, GA, Centers for Disease Control and Prevention, July 29, 2020. Available at: https://www.cdc.gov/hepatitis/hcv/guidelinesc.htm. Accessed July 21, 2022.

Centers for Disease Control and Prevention: Hepatitis B questions and answers for health professionals, in Viral Hepatitis. Atlanta, GA, Centers for Disease Control and Prevention, March 30, 2022. Available at: https://www.cdc.gov/hepatitis/hbv/hbvfaq.htm. Accessed July 21, 2022.

Centers for Disease Control and Prevention: Types of HIV tests, in HIV: Testing. Atlanta, GA, Centers for Disease Control and Prevention, June 22, 2022. Available at: https://www.cdc.gov/hiv/basics/hiv-testing/test-types.html. Accessed July 21, 2022.

Centers for Disease Control and Prevention: HIV and COVID-19 basics, in HIV. Atlanta, GA, Centers for Disease Control and Prevention, July 12, 2022. Available at: https://www.cdc.gov/hiv/basics/covid-19.html. Accessed July 21, 2022.

Chaconas G, Castellanos M, Verhey TB: Changing of the guard: how the Lyme disease spirochete subverts the host immune response. J Biol Chem 295(2):301–313, 2020

Chalasani NP, Maddur H, Russo MW, et al: Practice Parameters Committee of the American College of Gastroenterology: ACG Clinical Guideline: diagnosis and management of idiosyncratic drug-induced liver injury. Am J Gastroenterol 116(5):878–898, 2021

Chandra SV: Psychiatric illness due to manganese poisoning. Acta Psychiatr Scand Suppl 303:49–54, 1983

Charmandari E, Nicolaides NC, Chrousos GP: Adrenal insufficiency. Lancet 383(9935):2152–2167, 2014

Chaumont H, Meppiel E, Roze E, et al: Long-term outcomes after NeuroCOVID: a 6-month follow-up study on 60 patients. Rev Neurol (Paris) 178(1–2):137–143, 2022

Chiovato L, Magri F, Carlé A: Hypothyroidism in context: where we've been and where we're going. Adv Ther 36(Suppl 2):47–58, 2019

Chiveri L, Verrengia E, Muscia F, et al: Limbic encephalitis in a COVID-19 patient? J Neurovirol 27(3):498–500, 2021

Cho YT, Yang CW, Chu CY: Drug reaction with eosinophilia and systemic symptoms (DRESS): an interplay among drugs, viruses, and immune system. Int J Mol Sci 18(6):1243, 2017

Choi JW, Son HJ, Lee SS, et al: Acute hepatitis E virus superinfection increases mortality in patients with cirrhosis. BMC Infect Dis 22(1):62, 2022

Chow F: Brain and spinal epidural abscess. Continuum (Minneap Minn) 24(5, Neuroinfectious Disease):1327–1348, 2018

Christopoulou F, Rizos EC, Kosta P, et al: Does this patient have hypertensive encephalopathy? J Am Soc Hypertens 10(5):399–403, 2016

Chrostek L, Cylwik B, Szmitkowski M, et al: The diagnostic accuracy of carbohydrate-deficient transferrin, sialic acid and commonly used markers of alcohol abuse during abstinence. Clin Chim Acta 364(1–2):167–171, 2006

Chrysant SG, Chrysant GS: Adverse cardiovascular and blood pressure effects of drug-induced hypomagnesemia. Expert Opin Drug Saf 19(1):59–67, 2020

Chrysant SG: The current debate over treatment of subclinical hypothyroidism to prevent cardiovascular complications. Int J Clin Pract 74(7):e13499, 2020

Chung F, Abdullah HR, Liao P: STOP-Bang questionnaire: a practical approach to screen for obstructive sleep apnea. Chest 149(3):631–638, 2016

Churilov LP, Sobolevskaia PA, Stroev YI: Thyroid gland and brain: enigma of Hashimoto's encephalopathy. Best Pract Res Clin Endocrinol Metab 33(6):101364, 2019

Ciocan C, Mansour I, Beneduce A, et al: Lead poisoning from Ayurvedic treatment: a further case. Med Lav 112(2):162–167, 2021

Cipriani G, Danti S, Nuti A, et al: Is that schizophrenia or frontotemporal dementia? Supporting clinicians in making the right diagnosis. Acta Neurol Belg 120(4):799–804, 2020

Clarke BL, Brown EM, Collins MT, et al: Epidemiology and diagnosis of hypoparathyroidism. J Clin Endocrinol Metab 101(6):2284–2299, 2016

Clarke BL: Asymptomatic primary hyperparathyroidism. Front Horm Res 51:13–22, 2019

Clyne B, Jerrard DA: Syphilis testing. J Emerg Med 18:361–367, 2000

Cohen BM, Sommer BR, Vuckovic A: Antidepressant-resistant depression in patients with comorbid subclinical hypothyroidism or high-normal TSH levels. Am J Psychiatry 175(7):598–604, 2018

Colvin MK, Stern TA: Diagnosis, evaluation, and treatment of attention-deficit/hyperactivity disorder. J Clin Psychiatry 76(9):e1148, 2015

Cooper MS, Gittoes NJ: Diagnosis and management of hypocalcaemia. BMJ 336(7656):1298–1302, 2008

Cortese I, Reich DS, Nath A: Progressive multifocal leukoencephalopathy and the spectrum of JC virus-related disease. Nat Rev Neurol 17(1):37–51, 2021

Coughlin JM, Yang T, Rebman AW, et al: Imaging glial activation in patients with post-treatment Lyme disease symptoms: a pilot study using [11C]DPA-713 PET. J Neuroinflammation 15(1):346, 2018

Cousins Z, Forbes M, Coulson B: Chronic subdural haematoma in an elderly patient with a manic episode. Aust N Z J Psychiatry 55(6):632–633, 2021

Crossgrove J, Zheng W: Manganese toxicity upon overexposure. NMR Biomed 17(8):544–553, 2004

Crotty GF, Doherty C, Solomon IH, et al: Learning from history: Lord Brain and Hashimoto's encephalopathy. Pract Neurol 19(4):316–320, 2019

Dadiomov D: Laboratory testing for substance use disorders, in Absolute Addiction Psychiatry Review. Edited by Marienfeld C. Cham, Switzerland, Springer, 2020, pp 17–30

Dalmau J, Armangué T, Planagumà J, et al: An update on anti-NMDA receptor encephalitis for neurologists and psychiatrists: mechanisms and models. Lancet Neurol 18(11):1045–1057, 2019

Dard R, Janel N, Vialard F: COVID-19 and Down's syndrome: are we heading for a disaster? Eur J Hum Genet 28(11):1477–1478, 2020

Dassanayake TL, Weerasinghe VS, Gawarammana I, et al: Subacute and chronic neuropsychological sequalae of acute organophosphate pesticide self-poisoning: a prospective cohort study from Sri Lanka. Clin Toxicol (Phila) 59(2):118–130, 2021

Dave HN, Eugene Ramsay R, Khan F, et al: Pyridoxine deficiency in adult patients with status epilepticus. Epilepsy Behav 52(Pt A):154–158, 2015

Davies R, Ahmed G, Freer T: Psychiatric aspects of chronic exposure to organophosphates: diagnosis and management. Advances in Psychiatric Treatment 6(5):356–361, 2000

Davies RW, Fiksinski AM, Breetvelt EJ, et al: Using common genetic variation to examine phenotypic expression and risk prediction in 22q11.2 deletion syndrome. Nat Med 26(12):1912–1918, 2020

de Filippis R, Soldevila-Matías P, De Fazio P, et al: Clozapine-related drug reaction with eosinophilia and systemic symptoms (DRESS) syndrome: a systematic review. Expert Rev Clin Pharmacol 13(8):875–883, 2020

de Filippis R, Soldevila-Matías P, Guinart D, et al: Unravelling cases of clozapine-related drug reaction with eosinophilia and systemic symptoms (DRESS) in patients reported otherwise: a systematic review. J Psychopharmacol 35(9):1062–1073, 2021

de Leon MJ, DeSanti S, Zinkowski R, et al: MRI and CSF studies in the early diagnosis of Alzheimer's disease. J Intern Med 256:205–223, 2004

de Oliveira L, Melhem MSC, Buccheri R, et al: Early clinical and microbiological predictors of outcome in hospitalized patients with cryptococcal meningitis. BMC Infect Dis 22(1):138, 2022

de Vries Lentsch S, Louter MA, van Oosterhout W, et al: Depressive symptoms during the different phases of a migraine attack: a prospective diary study. J Affect Disord 297:502–507, 2022

DeDios-Stern S, Gotra MY, Soble JR: Comprehensive neuropsychological findings in a case of Marchiafava-Bignami disease. Clin Neuropsychol 35(6):1191–1202, 2021

Deng J, Zhou F, Hou W, et al: The prevalence of depression, anxiety, and sleep disturbances in COVID-19 patients: a meta-analysis. Ann N Y Acad Sci 1486(1):90–111, 2021

Devreese K, Hoylaerts MF: Challenges in the diagnosis of the antiphospholipid syndrome. Clin Chem 56:930–940, 2010

Dharel N, Bajaj JS: Definition and nomenclature of hepatic encephalopathy. J Clin Exp Hepatol 5(Suppl 1):S37–S41, 2015

Dheda K, Barry CE III, Maartens G: Tuberculosis. Lancet 387(10024):1211–1226, 2016

Dhir S, Tarasenko M, Napoli E, et al: Neurological, psychiatric, and biochemical aspects of thiamine deficiency in children and adults. Front Psychiatry 10:207, 2019

Dias CL, Fonseca L, Gadelha A, et al: Clozapine-induced hepatotoxicity: a life-threatening situation. Schizophr Res 235:3–4, 2021

DiNicolantonio JJ, Liu J, O'Keefe JH: Thiamine and cardiovascular disease: a literature review. Prog Cardiovasc Dis 61(1):27–32, 2018

Divani AA, Andalib S, Biller J, et al: Central nervous system manifestations associated with COVID-19. Curr Neurol Neurosci Rep 20(12):60, 2020

Dobrescu SR, Dinkler L, Gillberg C, et al: Anorexia nervosa: 30-year outcome. Br J Psychiatr 216(2):97–104, 2020

Dobs AS: The role of accurate testosterone testing in the treatment and management of male hypogonadism. Steroids 73(13):1305–1310, 2008

Donegan D: Opioid induced adrenal insufficiency: what is new? Curr Opin Endocrinol Diabetes Obes 26(3):133–138, 2019

Dong X, Bai C, Nao J: Clinical and radiological features of Marchiafava-Bignami disease. Medicine (Baltimore) 97(5):e9626, 2018

Dörner T, Furie R: Novel paradigms in systemic lupus erythematosus. Lancet 393(10188):2344–2358, 2019

Dos Santos DT, Imthon AK, Strelow MZ, et al: Parkinsonism-hyperpyrexia syndrome after amantadine withdrawal: case report and review of the literature. Neurologist 26(4):149–152, 2021

Dowsett J, Didriksen M, von Stemann JH, et al: Chronic inflammation markers and cytokine-specific autoantibodies in Danish blood donors with restless legs syndrome. Sci Rep 12(1):1672, 2022

Dregan A, Rayner L, Davis KAS, et al: Associations between depression, arterial stiffness, and metabolic syndrome among adults in the UK Biobank Population Study: a mediation analysis. JAMA Psychiatry 77(6):598–606, 2020

Druschky K, Toto S, Bleich S, et al: Severe drug-induced liver injury in patients under treatment with antipsychotic drugs: data from the AMSP study. World J Biol Psychiatry 22(5):373–386, 2021

Dumes AA: Lyme disease and the epistemic tensions of "medically unexplained illnesses." Med Anthropol 39(6):441–456, 2020

Dunphy L, Kothari T, Ford J: Posterior reversible encephalopathy syndrome in the puerperium: a case report. BMJ Case Rep 15(1):e246570, 2022

Duntas LH, Yen PM: Diagnosis and treatment of hypothyroidism in the elderly. Endocrine 66(1):63–69, 2019

Duque-Serrano L, Patarroyo-Rodriguez L, Gotlib D, et al: Psychiatric aspects of acute porphyria: a comprehensive review. Curr Psychiatry Rep 20(1):5, 2018

Dutra BG, da Rocha AJ, Nunes RH, et al: Neuromyelitis optica spectrum disorders: spectrum of MR imaging findings and their differential diagnosis. Radiographics 38(1):169–193, 2018

Eddy KT, Tabri N, Thomas JJ, et al: Recovery from anorexia nervosa and bulimia nervosa at 22-year follow-up. J Clin Psychiatry 78(2):184–189, 2017

Edwin TH, Henjum K, Nilsson LNG, et al: A high cerebrospinal fluid soluble TREM2 level is associated with slow clinical progression of Alzheimer's disease. Alzheimers Dement (Amst) 12(1):e12128, 2020

Ekino S, Susa M, Ninomiya T, et al: Minamata disease revisited: an update on the acute and chronic manifestations of methyl mercury poisoning. J Neurol Sci 262(1–2):131–144, 2007

Elliott TL, Braun M: Electrolytes: potassium disorders. FP Essent 459:21–28, 2017

Ellison DH, Berl T: Clinical practice: the syndrome of inappropriate antidiuresis. N Engl J Med 356(20):2064–2072, 2007

Endres D, Pollak TA, Bechter K, et al: Immunological causes of obsessive-compulsive disorder: is it time for the concept of an "autoimmune OCD" subtype? Transl Psychiatry 12(1):5, 2022

Ensrud KE, Crandall CJ: Osteoporosis. Ann Intern Med 167(3):ITC17–ITC32, 2017

Environmental Working Group: EWG's Consumer Guide to Seafood. Washington, DC, Environmental Working Group, 2020. Available at: https://www.ewg.org/consumer-guides/ewgs-consumer-guide-seafood. Accessed July 21, 2022.

Epstein S, Xia Z, Lee AJ, et al: Vaccination against SARS-CoV-2 in neuroinflammatory disease: early safety/tolerability data. Mult Scler Relat Disord 57:103433, 2022

Erkan D, Lockshin MD: Non-criteria manifestations of antiphospholipid syndrome. Lupus 19(4):424–427, 2010

Esumi R, Suzuki K, Ishikura K, et al: Challenges in diagnosing comatose patients with ethylene glycol poisoning. Am J Med 134(2):e127–e128, 2021

Etemadifar M, Abhari AP, Nouri H, et al: Does COVID-19 increase the long-term relapsing-remitting multiple sclerosis clinical activity? A cohort study. BMC Neurol 22(1):64, 2022

Etemadifar M, Ashourizadeh H, Nouri H, et al: MRI signs of CNS demyelinating diseases. Mult Scler Relat Disord 47:102665, 2021

European Association for Study of Liver: EASL clinical practice guidelines: Wilson's disease. J Hepatol 56(3):671–685, 2012

European Association for the Study of the Liver: EASL clinical practice guidelines: drug-induced liver injury. J Hepatol 70(6):1222–1261, 2019

Factora R, Luciano M: When to consider normal pressure hydrocephalus in the patient with gait disturbance. Geriatrics 63(2):32–37, 2008

Fallon BA, Madsen T, Erlangsen A, et al: Lyme borreliosis and associations with mental disorders and suicidal behavior: a nationwide Danish cohort study. Am J Psychiatry 178(10):921–931, 2021

Farrugia FA, Charalampopoulos A: Pheochromocytoma. Endocr Regul 53(3):191–212, 2019

Felsenfeld AJ, Levine BS, Rodriguez M: Pathophysiology of calcium, phosphorus, and magnesium dysregulation in chronic kidney disease. Semin Dial 28(6):564–577, 2015

Fernandez BA, Scherer SW: Syndromic autism spectrum disorders: moving from a clinically defined to a molecularly defined approach. Dialogues Clin Neurosci 19(4):353–371, 2017

Fevang B, Wyller VBB, Mollnes TE, et al: Lasting immunological imprint of primary Epstein-Barr virus infection with associations to chronic low-grade inflammation and fatigue. Front Immunol 12:715102, 2021

Figgie MP Jr, Appleby BS: Clinical use of improved diagnostic testing for detection of prion disease. Viruses 13(5):789, 2021

Fihn SD: Clinical practice: acute uncomplicated urinary tract infection in women. N Engl J Med 349(3):259–266, 2003

Filippatos TD, Makri A, Elisaf MS, et al: Hyponatremia in the elderly: challenges and solutions. Clin Interv Aging 12:1957–1965, 2017

Filis AK, Aghayev K, Vrionis FD: Cerebrospinal fluid and hydrocephalus: physiology, diagnosis, and treatment. Cancer Control 24(1):6–8, 2017

Fischer M, Schmutzhard E: Posterior reversible encephalopathy syndrome. J Neurol 264(8):1608–1616, 2017

Fitzgerald K, Mikalunas V, Rubin H, et al: Hypermanganesemia in patients receiving total parenteral nutrition. JPEN J Parenter Enteral Nutr 23(6):333–336, 1999

Fong J, Khan A: Hypocalcemia: updates in diagnosis and management for primary care. Can Fam Physician 58(2):158–162, 2012

Fontana RJ, Engle RE, Gottfried M, et al: Role of hepatitis E virus infection in North American patients with severe acute liver injury. Clin Transl Gastroenterol 11(11):e00273, 2020

Forsmark CE, Vege SS, Wilcox CM: Acute pancreatitis. N Engl J Med 375(20):1972–1981, 2016

Foster E, Carney P, Liew D, et al: First seizure presentations in adults: beyond assessment and treatment. J Neurol Neurosurg Psychiatry 90(9):1039–1045, 2019

Francis A: Catatonia: diagnosis, classification and treatment. Curr Psychiatry Rep 12(3):180–185, 2010

Fujii Y, Mizoguchi Y, Masuoka J, et al: Cushing's syndrome and psychosis: a case report and literature review. Prim Care Companion CNS Disord 20(5):18br02279, 2018

Fukatsu T, Kanemoto K: Phantom boarder symptom in elderly Japanese. Psychogeriatrics 22(1):108–112, 2022

Fumagalli F, Zambon AA, Rancoita PMV, et al: Metachromatic leukodystrophy: a single-center longitudinal study of 45 patients. J Inherit Metab Dis 44(5):1151–1164, 2021

Fung WL, Butcher NJ, Costain G, et al: Practical guidelines for managing adults with 22q11.2 deletion syndrome. Genet Med 17(8):599–609, 2015

Furin J, Cox H, Pai M: Tuberculosis. Lancet 393(10181):1642–1656, 2019

Fuster D, Samet JH: Alcohol use in patients with chronic liver disease. N Engl J Med 379(13):1251–1261, 2018

Gaebel W, Zielasek J: Schizophrenia in 2020: trends in diagnosis and therapy. Psychiatry Clin Neurosci 69(11):661–673, 2015

Gafni RI, Collins MT: Hypoparathyroidism. N Engl J Med 380(18):1738–1747, 2019

Gafter-Gvili A, Schechter A, Rozen-Zvi B: Iron deficiency anemia in chronic kidney disease. Acta Haematol 2019;142(1):44–50, 2019

Galati SJ, Rayfield EJ: Approach to the patient with postprandial hypoglycemia. Endocr Pract 20(4):331–340, 2014

Gale SA, Acar D, Daffner KR: Dementia. Am J Med 131(10):1161–1169, 2018

Galimberti F, Mesinkovska NA: Skin findings associated with nutritional deficiencies. Cleve Clin J Med 83(10):731–739, 2016

Gama Marques J: Pellagra with casal necklace causing secondary schizophrenia with Capgras syndrome in a homeless man. Prim Care Companion CNS Disord 24(2):21cr03014, 2022

Garber JR, Cobin RH, Gharib H, et al: Clinical practice guidelines for hypothyroidism in adults: cosponsored by the American Association of Clinical Endocrinologists and the American Thyroid Association. Endocr Pract 18(6):988–1028, 2012

Garcia D, Erkan D: Diagnosis and management of the antiphospholipid syndrome. N Engl J Med 378(21):2010–2021, 2018

Garcia-Malo C, Romero-Peralta S, Cano-Pumarega I: Restless legs syndrome: clinical features. Sleep Med Clin 16(2):233–247, 2021

Gardner TB, Adler DG, Forsmark CE, et al: ACG clinical guideline: chronic pancreatitis. Am J Gastroenterol 115(3):322–339, 2020

Garrett C, Doherty A: Diabetes and mental health. Clin Med (Lond) 14(6):669–672, 2014

Gasperi V, Sibilano M, Savini I, et al: Niacin in the central nervous system: an update of biological aspects and clinical applications. Int J Mol Sci 20(4):974, 2019

Gelisse P, Crespel A, Luigi Gigli G, et al: Stimulus-induced rhythmic or periodic intermittent discharges (SIRPIDs) in patients with triphasic waves and Creutzfeldt-Jakob disease. Clin Neurophysiol 132(8):1757–1769, 2021

Getachew M, Yeshigeta R, Tiruneh A, et al: Soil-transmitted helminthic infections and geophagia among pregnant women in Jimma Town health institutions, Southwest Ethiopia. Ethiop J Health Sci 31(5):1033–1042, 2021

Gewirtz AN, Gao V, Parauda SC, et al: Posterior reversible encephalopathy syndrome. Curr Pain Headache Rep 25(3):19, 2021

Ghavanini AA, Kimpinski K: Revisiting the evidence for neuropathy caused by pyridoxine deficiency and excess. J Clin Neuromuscul Dis 16(1):25–31, 2014

Ghosh R, Tabrizi SJ: Clinical features of Huntington's disease. Adv Exp Med Biol 1049:1–28, 2018

Giagulli VA, Campone B, Castellana M, et al: Neuropsychiatric aspects in men with Klinefelter's syndrome. Endocr Metab Immune Disord Drug Targets 19(2):109–115, 2019

Giau VV, Bagyinszky E, An SSA: Potential fluid biomarkers for the diagnosis of mild cognitive impairment. Int J Mol Sci 20(17):4149, 20109

Gibbons E, Whittam D, Jacob A, et al: Images of the month 1: trident sign and neurosarcoidosis. Clin Med (Lond) 21(6):e667–e668, 2021

Gibson D, Workman C, Mehler PS: Medical complications of anorexia nervosa and bulimia nervosa. Psychiatr Clin North Am 42(2):263–274, 2019

Gibson GE, Hirsch JA, Fonzetti P, et al: Vitamin B1 (thiamine) and dementia. Ann N Y Acad Sci 1367(1):21–30, 2016

Gifford RW Jr, Westbrook E: Hypertensive encephalopathy: mechanisms, clinical features, and treatment. Prog Cardiovasc Dis 17(2):115–124, 1974

Ginès P, Krag A, Abraldes JG, et al: Liver cirrhosis. Lancet 398(10308):1359–1376, 2021

Giri S, Tronvik EA, Hagen K: The bidirectional temporal relationship between headache and affective disorders: longitudinal data from the HUNT studies. J Headache Pain 23(1):14, 2022

Giusti F, Brandi ML: Clinical presentation of hypoparathyroidism. Front Horm Res 51:139–146, 2019

Godler DE, Butler MG: Special issue: genetics of Prader-Willi syndrome. Genes (Basel) 12(9):1429, 2021

Golden EC, Lipford MC: Narcolepsy: diagnosis and management. Cleve Clin J Med 85(12):959–969, 2018

Golfeyz S, Lewis S, Weisberg IS: Hemochromatosis: pathophysiology, evaluation, and management of hepatic iron overload with a focus on MRI. Expert Rev Gastroenterol Hepatol 12(8):767–778, 2018

Gomes F, Bergeron G, Bourassa MW, et al: Thiamine deficiency unrelated to alcohol consumption in high-income countries: a literature review. Ann N Y Acad Sci 1498(1):46–56, 2021

Gonzalez H, Koralnik IJ, Marra CM: Neurosyphilis. Semin Neurol 39(4):448–455, 2019

Goo YJ, Song SH, Kwon OI, et al: Venous thromboembolism and severe hypernatremia in a patient with lithium-induced nephrogenic diabetes insipidus and acute kidney injury: a case report. December 15, 2021 Ann Palliat Med [Epub ahead of print]

Goodman WK, Grice DE, Lapidus KA, et al: Obsessive-compulsive disorder. Psychiatr Clin North Am 37(3):257–267, 2014

Gorelick PB, Scuteri A, Black SE, et al: Vascular contributions to cognitive impairment and dementia: a statement for healthcare professionals from the American Heart Association/American Stroke Association. Stroke 42(9):2672–2713, 2011

Gossard TR, Trotti LM, Videnovic A, et al: Restless legs syndrome: contemporary diagnosis and treatment. Neurotherapeutics 18(1):140–155, 2021

Gothelf D: Velocardiofacial syndrome. Child Adolesc Psychiatr Clin N Am 16(3):677–693, 2007

Goullé JP, Grangeot-Keros L: Aluminum and vaccines: current state of knowledge. Med Mal Infect 50(1):16–21, 2020

Grasso EA, Cacciatore M, Gentile C, et al: Epilepsy in systemic lupus erythematosus. Clin Exp Rheumatol 39(3):651–659, 2021

Graus F, Titulaer MJ, Balu R, et al: A clinical approach to diagnosis of autoimmune encephalitis. Lancet Neurol 15(4):391–404, 2016

Gravholt CH, Chang S, Wallentin M, et al: Klinefelter's syndrome: integrating genetics, neuropsychology, and endocrinology. Endocr Rev 39(4):389–423, 2018

Grebenciucova E, Berger JR: Progressive multifocal leukoencephalopathy. Neurol Clin 36(4):739–750, 2018

Green R, Miller JW: Vitamin B12 deficiency. Vitam Horm 119:405–439, 2022

Green T, Gothelf D, Glaser B, et al: Psychiatric disorders and intellectual functioning throughout development in velocardiofacial (22q11.2 deletion) syndrome. J Am Acad Child Adolesc Psychiatry 48(11):1060–1068, 2009

Gregory S, Scahill RI: Functional magnetic resonance imaging in Huntington's disease. Int Rev Neurobiol 142:381–408, 2018

Grigsby J, Brega AG, Bennett RE, et al: Clinically significant psychiatric symptoms among male carriers of the fragile X premutation, with and without FXTAS, and the mediating influence of executive functioning. Clin Neuropsychol 30(6):944–959, 2016

Gris JC, Nobile B, Bouvier S: Neuropsychiatric presentations of antiphospholipid antibodies. Thromb Res 135(Suppl 1):S56–S59, 2015

Groth KA, Skakkebæk A, Høst C, et al: Clinical review: Klinefelter's syndrome—a clinical update. J Clin Endocrinol Metab 98(1):20–30, 2013

Grunberger G, Weiner JL, Silverman R, et al: Factitious hypoglycemia due to surreptitious administration of insulin: diagnosis, treatment, and long-term follow-up. Ann Intern Med 108(2):252–257, 1988

Guinart D, Misawa F, Rubio JM, et al: A systematic review and pooled, patient-level analysis of predictors of mortality in neuroleptic malignant syndrome. Acta Psychiatr Scand 144(4):329–341, 2021

Guinart D, Misawa F, Rubio JM, et al: Outcomes of neuroleptic malignant syndrome with depot versus oral antipsychotics: a systematic review and pooled, patient-level analysis of 662 case reports. J Clin Psychiatry 82(1):20r13272, 2020

Guinart D, Taipale H, Rubio JM, et al: Risk factors, incidence, and outcomes of neuroleptic malignant syndrome on long-acting injectable vs oral antipsychotics in a nationwide schizophrenia cohort. Schizophr Bull 47(6):1621–1630, 2021

Guise TA, Wysolmerski JJ: Cancer-associated hypercalcemia. N Engl J Med 386(15):1443–1451, 2022

Guziejko K, Czupryna P, Zielenkiewicz-Madejska EK, et al: Pneumococcal meningitis and COVID-19: dangerous coexistence: a case report. BMC Infect Dis 22(1):182, 2022

Hadtstein F, Vrolijk M: Vitamin B-6-induced neuropathy: exploring the mechanisms of pyridoxine toxicity. Adv Nutr 12(5):1911–1929, 2021

Hagerman RJ, Hagerman P: Fragile X-associated tremor/ataxia syndrome: features, mechanisms and management. Nat Rev Neurol 12(7):403–412, 2016

Hagerman RJ, Jackson C, Amiri K, et al: Girls with fragile X syndrome: physical and neurocognitive status and outcome. Pediatrics 89(3):395–400, 1992

Hainer BL, Matheson EM: Approach to acute headache in adults. Am Fam Physician 87(10):682–687, 2013

Hakami Y, Khan A: Hypoparathyroidism. Front Horm Res 51:109–126, 2019

Hall DA, Berry-Kravis E: Fragile X syndrome and fragile X-associated tremor ataxia syndrome. Handb Clin Neurol 147:377–391, 2018

Hall SA, Esche GR, Araujo AB, et al: Correlates of low testosterone and symptomatic androgen deficiency in a population-based sample. J Clin Endocrinol Metab 93(10):3870–3877, 2008

Hallab A, Naveed S, Altibi A, et al: Association of psychosis with antiphospholipid antibody syndrome: a systematic review of clinical studies. Gen Hosp Psychiatry 50:137–147, 2018

Hamada Y, Hirano E, Sugimoto K, et al: A farewell to phlebotomy-use of placenta-derived drugs Laennec and Porcine for improving hereditary hemochromatosis without phlebotomy: a case report. J Med Case Rep 16(1):26, 2022

Hamaguchi M, Fujita H, Suzuki T, et al: Sick sinus syndrome as the initial manifestation of neuromyelitis optica spectrum disorder: a case report. BMC Neurol 22(1):56, 2022

Hamed S, Mohamed K, Abd Elhameed S, et al: Movement disorders due to selective basal ganglia lesions with uremia. Can J Neurol Sci 47(3):350–365, 2020

Hamed SA: Brain injury with diabetes mellitus: evidence, mechanisms and treatment implications. Expert Rev Clin Pharmacol 10(4):409–428, 2017

Hamed SA: Neurologic conditions and disorders of uremic syndrome of chronic kidney disease: presentations, causes, and treatment strategies. Expert Rev Clin Pharmacol 12(1):61–90, 2019

Hanin C, Arnulf I, Maranci JB, et al: Narcolepsy and psychosis: a systematic review. Acta Psychiatr Scand 144(1):28–41, 2021

Harciarek M, Mankowska A: Hemispheric stroke: mood disorders. Handb Clin Neurol 183:155–167, 2021

Harrington BC, Jimerson M, Haxton C, et al: Initial evaluation, diagnosis, and treatment of anorexia nervosa and bulimia nervosa. Am Fam Physician 91(1):46–52, 2015

Hartmann AS: Pica behaviors in a German community-based online adolescent and adult sample: an examination of substances, triggers, and associated pathology. Eat Weight Disord 25(3):811–815, 2020

Hawkins M, Sockalingam S, Bonato S, et al: A rapid review of the pathoetiology, presentation, and management of delirium in adults with COVID-19. J Psychosom Res 141:110350, 2020

Hay AD, Fahey T: Clinical diagnosis of urinary tract infection. JAMA 288:1229, author reply 1230–1231, 2002

Hay P: Current approach to eating disorders: a clinical update. Intern Med J 50(1):24–29, 2020

Hayes MT: Parkinson's disease and Parkinsonism. Am J Med 132(7):802–807, 2019

Hedera P: Wilson's disease: a master of disguise. Parkinsonism Relat Disord 59:140–145, 2019

Helander A, Böttcher M, Dahmen N, et al: Elimination characteristics of the alcohol biomarker phosphatidylethanol (PEth) in blood during alcohol detoxification. Alcohol Alcohol 54(3):251–257, 2019

Heller HM, Gonzalez RG, Edlow BL, et al: Case 40–2020: a 24-year-old man with headache and Covid-19. N Engl J Med 383(26):2572–2580, 2020

Hidese S, Saito K, Asano S, et al: Association between iron-deficiency anemia and depression: a web-based Japanese investigation. Psychiatry Clin Neurosci 72(7):513–521, 2018

Hilbert K, Lueken U, Muehlhan M, et al: Separating generalized anxiety disorder from major depression using clinical, hormonal, and structural MRI data: a multimodal machine learning study. Brain Behav 7(3):e00633, 2017

Hillbom M, Saloheimo P, Fujioka S, et al: Diagnosis and management of Marchiafava-Bignami disease: a review of CT/MRI confirmed cases. J Neurol Neurosurg Psychiatry 85(2):168–173, 2014

Hinds K, Sutcliffe K: Heterodox and orthodox discourses in the case of Lyme disease: a synthesis of arguments. Qual Health Res 29(11):1661–1673, 2019

Hirst RB, Beard CL, Colby KA, et al: Anorexia nervosa and bulimia nervosa: a meta-analysis of executive functioning. Neurosci Biobehav Rev 83:678–690, 2017

HIV.gov: U.S. statistics, in HIV Basics, Overview: Data and Trends. Washington, DC, U.S. Department of Health and Human Services, 2022. Available at: https://www.hiv.gov/hiv-basics/overview/data-and-trends/statistics. Accessed July 21, 2022.

HIVinfo: HIV overview: HIV testing, in Understanding HIV: Facts Sheets. Bethesda, MD, National Institutes of Health, 2021. Available at: https://hivinfo.nih.gov/understanding-hiv/fact-sheets/hiv-testing. Accessed July 21, 2022.

Hobbs E, Vera JH, Marks M, et al: Neurosyphilis in patients with HIV. Pract Neurol 18(3):211–218, 2018

Holingue C, Wennberg A, Berger S, et al: Disturbed sleep and diabetes: a potential nexus of dementia risk. Metabolism 84:85–93, 2018

Hollander-Rodriguez JC, Calvert JF Jr: Hyperkalemia. Am Fam Physician 73(2):283–290, 2006

Holroyd KB, Manzano GS, Levy M: Update on neuromyelitis optica spectrum disorder. Curr Opin Ophthalmol 31(6):462–468, 2020

Holubiac IS, Leuciuc FV, Craciun DM, et al: Effect of strength training protocol on bone mineral density for postmenopausal women with osteopenia/osteoporosis assessed by dual-energy X-ray absorptiometry (DEXA). Sensors (Basel) 22(5):1904, 2022

Homme KG, Kern JK, Haley BE, et al: New science challenges old notion that mercury dental amalgam is safe. Biometals 27(1):19–24, 2014

Hoorn EJ, Zietse R: Diagnosis and treatment of hyponatremia: compilation of the guidelines. J Am Soc Nephrol 28(5):1340–1349, 2017

Hori M, Maekawa T, Kamiya K, et al: Advanced diffusion MR imaging for multiple sclerosis in the brain and spinal cord. Magn Reson Med Sci 21(1):58–70, 2022

Hshieh TT, Inouye SK, Oh ES: Delirium in the elderly. Clin Geriatr Med 36(2):183–199, 2020

Hsu WY, Chang TG, Chang CC, et al: Suicide ideation among outpatients with alcohol use disorder. Behav Neurol 2022:4138629, 2022

Hu LY, Shen CC, Hu YW, et al: Hyperthyroidism and risk for bipolar disorders: a nationwide population-based study. PLoS One 8(8):e73057, 2013

Hu XF, Lowe M, Chan HM: Mercury exposure, cardiovascular disease, and mortality: a systematic review and dose-response meta-analysis. Environ Res 193:110538, 2021

Huda S, Whittam D, Bhojak M, et al: Neuromyelitis optica spectrum disorders. Clin Med (Lond) 19(2):169–176, 2019

Hum RM, Ho P: Hereditary haemochromatosis presenting to rheumatology clinic as inflammatory arthritis. BMJ Case Rep 15(1):e246236, 2022

Hung DZ, Yang KW, Wu CC, et al: Lead poisoning due to incense burning: an outbreak in a family. Clin Toxicol (Phila) 59(8):756–759, 2021

Hur W, Chung JY, Choi PK, et al: Uremia presented as acute cranial neuropathy. Neurol Sci 40(7):1487–1489, 2019

Hvas AM, Nexo E: Diagnosis and treatment of vitamin B12 deficiency: an update. Haematologica 91(11):1506–1512, 2006

Iannella G, Magliulo G, Greco A, et al: Obstructive sleep apnea syndrome: from symptoms to treatment. Int J Environ Res Public Health 19(4):2459, 2022

Ibitoye RT, Wilkins A, Scolding NJ: Neurosarcoidosis: a clinical approach to diagnosis and management. J Neurol 264(5):1023–1028, 2017

Iglesias P, Devora O, Garcia J, et al: Severe hyperthyroidism: aetiology, clinical features and treatment outcome. Clin Endocrinol (Oxf) 72(4):551–557, 2010

Ijaz S, Bolea B, Davies S, et al: Antipsychotic polypharmacy and metabolic syndrome in schizophrenia: a review of systematic reviews. BMC Psychiatry 18(1):275, 2018

Insogna KL: Primary hyperparathyroidism. N Engl J Med 379(11):1050–1059, 2018

Ioachimescu AG: Hypercalcemia and its multiple facets. Endocrinol Metab Clin North Am 50(4):xiii–xiv, 2021

Isaacs M, Cardones AR, Rahnama-Moghadam S: DRESS syndrome: clinical myths and pearls. Cutis 102(5):322–326, 2018

Jackson AC: Chronic neurological disease due to methylmercury poisoning. Can J Neurol Sci 45(6):620–623, 2018

Jackson GH, Meyer A, Lippmann S: Wilson's disease: psychiatric manifestations may be the clinical presentation. Postgrad Med 95(8):135–138, 1994

Jacobson S, Jerrier H: EEG in delirium. Semin Clin Neuropsychiatry 5(2):86–92, 2000

Jadresic DP: Psychiatric aspects of hyperthyroidism. J Psychosom Res 34(6):603–615, 1990

Jain R, Jain S, Montano CB: Addressing diagnosis and treatment gaps in adults with attention-deficit/hyperactivity disorder. Prim Care Companion CNS Disord 19(5):17nr02153, 2017

Jarius S, Paul F, Weinshenker BG, et al: Neuromyelitis optica. Nat Rev Dis Primers 6(1):85, 2020

Jauhar S, Johnstone M, McKenna PJ: Schizophrenia. Lancet 399(10323):473–486, 2022

Javelot H, Weiner L: Panic and pandemic: narrative review of the literature on the links and risks of panic disorder as a consequence of the SARS-CoV-2 pandemic. Encephale 47(1):38–42, 2021

Jeon C, Gough K: Neurosyphilis presenting as hypomania. CMAJ 193(30):E1177, 2021

Jeon SW, Kim YK: Unresolved issues for utilization of atypical antipsychotics in schizophrenia: antipsychotic polypharmacy and metabolic syndrome. Int J Mol Sci 18(10):2174, 2017

Jevtic D, Dumic I, Nordin T, et al: Less known gastrointestinal manifestations of drug reaction with eosinophilia and systemic symptoms (DRESS) syndrome: a systematic review of the literature. J Clin Med 10(18):4287, 2021

Jha AK, Kumar G, Dayal VM, et al: Neurological manifestations of hepatitis E virus infection: an overview. World J Gastroenterol 27(18):2090–2104, 2021

Jiménez-Fernández S, Solis MO, Martínez-Reyes I, et al: Secondary mania in an elderly patient during SARS-CoV-2 infection with complete remission: a 1-year follow-up. Psychiatr Danub 33(3):418–420, 2021

John TM, Taege AJ: Appropriate laboratory testing in Lyme disease. Cleve Clin J Med 86(11):751–759, 2019

Johnson CD, Besselink MG, Carter R: Acute pancreatitis. BMJ 349:g4859, 2014

Johnson EB, Gregory S: Huntington's disease: brain imaging in Huntington's disease. Prog Mol Biol Transl Sci 165:321–369, 2019

Johnson EB, Ziegler G, Penny W, et al: Dynamics of cortical degeneration over a decade in Huntington's disease. Biol Psychiatry 89(8):807–816, 2021

Johnson EL: Seizures and epilepsy. Med Clin North Am 103(2):309–324, 2019

Johnson K, Herring J, Richstein J: Fragile X premutation associated conditions (FXPAC). Front Pediatr 8:266, 2020

Johnson-Arbor K, Schultz B: Effective decontamination and remediation after elemental mercury exposure: a case report in the United States. J Prev Med Public Health 54(5):376–379, 2021

Johnston CB, Dagar M: Osteoporosis in older adults. Med Clin North Am 104(5):873–884, 2020

Jokanovic M: Neurotoxic effects of organophosphorus pesticides and possible association with neurodegenerative diseases in man: a review. Toxicology 410:125–131, 2018

Jones CA, Colletti CM, Ding MC: Post-stroke dysphagia: recent insights and unanswered questions. Curr Neurol Neurosci Rep 20(12):61, 2020

Jones MR, Urits I, Wolf J, et al: Drug-induced peripheral neuropathy: a narrative review. Curr Clin Pharmacol 15(1):38–48, 2020

Jongsiriyanyong S, Limpawattana P: Mild cognitive impairment in clinical practice: a review article. Am J Alzheimers Dis Other Demen 33(8):500–507, 2018

Jordan AS, McSharry DG, Malhotra A: Adult obstructive sleep apnoea. Lancet 383(9918):736–747, 2014

Jovicevic V, Ivanovic J, Andabaka M, et al: COVID-19 and vaccination against SARS-CoV-2 in patients with neuromyelitis optica spectrum disorders. Mult Scler Relat Disord 57:103320, 2022

Julian T, Glascow N, Syeed R, et al: Alcohol-related peripheral neuropathy: a systematic review and meta-analysis. J Neurol 266(12):2907–2919, 2019

Jum'ah A, Aboul Nour H, Alkhoujah M, et al: Neurosyphilis in disguise. Neuroradiology 64(3):433–441, 2022

Juo YY, Livingston EH: Testing for nonalcoholic fatty liver disease. JAMA 322(18):1836, 2019

Kachian ZR, Cohen-Zimerman S, Bega D, et al: Suicidal ideation and behavior in Huntington's disease: systematic review and recommendations. J Affect Disord 250:319–329, 2019

Kahn RS, Sommer IE, Murray RM, et al: Schizophrenia. Nat Rev Dis Primers 1:15067, 2015

Kakkar C, Prakashini K, Polnaya A: Acute Marchiafava-Bignami disease: clinical and serial MRI correlation. BMJ Case Rep 2014:bcr2013203442, 2014

Kam T, Alexander M: Drug-induced immune thrombocytopenia. J Pharm Pract 27(5):430–439, 2014

Kameda M, Kajimoto Y, Kambara A, et al: Evaluation of the effectiveness of the tap test by combining the use of functional gait assessment and global rating of change. Front Neurol 13:846429, 2022

Kamel KS, Schreiber M, Harel Z: Hypernatremia. JAMA 327(8):774–775, 2022

Kanakis GA, Nieschlag E: Klinefelter's syndrome: more than hypogonadism. Metabolism 86:135–144, 2018

Kane SF, Roberts C, Paulus R: Hereditary hemochromatosis: rapid evidence review. Am Fam Physician 104(3):263–270, 2021

Kao YC, Lin MI, Weng WC, Lee WT: Neuropsychiatric disorders due to limbic encephalitis: immunologic aspect. Int J Mol Sci 22(1):389, 2020

Karanfilian BV, Park T, Senatore F, et al: Minimal hepatic encephalopathy. Clin Liver Dis 24(2):209–218, 2020

Katarey D, Verma S: Drug-induced liver injury. Clin Med (Lond) 16(Suppl 6):s104–s109, 2016

Katz DI, Bernick C, Dodick DW, et al: National Institute of Neurological Disorders and Stroke consensus diagnostic criteria for traumatic encephalopathy syndrome. Neurology 96(18):848–863, 2021

Kazamel M, Stino AM, Smith AG: Metabolic syndrome and peripheral neuropathy. Muscle Nerve 63(3):285–293, 2021

Kennedy PGE, Quan PL, Lipkin WI: Viral encephalitis of unknown cause: current perspective and recent advances. Viruses 9(6):138, 2017

Keshavan MS, Kaneko Y: Secondary psychoses: an update. World Psychiatry 12(1):4–15, 2013

Khan AA, Hanley DA, Rizzoli R, et al: Primary hyperparathyroidism: review and recommendations on evaluation, diagnosis, and management. A Canadian and international consensus. Osteoporos Int 28(1):1–19, 2017

Khan F, Sharma N, Ud Din M, et al: Clinically isolated brainstem progressive multifocal leukoencephalopathy: diagnostic challenges. Am J Case Rep 23:e935019, 2022

Khera M, Broderick GA, Carson CC III, et al: Adult-onset hypogonadism. Mayo Clin Proc 91(7):908–926, 2016

Kho J, Mandal AKJ, Geraldes R, et al: COVID-19 encephalitis and Wernicke's encephalopathy. J Med Virol 93(9):5248–5251, 2021

Kimoto S, Yamamuro K, Kishimoto T: Acute psychosis in patients with subclinical hyperthyroidism. Psychiatry Clin Neurosci 73(6):348–349, 2019

Kinsley S, Giovane RA, Daly S, et al: Rare case of Marchiafava-Bignami disease due to thiamine deficiency and malnutrition. BMJ Case Rep 13(12):e238187, 2020

Kiriakidou M, Ching CL: Systemic lupus erythematosus. Ann Intern Med 172(11):ITC81–ITC96, 2020

Kleeff J, Whitcomb DC, Shimosegawa T, et al: Chronic pancreatitis. Nat Rev Dis Primers 3:17060, 2017

Klevebrant L, Frick A: Effects of caffeine on anxiety and panic attacks in patients with panic disorder: a systematic review and meta-analysis. Gen Hosp Psychiatry 74:22–31, 2022

Klimiec-Moskal E, Slowik A, Dziedzic T: Delirium and subsyndromal delirium are associated with the long-term risk of death after ischaemic stroke. Aging Clin Exp Res 34(6):1459–1462, 2022

Klineova S, Lublin FD: Clinical course of multiple sclerosis. Cold Spring Harb Perspect Med 8(9):a028928, 2018

Klingelhoefer L, Bhattacharya K, Reichmann H: Restless legs syndrome. Clin Med (Lond) 16(4):379–382, 2016

Klotz K, Weistenhöfer W, Neff F, et al: The health effects of aluminum exposure. Dtsch Arztebl Int 114(39):653–659, 2017

Knight-Greenfield A, Nario JJQ, Gupta A: Causes of acute stroke: a patterned approach. Radiol Clin North Am 57(6):1093–1108, 2019

Kohil A, Jemmieh S, Smatti MK, et al: Viral meningitis: an overview. Arch Virol 166(2):335–345, 2021

Köhler W, Curiel J, Vanderver A: Adulthood leukodystrophies. Nat Rev Neurol 14(2):94–105, 2018

Kohnke S, Meek CL: Don't seek, don't find: the diagnostic challenge of Wernicke's encephalopathy. Ann Clin Biochem 58(1):38–46, 2021

Kolipinski M, Subramanian M, Kristen K, et al: Sources and toxicity of mercury in the San Francisco Bay area, spanning California and beyond. J Environ Public Health 2020:8184614, 2020

Kopel D, Peeler C, Zhu S: Headache emergencies. Neurol Clin 39(2):355–372, 2021

Kornum BR: Narcolepsy Type I as an autoimmune disorder. Handb Clin Neurol 181:161–172, 2021

Kotfis K, Williams Roberson S, Wilson J, et al: COVID-19: What do we need to know about ICU delirium during the SARS-CoV-2 pandemic? Anaesthesiol Intensive Ther 52(2):132–138, 2020

Krahn LE, Zee PC, Thorpy MJ: Current understanding of narcolepsy 1 and its comorbidities: what clinicians need to know. Adv Ther 39(1):221–243, 2022

Kreiman BL, Boles RG: State of the art of genetic testing for patients with autism: a practical guide for clinicians. Semin Pediatr Neurol 34:100804, 2020

Krishnan D, Zaini SS, Latif KA, et al: Neurosyphilis presenting as acute ischemic stroke. Clin Med (Lond) 20(1):95–97, 2020

Kromm JA, Power C, Blevins G, et al: Rapid multifocal neurologic decline in an immunocompromised patient. JAMA Neurol 73(2):226–231, 2016

Kugler JP, Hustead T: Hyponatremia and hypernatremia in the elderly. Am Fam Physician 61:3623–3630, 2000

Kullmann F, Hollerbach S, Lock G, et al: Brain electrical activity mapping of EEG for the diagnosis of (sub)clinical hepatic encephalopathy in chronic liver disease. Eur J Gastroenterol Hepatol 13:513–522, 2001

Kumachev A, Wu PE: Drug-induced liver injury. CMAJ 193(9):E310, 2021

Kumar M, Nayak PK: Psychological sequelae of myocardial infarction. Biomed Pharmacother 95:487–496, 2017

Kumrungsee T, Peipei Zhang, Yanaka N, et al: Emerging cardioprotective mechanisms of vitamin B6: a narrative review. Eur J Nutr 2022;61(2):605–613, 2022

Lajiness-O'Neill R, Beaulieu I, Asamoah A, et al: The neuropsychological phenotype of velocardiofacial syndrome (VCFS): relationship to psychopathology. Arch Clin Neuropsychol 21(2):175–184, 2006

Lala A, Johnson KW, Januzzi JL, et al: Prevalence and impact of myocardial injury in patients hospitalized with COVID-19 infection. J Am Coll Cardiol 76(5):533–546, 2020

Lambeck J, Hieber M, Dreßing A, et al: Central pontine myelinosis and osmotic demyelination syndrome. Dtsch Arztebl Int 116(35–36):600–606, 2019

Langan RC, Goodbred AJ: Hepatitis A. Am Fam Physician 104(4):368–374, 2021

Langan RC, Goodbred AJ: Vitamin B12 deficiency: recognition and management. Am Fam Physician 96(6):384–389, 2017

Languren G, Montiel T, Julio-Amilpas A, et al: Neuronal damage and cognitive impairment associated with hypoglycemia: an integrated view. Neurochem Int 63(4):331–343, 2013

Lantos PM, Rumbaugh J, Bockenstedt LK, et al: Clinical practice guidelines by the Infectious Diseases Society of America (IDSA), American Academy of Neurology (AAN), and American College of Rheumatology (ACR): 2020 guidelines for the prevention, diagnosis, and treatment of Lyme disease. Arthritis Care Res (Hoboken) 73(1):1–9, 2021

Lantos PM: Chronic Lyme disease. Infect Dis Clin North Am 29(2):325–340, 2015

Lappin JM, Darke S, Farrell M: Stroke and methamphetamine use in young adults: a review. J Neurol Neurosurg Psychiatry 88(12):1079–1091, 2017

Laratta CR, Ayas NT, Povitz M, et al: Diagnosis and treatment of obstructive sleep apnea in adults. CMAJ 189(48):E1481–E1488, 2017

Lau KHV: Laboratory evaluation of peripheral neuropathy. Semin Neurol 39(5):531–541, 2019

Laurent C, Capron J, Quillerou B, et al: Steroid-responsive encephalopathy associated with autoimmune thyroiditis (SREAT): characteristics, treatment and outcome in 251 cases from the literature. Autoimmun Rev 15(12):1129–1133, 2016

Lawlor BA: Hypocalcemia, hypoparathyroidism, and organic anxiety syndrome. J Clin Psychiatry 49(8):317–318, 1988

Lee BT, Odin JA, Grewal P: An approach to drug-induced liver injury from the geriatric perspective. Curr Gastroenterol Rep 23(4):6, 2021

Lee EJ, Lee AI: Thrombocytopenia. Prim Care 43(4):543–557, 2016

Leibetseder A, Eisermann M, LaFrance WC Jr, et al: How to distinguish seizures from nonepileptic manifestations. Epileptic Disord 22(6):716–738, 2020

Leung W, Singh I, McWilliams S, et al: Iron deficiency and sleep: a scoping review. Sleep Med Rev 51:101274, 2020

Leys F, Wenning GK, Fanciulli A: The role of cardiovascular autonomic failure in the differential diagnosis of α-synucleinopathies. Neurol Sci 43(1):187–198, 2022

Li W, Ran C, Ma J: Diverse MRI findings and clinical outcomes of acute Marchiafava-Bignami disease. Acta Radiol 62(7):904–908, 2021

Li X, Yuan J, Liu L, et al: Antibody-LGI 1 autoimmune encephalitis manifesting as rapidly progressive dementia and hyponatremia: a case report and literature review. BMC Neurol 19(1):19, 2019

Liamis G, Filippatos TD, Elisaf MS: Evaluation and treatment of hypernatremia: a practical guide for physicians. Postgrad Med 128(3):299–306, 2016

Lien YH, Shapiro JI: Hyponatremia: clinical diagnosis and management. Am J Med 120:653–658, 2007

Lim EJ, Son CG: Review of case definitions for myalgic encephalomyelitis/chronic fatigue syndrome (ME/CFS). J Transl Med 2020;18(1):289, 2020

Lin SY, Lee HH, Lee JF, et al: Urine specimen validity test for drug abuse testing in workplace and court settings. J Food Drug Anal 26(1):380–384, 2018

Linder KA, Malani PN: Hepatitis A. JAMA 318(23):2393, 2017

Lintas C, Persico AM: Autistic phenotypes and genetic testing: state-of-the-art for the clinical geneticist. J Med Genet 46(1):1–8, 2009

Lintel H, Corpuz T, Paracha SU, et al: Mood disorders and anxiety in Parkinson's disease: current concepts. J Geriatr Psychiatry Neurol 34(4):280–288, 2021

Littmann L, Gibbs MA: Electrocardiographic manifestations of severe hyperkalemia. J Electrocardiol 51(5):814–817, 2018

Liu YS, Lin KY, Masur J, et al: Outcomes after recurrent intentional methanol exposures not treated with alcohol dehydrogenase inhibitors or hemodialysis. J Emerg Med 58(6):910–916, 2020

Livingston M, Kalansooriya A, Hartland AJ, et al: Serum testosterone levels in male hypogonadism: why and when to check: a review. Int J Clin Pract 71(11):e12995, 2017

Llansó L, Bartolomé-Solanas A, Renú A: Wernicke's encephalopathy following hyperemesis gravidarum. Pract Neurol practneurol-2021–003241, 2022

Lonser RR, Nieman L, Oldfield EH: Cushing's disease: pathobiology, diagnosis, and management. J Neurosurg 126(2):404–417, 2017

Loomba R, Adams LA: Advances in non-invasive assessment of hepatic fibrosis. Gut 69(7):1343–1352, 2020

Lord C, Elsabbagh M, Baird G, et al: Autism spectrum disorder. Lancet 392(10146):508–520, 2018

Lorincz MT: Neurologic Wilson's disease. Ann N Y Acad Sci 1184:173–187, 2010

Louis DN, Perry A, Wesseling P, et al: The 2021 WHO classification of tumors of the central nervous system: a summary. Neuro Oncol 23(8):1231–1251, 2021

Luthe SK, Sato R: Alcoholic pellagra as a cause of altered mental status in the emergency department. J Emerg Med 53(4):554–557, 2017

Machado S, Sancassiani F, Paes F, et al: Panic disorder and cardiovascular diseases: an overview. Int Rev Psychiatry 29(5):436–444, 2017

Magnin E, Maurs C: Attention-deficit/hyperactivity disorder during adulthood. Rev Neurol (Paris) 173(7–8):506–515, 2017

Mahawish K, Teinert L, Cavanagh K, et al: Limbic encephalitis. BMJ Case Rep 2014:bcr2014204591, 2014

Maheshwari M, Athiraman H: Whippets causing vitamin B12 deficiency. Cureus 14(3):e23148, 2022

Mahoney CE, Cogswell A, Koralnik IJ, et al: The neurobiological basis of narcolepsy. Nat Rev Neurosci 20(2):83–93, 2019

Mak CM, Lam CW: Diagnosis of Wilson's disease: a comprehensive review. Crit Rev Clin Lab Sci 45(3):263–290, 2008

Mak E, Su L, Williams GB, et al: Neuroimaging correlates of cognitive impairment and dementia in Parkinson's disease. Parkinsonism Relat Disord 21(8):862–870, 2015

Makin SD, Turpin S, Dennis MS, et al: Cognitive impairment after lacunar stroke: systematic review and meta-analysis of incidence, prevalence and comparison with other stroke subtypes. J Neurol Neurosurg Psychiatry 84(8):893–900, 2013

Malhotra A, Mongelluzzo G, Wu X, et al: Ethylene glycol toxicity: MRI brain findings. Clin Neuroradiol 27(1):109–113, 2017

Mana J, Vaneckova M, Klempír J, et al: Methanol poisoning as an acute toxicological basal ganglia lesion model: evidence from brain volumetry and cognition. Alcohol Clin Exp Res 43(7):1486–1497, 2019

Manconi M, Garcia-Borreguero D, Schormair B, et al: Restless legs syndrome. Nat Rev Dis Primers 7(1):80, 2021

Manning T, Bartow C, Dunlap M, et al: Reversible cerebral vasoconstriction syndrome associated with fluoxetine. J Acad Consult Liaison Psychiatry 62(6):634–644, 2021

Mannstadt M, Bilezikian JP, Thakker RV, et al: Hypoparathyroidism. Nat Rev Dis Primers 3:17055, 2017

Marcantonio ER: Delirium in hospitalized older adults. N Engl J Med 377(15):1456–1466, 2017

Marder SR, Cannon TD: Schizophrenia. N Engl J Med 381(18):1753–1761, 2019

Mariani M, Alosco ML, Mez J, et al: Clinical presentation of chronic traumatic encephalopathy. Semin Neurol 40(4):370–383, 2020

Marik PE, Bellomo R: Stress hyperglycemia: an essential survival response! Crit Care 17(2):305, 2013

Maron E, Nutt D: Biological markers of generalized anxiety disorder. Dialogues Clin Neurosci 19(2):147–158, 2017

Marques AR: Laboratory diagnosis of Lyme disease: advances and challenges. Infect Dis Clin North Am 29(2):295–307, 2015

Marsh L: Depression and Parkinson's disease: current knowledge. Curr Neurol Neurosci Rep 13(12):409, 2013

Martiniakova M, Babikova M, Mondockova V, et al: The role of macronutrients, micronutrients and flavonoid polyphenols in the prevention and treatment of osteoporosis. Nutrients 14(3):523, 2022

Masi L: Primary hyperparathyroidism. Front Horm Res 51:1–12, 2019

Masingue M, Benoist JF, Roze E, et al: Cerebral folate deficiency in adults: a heterogeneous potentially treatable condition. J Neurol Sci 396:112–118, 2019

Mathur A, Samaranayake S, Storrar NP, et al: Investigating thrombocytosis. BMJ 366:l4183, 2019

Matthews M, Nigg JT, Fair DA: Attention deficit hyperactivity disorder. Curr Top Behav Neurosci 16:235–266, 2014

Mattison MLP: Delirium. Ann Intern Med 173(7):ITC49–ITC64, 2020

Mattozzi S, Sabater L, Escudero D, et al: Hashimoto encephalopathy in the 21st century. Neurology 94(2):e217–e224, 2020

Mayo Clinic: Medical Professionals. Rochester, MN, Mayo Clinic, 2022. Available at: https://www.mayoclinic.org/medical-professionals. Accessed July 21, 2022.

Mazereel V, Detraux J, Vancampfort D, et al: Impact of psychotropic medication effects on obesity and the metabolic syndrome in people with serious mental illness. Front Endocrinol (Lausanne) 11:573479, 2020

McAllister B, Gusella JF, Landwehrmeyer GB, et al: Timing and impact of psychiatric, cognitive, and motor abnormalities in Huntington disease. Neurology 96(19):e2395–e2406, 2021

McColgan P, Tabrizi SJ: Huntington's disease: a clinical review. Eur J Neurol 25(1):24–34, 2018

McCutcheon RA, Reis Marques T, Howes OD: Schizophrenia: an overview. JAMA Psychiatry 77(2):201–210, 2020

McDonald-McGinn DM, Sullivan KE, Marino B, et al: 22q11.2 deletion syndrome. Nat Rev Dis Primers 1:15071, 2015

McFaline-Figueroa JR, Lee EQ: Brain tumors. Am J Med 131(8):874–882, 2018

McGill MR, Jaeschke H: Biomarkers of drug-induced liver injury. Adv Pharmacol 85:221–239, 2019

McKee AC, Stern RA, Nowinski CJ, et al: The spectrum of disease in chronic traumatic encephalopathy. Brain 136(Pt 1):43–64, 2013

McKeith IG: Consensus guidelines for the clinical and pathologic diagnosis of dementia with Lewy bodies (DLB): report of the Consortium on DLB International Workshop. J Alzheimers Dis 9(5):417–423, 2006

McKeith IG, Boeve BF, Dickson DW, et al: Diagnosis and management of dementia with Lewy bodies: Fourth consensus report of the DLB Consortium. Neurology 89(1):88–100, 2017

McKhann GM, Knopman DS, Chertkow H, et al: The diagnosis of dementia due to Alzheimer's disease: recommendations from the National Institute on Aging-Alzheimer's Association workgroups on diagnostic guidelines for Alzheimer's disease. Alzheimers Dement 7(3):263–269, 2011

McNay EC, Cotero VE: Mini-review: impact of recurrent hypoglycemia on cognitive and brain function. Physiol Behav 100(3):234–238, 2010

McPherson RA, Pincus MR: Henry's Clinical Diagnosis and Management by Laboratory Methods, 24th Edition. Philadelphia, PA, Elsevier, 2022

Mead P, Petersen J, Hinckley A: Updated CDC recommendation for serologic diagnosis of Lyme disease. MMWR Morb Mortal Wkly Rep 68(32):703, 2019

Méchaï F, Bouchaud O: Tuberculous meningitis: challenges in diagnosis and management. Rev Neurol (Paris) 175(7–8):451–457, 2019

Mehnert-Kay SA: Diagnosis and management of uncomplicated urinary tract infections. Am Fam Physician 72(3):451–456, 2005

Mehrpour O, Sadeghi M: Toll of acute methanol poisoning for preventing COVID-19. Arch Toxicol 94(6):2259–2260, 2020

Mehta LS, Beckie TM, DeVon HA, et al: Acute myocardial infarction in women: a scientific statement from the American Heart Association. Circulation 133(9):916–947, 2016

Mehta V, Harward SC, Sankey EW, et al: Evidence based diagnosis and management of chronic subdural hematoma: a review of the literature. J Clin Neurosci 50:7–15, 2018

Mendez MF, Parand L, Akhlaghipour G: Bipolar disorder among patients diagnosed with frontotemporal dementia. J Neuropsychiatry Clin Neurosci 32(4):376–384, 2020

Meuret AE, Kroll J, Ritz T: Panic disorder comorbidity with medical conditions and treatment implications. Annu Rev Clin Psychol 13:209–240, 2017

Meyer TW, Hostetter TH: Uremia. N Engl J Med 357(13):1316–1325, 2007

Mez J, Daneshvar DH, Kiernan PT, et al: Clinicopathological evaluation of chronic traumatic encephalopathy in players of American football. JAMA 318(4):360–370, 2017

Mez J, Stern RA, McKee AC: Chronic traumatic encephalopathy. Semin Neurol 40(4):351–352, 2020

Michelena G, Casas M, Eizaguirre MB, et al: Can COVID-19 exacerbate multiple sclerosis symptoms? A case series analysis. Mult Scler Relat Disord 57:103368, 2022

Micoulaud-Franchi JA, Kotwas I, Arthuis M, et al: Screening for epilepsy-specific anxiety symptoms: French validation of the EASI. Epilepsy Behav 128:108585, 2022

Mignot E, Black S: Narcolepsy risk and COVID-19. J Clin Sleep Med 16(10):1831–1833, 2020

Miller JB, Suchdev K, Jayaprakash N, et al: New developments in hypertensive encephalopathy. Curr Hypertens Rep 20(2):13, 2018

Miller MA, Cappuccio FP: A systematic review of COVID-19 and obstructive sleep apnoea. Sleep Med Rev 55:101382, 2021

Mills K, Akintayo O, Egbosiuba L, et al: Chronic diarrhea in a drinker: a breakthrough case of pellagra in the US South. J Investig Med High Impact Case Rep 8:2324709620941305, 2020

Minisola S, Pepe J, Piemonte S, et al: The diagnosis and management of hypercalcaemia. BMJ 350:h2723, 2015

Miola A, Dal Porto V, Meda N, et al: Secondary mania induced by TNF-α inhibitors: a systematic review. Psychiatry Clin Neurosci 76(1):15–21, 2022

Misawa F, Okumura Y, Takeuchi Y, et al: Neuroleptic malignant syndrome associated with long-acting injectable versus oral second-generation antipsychotics: analyses based on a spontaneous reporting system database in Japan. Schizophr Res 231:42–46, 2021

Mitchell JE, Peterson C: Anorexia nervosa. N Engl J Med 382(14):1343–1351, 2020

Mitra P, Sharma S, Purohit P, et al: Clinical and molecular aspects of lead toxicity: an update. Crit Rev Clin Lab Sci 54(7–8):506–528, 2017

Mody L, Juthani-Mehta M: Urinary tract infections in older women: a clinical review. JAMA 311(8):844–854, 2014

Moeller KE, Kissack JC, Atayee RS, et al: Clinical interpretation of urine drug tests: what clinicians need to know about urine drug screens. Mayo Clin Proc 92(5):774–796, 2017

Mogavero MP, Mezzapesa DM, Savarese M, et al: Morphological analysis of the brain subcortical gray structures in restless legs syndrome. Sleep Med 88:74–80. 2021

Mohseni S: Neurologic damage in hypoglycemia. Handb Clin Neurol 126:513–532, 2014

Montaño A, Hanley DF, Hemphill JC 3rd: Hemorrhagic stroke. Handb Clin Neurol 176:229–248, 2021

Montford JR, Linas S: How dangerous is hyperkalemia? J Am Soc Nephrol 28(11):3155–3165, 2017

Moore A, Nelson C, Molins C, et al: Current guidelines, common clinical pitfalls, and future directions for laboratory diagnosis of Lyme disease, United States. Emerg Infect Dis 22(7):1169–1177, 2016

Moreira-de-Oliveira ME, de Menezes GB, Loureiro CP, et al: The impact of COVID-19 on patients with OCD: a one-year follow-up study. J Psychiatr Res 147:307–312, 2022

Moro C, Nunes C, Onzi G, et al: Gastrointestinal: life-threatening diarrhea due to pellagra in an elderly patient. J Gastroenterol Hepatol 35(9):1465, 2020

Morozova A, Zorkina Y, Abramova O, et al: Neurobiological highlights of cognitive impairment in psychiatric disorders. Int J Mol Sci 23(3):1217, 2022

Moulton CD, Pickup JC, Ismail K: The link between depression and diabetes: the search for shared mechanisms. Lancet Diabetes Endocrinol 3(6):461–471, 2015

Mouri M, Badireddy M: Hyperglycemia, in StatPearls. Treasure Island, FL, StatPearls Publishing, 2022. Available at: https://www.ncbi.nlm.nih.gov/books/NBK430900. Accessed April 2, 2022.

Mufson EJ, Kelley C, Perez SE: Chronic traumatic encephalopathy and the nucleus basalis of Meynert. Handb Clin Neurol 182:9–29, 2021

Muhsin SA, Mount DB: Diagnosis and treatment of hypernatremia. Best Pract Res Clin Endocrinol Metab 30(2):189–203, 2016

Mulholland PJ: Susceptibility of the cerebellum to thiamine deficiency. Cerebellum 5(1):55–63, 2006

Muneer M: Hypoglycaemia. Adv Exp Med Biol 1307:43–69, 2021

Muñoz-Quezada MT, Lucero BA, Iglesias VP, et al: Chronic exposure to organophosphate (OP) pesticides and neuropsychological functioning in farm workers: a review. Int J Occup Environ Health 22(1):68–79, 2016

Murad MH, Coto-Yglesias F, Wang AT, et al: Clinical review: drug-induced hypoglycemia. A systematic review. J Clin Endocrinol Metab 94:741–745, 2009

Murata T, Sugimoto A, Inagaki T, et al: Molecular basis of Epstein-Barr virus latency establishment and lytic reactivation. Viruses 13(12):2344, 2021

Murphy R, O'Donoghue S, Counihan T, et al: Neuropsychiatric syndromes of multiple sclerosis. J Neurol Neurosurg Psychiatry 88(8):697–708, 2017

Murt A, Eskazan AE, Yılmaz U, et al: COVID-19 presenting with immune thrombocytopenia: a case report and review of the literature. J Med Virol 93(1):43–45, 2021

Muscal E, Brey RL: Antiphospholipid syndrome and the brain in pediatric and adult patients. Lupus 19(4):406–411, 2010

Na D, Tao G, Shu-Ying L, et al: Association between hypomagnesemia and severity of primary hyperparathyroidism: a retrospective study. BMC Endocr Disord 21(1):170, 2021

Nagamine T: Beware of neuroleptic malignant syndrome in COVID-19 pandemic. Innov Clin Neurosci 18(7–9):9–10, 2021

Nagano M, Kobayashi K, Yamada-Otani M, et al: Hashimoto's encephalopathy presenting with smoldering limbic encephalitis. Intern Med 58(8):1167–1172, 2019

Nakajima M, Yamada S, Miyajima M, et al: Guidelines for management of idiopathic normal pressure hydrocephalus (third edition): endorsed by the Japanese society of normal pressure hydrocephalus. Neurol Med Chir (Tokyo) 61(2):63–97, 2021

Nakhleh R, Tessema ST, Mahgoub A: Creutzfeldt-Jakob disease as a cause of dementia. BMJ Case Rep 14(5):e240020, 2021

Nakiyemba O, Obore S, Musaba M, et al: Covariates of pica among pregnant women attending antenatal care at Kawempe hospital, Kampala, Uganda: a cross-sectional Study. Am J Trop Med Hyg 105(4):909–914, 2021

Namekawa M, Nakamura Y, Nakano I: Cortical involvement in Marchiafava-Bignami disease can be a predictor of a poor prognosis: a case report and review of the literature. Intern Med 52(7):811–813, 2013

Nardone R, Sebastianelli L, Versace V, et al: Involvement of central sensory pathways in subjects with restless legs syndrome: a neurophysiological study. Brain Res 1772:147673, 2021

Natelson BH: Myalgic encephalomyelitis/chronic fatigue syndrome and fibromyalgia: definitions, similarities, and differences. Clin Ther 41(4):612–618, 2019

National Institute of Diabetes and Digestive and Kidney Diseases: LiverTox. Bethesda, MD, National Institute of Diabetes and Digestive and Kidney Diseases, 2012. Available at: https://www.ncbi.nlm.nih.gov/books/NBK547852. Accessed July 21, 2022.

National Institutes of Health Office of Dietary Supplements: Niacin: fact sheet for health professionals, in Health Information: Dietary Supplement Fact Sheets. Bethesda, MD, National Institutes of Health, March 26, 2021. Available at: https://ods.od.nih.gov/factsheets/Niacin-HealthProfessional. Accessed July 21, 2022.

Naughton SX, Terry AV Jr: Neurotoxicity in acute and repeated organophosphate exposure. Toxicology 408:101–112, 2018

Neary NM, King KS, Pacak K: Drugs and pheochromocytoma—don't be fooled by every elevated metanephrine. N Engl J Med 364(23):2268–2270, 2011

Neumann HPH, Young WF Jr, Eng C: Pheochromocytoma and paraganglioma. N Engl J Med 381(6):552–565, 2019

Neumann J, Beck O, Helander A, et al: Performance of PEth compared with other alcohol biomarkers in subjects presenting for occupational and pre-employment medical examination. Alcohol Alcohol 55(4):401–408, 2020

Neuschwander-Tetri BA: Non-alcoholic fatty liver disease. BMC Med 15(1):45, 2017

Ng E, Neff M: Recognising the return of nutritional deficiencies: a modern pellagra puzzle. BMJ Case Rep 11(1):e227454, 2018

Nguyen VL, Haber PS, Seth D: Applications and challenges for the use of phosphatidylethanol testing in liver disease patients (mini review). Alcohol Clin Exp Res 42(2):238–243, 2018

Nicolli A, Mina GG, De Nuzzo D, et al: Unusual domestic source of lead poisoning. Int J Environ Res Public Health 17(12):4374, 2020

Nielsen RE, Banner J, Jensen SE: Cardiovascular disease in patients with severe mental illness. Nat Rev Cardiol 18(2):136–145, 2021

Nieman LK: Diagnosis of Cushing's syndrome in the modern era. Endocrinol Metab Clin North Am 47(2):259–273, 2018

Nigrovic LE, Lewander DP, Balamuth F, et al: The Lyme Disease Polymerase Chain Reaction Test has low sensitivity. Vector Borne Zoonotic Dis 20(4):310–313, 2020

Nikogosyan G, Orias D, Goebert D, et al: Acute aripiprazole-associated liver injury. J Clin Psychopharmacol 41(3):344–346, 2021

Niles JK, Gudin J, Radcliff J, et al: The opioid epidemic within the COVID-19 pandemic: drug testing in 2020. Popul Health Manag 24(S1):S43–S51, 2021

Nissen MS, Ryding M, Meyer M, et al: Autoimmune encephalitis: current knowledge on subtypes, disease mechanisms and treatment. CNS Neurol Disord Drug Targets 19(8):584–598, 2020

Njati SY, Maguta MM: Lead-based paints and children's PVC toys are potential sources of domestic lead poisoning: a review. Environ Pollut 249:1091–1105, 2019

Nobili F, Arbizu J, Bouwman F, et al: European Association of Nuclear Medicine and European Academy of Neurology recommendations for the use of brain 18F-fluorodeoxyglucose positron emission tomography in neurodegenerative cognitive impairment and dementia: Delphi consensus. Eur J Neurol 25(10):1201–1217, 2018

Noordam C, Höybye C, Eiholzer U: Prader-Willi syndrome and hypogonadism: a review article. Int J Mol Sci 22(5):2705, 2021

Novo-Veleiro I, Herrera-Flores J, Rosón-Hernández B, et al: Alcoholic liver disease among patients with Wernicke encephalopathy: a multicenter observational study. Drug Alcohol Depend 230:109186, 2022

Ntaios G, Michel P, Georgiopoulos G, et al: Characteristics and outcomes in patients with COVID-19 and acute ischemic stroke: the Global COVID-19 Stroke Registry. Stroke 51(9):e254–e258, 2020

Ntusi NAB: HIV and myocarditis. Curr Opin HIV AIDS 12(6):561–565, 2017

Nucifora FC Jr, Woznica E, Lee BJ, et al: Treatment resistant schizophrenia: clinical, biological, and therapeutic perspectives. Neurobiol Dis 131:104257, 2019

OneCare Media: Testing.com: Your Trusted Guide. Understand Your Tests, Empower Your Health. Seattle, WA, OneCare Media, 2022. Available at: https://www.testing.com. Accessed July 20, 2022.

Øie LR, Kurth T, Gulati S, et al: Migraine and risk of stroke. J Neurol Neurosurg Psychiatry 91(6):593–604, 2020

O'Keeffe ST: Thiamine deficiency in elderly people. Age Ageing 29:99–101, 2000

Olek MJ: Multiple sclerosis. Ann Intern Med 174(6):ITC81–ITC96, 2021

Ollila HM: Narcolepsy type 1: what have we learned from genetics? Sleep 43(11):zsaa099, 2020

Olney NT, Spina S, Miller BL: Frontotemporal dementia. Neurol Clin 35(2):339–374, 2017

Olszewska DA, Lonergan R, Fallon EM, et al: Genetics of frontotemporal dementia. Curr Neurol Neurosci Rep 16(12):107, 2016

Online Mendelian Inheritance in Man: Clinical features, in Prader-Willi Syndrome (#176270). Baltimore, MD, Johns Hopkins University, March 28, 2022. Available at: https://www.omim.org/entry/176270#clinicalFeatures. Accessed July 21, 2022.

Onyike CU, Huey ED: Frontotemporal dementia and psychiatry. Int Rev Psychiatry 25(2):127–129, 2013

O'Rourke L, Murphy KC: Recent developments in understanding the relationship between 22q11.2 deletion syndrome and psychosis. Curr Opin Psychiatry 32(2):67–72, 2019

Ostrom QT, Wright CH, Barnholtz-Sloan JS: Brain metastases: epidemiology. Handb Clin Neurol 149:27–42, 2018

Oudman E, Wijnia JW, Oey M, et al: Wernicke's encephalopathy in hyperemesis gravidarum: a systematic review. Eur J Obstet Gynecol Reprod Biol 236:84–93, 2019

Oudman E, Wijnia JW, Oey MJ, et al: Wernicke's encephalopathy in Crohn's disease and ulcerative colitis. Nutrition 86:111182, 2021

Ozsezen B, Emiralioglu N, Özön A, et al: Sleep disordered breathing in patients with Prader Willi syndrome: Impact of underlying genetic mechanism. Respir Med 187:106567, 2021

Pacei F, Tesone A, Laudi N, et al: The relevance of thiamine evaluation in a practical setting. Nutrients 12(9):2810, 2020

Palmer BF, Clegg DJ: Diagnosis and treatment of hyperkalemia. Cleve Clin J Med 84(12):934–942, 2017

Palmer BF, Clegg DJ: Electrolyte disturbances in patients with chronic alcohol-use disorder. N Engl J Med 377(14):1368–1377, 2017

Palmieri A, Valentinis L, Zanchin G: Update on headache and brain tumors. Cephalalgia 41(4):431–437, 2021

Pan LA, Martin P, Zimmer T, et al: Neurometabolic disorders: potentially treatable abnormalities in patients with treatment-refractory depression and suicidal behavior. Am J Psychiatry 174(1):42–50, 2017

Pandey A, Stoker T, Adamczyk LA, et al: Aseptic meningitis and hydrocephalus secondary to neurosarcoidosis. BMJ Case Rep 14(8):e242312, 2021

Pannu AK, Bhalla A, Vishnu RI, et al: Organophosphate induced delayed neuropathy after an acute cholinergic crisis in self-poisoning. Clin Toxicol (Phila) 59(6):488–492, 2021

Paquin V, Therriault J, Pascoal TA, et al: Frontal variant of Alzheimer disease differentiated from frontotemporal dementia using in vivo amyloid and tau imaging. Cogn Behav Neurol 33(4):288–293, 2020

Parashar S, Collins AB, Montaner JS, et al: Reducing rates of preventable HIV/AIDS-associated mortality among people living with HIV who inject drugs. Curr Opin HIV AIDS 11(5):507–513, 2016

Pardamean E, Roan W, Iskandar KTA, et al: Mortality from coronavirus disease 2019 (COVID-19) in patients with schizophrenia: a systematic review, meta-analysis and meta-regression. Gen Hosp Psychiatry 75:61–67, 2022

Park HY, Kim M, Suh CH, et al: Diagnostic value of diffusion-weighted brain magnetic resonance imaging in patients with sporadic Creutzfeldt-Jakob disease: a systematic review and meta-analysis. Eur Radiol 31(12):9073–9085, 2021

Park JH, Kummerlowe M, Gardea Resendez M, et al: First manic episode following COVID-19 infection. Bipolar Disord 23(8):847–849, 2021

Park M, Reynolds CF III: Depression among older adults with diabetes mellitus. Clin Geriatr Med 31(1):117-137, 2015

Park SH, Ishino R: Liver injury associated with antidepressants. Curr Drug Saf 8(3):207–223, 2013

Pascoe MC, Linden T: Folate and MMA predict cognitive impairment in elderly stroke survivors: a cross sectional study. Psychiatry Res 243:49–52, 2016

Patel A, Sul J, Gordon ML, et al: Progressive multifocal leukoencephalopathy in a patient with progressive multiple sclerosis treated with ocrelizumab monotherapy. JAMA Neurol 278(6):736–740, 2021

Patel D, Steinberg J, Patel P: Insomnia in the elderly: a review. J Clin Sleep Med 14(6):1017–1024, 2018

Patel SR: Obstructive sleep apnea. Ann Intern Med 171(11):ITC81–ITC96, 2019

Paul S, Mondal GP, Bhattacharyya R, et al: Neuromyelitis optica spectrum disorders. J Neurol Sci 420:117225, 2021

Pazderska A, Pearce SH: Adrenal insufficiency: recognition and management. Clin Med (Lond) 17(3):258–262, 2017

Pellikaan K, Rosenberg AGW, Kattentidt-Mouravieva AA, et al: Missed diagnoses and health problems in adults with Prader-Willi syndrome: recommendations for screening and treatment. J Clin Endocrinol Metab 105(12):e4671–e4687, 2020

Penninx BWJH, Lange SMM: Metabolic syndrome in psychiatric patients: overview, mechanisms, and implications. Dialogues Clin Neurosci 20(1):63–73, 2018

Pepe J, Colangelo L, Biamonte F, et al: Diagnosis and management of hypocalcemia. Endocrine 69(3):485–495, 2020

Perez A, Huse JT: The evolving classification of diffuse gliomas: World Health Organization Updates for 2021. Curr Neurol Neurosci Rep 21(12):67, 2021

Perez A, Jansen-Chaparro S, Saigi I, et al: Glucocorticoid-induced hyperglycemia. J Diabetes 6(1):9–20, 2014

Perez DL, LaFrance WC Jr: Nonepileptic seizures: an updated review. CNS Spectr 21(3):239–246, 2016

Perez MN, Salas RME: Insomnia. Continuum (Minneap Minn) 26(4):1003–1015, 2020

Peri A, Grohé C, Berardi R, et al: SIADH: differential diagnosis and clinical management. Endocrine 55(1):311–319, 2017

Periyasamy S, John S, Padmavati R, et al: Association of schizophrenia risk with disordered niacin metabolism in an Indian genome-wide association study. JAMA Psychiatry 76(10):1026–1034, 2019

Perlman DM, Sudheendra MT, Furuya Y, et al: Clinical presentation and treatment of high-risk sarcoidosis. Ann Am Thorac Soc 18(12):1935–1947, 2021

Petersen RC: Mild cognitive impairment. Continuum (Minneap Minn) 22(2):404–418, 2016

Petersmann A, Müller-Wieland D, Müller UA, et al: Definition, classification and diagnosis of diabetes mellitus. Exp Clin Endocrinol Diabetes 127(S01):S1–S7, 2019

Petri M: Antiphospholipid syndrome. Transl Res 225:70–81, 2020

Phillips J, Henderson AC: Hemolytic anemia: evaluation and differential diagnosis. Am Fam Physician 98(6):354–361, 2018

Phypers M, Harris T, Power C: CNS tuberculosis: a longitudinal analysis of epidemiological and clinical features. Int J Tuberc Lung Dis 10(1):99–103, 2006

Pinkhasov A, Xiong G, Bourgeois JA, et al: Management of SIADH-related hyponatremia due to psychotropic medications: an expert consensus from the Association of Medicine and Psychiatry. J Psychosom Res 151:110654, 2021

Pitrak D, Nguyen CT, Cifu AS: Diagnosis of Lyme disease. JAMA 327(7):676–677, 2022

Pivonello R, De Martino MC, De Leo M, et al: Cushing's disease: the burden of illness. Endocrine 56(1):10–18, 2017

Poirier-Blanchette L, Simard C, Schwartz BC: Spurious point-of-care lactate elevation in ethylene glycol intoxication: rediscovering a clinical pearl. BMJ Case Rep 14(2):e239936, 2021

Pope S, Artuch R, Heales S, et al: Cerebral folate deficiency: analytical tests and differential diagnosis. J Inherit Metab Dis 42(4):655–672, 2019

Popkirov S, Asadi-Pooya AA, Duncan R, et al: The aetiology of psychogenic non-epileptic seizures: risk factors and comorbidities. Epileptic Disord 21(6):529–547, 2019

Poplin V, Boulware DR, Bahr NC: Methods for rapid diagnosis of meningitis etiology in adults. Biomark Med 14(6):459–479, 2020

Portale S, Sculati M, Stanford FC, et al: Pellagra and anorexia nervosa: a case report. Eat Weight Disord 25(5):1493–1496, 2020

Porter KK, Cason DE, Morgan DE: Acute pancreatitis: how can MR imaging help. Magn Reson Imaging Clin N Am 26(3):439–450, 2018

Posada J, Mahan N, Abdel Meguid AS: Catatonia as a presenting symptom of isolated neurosarcoidosis in a woman with schizophrenia. J Acad Consult Liaison Psychiatry 62(5):546–550, 2021

Posner J, Polanczyk GV, Sonuga-Barke E: Attention-deficit hyperactivity disorder. Lancet 395(10222):450–462, 2020

Post JJ, Benfield T, Woolley I: When pandemics collide: measuring the impact of coronavirus disease 2019 on people with HIV. AIDS 36(3):473–474, 2022

Power C, Lawlor BA: The behavioral variant frontotemporal dementia phenocopy syndrome: a review. J Geriatr Psychiatry Neurol 34(3):196–208, 2021

Pratiwi C, Zulkifly S, Dahlan TF, et al: Hospital related hyperglycemia as a predictor of mortality in non-diabetes patients: a systematic review. Diabetes Metab Syndr 15(6):102309, 2021

Pressman PS, Matlock D, Ducharme S: Distinguishing behavioral variant frontotemporal dementia from primary psychiatric disorders: a review of recently published consensus recommendations from the Neuropsychiatric International Consortium for Frontotemporal Dementia. J Neuropsychiatry Clin Neurosci 33(2):152–156, 2021

Principi N, Esposito S: Aluminum in vaccines: does it create a safety problem? Vaccine 36(39):5825–5831, 2018

Qian Q: Hypernatremia. Clin J Am Soc Nephrol 14(3):432–434, 2019

Ragnarsson O: Cushing's syndrome: disease monitoring: recurrence, surveillance with biomarkers or imaging studies. Best Pract Res Clin Endocrinol Metab 34(2):101382, 2020

Rajan S, Kaas B, Moukheiber E: Movement disorders emergencies. Semin Neurol 39(1):125–136, 2019

Ramaekers V, Sequeira JM, Quadros EV: Clinical recognition and aspects of the cerebral folate deficiency syndromes. Clin Chem Lab Med 51(3):497–511, 2013

Ramanujam VS, Anderson KE: Porphyria diagnostics—Part 1: a brief overview of the porphyrias. Curr Protoc Hum Genet 86:17.20.1–17.20.26, 2015

Ramírez-Bermúdez J, Marrufo-Melendez O, Berlanga-Flores C, et al: White matter abnormalities in late onset first episode mania: a diffusion tensor imaging study. Am J Geriatr Psychiatry 29(12):1225–1236, 2021

Ramos-Casals M, Pérez-Alvarez R, Kostov B, et al: Clinical characterization and outcomes of 85 patients with neurosarcoidosis. Sci Rep 11(1):13735, 2021

Ran E, Wang M, Yi Y, et al: Mercury poisoning complicated by acquired neuromyotonia syndrome: a case report. Medicine (Baltimore) 100(32):e26910, 2021

Rangan GK, Dorani N, Zhang MM, et al: Clinical characteristics and outcomes of hyponatraemia associated with oral water intake in adults: a systematic review. BMJ Open 11(12):e046539, 2021

Rao S, Sunkara A, Ashwath A, et al: Lupus cerebritis refractory to guideline-directed therapy: a case report. J Investig Med High Impact Case Rep 9:23247096211008708, 2021

Rao SN, Chandak GR: Cardiac beriberi: often a missed diagnosis. J Trop Pediatr 56(4):284–285, 2010

Ray S, Agarwal P: Depression and anxiety in Parkinson disease. Clin Geriatr Med 36(1):93–104, 2020

Redford C, Vaidya B: Subclinical hypothyroidism: should we treat? Post Reprod Health 23(2):55–62, 2017

Refardt J, Winzeler B, Christ-Crain M: Copeptin and its role in the diagnosis of diabetes insipidus and the syndrome of inappropriate antidiuresis. Clin Endocrinol (Oxf) 91(1):22–32, 2019

Refardt J, Winzeler B, Christ-Crain M: Diabetes insipidus: an update. Endocrinol Metab Clin North Am 49(3):517–531, 2020

Reich SG, Savitt JM: Parkinson's disease. Med Clin North Am 103(2):337–350, 2019

Resende LL, de Paiva ARB, Kok F, et al: Adult leukodystrophies: a step-by-step diagnostic approach. Radiographics 39(1):153–168, 2019

Reuben A: Childhood lead exposure and adult neurodegenerative disease. J Alzheimers Dis 64(1):17–42, 2018

Reynolds EH: The neurology of folic acid deficiency. Handb Clin Neurol 120:927–943, 2014

Reynolds RM, Padfield PL, Seckl JR: Disorders of sodium balance. BMJ 332(7543):702–705, 2006

Ricci M, Cimini A, Chiaravalloti A, et al: Positron emission tomography (PET) and neuroimaging in the personalized approach to neurodegenerative causes of dementia. Int J Mol Sci 21(20):7481, 2020

Rice KM, Walker EM Jr, Wu M, et al: Environmental mercury and its toxic effects. J Prev Med Public Health 47(2):74–83, 2014

Richard-Eaglin A: Male and female hypogonadism. Nurs Clin North Am 53(3):395–405, 2018

Richter PMA, Ramos RT: Obsessive-compulsive disorder. Continuum (Minneap Minn) 24(3):828–844, 2018

Riemann D, Nissen C, Palagini L, et al: The neurobiology, investigation, and treatment of chronic insomnia. Lancet Neurol 14(5):547–558, 2015

Rigakos G, Liakou CI, Felipe N, et al: Clinical presentation, diagnosis, and radiological Findings of neoplastic meningitis. Cancer Control 24(1):9–21, 2017

Rinck D, Frieling H, Freitag A, et al: Combinations of carbohydrate-deficient transferrin, mean corpuscular erythrocyte volume, gamma-glutamyltransferase, homocysteine and folate increase the significance of biological markers in alcohol dependent patients. Drug Alcohol Depend 89(1):60–65, 2007

Robbins TW, Vaghi MM, Banca P: Obsessive-compulsive disorder: puzzles and prospects. Neuron 102(1):27–47, 2019

Robinson RG, Jorge RE: Post-stroke depression: a review. Am J Psychiatry 173(3):221–231, 2016

Rocha A, Trujillo KA: Neurotoxicity of low-level lead exposure: history, mechanisms of action, and behavioral effects in humans and preclinical models. Neurotoxicology 73:58–80, 2019

Roest AM, Zuidersma M, de Jonge P: Myocardial infarction and generalised anxiety disorder: 10-year follow-up. Br J Psychiatry 200(4):324–329, 2012

Rommel N, Hamdy S: Oropharyngeal dysphagia: manifestations and diagnosis. Nat Rev Gastroenterol Hepatol 13(1):49–59, 2016

Ropper AH: Neurosyphilis. N Engl J Med 381(14):1358–1363, 2019

Rose CF, Amodio P, Bajaj JS, et al: Hepatic encephalopathy: novel insights into classification, pathophysiology and therapy. J Hepatol 73(6):1526–1547, 2020

Rosen E, Bakshi N, Watters A, et al: Hepatic complications of anorexia nervosa. Dig Dis Sci 62(11):2977–2981, 2017

Rosner MH, Husain-Syed F, Reis T, et al: Uremic encephalopathy. Kidney Int 101(2):227–241, 2022

Ross DS, Burch HB, Cooper DS, et al: 2016 American Thyroid Association guidelines for diagnosis and management of hyperthyroidism and other causes of thyrotoxicosis. Thyroid 26(10):1343–1421, 2016

Rosso M, Fremion E, Santoro SL, et al: Down syndrome disintegrative disorder: a clinical regression syndrome of increasing importance. Pediatrics 145(6):e20192939, 2020

Roszali MA, Zakaria AN, Mohd Tahir NA: Parenteral nutrition-associated hyperglycemia: prevalence, predictors and management. Clin Nutr ESPEN 41:275–280, 2021

Roy A, Fuentes-Afflick E, Fernald LCH, et al: Pica is prevalent and strongly associated with iron deficiency among Hispanic pregnant women living in the United States. Appetite 120:163–170, 2018

Rudler M, Weiss N, Bouzbib C, et al: Diagnosis and management of hepatic encephalopathy. Clin Liver Dis 25(2):393–417, 2021

Rundo JV: Obstructive sleep apnea basics. Cleve Clin J Med 86(9 Suppl 1):2–9, 2019

Rushworth RL, Torpy DJ, Falhammar H: Adrenal crisis. N Engl J Med 381(9):852–861, 2019

Sachs KV, Harnke B, Mehler PS, et al: Cardiovascular complications of anorexia nervosa: a systematic review. Int J Eat Disord 49(3):238–248, 2016

Sahu P, Thippeswamy H, Chaturvedi SK: Neuropsychiatric manifestations in vitamin B12 deficiency. Vitam Horm 119:457–470, 2022

Sahyouni R, Goshtasbi K, Mahmoodi A, et al: Chronic subdural hematoma: a historical and clinical perspective. World Neurosurg 108:948–953, 2017

Said HM, Kaya D, Yavuz I, et al: A comparison of cerebrospinal fluid beta-amyloid and tau in idiopathic normal pressure hydrocephalus and neurodegenerative dementias. Clin Interv Aging 17:467–477, 2022

Sailer CO, Winzeler B, Nigro N, et al: Characteristics and outcomes of patients with profound hyponatraemia due to primary polydipsia. Clin Endocrinol (Oxf) 87(5):492–499, 2017

Salathe C, Blanc AL, Tagan D: SIADH and water intoxication related to ecstasy. BMJ Case Rep 2018:bcr2018224731, 2018

Salcedo-Arellano MJ, Dufour B, McLennan Y, et al: Fragile X syndrome and associated disorders: clinical aspects and pathology. Neurobiol Dis 136:104740, 2020

Salonia A, Rastrelli G, Hackett G, et al: Paediatric and adult-onset male hypogonadism. Nat Rev Dis Primers 5(1):38, 2019

Samarghandian S, Shirazi FM, Saeedi F, et al: A systematic review of clinical and laboratory findings of lead poisoning: lessons from case reports. Toxicol Appl Pharmacol 429:115681, 2021

Sami M, Khan H, Nilforooshan R: Late onset mania as an organic syndrome: a review of case reports in the literature. J Affect Disord 188:226–231, 2015

Sammaritano LR: Antiphospholipid syndrome. Best Pract Res Clin Rheumatol 34(1):101463, 2020

Sanchez-Meza F, Torre A, Castillo-Martinez L, et al: Evaluation of cerebral dysfunction in patients with chronic kidney disease using neuropsychometric and neurophysiological tests. Ren Fail 43(1):577–584, 2021

Sandler CX, Lloyd AR: Chronic fatigue syndrome: progress and possibilities. Med J Aust 212(9):428–433, 2020

Santoro JD, Pagarkar D, Chu DT, et al: Neurologic complications of Down syndrome: a systematic review. J Neurol 268(12):4495–4509, 2021

Santos A, Webb SM, Resmini E: Psychological complications of Cushing's syndrome. Curr Opin Endocrinol Diabetes Obes 28(3):325–329, 2021

Santos de Lima F, Issa N, Seibert K, et al: Epileptiform activity and seizures in patients with COVID-19. J Neurol Neurosurg Psychiatry 92(5):565–566, 2021

Santos E, Emeka-Nwonovo C, Wang JY, et al: Developmental aspects of FXAND in a man with the FMR1 premutation. Mol Genet Genomic Med 8(2):e1050, 2020

Sanvisens A, Zuluaga P, Pineda M, et al: Folate deficiency in patients seeking treatment of alcohol use disorder. Drug Alcohol Depend 180:417–422, 2017

Sanyal AJ, Van Natta ML, Clark J, et al: Prospective study of outcomes in adults with nonalcoholic fatty liver disease. N Engl J Med 385(17):1559–1569, 2021

Sapountzi P, Emanuele NV, Loutrianakis E, et al: Visual vignette. Diagnosis: hypocalcemia due to primary hypoparathyroidism. Endocr Pract 12:233, 2006

Saracino D, Ferrieux S, Noguès-Lassiaille M, et al: Primary progressive aphasia associated with GRN mutations: new insights into the nonamyloid logopenic variant. Neurology 97(1):e88–e102, 2021

Satyaputra F, Hendry S, Braddick M, et al: The laboratory diagnosis of syphilis. J Clin Microbiol 59(10):e0010021, 2021

Satzer D, Bond DJ: Mania secondary to focal brain lesions: implications for understanding the functional neuroanatomy of bipolar disorder. Bipolar Disord 18(3):205–220, 2016

Sawalha K, Kakkera K: Acute respiratory failure from hypermagnesemia requiring prolonged mechanical ventilation. J Investig Med High Impact Case Rep 8:2324709620984898, 2020

Sayar Z, Moll R, Isenberg D, et al: Thrombotic antiphospholipid syndrome: a practical guide to diagnosis and management. Thromb Res 198:213–221, 2021

Sazegar P: Cannabis essentials: tools for clinical practice. Am Fam Physician 104(6):598–608, 2021

Sbardella E, Grossman AB: Pheochromocytoma: an approach to diagnosis. Best Pract Res Clin Endocrinol Metab 34(2):101346, 2020

Scammell TE: Narcolepsy. N Engl J Med 373(27):2654–2662, 2015

Scarlett JA, Mako ME, Rubenstein AH, et al: Factitious hypoglycemia: diagnosis by measurement of serum C-peptide immunoreactivity and insulin-binding antibodies. N Engl J Med 297(19):1029–1032, 1977

Schafer AI: Thrombocytosis. JAMA 314(11):1171–1172, 2015

Scheen M, Giraud R, Bendjelid K: Stress hyperglycemia, cardiac glucotoxicity, and critically ill patient outcomes current clinical and pathophysiological evidence. Physiol Rep 9(2):e14713, 2021

Scherer JS, Combs SA, Brennan F: Sleep disorders, restless legs syndrome, and uremic pruritus: diagnosis and treatment of common symptoms in dialysis patients. Am J Kidney Dis 69(1):117–128, 2017

Schernthaner-Reiter MH, Stratakis CA, Luger A: Genetics of diabetes insipidus. Endocrinol Metab Clin North Am 46(2):305–334, 2017

Schiff D, Alyahya M: Neurological and medical complications in brain tumor patients. Curr Neurol Neurosci Rep 20(8):33, 2020

Schifman RB, Luevano DR: Aluminum toxicity: evaluation of 16-year trend among 14,919 patients and 45,480 results. Arch Pathol Lab Med 142(6):742–746, 2018

Schmidt C, Oxley Oxland J, et al: A rare case of hypokalaemia and hypophosphataemia secondary to geophagia. BMJ Case Rep 14(5):e239322, 2021

Schneider RB, Iourinets J, Richard IH: Parkinson's disease psychosis: presentation, diagnosis and management. Neurodegener Dis Manag 7(6):365–376, 2017

Schriefer ME: Lyme disease diagnosis: serology. Clin Lab Med 35(4):797–814, 2015

Schroeder ME, Manderski MT, Amro C, et al: Large gathering attendance is associated with increased odds of contracting COVID-19: a survey based study. J Prev 43(2):157–166, 2022

Schuster MP, Borkent J, Chrispijn M, et al: Increased prevalence of metabolic syndrome in patients with bipolar disorder compared to a selected control group: a Northern Netherlands LifeLines population cohort study. J Affect Disord 295:1161–1168, 2021

Schutzer SE, Body BA, Boyle J, et al: Direct diagnostic tests for Lyme disease. Clin Infect Dis 68(6):1052–1057, 2019

Schwartz L, Caixàs A, Dimitropoulos A, et al: Behavioral features in Prader-Willi syndrome (PWS): consensus paper from the International PWS Clinical Trial Consortium. J Neurodev Disord 13(1):25, 2021

Sealock JM, Lee YH, Moscati A, et al: Use of the PsycheMERGE network to investigate the association between depression polygenic scores and white blood cell count. JAMA Psychiatry 78(12):1365–1374, 2021

Sechi G, Serra A: Wernicke's encephalopathy: new clinical settings and recent advances in diagnosis and management. Lancet Neurol 6(5):442–455, 2007

Seeley WW: Behavioral variant frontotemporal dementia. Continuum (Minneap Minn) 25(1):76–100, 2019

Sefidbakht S, Lotfi M, Jalli R, et al: Methanol toxicity outbreak: when fear of COVID-19 goes viral. Emerg Med J 37(7):416, 2020

Sell J, Ramirez S, Partin M: Parathyroid disorders. Am Fam Physician 105(3):289–298, 2022

Selvarajah D, Kar D, Khunti K, et al: Diabetic peripheral neuropathy: advances in diagnosis and strategies for screening and early intervention. Lancet Diabetes Endocrinol 7(12):938–948, 2019

Semelka M, Wilson J, Floyd R: Diagnosis and treatment of obstructive sleep apnea in adults. Am Fam Physician 94(5):355–360, 2016

Seoud T, Syed A, Carleton N, et al: Depression before and after a diagnosis of pancreatic cancer: results from a national, population-based study. Pancreas 49(8):1117–1122, 2020

Seto N, Ishida M, Hamano T, et al: A case of Wernicke encephalopathy arising in the early stage after the start of hemodialysis. CEN Case Rep Jan 6, 2022 [Epub ahead of print]

Shaban A, Leira EC: Neurological complications in patients with systemic lupus erythematosus. Curr Neurol Neurosci Rep 19(12):97, 2019

Shabani M, Hadeiy SK, Parhizgar P, et al: Lead poisoning; a neglected potential diagnosis in abdominal pain. BMC Gastroenterol 20(1):134, 2020

Shah M, Dorman SE: Latent tuberculosis infection. N Engl J Med 385(24):2271–2280, 2021

Shapiro ED. Clinical practice: Lyme disease. N Engl J Med 370(18):1724–1731, 2014

Shapiro PA: Management of depression after myocardial infarction. Curr Cardiol Rep 17(10):80, 2015

Sheka AC, Adeyi O, Thompson J, et al: Nonalcoholic steatohepatitis: a review. JAMA 323(12):1175–1183, 2020

Shepshelovich D, Schechter A, Calvarysky B, et al: Medication-induced SIADH: distribution and characterization according to medication class. Br J Clin Pharmacol 83(8):1801–1807, 2017

Shela HM, Al-Najami I, Christensen HD, et al: Rapid diagnosis of ethylene glycol poisoning by urine microscopy. Am J Case Rep 19:689–693, 2018

Shribman S, Marjot T, Sharif A, et al: Investigation and management of Wilson's disease: a practical guide from the British Association for the Study of the Liver. Gastroenterol Hepatol 7(6):560–575, 2022

Siao P, Kaku M: A clinician's approach to peripheral neuropathy. Semin Neurol 39(5):519–530, 2019

Siblerud R, Mutter J, Moore E, et al: A hypothesis and evidence that mercury may be an etiological factor in Alzheimer's disease. Int J Environ Res Public Health 16(24):5152, 2019

Sigel K, Makinson A, Thaler J: Lung cancer in persons with HIV. Curr Opin HIV AIDS 12(1):31–38, 2017

Sillanaukee P: Laboratory markers of alcohol abuse. Alcohol Alcohol 31(6):613–616, 1996

Singh RD, van Dijck JTJM, van Essen TA, et al: Randomized Evaluation of Surgery in Elderly with Traumatic Acute SubDural Hematoma (RESET-ASDH trial): study protocol for a pragmatic randomized controlled trial with multicenter parallel group design. Trials 23(1):242, 2022

Singh VK, Yadav D, Garg PK: Diagnosis and management of chronic pancreatitis: a review. JAMA 322(24):2422–2434, 2019

Sinha S, Kataria A, Kolla BP, et al: Wernicke encephalopathy: clinical pearls. Mayo Clin Proc 94(6):1065–1072, 2019

Skakkebæk A, Wallentin M, Gravholt CH: Klinefelter's syndrome or testicular dysgenesis: genetics, endocrinology, and neuropsychology. Handb Clin Neurol 181:445–462, 2021

Sloan S, Dosumu-Johnson RT: A new onset of mania in a 49-year-old man: an interesting case of Wilson disease. J Psychiatr Pract 26(6):510–517, 2020

Smith A, Baumgartner K, Bositis C: Cirrhosis: diagnosis And Management. Am Fam Physician 100(12):759–770, 2019

Smith NS, Bauer BW, Capron DW: Comparing symptom networks of daytime and nocturnal panic attacks in a community-based sample. J Anxiety Disord 85:102514, 2022

Smith TJ, Johnson CR, Koshy R, et al: Thiamine deficiency disorders: a clinical perspective. Ann N Y Acad Sci 1498(1):9–28, 2021

Smock KJ, Perkins SL: Thrombocytopenia: an update. Int J Lab Hematol 36(3):269–278, 2014

Sobczynska-Malefora A, Harrington DJ: Laboratory assessment of folate (vitamin B9) status. J Clin Pathol 71(11):949–956, 2018

Sönmez E, Bulur O, Ertugrul DT, et al: Hyperthyroidism influences renal function. Endocrine 65(1):144–148, 2019

Sonneville R, Ruimy R, Benzonana N, et al: An update on bacterial brain abscess in immuno-competent patients. Clin Microbiol Infect 23(9):614–620, 2017

Srinutta T, Chewcharat A, Takkavatakarn K, et al: Proton pump inhibitors and hypomagnese-mia: a meta-analysis of observational studies. Medicine (Baltimore) 98(44):e17788, 2019

Stach K, Stach W, Augoff K: Vitamin B6 in health and disease. Nutrients 13(9):3229, 2021

Stallones L, Beseler CL: Assessing the connection between organophosphate pesticide poison-ing and mental health: a comparison of neuropsychological symptoms from clinical obser-vations, animal models and epidemiological studies. Cortex 74:405–416, 2016

Stanford Medicine: Liver disease, head to foot, in Stanford Medicine 25: Promoting the Culture of Bedside Medicine. Stanford, CA, Stanford Medicine, 2022. Available at: https://stanfordmedicine25.stanford.edu/the25/liverdisease.html. Accessed July 22, 2022.

Stauder R, Valent P, Theurl I: Anemia at older age: etiologies, clinical implications, and man-agement. Blood 131(5):505–514, 2018

Stein TD, Crary JF: Chronic traumatic encephalopathy and neuropathological comorbidities. Semin Neurol 40(4):384–393, 2020

Štepánek L, Nakládalová M, Klementa V, et al: Acute lead poisoning in an indoor firing range. Med Pr 71(3):375–379, 2020

Steriade C, Shumak SL, Feinstein A: A 54-year-old man with hallucinations and hearing loss. CMAJ 186(17):1315–1318, 2014

Stern BJ, Royal W III, Gelfand JM, et al: Definition and consensus diagnostic criteria for neuro-sarcoidosis: from the Neurosarcoidosis Consortium Consensus Group. JAMA Neurol 75(12):1546–1553, 2018

Sterns RH: Disorders of plasma sodium: causes, consequences, and correction. N Engl J Med 372(1):55–65, 2015

Stevens JS, Moses AA, Nickolas TL, et al: Increased mortality associated with hypermagnese-mia in severe COVID-19 illness. Kidney360 2(7):1087–1094, 2021

Stölzel U, Doss MO, Schuppan D: Clinical guide and update on porphyrias. Gastroenterology 157(2):365–381, 2019

Stratakis N, Conti DV, Borras E, et al: Association of fish consumption and mercury exposure during pregnancy with metabolic health and inflammatory biomarkers in children. JAMA Netw Open 3(3):e201007, 2020

Straus SE, Thorpe KE, Holroyd-Leduc J: How do I perform a lumbar puncture and analyze the results to diagnose bacterial meningitis? JAMA 296(16):2012–2022, 2006

Strumia R: Dermatologic signs in patients with eating disorders. Am J Clin Dermatol 6:165–173, 2005

Styles M, Alsharshani D, Samara M, et al: Risk factors, diagnosis, prognosis and treatment of autism. Front Biosci (Landmark Ed) 25:1682–1717, 2020

Suárez I, Fünger SM, Kröger S, et al: The diagnosis and treatment of tuberculosis. Dtsch Arztebl Int 116(43):729–735, 2019

Suh Y, Gandhi J, Seyam O, et al: Neurological and neuropsychiatric manifestations of por-phyria. Int J Neurosci 129(12):1226–1233, 2019

Sutton EL: Insomnia. Ann Intern Med 174(3):ITC33–ITC48, 2021

Suttrup I, Warnecke T: Dysphagia in Parkinson's disease. Dysphagia 31(1):24–32, 2016

Swain F, Bird R: How I approach new onset thrombocytopenia. Platelets 31(3):285–290, 2020

Swain S, Turner C, Tyrrell P, et al: Diagnosis and initial management of acute stroke and tran-sient ischaemic attack: summary of NICE guidance. BMJ 337:a786, 2008

Swift IJ, Sogorb-Esteve A, Heller C, et al: Fluid biomarkers in frontotemporal dementia: past, present and future. J Neurol Neurosurg Psychiatry 92(2):204–215, 2021

Takahashi M, Uchino N: Risk factors of hypermagnesemia in end-stage cancer patients hospitalized in a palliative care unit. Ann Palliat Med 9(6):4308–4314, 2020

Taleb S, Zgueb Y, Ouali U, et al: Drug reaction with eosinophilia and systemic symptoms syndrome related to aripiprazole therapy. J Clin Psychopharmacol 39(6):691–693, 2019

Tammimies K, Marshall CR, Walker S, et al: Molecular diagnostic yield of chromosomal microarray analysis and whole-exome sequencing in children with autism spectrum disorder. AMA 314(9):895–903, 2015

Tan YY, Tan K: Hypertensive brainstem encephalopathy: a diagnosis often overlooked. Clin Med (Lond) 19(6):511–513, 2019

Tang KL, Antshel KM, Fremont WP, et al: Behavioral and psychiatric phenotypes in 22q11.2 deletion syndrome. J Dev Behav Pediatr 36(8):639–650, 2015

Tang Q, Li S, Yang Z, Wu M, et al: A narrative review of multimodal imaging of white matter lesions in type-2 diabetes mellitus. Ann Palliat Med 10(12):12867–12876, 2021

Taylor JP, McKeith IG, Burn DJ, et al: New evidence on the management of Lewy body dementia. Lancet Neurol 19(2):157–169, 2020

Teisseyre M, Moranne O, Renaud S: Late diagnosis of chronic hypocalcemia due to autoimmune hypoparathyroidism. BMJ Case Rep 14(6):e243299, 2021

Tetens MM, Haahr R, Dessau RB, et al: Assessment of the risk of psychiatric disorders, use of psychiatric hospitals, and receipt of psychiatric medication among patients with Lyme neuroborreliosis in Denmark. JAMA Psychiatry 78(2):177–186, 2021

Thakur KT, Boubour A, Saylor D, et al: Global HIV neurology: a comprehensive review. AIDS 33(2):163–184, 2019

Thambisetty M, Biousse V, Newman NJ: Hypertensive brainstem encephalopathy: clinical and radiographic features. J Neurol Sci 208:93–99, 2003

Thapar A, Cooper M: Attention deficit hyperactivity disorder. Lancet 387(10024):1240–1250, 2016

Theologou M, Natsis K, Kouskouras K, et al: Cerebrospinal fluid homeostasis and hydrodynamics: a review of facts and theories. Eur Neurol April 11:1–13, 2022

Thihalolipavan S, Candalla BM, Ehrlich J: Examining pica in NYC pregnant women with elevated blood lead levels. Matern Child Health J 17(1):49–55, 2013

Thom RP, Levy-Carrick NC, Bui M, et al: Delirium. Am J Psychiatry 176(10):785–793, 2019

Thygesen K, Alpert JS, Jaffe AS, et al: Fourth universal definition of myocardial infarction. Circulation 138(20):e618–e651, 2018

Títoff V, Moury HN, Títoff IB, et al: Seizures, antiepileptic drugs, and CKD. Am J Kidney Dis 73(1):90–101, 2019

Tleyjeh IM, Saddik B, Ramakrishnan RK, et al: Long term predictors of breathlessness, exercise intolerance, chronic fatigue and well-being in hospitalized patients with COVID-19: a cohort study with 4 months median follow-up. J Infect Public Health 15(1):21–28, 2022

Tohen M, Shulman KI, Satlin A: First-episode mania in late life. Am J Psychiatry 151(1):130–132, 1994

Tokumaru AM, Saito Y, Murayma S: Diffusion-weighted imaging is key to diagnosing specific diseases. Magn Reson Imaging Clin N Am 29(2):163–183, 2021

Tolosa E, Garrido A, Scholz SW, et al: Challenges in the diagnosis of Parkinson's disease. Lancet Neurol 20(5):385–397, 2021

Tomasi J, Lisoway AJ, Zai CC, et al: Towards precision medicine in generalized anxiety disorder: Review of genetics and pharmaco(epi)genetics. J Psychiatr Res 119:33–47, 2019

Tonon CR, Silva TAAL, Pereira FWL, et al: A review of current clinical concepts in the pathophysiology, etiology, diagnosis, and management of hypercalcemia. Med Sci Monit 28:e935821, 2022

Torales J, González I, Barrios I, et al: Manic episodes due to medical illnesses: a literature review. J Nerv Ment Dis 206(9):733–738, 2018

Torosyan N, Spencer D, Penev S, et al: Psychogenic polydipsia in a woman with anorexia nervosa: case report and recommendations. Prim Care Companion CNS Disord 20(1):17l02120, 2018

Tracy JA, Dyck PJ: Porphyria and its neurologic manifestations. Handb Clin Neurol 120:839–849, 2014

Treasure J, Claudino AM, Zucker N: Eating disorders. Lancet 375(9714):583–593, 2010

Treasure J, Zipfel S, Micali N, et al: Anorexia nervosa. Nat Rev Dis Primers 1:15074, 2015

Treister-Goltzman Y, Yarza S, Peleg R: Lipid profile in mild subclinical hypothyroidism: systematic review and meta-analysis. Minerva Endocrinol (Torino) 46(4):428–440, 2021

Trenkwalder C, Allen R, Högl B, et al: Restless legs syndrome associated with major diseases: a systematic review and new concept. Neurology 86(14):1336–1343, 2016

Trenkwalder C, Allen R, Högl B, et al: Comorbidities, treatment, and pathophysiology in restless legs syndrome. Lancet Neurol 217(11):994–1005, 2018

Trimpou P, Olsson DS, Ehn O, et al: Diagnostic value of the water deprivation test in the polyuria-polydipsia syndrome. Hormones (Athens) 16(4):414–422, 2017

Tsai CH, Yu KT, Chan HY, et al: Hashimoto's encephalopathy presenting as catatonia in a bipolar patient. Asian J Psychiatr 66:102895, 2021

Tse L, Barr AM, Scarapicchia V, et al: Neuroleptic malignant syndrome: a review from a clinically oriented perspective. Curr Neuropharmacol 13(3):395–406, 2015

Tung CS, Wu SL, Tsou JC, et al: Marchiafava-Bignami disease with widespread lesions and complete recovery. AJNR Am J Neuroradiol 31(8):1506–1507, 2010

Turk KW, Geada A, Alvarez VE, et al: A comparison between tau and amyloid-β cerebrospinal fluid biomarkers in chronic traumatic encephalopathy and Alzheimer disease. Alzheimers Res Ther 14(1):28, 2022

Turner JJO: Hypercalcaemia: presentation and management. Clin Med (Lond) 17(3):270–273, 2017

Tyler KL: Acute viral encephalitis. N Engl J Med 379(6):557–566, 2018

U.S. Food and Drug Administration: Dental amalgam fillings, in Products and Medical Procedures: Dental Devices. Washington, DC, U.S. Food and Drug Administration, February 18, 2021. Available at: https://www.fda.gov/medical-devices/dental-devices/dental-amalgam-fillings. Accessed July 22, 2022.

Udani K, Chris-Olaiya A, Ohadugha C, et al: Cardiovascular manifestations in hospitalized patients with hemochromatosis in the United States. Int J Cardiol 342:117–124, 2021

Ueland PM, Ulvik A, Rios-Avila L, et al: Direct and functional biomarkers of vitamin B6 status. Annu Rev Nutr 35:33–70, 2015

Ueno A, Hamano T, Enomoto S, et al: Influences of vitamin B12 supplementation on cognition and homocysteine in patients with vitamin B12 deficiency and cognitive impairment. Nutrients 14(7):1494, 2022

Ulwelling W, Smith K: The PEth blood test in the security environment: what it is; why it is important; and interpretative guidelines. J Forensic Sci 63(6):1634–1640, 2018

Umpierrez G, Korytkowski M: Diabetic emergencies: ketoacidosis, hyperglycaemic hyperosmolar state and hypoglycaemia. Nat Rev Endocrinol 12(4):222–232, 2016

Ungprasert P, Matteson EL: Neurosarcoidosis. Rheum Dis Clin North Am 43(4):593–606, 2017

Uretsky M, Bouix S, Killiany RJ, et al: Association between antemortem FLAIR white matter hyperintensities and neuropathology in brain donors exposed to repetitive head impacts. Neurology 98(1):e27–e39, 2022

Uzomah UA, Rozen G, Mohammadreza Hosseini S, et al: Incidence of carditis and predictors of pacemaker implantation in patients hospitalized with Lyme disease. PLoS One 16(11):e0259123, 2021

Vaccarino V, Almuwaqqat Z, Kim JH, et al: Association of mental stress-induced myocardial ischemia with cardiovascular events in patients with coronary heart disease. JAMA 326(18):1818–1828, 2021

van den Broek J, Bischof D, Derron N, et al: Screening methanol poisoning with a portable breath detector. Anal Chem 93(2):1170–1178, 2021

van der Ende EL, Jackson JL, White A, et al: Unravelling the clinical spectrum and the role of repeat length in C9ORF72 repeat expansions. J Neurol Neurosurg Psychiatry 92(5):502–509, 2021

van der Plas E, Langbehn DR, Conrad AL, et al: Abnormal brain development in child and adolescent carriers of mutant huntingtin. Neurology 93(10):e1021–e1030, 2019

van Kempen TATG, Deixler E: SARS-CoV-2: influence of phosphate and magnesium, moderated by vitamin D, on energy (ATP) metabolism and on severity of COVID-19. Am J Physiol Endocrinol Metab 320(1):E2–E6, 2021

Van Laecke S: Hypomagnesemia and hypermagnesemia. Acta Clin Belg 74(1):41–47, 2019

van Rappard DF, Boelens JJ, Wolf NI: Metachromatic leukodystrophy: disease spectrum and approaches for treatment. Best Pract Res Clin Endocrinol Metab 29(2):261–273, 2015

van Rappard DF, Bugiani M, Boelens JJ, et al: Gallbladder and the risk of polyps and carcinoma in metachromatic leukodystrophy. Neurology 87(1):103–111, 2016

Van Someren EJW: Brain mechanisms of insomnia: new perspectives on causes and consequences. Physiol Rev 101(3):995–1046, 2021

Vargo MM: Brain tumors and metastases. Phys Med Rehabil Clin N Am 28(1):115–141, 2017

Vasilevska V, Guest PC, Bernstein HG, et al: Molecular mimicry of NMDA receptors may contribute to neuropsychiatric symptoms in severe COVID-19 cases. J Neuroinflammation 18(1):245, 2021

Veasey SC, Rosen IM: Obstructive sleep apnea in adults. N Engl J Med 380(15):1442–1449, 2019

Vege SS, Chari ST: Chronic pancreatitis. N Engl J Med 386(9):869–878, 2022

Venkatesan A, Tunkel AR, Bloch KC, et al: Case definitions, diagnostic algorithms, and priorities in encephalitis: consensus statement of the international encephalitis consortium. Clin Infect Dis 57(8):1114–1128, 2013

Viera AJ, Wouk N: Potassium disorders: hypokalemia and hyperkalemia. Am Fam Physician 92(6):487–495, 2015

Viering DHHM, de Baaij JHF, Walsh SB, et al: Genetic causes of hypomagnesemia, a clinical overview. Pediatr Nephrol 32(7):1123–1135, 2017

Vindegaard N, Petersen LV, Lyng-Rasmussen BI, et al: Infectious mononucleosis as a risk factor for depression: a nationwide cohort study. Brain Behav Immun 94:259–265, 2021

Vladimirov T, Dreikorn M, Stahl K: Central pontine myelinolysis in a patient with bulimia: case report and literature review. Clin Neurol Neurosurg 192:105722, 2020

Vo QT, Thompson DF: A review and assessment of drug-Induced thrombocytosis. Ann Pharmacother 53(5):523–536, 2019

Vogel EA, Chieng A, Robinson A, et al: Associations between substance use problems and stress during COVID-19. J Stud Alcohol Drugs 82(6):776–781, 2021

Voican CS, Corruble E, Naveau S, et al: Antidepressant-induced liver injury: a review for clinicians. Am J Psychiatry 171(4):404–415, 2014

Volkow ND, Swanson JM: Clinical practice: Adult attention deficit-hyperactivity disorder. N Engl J Med 369(20):1935–1944, 2013

Volpe U, Tortorella A, Manchia M, et al: Eating disorders: what age at onset? Psychiatry Res 238:225–227, 2016

Vulser H, Wiernik E, Hoertel N, et al: Association between depression and anemia in otherwise healthy adults. Acta Psychiatr Scand 134(2):150–160, 2016

Waddell LA, Greig J, Mascarenhas M, et al: The accuracy of diagnostic tests for Lyme disease in humans, a systematic review and meta-analysis of North American research. PLoS One 11(12):e0168613, 2016

Wade TD: Recent research on bulimia nervosa. Psychiatr Clin North Am 42(1):21–32, 2019

Wagner-Bartak NA, Baiomy A, Habra MA, et al: Cushing syndrome: diagnostic workup and imaging features, with clinical and pathologic correlation. AJR Am J Roentgenol 209(1):19–32, 2017

Wainberg M, Kloiber S, Diniz B, et al: Clinical laboratory tests and five-year incidence of major depressive disorder: a prospective cohort study of 433,890 participants from the UK Biobank. Transl Psychiatry 11(1):380, 2021

Waldemar G, Dubois B, Emre M, et al: Recommendations for the diagnosis and management of Alzheimer's disease and other disorders associated with dementia: EFNS guideline. Eur J Neurol 14(1):e1–e26, 2007

Walker MD, Bilezikian JP: Primary hyperparathyroidism: recent advances. Curr Opin Rheumatol 30(4):427–439, 2018

Walker P, Parnell S, Dillon RC: Epsom salt ingestion leading to severe hypermagnesemia necessitating dialysis. J Emerg Med 58(5):767–770, 2020

Wang C, Fipps DC: Primary CNS lymphoma and secondary causes of mania: a case report and literature review. J Neuropsychiatry Clin Neurosci 34(1):84–88, 2022

Wang X, Han D, Li G: Electrocardiographic manifestations in severe hypokalemia. J Int Med Res 48(1):300060518811058, 2020

Watson JC, Dyck PJ: Peripheral neuropathy: a practical approach to diagnosis and symptom management. Mayo Clin Proc 90(7):940–951, 2015

Wattjes MP, Ciccarelli O, Reich DS, et al: 2021 MAGNIMS-CMSC-NAIMS consensus recommendations on the use of MRI in patients with multiple sclerosis. Lancet Neurol 20(8):653–670, 2021

Weinbrenner T, Züger M, Jacoby GE, et al: Lipoprotein metabolism in patients with anorexia nervosa: a case-control study investigating the mechanisms leading to hypercholesterolaemia. Br J Nutr 91(6):959–969, 2004

Weissenborn K: Hepatic encephalopathy: definition, clinical grading and diagnostic principles. Drugs 79(Suppl 1):5–9, 2019

Wekking EM: Psychiatric symptoms in systemic lupus erythematosus: an update. Psychosom Med 55:219–228, 1993

West R, Kobokovich A, Connell N, et al: COVID-19 antibody tests: a valuable public health tool with limited relevance to individuals. Trends Microbiol 29(3):214–223, 2021

Westmoreland P, Krantz MJ, Mehler PS: Medical complications of anorexia nervosa and bulimia. Am J Med 129(1):30–37, 2016

White L, Jackson T: Delirium and COVID-19: a narrative review of emerging evidence. Anaesthesia 77(Suppl 1):49–58, 2022

Whittaker A, Anson M, Harky A: Neurological manifestations of COVID-19: a systematic review and current update. Acta Neurol Scand 142(1):14–22, 2020

Whooten R, Schmitt J, Schwartz A: Endocrine manifestations of Down syndrome. Curr Opin Endocrinol Diabetes Obes 25(1):61–66, 2018

Wiegersma AM, Dalman C, Lee BK, et al: Association of prenatal maternal anemia with neurodevelopmental disorders. JAMA Psychiatry 76(12):1294–1304, 2019

Wieting J, Eberlein C, Bleich S, et al: Behavioural change in Prader-Willi syndrome during COVID-19 pandemic. J Intellect Disabil Res 65(7):609–616, 2021

Wijdicks EF: Hepatic encephalopathy. N Engl J Med 375(17):1660–1670, 2016

Wilkinson JM, Codipilly DC, Wilfahrt RP: Dysphagia: evaluation and collaborative management. Am Fam Physician 103(2):97–106, 2021

Williams AL, Bevan J, Arnold MJ: Lyme disease: updated recommendations from the IDSA, AAN, and ACR. Am Fam Physician 104(6):652–654, 2021

Williams Barnhardt E, Jacque M, Sharma TR: Brief reversible psychosis and altered mental status in a patient with folate deficiency: a case report. Prim Care Companion CNS Disord 18(1):10.4088/PCC.15l01839, 2016

Wilson MP, Plecko B, Mills PB, et al: Disorders affecting vitamin B_6 metabolism. J Inherit Metab Dis 42(4):629–646, 2019

Wilson MR, Sample HA, Zorn KC, et al: Clinical metagenomic sequencing for diagnosis of meningitis and encephalitis. N Engl J Med 380(24):2327–2340, 2019

Winkelman JW: Clinical practice. Insomnia disorder. N Engl J Med 373(15):1437–1444, 2015

Wirth KJ, Scheibenbogen C, Paul F: An attempt to explain the neurological symptoms of myalgic encephalomyelitis/chronic fatigue syndrome. J Transl Med 19(1):471, 2021

Wise GJ, Schlegel PN: Sterile pyuria. N Engl J Med 372(11):1048–1054, 2015

Womack J, Jimenez M: Common questions about infectious mononucleosis. Am Fam Physician 91(6):372–376, 2015

Wong C, Benyaminov F, Block L: Reversible dementia in the setting of multiple medical comorbidities due to B12 deficiency. BMJ Case Rep 15(3):e248440, 2022

Wright WF, Pinto CN, Palisoc K, et al: Viral (aseptic) meningitis: a review. J Neurol Sci 398:176–183, 2019

Xing XW, Zhang JT, Ma YB, et al: Metagenomic next-generation sequencing for diagnosis of infectious encephalitis and meningitis: a large, prospective case series of 213 patients. Front Cell Infect Microbiol 10:88, 2020

Yamaguchi H, Shimada H, Yoshita K, et al: Severe hypermagnesemia induced by magnesium oxide ingestion: a case series. CEN Case Rep 8(1):31–37, 2019

Yasuda M, Chen B, Desnick RJ: Recent advances on porphyria genetics: inheritance, penetrance and molecular heterogeneity, including new modifying/causative genes. Mol Genet Metab 128(3):320–331, 2019

Yelehe-Okouma M, Czmil-Garon J, Pape E, et al: Drug-induced aseptic meningitis: a mini-review. Fundam Clin Pharmacol 32(3):252–260, 2018

Yelnik CM, Kozora E, Appenzeller S: Cognitive disorders and antiphospholipid antibodies. Autoimmun Rev 15(12):1193–1198, 2016

Yelnik CM, Kozora E, Appenzeller S: Non-stroke central neurologic manifestations in antiphospholipid syndrome. Curr Rheumatol Rep 18(2):11, 2016

Yew KS, Cheng E: Acute stroke diagnosis. Am Fam Physician 80(1):33–40, 2009

Yik JT, Becquart P, Gill J, et al: Serum neurofilament light chain correlates with myelin and axonal magnetic resonance imaging markers in multiple sclerosis. Mult Scler Relat Disord 7:103366, 2022

Yip L, Bixler D, Brooks DE, et al: Serious adverse health events, including death, associated with ingesting alcohol-based hand sanitizers containing methanol: Arizona and New Mexico, May–June 2020. MMWR Morb Mortal Wkly Rep 69(32):1070–1073, 2020

Yocum AD, Dennison JL, Simon EL: Esophageal obstruction and death in a nonverbal patient. J Emerg Med 60(5):e109-e113, 2021

Younes K, Miller BL: Frontotemporal dementia: neuropathology, genetics, neuroimaging, and treatments. Psychiatr Clin North Am 43(2):331–344, 2020

Young H: Guidelines for serological testing for syphilis. Sex Transm Infect 76:403–405, 2000

Young JL, Goodman DW: Adult attention-deficit/hyperactivity disorder diagnosis, management, and treatment in the DSM-5 era. Prim Care Companion CNS Disord 18(6):10.4088/PCC.16r02000, 2016

Younossi ZM, Felix S, Jeffers T, et al: Performance of the Enhanced Liver Fibrosis Test to estimate advanced fibrosis among patients with nonalcoholic fatty liver disease. JAMA Netw Open 4(9):e2123923, 2021

Yousaf T, Dervenoulas G, Valkimadi PE, et al: Neuroimaging in Lewy body dementia. J Neurol 266(1):1–26, 2019

Yousaf Z, Al-Shokri SD, Al-Soub H, et al: COVID-19-associated SIADH: a clue in the times of pandemic! Am J Physiol Endocrinol Metab 318(6):E882–E885, 2020

Yuen KCJ, Sharf V, Smith E, et al: Sodium and water perturbations in patients who had an acute stroke: clinical relevance and management strategies for the neurologist. Stroke Vasc Neurol 7(3):258–266, 2021

Yuh EL, Jain S, Sun X, et al: Pathological computed tomography features associated with adverse outcomes after mild traumatic brain injury: a TRACK-TBI study with external validation in CENTER-TBI. JAMA Neurol 78(9):1137–1148, 2021

Yusim A, Anbarasan D, Bernstein C, et al: Normal pressure hydrocephalus presenting as Othello syndrome: case presentation and review of the literature. Am J Psychiatry 165(9):1119–1125, 2008

Zai G: Pharmacogenetics of obsessive-compulsive disorder: an evidence-update. Curr Top Behav Neurosci 49:385–398, 2021

Zakharov S, Pelclova D, Navratil T, et al: Fomepizole versus ethanol in the treatment of acute methanol poisoning: comparison of clinical effectiveness in a mass poisoning outbreak. Clin Toxicol (Phila) 53(8):797–806, 2015

Zgaljardic DJ, Seale GS, Schaefer LA, et al: Psychiatric disease and post-acute traumatic brain injury. J Neurotrauma 32(23):1911–1925, 2015

Zhang L, Fu T, Yin R, et al: Prevalence of depression and anxiety in systemic lupus erythematosus: a systematic review and meta-analysis. BMC Psychiatry 17(1):70, 2017

Zhang M, Chen J, Yin Z, et al: The association between depression and metabolic syndrome and its components: a bidirectional two-sample Mendelian randomization study. Transl Psychiatry 11(1):633, 2021

Zhou JY, Xu B, Lopes J, et al: Hashimoto encephalopathy: literature review. Acta Neurol Scand 135(3):285–290, 2017

Zipfel S, Giel KE, Bulik CM, et al: Anorexia nervosa: aetiology, assessment, and treatment. Lancet Psychiatry 2(12):1099–1111, 2015

Zitzmann M, Aksglaede L, Corona G, et al: European academy of andrology guidelines on Klinefelter's syndrome. Andrology 9(1):145–167, 2021

Psychotropic Medications Section

American Society of Health-System Pharmacists: AHFS Drug Information. Bethesda, MD, American Society of Health-System Pharmacists, 2016

U.S. National Library of Medicine: DailyMed. Available at: https://dailymed.nlm.nih.gov/dailymed.

Index

Page numbers in **boldface** refer to primary discussions. For interpretation of abbreviations, such as ACTH, see the guide printed on the volume endpapers.